RECENT ADVANCES IN CARDIOVASCULAR RISK FACTORS

Edited by **Mehnaz Atiq**

Recent Advances in Cardiovascular Risk Factors
Edited by Mehnaz Atiq

Published by InTech
Janeza Trdine 9, 51000 Rijeka, Croatia

Publishing Process Manager Silvia Vlase

Technical Editor Teodora Smiljanic

Cover Designer InTech Design Team

Additional hard copies can be obtained from orders@intechopen.com

Recent Advances in Cardiovascular Risk Factors, Edited by Mehnaz Atiq
p. cm.
ISBN 978-953-51-0321-9

For EU product safety concerns:
IN TECH d.o.o., Prolaz Marije Krucifikse Kozulić 3, 51000 Rijeka, Croatia,
info@intechopen.com or visit our website at intechopen.com.

Meet the editor

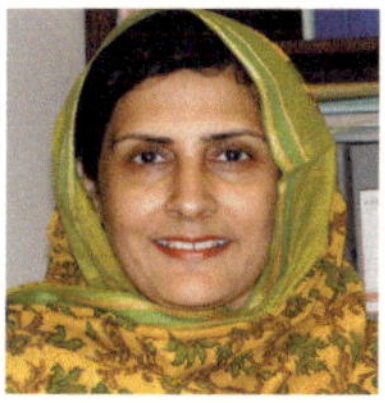

Dr Mehnaz Atiq is a Paediatric Cardiologist at the Aga Khan University hospital, Karachi, Pakistan. This is a tertiary care hospital with a reputed cardiology service, adult and congenital. The center provides state of art care to sick cardiac patients. These include General and Interventional cardiology for children and adults, nuclear studies, electrophysiology, cardiac magnetic resonance and computerized tomographic angiography for adults and children with heart disease. Dr Mehnaz Atiq did her undergraduate medical school from India and then migrated to Pakistan. She trained in Pediatric Cardiology locally and in Gothenburg, Sweden. Thereafter she pursued training in Interventional cardiology in the Hospital for Sick children, Toronto, Canada. She was the first to start fetal cardiology service in the country. Dr Mehnaz Atiq is presently a Professor in Pediatric Cardiology and runs a fellowship training program.

Contents

Preface

Among the non-communicable diseases, cardiovascular disorders are the leading cause of morbidity and mortality in both the developed and the developing countries. The spectrum of risk factors is wide and their understanding is imperative to prevent the first and recurrent episodes of myocardial infarction, stroke or peripheral vascular disease which may prove fatal or disabling.

There is ample evidence from longitudinal studies to prove that cardiovascular diseases are preventable. Individuals with low levels of risk factors generally have a healthy lifestyle. Genetic factors have to be kept in mind when risk stratification is done for cardiovascular diseases. Despite our knowledge of risk factors, huge differences exist in the prevalence between populations within the same region, between men and women and in the racial and ethnic subgroups. Much of this variability is explained on the basis of behavioral and cultural differences rather than genetic or clinical reason. Moreover, risk factors are frequently redefined as newer research throws light on interventions and their results.

This book has tried to present an update on risk factors incorporating new research which has thrown more light on the existing knowledge. It has also tried to highlight regional diversity addressing such issues. It will hopefully be resourceful to the cardiologists, general practitioners, family physicians, researchers, graduate students committed to cardiovascular risk prevention.

Dr. Mehnaz Atiq
Division of Cardiac Services
Aga Khan University Hospital
Karachi, Pakistan

1

Lipoprotein (a) and Cardiovascular Risk

José Antonio Díaz Peromingo
Short Stay Medical Unit, Department of Internal Medicine,
Hospital Clínico Universitario, Santiago de Compostela,
Spain

1. Introduction

First epidemiological studies of Lp(a) and CHD were reported at the end of the last century (1-3) but the investigation of this lipoprotein as a potential cardiovascular risk factor has been hampered by the lack of consistent approaches to its measurement for decades. Lp(a) laboratory standardization emerged in 2000 (4) and was accepted by the World Health Organization in 2004 (5). Another challenge associated to its measurement is the fact that population differences can also contribute to variation in Lp(a) serum concentration (6). Since Lp(a) characterization, evidences favoring its association with cardiovascular risk have been reported. At the same time, studies against this association have also been published leading to some confusion regarding to the possible role of Lp(a) in cardiovascular disease. The last years have clarified somewhat this issue and evidences of Lp(a) as an independent cardiovascular risk factor have been proposed (7-13). Several key points such as its homology with plasminogen, differences among the apo(a) isoforms, genetic considerations as well as special circumstances such as the relationship of Lp(a) and atrial fibrillation, dialysis, alcohol consumption and blood coagulation have been investigated. In this chapter, Lp(a) metabolism, epidemiological and genetic considerations, association with coronary heart disease and stroke, special situations as well as controversies and current treatment options are related.

2. Lipoprotein (a) metabolism

Lipoprotein (a), Lp (a), is a low density lipoprotein (LDL)-like particle synthesized in the liver by hepatocytes and then secreted into plasma. It was first described by Berg in 1963 (14). It consists of an apolipoprotein B100 (apoB100) molecule that is linked covalently by a disulfide bond to a large glycoprotein known as apolipoprotein (a), [apo(a)] (15). Lp(a) metabolic route is shown in figure 1. Its molecular weight ranges from 200 kDa to more than 800 kDa (16). The apo(a) gene (*LPA*) is a major determinant of the plasma concentration of Lp(a), including variations in the kringle region-coding repeats, with accounts for the size polymorphism of apo(a) leading to different apo(a) sizes (17). This fact is very important because small size isofoms seem to be associated to worse cardiovascular profile. Apo(a) chain contains 5 cysteine-rich domains known as kringles, and especially Kringle IV (KIV) is very similar to plasminogen (18,19). This particle is not only located in the plasma but also has been shown to enter the arterial intima of humans and has an increased affinity by the extracellular matrix (20). This issue confers a greater opportunity to Lp(a) oxidation (21) and interaction of Lp(a) with macrophages (22,23). Recently, it has been suggested that Lp(a) could be a preferential carrier of oxidized phospholipids in human plasma (24). These oxidized Lp(a) have a greater atherosclerotic effect as compared to native Lp(a) and this action may be increased by hyperglucemia (25). Different Lp(a) subtypes have been proposed regarding to apo(a) isoforms and these apo(a) isoforms predict the risk for CHD independently of the ethnic group (26). These isoforms are classified in order to their different size (16). Table 1 shows classification of these isoforms and its relation with KIV repeats.

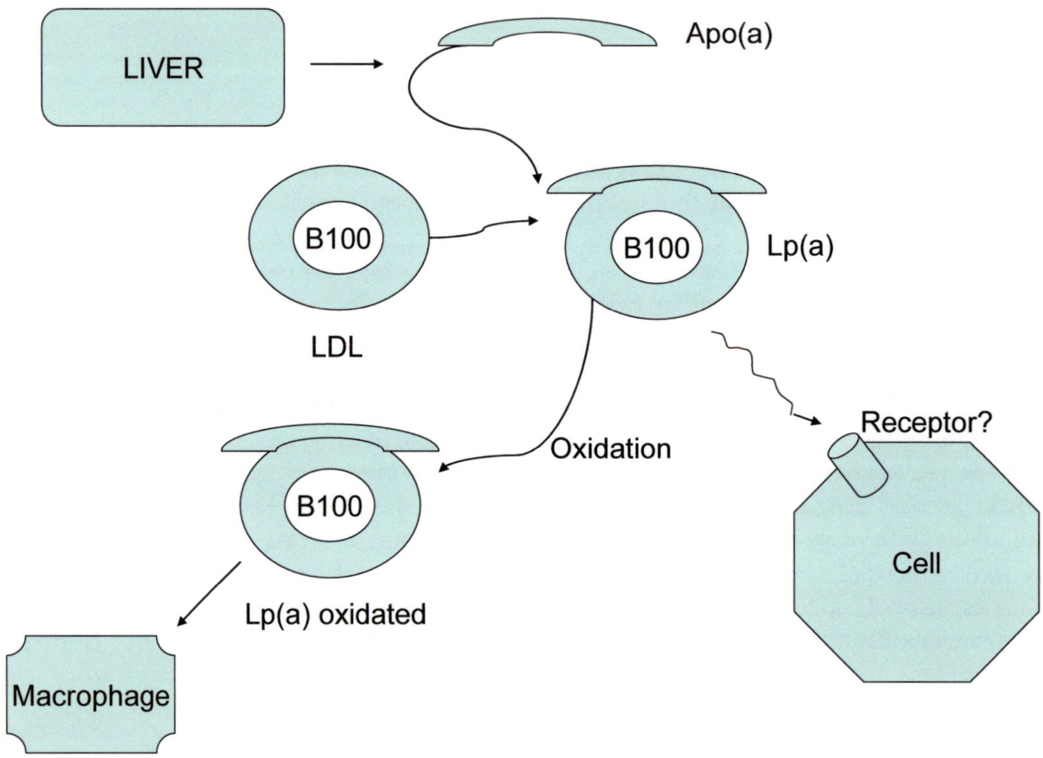

Fig. 1. Metabolic route of Lp(a).

3. Epidemiological aspects

Plasma levels of Lp(a) show great diversity regarding to different ethnical groups but a plasmatic concentration greater than 30 mg/dl is currently considered an independent cardiovascular risk factor (27). In this sense, African-Americans have higher Lp(a) concentrations than Caucasians. These levels may also be very different even in individuals carrying apo(a) of the same size polymorphism. It has been suggested the possibility of the presence of additional factors affecting this ethnical differences or the existence of high risk-Lp(a) or low risk-Lp(a) (28,29). By the other hand, not all ethnic groups show the same relation with Lp(a). In American-Indians, Lp(a) level has been reported to be low and non independently associated with cardiovascular disease (30).

Repeats (No.)	*Molecular weight (kDa)*
5-12	<400
13-20	400-500
20-25	500-650
>25	>700

Table 1. Relation between KIV_2 repeats and apo(a) isoforms size

Respecting to apo(a) isofoms, it has been suggested a most important pathogenic role of Lp(a) particles with smaller apo(a) isoforms (18,31). This is probably due to several factors. First, an increased capacity to bind oxidized phospholipids, second, the ability to localize in blood vessel walls, and eventually related to its thrombogenic effect by increasing inhibition of plasmin activity. Apo(a) size heterogeneity is related to a copy number variation in the protein domain kringle IV type 2 (KIV_2) (32) (Table 1). This copy number variation (5-50 identically repeated copies) confers heterogeneity in the molecular mass of apo(a) ranging between 200 and 800 kDa. Ethnical differences in the frequency distribution of apo(a) KIV repeated alleles have been reported (33,34). In all ethnic groups, Caucasians, Asians and African-Americans, higher levels of circulating Lp(a) concentrations tend to be associated with smaller apo(a) isoforms (35,36). This finding could explain partially the association of higher Lp(a) levels and cardiovascular disease. People with smaller apo(a) isoforms have an approximately 2-fold higher risk of coronary artery disease and ischemic stroke than those with larger apo(a) isoforms. Furthermore, isoforms with less KIV repetitions (isoforms F, B, S1 and S2) have the greater analogy with plasminogen being associated with higher coronary risk (37,38).

4. Genetic considerations

Apo(a) gen (6q2.6-q2.7) (39,40) have different kringle domains that show a high degree of homology to the kringle domains IV and V of plasminogen (41).

Genetic variants associated with Lp(a) level have been associated with coronary disease (42). More specifically, the apo(a) gen is the major determinant of variation in some populations like African-Americans modulating the plasmatic concentration of Lp(a) (43). It has been reported that apo(a) gene accounts for greater than 90% of the variation of plasmatic Lp(a) concentrations (28). Apo(a) gen polymorphisoms as well certain gene cluster associated to *LPA* have been shown to modulate Lp(a) concentrations leading to an increase in the risk for coronary artery disease (44). The genetic basis for apo(a) isoform variation is a segment existing in multiple repeats (KIV_2 polymorphism) located in the *LPA* gene (41). Variations in nucleotide polymorphisms in *LPA* may be an important contributor to the observed Lp(a) between-population variance and increase Lp(a) level in some populations (45-47). Once again, ethnical differences have been reported in people of European continental ancestry where apo(a) isoform polymorphism contributes between 40% and 70% of the variation of Lp(a) concentration showing fewer number of KIV_2 repeats (41,46), (Table 1).

5. Evidences favoring association with cardiovascular disease

- **Coronary heart disease:** Circulating Lp(a) concentration is associated with risk of coronary heart disease (CHD) independently from other conventional risk factors including total cholesterol concentration. Lp(a) excess has been independently associated to myocardial infarction and unstable angina (48), restenosis after coronary angioplasty (49), and coronary bypass grafting (50) respectively. Prospective epidemiological studies have reported positive association of baseline Lp(a) concentration with CHD risk . Based on this epidemiological data, a relative risk or 1.5 has been reported involving those patients with mean Lp(a) values of 50 mg/dL, especially in patients with premature coronary disease (51). Continuous associations of Lp(a) with the risk of coronary artery disease have been reported and this association is similar regarding to coronary death and non-fatal myocardial infarction (52-54). This association is not significantly affected by sex, non-HDL or HDL cholesterol, triglycerides, blood pressure, diabetes, of body mass index. These results are consistent mainly in Caucasians but studies in non-Caucasians are needed to corroborate also this issue in other populations (33). The association of Lp(a) concentrations with CHD is only slightly reduced after adjustment for long-term average levels of lipids and other established risk factors. This situation increases the likelihood that Lp(a) is an independent risk factor for CHD (53). The strength of Lp(a) as coronary risk factor is relatively modest as compared with non-HDL cholesterol. This is somewhat different when the level of Lp(a) is very high leading to a proportionally most important role for Lp(a) as CHD risk factor (52). Trying to associate fibrinolysis and myocardial ischemic disease, it has been suggested that Lp(a) may inhibit fibrinolysis of coronary artery thrombus (55). This is because higher levels of Lp(a) have been reported in survivors of myocardial infarction in whom recanalization of infarct artery failed as compared with patients with a patent artery (56). Other prospective studies have not shown relationship between high levels of Lp(a) or apo(a) isoforms and cardiovascular risk (57-59) contributing to some degree of controversy.
- **Stroke:** Serum Lp(a) concentration is also associated independently with risk of ischemic stroke (60,61). Current data in relation to Lp(a) concentration and stroke are sparse but seem to be similar than those for CHD. Serum Lp(a) level was demonstrated to predict stroke in elderly people in a large longitudinal (62) and in a case-control study (63). It has been shown that high levels of Lp(a) are associated with ischemic stroke in patients with atrial fibrillation especially when left atrial thrombus is present (64). Unhealthy dietary fat intake and a high serum Lp(a) level have been shown to predict fatal and nonfatal stroke of transient ischemic attack independently of established risk factors in a study of a community-based sample of middle-age men (65). Lp(a) has also been detected in intraparenchymal cerebral vessels suggesting a potential imflammatory role in acute stroke for Lp(a) (66). Other studies have not found statistical relationship between higher level of Lp(a) and thrombotic stroke (67).

6. Special situations

There are some common medical conditions that may be influenced by the level of Lp(a). Conversely, serum Lp(a) levels can be modified by the existence of some medical disorders. These medical conditions are summarized as follows:

- **Lp(a) and dialysis:** It is well known than atherosclerosis is more prevalent among patients with end-stage renal disease (68). Hemodialysis procedure "per se" has been shown to modify serum levels of Lp(a) increasing them after hemodialysis procedure (69). It has been proposed that inflammation, a very important condition in hemodialysis patients, could play an important role in this Lp(a) increase (70-72). Basal serum levels of Lp(a) are increased in dialysis patients and the level is elevated in almost 70% of patients (73). Even more, in patients with continuous ambulatory peritoneal dialysis, Lp(a) level is significantly higher as compared with patients on hemodialysis (74) pointing to a possible modulating effect of Lp(a) concentration by the different dialysis procedures. Particularly, high serum Lp(a) levels and the low molecular weight apo(a) phenotype have been associated with adverse clinical outcomes in dialysis patients (75).
- **Lp(a) and atrial fibrillation:** Higher serum Lp(a) level in ischemic stroke patients associated with atrial fibrillation and left atrial thrombus formation or in acute myocardial infarction has been reported (76,77). Lp(a) elevation and reduced left atrial appendage flow velocities have been shown to be independently risk factors for thromboembolism in chronic nonvalvular atrial fibrillation (55). Probably, the association of Lp(a) is stronger in the presence of atrial thrombus instead of atrial fibrillation itself, because of the plasminogen inhibitory action of Lp(a) (64). In this sense, other studies have not found association between higher levels of Lp(a) and non-valvular atrial fibrillation (78).
- **Lp(a) and blood coagulation:** the genetic homology in the cDNA sequence of human apo(a) with plasminogen, the zymogen for the major fibrinolytic serine protease plasmin (79), has been related with the cardiovascular pathogenicity of Lp(a) (80). There is a major difference in the kringle structure between plasminogen and Lp(a) that is a single aminoacid exchange (R560S) that prevents apo(a) from enzymatic cleaveage such as the action of tissue-type plasminogen activator (t-PA) or urokinase plasminogen activator (u-PA). This molecular mimicry between plasminogen and Lp(a) contribute to the role of Lp(a) in atherogenesis binding Lp(a) to the tissue factor pathway inhibitor (TFPI), docking to diverse lipoprotein receptors (especially those affecting LDL or very low density lipoprotein (VLDL) and by the entrapment of Lp(a) into matricellular proteins (81). This situation leads to a retention of Lp(a) and recruitment of monocytes, upregulating the expression of the plasminogen activator inhibitor 2 in these monocytes (82). It has also been reported that Lp(a) modulates endothelial cell surface fibrinolysis contributing to the increase in atherosclerotic risk (83).
- **Lp(a) and alcohol intake:** Many epidemiological and clinical studies have shown that light-to-moderate alcohol consumption is associated with reduced risk of CHD and total mortality in the middle-age and elderly of both genders (84,85). Lipid levels are modified by alcohol in different forms but it is not completely clear the way they are. In alcohol abuse patients, levels of Lp(a) have been reported to decrease and this has been related to the time of abstinence (86). In other study an increased level among table wine drinkers has been described (87). A special situation is the association of alcohol intake, Lp(a) level and vascular disease. In this sense, high serum Lp(a) concentration and heavy drinking were found independently associated with larger infrarenal aortic diameters (88) and abdominal aortic aneurysms (89), probably due to the capability of Lp(a) to inhibit elastolysis in the vessels wall (90).

7. Treatment

Treatment possibilities are scarce at present when the aim is to reduce Lp(a) plasma concentration. Only niacin, in a dose dependent fashion, and certain inhibitors of cholesteryl ester transfer protein have shown limited effect ranging between 20%-40% lowering from baseline levels (91,92). Other drugs such as acetylsalicylic acid and L-carnitine can decrease mildly elevated Lp(a) concentrations (91,93,94). Contradictory findings have been reported with statins (95-98). Promising molecules like mipomersen, an antisense oligonucleotide directed to human $apoB_{100}$ have been shown to reduce Lp(a) concentrations by 70% in transgenic mice (99). Similar molecules such as eprotirone, tibolone and proprotein convertase subtilisin/kexin type 9 (PCSK-9) inhibitors can also decrease Lp(a) concentrations being currently under development (91,100-102). Nevertheless, the most dramatic change in Lp(a) concentrations can be achieved with regular lipid apheresis (103,104). Table 2 shows the efficacy of different treatment options in reducing Lp(a) plasmatic level.

Treatment	*Change in Lp(a) concentration (%)*
Diet and exercise	0
Resins	0
Fibrates	5-10
Statins	5
Nicotinic acid	35
Neomicine	25
Estrogen substitutive therapy	15-40
Apheresis	40-60

Table 2. Effect of different pharmacological therapies on Lp(a) serum concentration.

8. Controversies

The risk associated to Lp(a) concentration is only about one-quarter of that seen with LDL cholesterol so any clinical implication of this moderate association currently appeared limited. The role of specific Lp(a) subtypes could help to clarify the vascular risk. Particularly, smaller apo(a) isoforms could act associated with other factors such as small-dense LDL and oxidized LDL particles in the vessel wall increasing inflammation and accelerating atherosclerotic disease. This fact needs for more investigation.

Studies reporting association of apo(a) isoforms size variations with the risk of vascular disease have reported divergent relative risks, involve wide confidence intervals and the number of individuals included has been small. If smaller apo(a) isoforms are relevant to vascular disease independent from Lp(a) concentration is not completely clear at present. Moreover, many studies have used different cut-offs to define smaller apo(a) size.

The effect of the change in Lp(a) level and its relation with inflammation as well as its influence on endothelial function are unknown at present.

It has been suggested that Lp(a) is associated with CHD only at very high concentrations but this affirmation remains somewhat controversial making very important to identify possible ethnical differences as well as an adequate cut-off level we can rely on.

9. Conclusions

Lp(a) results from the association of apo(a) and LDL particles. Since first studies linking Lp(a) and cardiovascular disease, an important amount of clinical and laboratory evidences have supported the fact that Lp(a) is and independent cardiovascular risk factor, especially in younger people with premature cardiovascular disease.

Many ethnical differences and variations in apo(a) size have been reported. Moreover, small apo(a) size isoforms have been related with an increased cardiovascular risk. Its relation with the number of KIV repeats determines genetically variation in apo(a) size. Several studies including methanalysis have related higher levels of Lp(a) with CHD and stroke.

It seems also that Lp(a) is elevated in patients under dialysis, and possibly in those with atrial fibrillation increasing the cardiovascular risk of these patients, normally already high.

An interesting link between laboratory and clinical effects of Lp(a) is its action modulating the fibrinolytic system because of the great homology between Lp(a) and plasminogen.

The association between higher levels of Lp(a) and alcohol intake remains more controversial at present.

Current treatment options are not very useful except for niacin and plasma apheresis but both therapies are not easy to use because of toxicity, tolerability and availability.

Finally, large prospective studies are needed focusing on Lp(a)-associated small apo(a) isoforms and cardiovascular disease, and also in order to ensure treatment approaches.

10. References

[1] Schriewer H, Assmann G, Sandkamp M, Schulte H. The relationship of lipoprotein (a) (Lp(a)) to risk factors of coronary heart disease: initial results of the prospective epidemiological study on company employees in Westfalia. J Clin Chem Clin Biochem. 1984;22:591-596.

[2] Schernthaner G, Kostner GM, Dieplinger H, Prager R, Mühlhauser I. Apolipoproteins (A-I, A-II, B), Lp(a) lipoprotein and lecithin: cholesterol acyltransferase activity in diabetes mellitus. Atherosclerosis. 1983;49:277-293.

[3] Murai A, Miyahara T, Fujimoto N, Matsuda M, Kameyama M. Lp(a) lipoprotein as a risk factor for coronary heart disease and cerebral infarction. Atherosclerosis. 1986;59:199-204.

[4] Marcovina SM, Albers JJ, Scanu AM, Kennedy H, Giaculli F, Berg K, Couderc R, Dati F, Rifai N, Sakurabayashi I, Tate JR, Steinmetz A. Use of a reference material proposed by the International Federation of Clinical Chemistry and Laboratory Medicine to evaluate analytical methods for the determination of plasma lipoprotein(a). Clin Chem. 2000;46:1956-1967.

[5] Dati F, Tate JR, Marcovina SM, Steinmetz A; International Federation of Clinical Chemistry and Laboratory Medicine; IFCC Working Group for Lipoprotein(a) Assay Standardization. First WHO/IFCC International Reference Reagent for Lipoprotein(a) for Immunoassay--Lp(a) SRM 2B. Clin Chem Lab Med. 2004;42:670-676.

[6] Scanu AM, Lawn RM, Berg K. Lipoprotein(a) and atherosclerosis. Ann Intern Med. 1991;115:209-218.

[7] Orsó E, Ahrens N, Kilalić D, Schmitz G. Familial hypercholesterolemia and lipoprotein(a) hyperlipidemia as independent and combined cardiovascular risk factors. Atheroscler Suppl. 2009;10:74-78.

[8] Ariyo AA, Thach C, Tracy R; Cardiovascular Health Study Investigators. Lp(a) lipoprotein, vascular disease, and mortality in the elderly. N Engl J Med. 2003;349:2108-2115.

[9] Nordestgaard BG, Chapman MJ, Ray K, Borén J, Andreotti F, Watts GF, Ginsberg H, Amarenco P, Catapano A, Descamps OS, Fisher E, Kovanen PT, Kuivenhoven JA, Lesnik P, Masana L, Reiner Z, Taskinen MR, Tokgözoglu L, Tybjærg-Hansen A; European Atherosclerosis Society Consensus Panel. Lipoprotein(a) as a cardiovascular risk factor: current status. Eur Heart J. 2010;31:2844-2853.

[10] Marcovina SM, Koschinsky ML, Albers JJ, Skarlatos S. Report of the National Heart, Lung, and Blood Institute Workshop on Lipoprotein(a) and Cardiovascular Disease: recent advances and future directions. Clin Chem. 2003;49:1785-1796.

[11] Boffa MB, Marcovina SM, Koschinsky ML. Lipoprotein(a) as a risk factor for atherosclerosis and thrombosis: mechanistic insights from animal models. Clin Biochem. 2004;37:333-343.

[12] Emerging Risk Factors Collaboration, Erqou S, Kaptoge S, Perry PL, Di Angelantonio E, Thompson A, White IR, Marcovina SM, Collins R, Thompson SG, Danesh J. Lipoprotein(a) concentration and the risk of coronary heart disease, stroke, and nonvascular mortality. JAMA. 2009;302:412-423.

[13] Anuurad E, Boffa MB, Koschinsky ML, Berglund L. Lipoprotein(a): a unique risk factor for cardiovascular disease. Clin Lab Med. 2006;26:751-772.

[14] Berg K. A new serum type system in man. The LP system. Acta Pathol Microbiol Scand. 1963;59:369-382.

[15] Utermann G. The mysteries of lipoprotein(a). Science. 1989;246:904-910.

[16] Erqou S, Thompson A, Di Angelantonio E, Saleheen D, Kaptoge S, Marcovina S, Danesh J. Apolipoprotein(a) isoforms and the risk of vascular disease: systematic review of 40 studies involving 58,000 participants. J Am Coll Cardiol. 2010;55:2160-2167.

[17] Rubin J, Kim HJ, Pearson TA, Holleran S, Berglund L, Ramakrishnan R. The apolipoprotein(a) gene: linkage disequilibria at three loci differs in African Americans and Caucasians. Atherosclerosis. 2008;201:138-147.

[18] Simó JM, Joven J, Vilella E, Ribas M, Pujana MA, Sundaram IM, Hammel JP, Hoover-Plow JL. Impact of apolipoprotein(a) isoform size heterogeneity on the lysine

binding function of lipoprotein(a) in early onset coronary artery disease. Thromb Haemost. 2001;85:412-417.
[19] Kraft HG, Lingenhel A, Pang RW, Delport R, Trommsdorff M, Vermaak H, Janus ED, Utermann G. Frequency distributions of apolipoprotein(a) kringle IV repeat alleles and their effects on lipoprotein(a) levels in Caucasian, Asian, and African populations: the distribution of null alleles is non-random. Eur J Hum Genet. 1996;4:74-87.
[20] Williams KJ, Flees GM, Petrie KA, Snyder ML, Brocia RW, Swenson TL. Mechanisms by which lipoprotein lipase alters cellular metabolism of lipoprotein(a), low density lipoprotein, and nascent lipoproteins. Roles for low density lipoprotein receptors and heparin sulfate proteoglycans. J Biol Chem. 1992;267:13284-13292.
[21] Naruscewicz M, Selinger E, Davignon J. Oxidative modification of lipoprotein(a) and the effect of beta-carotene. Metabolism. 1992;41:1215-1224.
[22] Zioncheck TF, Powell LM, Rice GC, Eaton DL, Lawn RM. Interaction of recombinant apolipoprotein(a) and lipoprotein(a) with macrophages. J Clin Invest. 1991;87:767-771.
[23] Tsimikas S, Witztum JL. The role of oxidized phospholipids in mediating lipoprotein(a) atherogenicity. Curr Opin Lipidol. 2008;19:369-377.
[24] Bergmark C, Dewan A, Orsoni A, Merki E, Miller ER, Shin MJ, Binder CJ, Hörkkö S, Krauss RM, Chapman MJ, Witztum JL, Tsimikas S. A novel function of lipoprotein [a] as a preferential carrier of oxidized phospholipids in human plasma. J Lipid Res. 2008;49:2230-2239.
[25] Kotani K, Yamada S, Uurtuya S, Yamada T, Taniguchi N, Sakurabayashi I. The association between blood glucose and oxidized lipoprotein(a) in healthy young women. Lipids Health Dis. 2010;9:103.
[26] Sandholzer C, Saha N, Kark JD, Rees A, Jaross W, Dieplinger H, Hoppichler F, Boerwinkle E, Utermann G. Apo(a) isoforms predict risk for coronary heart disease. A study in six populations. Arterioscler Thromb. 1992;12:1214-1226.
[27] Wittrup HH, Tybjaerd-Hansen A, Nordestgaard BG. Lipoprotein lipase mutations, plasma lipids and lipoproteins, and risk of ischaemic heart disease. A meta-analysis. Circulation. 1999;99:2901-2907.
[28] Boerwinkle E, Leffert CC, Lin J, Lackner C, Chiesa G, Hobbs HH. Apolipoprotein(a) gene accounts for greater than 90% of the variation in plasma lipoprotein(a) concentrations. J Clin Invest. 1992;90:52-60.
[29] Mooser V, Scheer D, Marcovina SM, Wang J, Guerra R, Cohen J, Hobbs HH. The Apo(a) gene is the major determinant of variation in plasma Lp(a) levels in African Americans. Am J Hum Genet. 1997;61:402-417.
[30] Wang W, Hu D, Lee ET, Fabsitz RR, Welty TK, Robbins DC, J L Yeh, Howard BV. Lipoprotein(a) in American Indians is low and not independently associated with cardiovascular disease. The Strong Heart Study. Ann Epidemiol. 2002;12:107-114.
[31] Zeljkovic A, Bogavac-Stanojevic N, Jelic-Ivanovic Z, Spasojevic-Kalimanovska V, Vekic J, Spasic S. Combined effects of small apolipoprotein (a) isoforms and small, dense LDL on coronary artery disease risk. Arch Med Res. 2009;40:29-35.
[32] Kraft HG, Lingenhel A, Pang RW, Delport R, Trommsdorff M, Vermaak H, Janus ED, Utermann G. Frequency distributions of apolipoprotein(a) kringle IV repeat alleles and their effects on lipoprotein(a) levels in Caucasian, Asian, and African

populations: the distribution of null alleles is non-random. Eur J Hum Genet. 1996;4:74-87.

[33] Guyton JR, Dahlen GH, Patsch W, Kautz JA, Gotto AM Jr. Relationship of plasma lipoprotein Lp(a) levels to race and to apolipoprotein B. Arteriosclerosis. 1985;5:265-272.

[34] Chiu L, Hamman RF, Kamboh MI. Apolipoprotein A polymorphisms and plasma lipoprotein(a) concentrations in non-Hispanic Whites and Hispanics. Hum Biol. 2000;72:821-835.

[35] Boomsma DI, Knijff P, Kaptein A, Labeur C, Martin NG, Havekes LM, Princen HM. The effect of apolipoprotein(a)-, apolipoprotein E-, and apolipoprotein A4-polymorphisms on quantitative lipoprotein(a) concentrations. Twin Res. 2000;3:152-158.

[36] Paultre F, Pearson TA, Weil HF, Tuck CH, Myerson M, Rubin J, Francis CK, Marx HF, Philbin EF, Reed RG, Berglund L. High levels of Lp(a) with a small apo(a) isoform are associated with coronary artery disease in African American and white men. Arterioscler Thromb Vasc Biol. 2000;20:2619-2624.

[37] Seman LJ, McNamara JR, Schaefer EJ. Lipoprotein(a), homocysteine, and remnantlike particles: emerging risk factors. Curr Opin Cardiol. 1999;14:186-191.

[38] Lamon-Fava S, Marcovina SM, Albers JJ, Kennedy H, Deluca C, White CC, Cupples LA, McNamara JR, Seman LJ, Bongard V, Schaefer EJ. Lipoprotein(a) levels, apo(a) isoform size, and coronary heart disease risk in the Framingham Offspring Study. J Lipid Res. 2011;52:1181-1187.

[39] Kraft HG, Köchl S, Menzel HJ, Sandholzer C, Utermann G. The apolipoprotein (a) gene: a transcribed hypervariable locus controlling plasma lipoprotein (a) concentration. Hum Genet. 1992;90:220-30.

[40] Ober C, Nord AS, Thompson EE, Pan L, Tan Z, Cusanovich D, Sun Y, Nicolae R, Edelstein C, Schneider DH, Billstrand C, Pfaffinger D, Phillips N, Anderson RL, Philips B, Rajagopalan R, Hatsukami TS, Rieder MJ, Heagerty PJ, Nickerson DA, Abney M, Marcovina S, Jarvik GP, Scanu AM, Nicolae DL. Genome-wide association study of plasma lipoprotein(a) levels identifies multiple genes on chromosome 6q. J Lipid Res. 2009;50:798-806.

[41] Crawford DC, Peng Z, Cheng JF, Boffelli D, Ahearn M, Nguyen D, Shaffer T, Yi Q, Livingston RJ, Rieder MJ, Nickerson DA. LPA and PLG sequence variation and kringle IV-2 copy number in two populations. Hum Hered. 2008;66:199-209.

[42] Clarke R, Peden JF, Hopewell JC, Kyriakou T, Goel A, Heath SC, Parish S, Barlera S, Franzosi MG, Rust S, Bennett D, Silveira A, Malarstig A, Green FR, Lathrop M, Gigante B, Leander K, de Faire U, Seedorf U, Hamsten A, Collins R, Watkins H, Farrall M; PROCARDIS Consortium. Genetic variants associated with Lp(a) lipoprotein level and coronary disease. N Engl J Med. 2009;361:2518-2528.

[43] Mooser V, Scheer D, Marcovina SM, Wang J, Guerra R, Cohen J, Hobbs HH. The Apo(a) gene is the major determinant of variation in plasma Lp(a) levels in African Americans. Am J Hum Genet. 1997;61:402-417.

[44] Marcovina SM, Albers JJ, Wijsman E, Zhang Z, Chapman NH, Kennedy H. Differences in Lp[a] concentrations and apo[a] polymorphs between black and white Americans. J Lipid Res. 1996;37:2569-2585.

[45] Chretien JP, Coresh J, Berthier-Schaad Y, Kao WH, Fink NE, Klag MJ, Marcovina SM, Giaculli F, Smith MW. Three single-nucleotide polymorphisms in LPA account for most of the increase in lipoprotein(a) level elevation in African Americans compared with European Americans. J Med Genet. 2006;43:917-923.
[46] Dumitrescu L, Glenn K, Brown-Gentry K, Shephard C, Wong M, Rieder MJ, Smith JD, Nickerson DA, Crawford DC. Variation in LPA is associated with Lp(a) levels in three populations from the Third National Health and Nutrition Examination Survey. PLoS One. 2011;6:e16604.
[47] Kraft HG, Haibach C, Lingenhel A, Brunner C, Trommsdorff M, Kronenberg F, Müller HJ, Utermann G. Sequence polymorphism in kringle IV 37 in linkage disequilibrium with the apolipoprotein (a) size polymorphism. Hum Genet. 1995;95:275-282.
[48] Dangas G, Ambrose JA, D'Agate DJ, Shao JH, Chockalingham S, Levine D, Smith DA. Correlation of serum lipoprotein(a) with the angiographic and clinical presentation of coronary artery disease. Am J Cardiol. 1999;83:583-585.
[49] Desmarais RL, Sarembock IJ, Ayers CR, Vernon SM, Powers ER, Gimple LW. Elevated serum lipoprotein(a) is a risk factor for clinical recurrence after coronary balloon angioplasty. Circulation. 1995;91:1403-1409.
[50] Hoff HF, Beck GJ, Skibinski CI, Jürgens G, O'Neil J, Kramer J, Lytle B. Serum Lp(a) level as a predictor of vein graft stenosis after coronary artery bypass surgery in patients. Circulation. 1988;77:1238-1244.
[51] Bostom AG, Cupples LA, Jenner JL, Ordovas JM, Seman LJ, Wilson PW, Schaefer EJ, Castelli WP. Elevated plasma lipoprotein(a) and coronary heart disease in men aged 55 years and younger. A prospective study. JAMA. 1996;276:544-548.
[52] Bennet A, Di Angelantonio E, Erqou S, Eiriksdottir G, Sigurdsson G, Woodward M, Rumley A, Lowe GD, Danesh J, Gudnason V. Lipoprotein(a) levels and risk of future coronary heart disease: large-scale prospective data. Arch Intern Med. 2008;168:598-608.
[53] Danesh J, Collins R, Peto R. Lipoprotein(a) and coronary heart disease. Meta-analysis of prospective studies. Circulation. 2000;102:1082-1085.
[54] Marcovina SM, Koschinsky ML. A critical evaluation of the role of Lp(a) in cardiovascular disease: can Lp(a) be useful in risk assessment? Semin Vasc Med. 2002;2:335-344.
[55] Igarashi Y, Kasai H, Yamashita F, Sato T, Inuzuka H, Ojima K, Aizawa Y. Lipoprotein(a), left atrial appendage function and thromboembolic risk in patients with chronic nonvalvular atrial fibrillation. Jpn Circ J. 2000;64:93-98.
[56] Moliterno DJ, Lange RA, Meidell RS, Willard JE, Leffert CC, Gerard RD, Boerwinkle E, Hobbs HH, Hillis LD. Relation of plasma lipoprotein(a) to infarct artery patency in survivors of myocardial infarction. Circulation. 1993;88:935-940.
[57] Ridker PM, Stampfer MJ, Rifai N. Novel risk factors for systemic atherosclerosis: a comparison of C-reactive protein, fibrinogen, homocysteine, lipoprotein(a), and standard cholesterol screening as predictors of peripheral arterial disease. JAMA. 2001;285:2481-2485.
[58] Moliterno DJ, Jokinen EV, Miserez AR, Lange RA, Willard JE, Boerwinkle E, Hillis LD, Hobbs HH. No association between plasma lipoprotein(a) concentrations and the

presence or absence of coronary atherosclerosis in African-Americans. Arterioscler Thromb Vasc Biol. 1995;15:850-855.
[59] Akanji AO. Apo(a) isoforms do not predict risk for coronary heart disease in a Gulf Arab population. Ann Clin Biochem. 2000;37(Pt 3):360-366.
[60] Smolders B, Lemmens R, Thijs V. Lipoprotein (a) and stroke: a meta-analysis of observational studies. Stroke. 2007;38:1959-1966.
[61] Shintani S, Kikuchi S, Hamaguchi H, Shiigai T. High serum lipoprotein(a) levels are an independent risk factor for cerebral infarction. Stroke. 1993;24:965-969.
[62] Ariyo AA, Thach C, Tracy R; Cardiovascular Health Study Investigators. Lp(a) lipoprotein, vascular disease, and mortality in the elderly. N Engl J Med. 2003;349:2108-2115.
[63] Milionis HJ, Filippatos TD, Loukas T, Bairaktari ET, Tselepis AD, Elisaf MS. Serum lipoprotein(a) levels and apolipoprotein(a) isoform size and risk for first-ever acute ischaemic nonembolic stroke in elderly individuals. Atherosclerosis. 2006l;187:170-176.
[64] Okura H, Inoue H, Tomon M, Nishiyama S, Yoshikawa T. Increased plasma lipoprotein(a) level in cardioembolic stroke with non-valvular atrial fibrillation. Intern Med. 1998;37:995.
[65] Wiberg B, Sundström J, Arnlöv J, Terént A, Vessby B, Zethelius B, Lind L. Metabolic risk factors for stroke and transient ischemic attacks in middle-aged men: a community-based study with long-term follow-up. Stroke. 2006;37:2898-2903.
[66] Jamieson DG, Fu L, Usher DC, Lavi E. Detection of lipoprotein(a) in intraparenchymal cerebral vessels: correlation with vascular pathology and clinical history. Exp Mol Pathol. 2001;71:99-105.
[67] Nagaraj SK, Pai P, Bhat G, Hemalatha A. Lipoprotein (a) and other Lipid Profile in Patients with Thrombotic Stroke: Is it a Reliable Marker? J Lab Physicians. 2011;3:28-32.
[68] Coresh J, Longenecker JC, Miller ER 3rd, Young HJ, Klag MJ. Epidemiology of cardiovascular risk factors in chronic renal disease. J Am Soc Nephrol. 1998;9(12 Suppl):S24-30.
[69] Díaz-Peromingo JA, Carbajal DG, Albán-Salgado A. Lipoprotein (a) in patients on hemodialysis. Acta Med Austriaca. 2004;31:73-75.
[70] Dejanova B, Filipce V, Dejanov P, Sikole A, Grozdanovski R, Maleska V. Atherosclerosis risk factors related to hemodialysis duration and erythropoietin therapy. Clin Chem Lab Med. 2001;39:484-486.
[71] Kaysen GA. Lipid and lipoprotein metabolism in chronic kidney disease. J Ren Nutr. 2009;19:73-77.
[72] Hoover-Plow J, Hart E, Gong Y, Shchurin A, Schneeman T. A physiological function for apolipoprotein(a): a natural regulator of the inflammatory response. Exp Biol Med (Maywood). 2009;234:28-34.
[73] Fleischmann EH, Bower JD, Salahudeen AK. Are conventional cardiovascular risk factors predictive of two-year mortality in hemodialysis patients? Clin Nephrol. 2001;56:221-230.
[74] Ozdemir FN, Güz G, Sezer S, Arat Z, Turan M, Haberal M. Atherosclerosis risk is higher in continuous ambulatory peritoneal dialysis patients than in hemodialysis patients. Artif Organs. 2001;25:448-452.

[75] Kronenberg F, Lingenhel A, Neyer U, Lhotta K, König P, Auinger M, Wiesholzer M, Andersson H, Dieplinger H. Prevalence of dyslipidemic risk factors in hemodialysis and CAPD patients. Kidney Int Suppl. 2003;84:113-116.
[76] Igarashi Y, Yamaura M, Ito M, Inuzuka H, Ojima K, Aizawa Y. Elevated serum lipoprotein(a) is a risk factor for left atrial thrombus in patients with chronic atrial fibrillation: a transesophageal echocardiographic study. Am Heart J. 1998;136:965-971.
[77] Celik S, Baykan M, Orem C, Kilinç K, Orem A, Erdöl C, Kaplan S. Serum lipoprotein(a) and its relation to left ventricular thrombus in patients with acute myocardial infarction. Jpn Heart J. 2001;42:5-14.
[78] Díaz-Peromingo JA, Albán-Salgado A, García-Suárez F, Sánchez-Leira J, Saborido-Froján J, Iglesias-Gallego M. Lipoprotein(a) and lipid profile in patients with atrial fibrillation. Med Sci Monit. 2006;12:122-125.
[79] McLean JW, Tomlinson JE, Kuang WJ, Eaton DL, Chen EY, Fless GM, Scanu AM, Lawn RM. cDNA sequence of human apolipoprotein(a) is homologous to plasminogen. Nature. 1987;330:132-137.
[80] Loscalzo J, Weinfeld M, Fless GM, Scanu AM. Lipoprotein(a), fibrin binding, and plasminogen activation. Arteriosclerosis. 1990;10:240-245.
[81] Caplice NM, Panetta C, Peterson TE, Kleppe LS, Mueske CS, Kostner GM, Broze GJ Jr, Simari RD. Lipoprotein (a) binds and inactivates tissue factor pathway inhibitor: a novel link between lipoproteins and thrombosis. Blood. 2001;98:2980-2987.
[82] Buechler C, Ullrich H, Ritter M, Porsch-Oezcueruemez M, Lackner KJ, Barlage S, Friedrich SO, Kostner GM, Schmitz G. Lipoprotein (a) up-regulates the expression of the plasminogen activator inhibitor 2 in human blood monocytes. Blood. 2001;97:981-986.
[83] Hajjar KA, Gavish D, Breslow JL, Nachman RL. Lipoprotein(a) modulation of endothelial cell surface fibrinolysis and its potential role in atherosclerosis. Nature. 1989;339:303-305.
[84] Rimm EB, Williams P, Fosher K, Criqui M, Stampfer MJ. Moderate alcohol intake and lower risk of coronary heart disease: meta-analysis of effects on lipids and haemostatic factors. BMJ. 1999;319:1523-1528.
[85] Rehm J, Gmel G, Sempos CT, Trevisan M. Alcohol-related morbidity and mortality. Alcohol Res Health. 2003;27:39-51.
[86] Kolovou GD, Salpea KD, Anagnostopoulou KK, Mikhailidis DP. Alcohol use, vascular disease, and lipid-lowering drugs. J Pharmacol Exp Ther. 2006;318:1-7.
[87] Böhm M, Rosenkranz S, Laufs U. Alcohol and red wine: impact on cardiovascular risk. Nephrol Dial Transplant. 2004;19:11-6.
[88.] Wang JA, Chen XF, Yu WF, Chen H, Lin XF, Xiang MJ, Fang CF, Du YX, Wang B. Relationship of heavy drinking, lipoprotein (a) and lipid profile to infrarenal aortic diameter. Vasc Med. 2009;14:323-329.
[89] Sofi F, Marcucci R, Giusti B, Pratesi G, Lari B, Sestini I, Lo Sapio P, Pulli R, Pratesi C, Abbate R, Gensini GF. High levels of homocysteine, lipoprotein (a) and plasminogen activator inhibitor-1 are present in patients with abdominal aortic aneurysm. Thromb Haemost. 2005;94:1094-1098.
[90] Petersen E, Wågberg F, Angquist KA. Does lipoprotein(a) inhibit elastolysis in abdominal aortic aneurysms? Eur J Vasc Endovasc Surg. 2003;26:423-428.

[91] Parhofer KG. Lipoprotein(a): medical treatment options for an elusive molecule. Curr Pharm Des. 2011;17:871-876.

[92] McKenney J. New perspectives on the use of niacin in the treatment of lipid disorders. Arch Intern Med. 2004;164:697-705.

[93] Chasman DI, Shiffman D, Zee RY, Louie JZ, Luke MM, Rowland CM, Catanese JJ, Buring JE, Devlin JJ, Ridker PM. Polymorphism in the apolipoprotein(a) gene, plasma lipoprotein(a), cardiovascular disease, and low-dose aspirin therapy. Atherosclerosis. 2009;203:371-376.

[94] Galvano F, Li Volti G, Malaguarnera M, Avitabile T, Antic T, Vacante M, Malaguarnera M. Effects of simvastatin and carnitine versus simvastatin on lipoprotein(a) and apoprotein(a) in type 2 diabetes mellitus. Expert Opin Pharmacother. 2009;10:1875-1882.

[95] McKenney JM, Jones PH, Bays HE, Knopp RH, Kashyap ML, Ruoff GE, McGovern ME. Comparative effects on lipid levels of combination therapy with a statin and extended-release niacin or ezetimibe versus a statin alone (the COMPELL study). Atherosclerosis. 2007;192:432-437.

[96] Gonbert S, Malinsky S, Sposito AC, Laouenan H, Doucet C, Chapman MJ, Thillet J. Atorvastatin lowers lipoprotein(a) but not apolipoprotein(a) fragment levels in hypercholesterolemic subjects at high cardiovascular risk. Atherosclerosis. 2002;164:305-311.

[97] Pan J, Van JT, Chan E, Kesala RL, Lin M, Charles MA. Extended-release niacin treatment of the atherogenic lipid profile and lipoprotein(a) in diabetes. Metabolism. 2002;51:1120-1127.

[98] Schaefer EJ, McNamara JR, Tayler T, Daly JA, Gleason JL, Seman LJ, Ferrari A, Rubenstein JJ. Comparisons of effects of statins (atorvastatin, fluvastatin, lovastatin, pravastatin, and simvastatin) on fasting and postprandial lipoproteins in patients with coronary heart disease versus control subjects. Am J Cardiol. 2004 Jan 1;93(1):31-9.

[99] Bell DA, Hooper AJ, Burnett JR. Mipomersen, an antisense apolipoprotein B synthesis inhibitor. Expert Opin Investig Drugs. 2011;20:265-272.

[100] Angelin B, Rudling M. Lipid lowering with thyroid hormone and thyromimetics. Curr Opin Lipidol. 2010;21:499-506.

[101] Perrone G, Capri O, Galoppi P, Brunelli R, Bevilacqua E, Ceci F, Ciarla MV, Strom R. Effects of either tibolone or continuous combined transdermal estradiol with medroxyprogesterone acetate on coagulatory factors and lipoprotein(a) in menopause. Gynecol Obstet Invest. 2009;68:33-39.

[102] Daher R, Al-Amin H, Beaini M, Usta I. Effect of tibolone therapy on lipids and coagulation indices. Clin Chem Lab Med. 2006;44:1498-1499.

[103] Tselmin S, Schmitz G, Julius U, Bornstein SR, Barthel A, Graessler J. Acute effects of lipid apheresis on human serum lipidome. Atheroscler Suppl. 2009;10:27-33.

[104] Jaeger BR, Richter Y, Nagel D, Heigl F, Vogt A, Roeseler E, Parhofer K, Ramlow W, Koch M, Utermann G, Labarrere CA, Seidel D; Group of Clinical Investigators. Longitudinal cohort study on the effectiveness of lipid apheresis treatment to reduce high lipoprotein(a) levels and prevent major adverse coronary events. Nat Clin Pract Cardiovasc Med. 2009;6:229-239.

2

Remnant Lipoproteins are a Stronger Risk Factor for Cardiovascular Events than LDL-C – From the Studies of Autopsies in Sudden Cardiac Death Cases

Katsuyuki Nakajima[1,2] and Masaki Q. Fujita[2]
[1]*Graduate School of Health Sciences, Gunma University, Maebashi, Gunma,*
[2]*Department of Legal Medicine (Forensic Medicine), Keio University School of Medicine, Shinjuku-ku, Tokyo, Japan*

1. Introduction

Plasma LDL-C level is the most well established risk factor for coronary heart disease (CHD) (1). Accordingly, the numerous studies have shown that the LDL-C lowering drugs, statins significantly reduced plasma LDL-C together with approximately 30% reduction in cardiovascular events (2). Therefore, it has been generally believed that the cardiovascular events are directly associated with the elevated LDL-C or its modified oxidized LDL (3). In this manuscript, we have reviewed the patho-physiological role of LDL-C and remnant lipoproteins at cardiovascular events in Japanese sudden cardiac death (SCD) cases (Table 1), especially in SCD cases with nearly normal coronary arteries (coronary atherosclerosis grade (-) and (±), namely Pokkuri Death Syndrome (PDS). As the formation and physiological role of LDL in liver and plasma has been well established, those of remnant lipoproteins (RLP) have also been established recently as a risk for CHD (4-6). As shown in Figure 1, TG-rich lipoprotein (TRL) remnants are formed in the circulation when apoB-48 containing chylomicrons (CM) of intestinal origin or apoB-100 containing VLDL of hepatic origin are converted by lipoprotein lipase (and to a lesser extent by hepatic lipase) into smaller and denser particles of LDL. Compared with their nascent precursors, TRL remnants are depleted of triglycerides, phospholipids, apoA-I and apoA-IV in the case of CM and are enriched in cholesteryl esters, apoCs and apoE (6). They can thus be identified, separated, or quantified in plasma on the basis of their density, charge, size, specific lipid components, apolipoprotein composition and apolipoprotein immunospecificity. This should mean that we have now two identified cardiovascular risk factors, LDL and RLP (CM remnants and VLDL remnants) (Figure 1), in SCD and PDS cases and attempted to understand the differences in their contributions to CHD.

Recent evidences have suggested that elevated plasma levels of remnant lipoprotein – cholesterol (RLP-C) and reduced lipoprotein lipase (LPL) activity relate to the promotion of coronary artery events associated with spasm (7-9), which has been often observed as a major risk of sudden cardiac death (10). Likewise, we previously reported a significant association between sudden cardiac death and plasma levels of RLP-C and RLP-triglyceride (RLP-TG), especially in cases of Pokkuri death (11). Pokkuri death in Japanese refers the cases who "die suddenly and unexpectedly", and had not taken any medications prior to death. PDS has been categorized as one type of SCD syndrome, but not having coronary atherosclerosis and without cardiac hyperplasia. Most of such cases have been observed in Asian young males, and as yet, no report of PDS is seen in Caucasians.

	Control (n=76)			SCD (n=165)		
	mean±SD			mean±SD		
	Non-athero (n=49)	Athero (n=27)	P value	Non-athero (n=48)	Athero (n=117)	P value
Age in years	42.7±16.5	51.3±14.5	< 0.01	37.5±13.1	54.5±10.5	< 0.0001
Male/Female	41/8	24/3	NS	43/5	90/27	NS
Heart weight (g)	358±86	387±80	NS	356±82	414±91	< 0.001
Body weight (kg)	61.7±11.7	62.9±9.5	NS	65.2±11.9	63.9±12.7	NS
Body height (cm)	165±8.2	164±9.1	NS	168±9.6	164±8.5	NS
BMI	22.6±4.8	23.5±3.3	NS	22.9±3.5	23.8±3.7	NS
Postmortem period (h)	8.7±2.9	8.6±3.5	NS	8.9±3.3	8.2±3.4	NS

SCD cases without atherosclerosis (Non-athero; n=48) are categorized as PDS in this manuscript.

Table 1. Demography data of sudden cardiac death and control death cases with and without coronary artery atherosclerosis

Both SCD with coronary atherosclerosis and PDS without coronary atherosclerosis showed abnormally high plasma RLP-C and RLP-TG level, namely postprandial remnant hyperlipoproteinemia in postmortem plasma (11-14) (Table 2). RLP isolated from postmortem plasma by an immunoaffinity gel separation method (15) showed atherogenic and inflammatory effects (16, 17) similar to the RLP isolated from plasma of living subjects (6). In particular, Shimokawa and colleagues (18) reported that RLP isolated from plasma of SCD cases induced strong spasm in in-vivo setting by up-regulating the Rho-kinase pathway in healthy porcine coronary arteries, which might mimic the etiological phenomenon of PDS. But LDL (or Ox-LDL) did not enhance the formation of coronary vascular lesions in regions where coronary spasm could be induced in the same experimental model (19).

Further, Takeichi et al. (11-13) suggested RLP as one of the major risk factors in SCD and PDS. Although LDL-C levels were also elevated in parallel with the majority of SCD cases who have severe coronary atherosclerosis, the role of LDL-C in fatal clinical events was not fully understood in these cases. Therefore, the relationship between plasma levels of RLP-C, RLP-TG, LDL-C and the incidence of cardiovascular events has been studied in SCD cases with and without coronary atherosclerosis as well as in control death cases (Table2). In particular, we were interested in PDS cases among SCD cases as a disease model of coronary artery events which were neither associated with the severity of coronary artery atherosclerosis nor plaque ruptures (20).

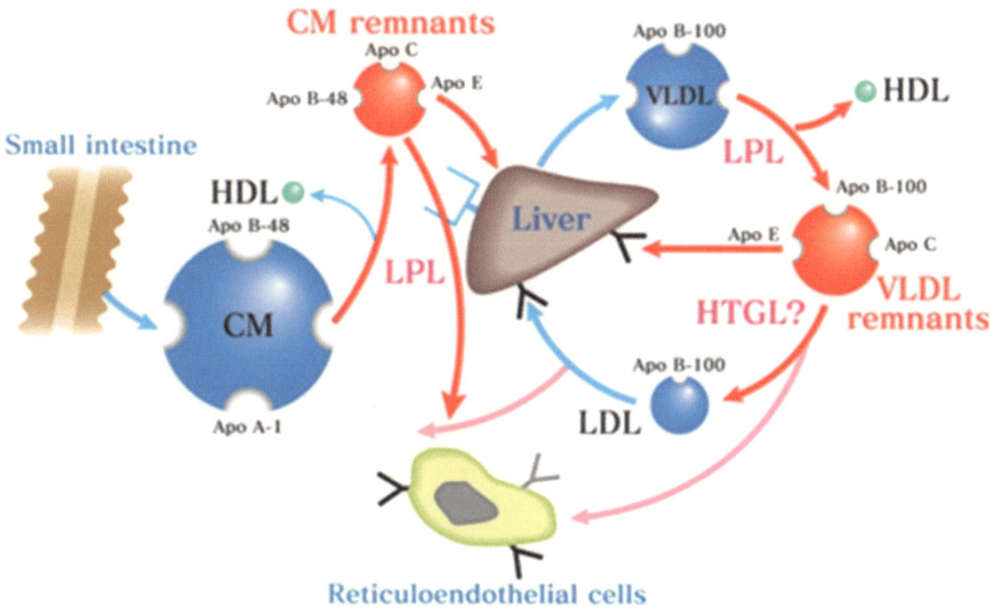

Fig. 1. Metabolic map of lipoproteins. After fat intake, the intestine secretes chylomicrons (CM), the triglycerides of which are lipolyzed by lipoprotein lipase (LPL). The LPL reaction constitutes the initial process in the formation of triglyceride-rich lipoprotein (TRL) remnants (CM remnants and VLDL remnants) . The VLDL secretion process is partly regulated by the rate of FFA influx to the liver. VLDL triglycerides are lipolyzed by endothelial-bound lipoprotein lipase and VLDL remnant particles are formed. The final TRL remnant composition is modulated by the cholesterol ester transfer protein (CETP) reaction with HDL, hepatic lipase (HL), and the exchange of soluble apolipoproteins such as C-I, C-II, C-III and E. The great majority of the remnants are removed from plasma by receptor-mediated processes and the principal receptors are the LDL receptor and the LDL-receptor-related protein (LRP) in liver. It is probable that the CM remnants use both of these routes, whereas the VLDL remnants are more likely to use only the LDL receptor.

	Control (n = 76)		SCD(n = 165)		
	median	25-75% tile	median	25-75% tile	P value[a]
Total cholesterol (mg/dl)	177	134-209	211	175-243	< 0.0001
Triglyceride (mg/dl)	116	81-157	148	100-230	< 0.001
VLDL-C (mg/dl)	20.3	6.0-35.6	27.0	16.1-47.6	< 0.001
LDL-C (mg/dl)	92	67-132	134	99-167	< 0.0001
HDL-C (mg/dl)	42	31-60	41	33-53	NS
RLP-C (mg/dl)	9.1	5.4-13.8	16.4	10.0-26.9	< 0.001
RLP-TG (mg/dl)	49	33-78	81	51-132	< 0.001

Table 2(a). Plasma lipid and lipoprotein levels in total cases of sudden cardiac death (SCD) and control death.

	Control (n = 49)		Pokkuri (n = 48)		
	median	25-75% tile	median	25-75% tile	P value[a]
Total cholesterol (mg/dl)	165	121-205	182	149-221	< 0.01
Triglyceride (mg/dl)	114	75-129	120	96-216	< 0.005
VLDL-C (mg/dl)	20.3	5.1-35.2	27.0	16.2-43.7	NS
LDL-C (mg/dl)	89	67-130	118	83-140	< 0.001
HDL-C (mg/dl)	39	30-59	41	34-56	NS
RLP-C (mg/dl)	7.1	5.1-10.1	14.3	9.5-26.4	< 0.001
RLP-TG (mg/dl)	48	33-67	78	50-117	< 0.001

Table 2(b). Plasma lipid and lipoprotein levels in cases of Pokkuri death and control death (without coronary artery atherosclerosis).

	Control (n = 27)		SCD(n = 117)		
	median	25-75% tile	median	25-75% tile	P value[a]
Total cholesterol (mg/dl)	203	171-216	219	185-248	< 0.05
Triglyceride (mg/dl)	120	82-188	154	106-232	< 0.05
VLDL-C (mg/dl)	21.5	7.0-39.0	26.9	15.8-49.4	NS
LDL-C (mg/dl)	95	69-136	148	103-179	< 0.01
HDL-C (mg/dl)	45	34-63	41	33-51	NS
RLP-C (mg/dl)	12.5	10.1-18.5	17.2	11.4-46.8	< 0.05
RLP-TG (mg/dl)	55	38-84	83	51-142	< 0.05

Table 2(c). Plasma lipid and lipoprotein levels in cases of sudden cardiac death (SCD) and control death(with coronary artery atherosclerosis).

We have established the cut-off values and the likelihood ratios of total cholesterol (TC), TG, RLP-C, RLP-TG and LDL-C in plasma of SCD and control death cases with and without coronary atherosclerosis after adjusting for the postmortem conditions (Table 3) (21). The cut-off values and likelihood ratios of these major plasma lipids and lipoproteins were calculated by using an ROC analysis model for predicting the risk of fatal clinical events with and without coronary atherosclerosis. In approximately two-third of sudden cardiac death cases, we found postprandial remnant hyperlipoproteinemia, especially rich in very low density lipoprotein (VLDL) remnants (14) and significantly elevated LDL-C. Both lipoproteins were significantly elevated in SCD, but LDL-C in PDS cases was within the normal range, together with significantly elevated remnant lipoproteins in fatal clinical events. Therefore, we found that PDS cases were a good disease model to distinguish the role of LDL and RLP as cardiovascular risk factors.

	Cut-off (mg/dl)	Sensitivity (%)	Specificity (%)	PPV Positive predictive value	NPV Negative predictive value	Likelihood ratio
(1) Total (SCD : Control)						
RLP-C	12.8	67.9	68.2	84.4	45.7	2.12
RLP-TG	53.3	72.9	60.8	82.5	46.9	1.86
LDL-C	92.5	79.4	52.7	81.0	50.2	1.68
Total Cholesterol	181	69.3	49.3	77.6	38.7	1.37
Triglycerides	117	66.3	49.3	76.8	36.6	1.31
(2) Non-athero (Pokkuri: Control)						
RLP-C	10.1	70.2	77.5	75.4	72.7	3.13
RLP-TG	67	66.7	75.6	72.8	62.9	2.73
LDL-C	106	58.3	61.7	59.9	60.2	1.52
Total Cholesterol	165	63.8	51.1	56.1	59.0	1.30
Triglycerides	113	53.3	50.0	51.1	52.2	1.07
(3) Athero (SCD : Control)						
RLP-C	13.4	65.3	69.2	90.2	31.5	2.12
RLP-TG	79.4	52.5	72.4	89.2	26.0	1.90
LDL-C	102	79.7	57.1	89.0	39.4	1.86
Total Cholesterol	217	55.2	78.6	91.8	28.8	2.58
Triglycerides	131	64.9	64.3	88.7	29.7	1.82

Number of cases are as follows: (1) total SCD; SCD (n=165) and Control (n=76) : (2) Non-athero; Pokkuri (Non-athero SCD) (n=48) and Non-athero control (n=49): (3) Athero; Athero SCD (n=117) and Athero-control (n=27).

Table 3. Cut-off value of RLP-C and RLP-TG from ROC analysis in predicting sudden cardiac death

2. Role of plasma LDL and remnant lipoproteins at coronary atherosclerosis and cardiovascular events

Based on our autopsy studies, more than two thirds of SCD cases were found to be associated with postprandial remnant hyperlipoproteinemia [11-15]. If severe spasm of the coronary artery is to be a crucial event prior to cardiac death in PDS, we may say that the vasospasm is not very likely to occur in coronary arteries with severe coronary artery atherosclerotic lesions due to reduced elasticity and increased stiffness or hardness of the vascular wall. Caucasians experience more severe coronary atherosclerosis than Japanese or other Southeastern Asians. Accordingly, this might be one explanation why PDS is uncommon among Caucasians. In view of this background, PDS could be an interesting disease case to study coronary heart disease (CHD), which is independent of severity of coronary atherosclerosis and plaque ruptures in spite of remnant hyperlipoproteinemia. Significantly younger age of PDS cases compared to the other SCD cases may be one of the reasons why PDS cases were not associated with severe coronary atherosclerosis. The prevalence of severe coronary atherosclerosis is known to be strongly associated with age (Table1). We found that plasma lipid (TC, TG) and lipoprotein (LDL-C, RLP-C, and RLP-TG) levels were significantly elevated in these sudden cardiac death cases as compared with those in control death cases when coronary atherosclerosis was pathologically graded above (1+), reflecting the clinical feature of severe coronary atherosclerosis (11-13). Most of the coronary arteries in PDS cases were pathologically graded as (−) and (±), indicating no coronary atherosclerosis [11]. Plasma LDL-C in SCD cases was shown to be correlated with the severity of coronary artery atherosclerosis [13]. This is in line with the perception (albeit by implication) that LDL-C plays a major role in the progression of coronary atherosclerosis in CHD patients. We found that the incidence of elevated plasma LDL-C was significantly greater in SCD cases with coronary atherosclerosis compared with than in controls and PDS cases. However, plasma LDL-C levels were all within normal range in PDS cases (22). Hence, LDL-C did not seem to play a significant role at cardiovascular events in PDS, despite being elevated within normal range , rather the data strongly indicated an association between plasma LDL-C and the progression of coronary atherosclerosis in SCD cases.

Elevated plasma remnant lipoproteins (RLP) levels were the most striking observation in PDS (RLP-C likelihood ratio; 3.13, RLP-TG; 2.73, LDL-C; 1.52, TC; 1.30, TG; 1.07) for predicting sudden cardiac death (Table 3). Despite the high plasma concentration of RLPs in PDS cases, the progression of atherosclerosis at coronary arteries was not observed. It might be valid to say that increased plasma RLPs may initiate the vascular endothelial damage and this is followed by an influx of large amounts of LDL into the vascular wall. Then it follows to form an advanced atherosclerotic lesion with macrophages and smooth muscle cells as Nakajima et al reviewed previously (6, 23). PDS cases may be in the early stage of atherosclerosis, which can lead cardiovascular events under certain conditions such as with severe stress without strong morphological changes. Therefore, the authors proposed that the occurrence of cardiovascular events at coronary arteries and the severity of atherosclerotic lesions in CHD should be considered as separate factors. Therefore, the intervention should be targeted to suppress the cardiovascular events more aggressively than to slow down the progression of atherosclerosis. Takeichi and Fujita did not observe frequent plaque ruptures in coronary arteries at autopsy in Japanese SCD cases [24].

The literature on atherosclerosis has long been dominated by data in Caucasian patients who in most cases had severe atherosclerosis at the time of fatal clinical events. Hence, fatal clinical events have been believed to occur in relation to the severity of atherosclerosis in coronary arteries. In contrast, fatal clinical events of PDS cases had occurred in the absence of coronary atherosclerosis or plaque rupture. Plasma LDL-C levels were also within normal range associated with no coronary atherosclerosis in PDS cases. This again puts more weight on RLP as the causative factor of cardiovascular events. Interestingly, we found that RLP-TG (TG concentration in remnant lipoproteins) was not an indicator for predicting the presence or progression of coronary atherosclerosis even in SCD [22]; however, it was significantly associated with fatal clinical events in SCD including PDS (Table 2). The bioactive components co-localized with triglycerides in RLP such as oxidized phospholipids or their metabolites [25] may enhance the formation of coronary vascular lesions and may induce severe spasm in coronary arteries. These results also suggested that triglycerides in RLP were not associated with the progression of atherosclerotic plaques, but cholesterol in RLP was strongly associated with the severity of atherosclerosis [13, 22]. Therefore RLP-TG could be an appropriate diagnostic marker for predicting cardiovascular events but not the severity of coronary atherosclerosis, whereas RLP-C could be a marker for predicting both cardiovascular events and the severity of coronary atherosclerosis. LDL-C could be a marker for predicting the severity of coronary atherosclerosis, but not cardiovascular events. Elevated Oxidized LDL seems to be associated with the presence of vulnerable plaque at blood vessels (6), not a causative factor for the formation or initiation of atherosclerosis because of it low concentration in plasma.

3. Postprandial remnant hyperlipoproteinemia as a risk for sudden cardiac death

Several clinical studies have shown that elevated plasma TG levels greatly increase the risk of sudden cardiac death. Results from the Paris Prospective Study (26) and The Apolipoprotein Related Mortality Risk Study (AMORIS) in Sweden (27) demonstrated that increased TG was a strong risk factor for fatal myocardial infarction. However, plasma TG levels can alter very easily within a short time. Therefore it has been difficult to identify the clinical events of elevated TG in the long term prospective studies until recently (28-30).

If the lipid and lipoprotein levels in postmortem plasma correctly reflected the antemortem levels, these data could probably provide the same values with the results obtained from the prospective studies, which require long-term observation for evaluation. The plasma levels of lipids and lipoproteins in sudden death cases may reflect the feature at the moment of fatal clinical events followed by certain inevitable postmortem alterations, but still may reflect the physiological conditions when the cardiac events had occurred. Therefore, we analyzed postmortem plasma under well-controlled conditions to clarify the cause of sudden cardiac death. Plasma RLP-C and RLP-TG levels vary greatly within a short time as the TG levels, compared with other stable plasma markers such as HDL-C and LDL-C. Hence, we believe that the cross-sectional study of RLPs at the moment of sudden death is a superior analytical method than a prospective study of RLP (31) to identify potential risks of CHD. During the investigations of sudden death cases, we found that the postmortem alterations of lipids and lipoproteins in plasma were unexpectedly slight (21) compared with proteins or other bio-markers. Moreover, these plasma lipoprotein levels were very similar to those determined in living patients from the studies in our laboratory.

Remnant lipoproteins are known to increase postprandially as chylomicron (CM) remnants, but very low density lipoprotein (VLDL) remnants also increase at the same time. The remarkable close correlation between the increment in the concentration of TG-rich lipoprotein (TRL) apoB-48 (CM) and apoB-100 (VLDL) after a fat meal indicates that reduced efficiency of CM particle clearance is closely coupled to the accumulation of VLDL particles as proposed by Karpe et al (32). Delayed clearance of CM particles, as evidently occurs in many hypertriglyceridemic states, may thus contribute to the elevation of apoB-100 in TRL. More than two thirds of the SCD including PDS case observed in this study showed stomach full, indicating the strong association with postprandial remnant hyperlipoproteinemia. Significant remnant hyperlipoproteinemia was observed in the plasma of SCD cases compared with the control death cases.

The postprandial increase of apoB-48-carrying CM and CM remnants after fat load is known to correlate well with the increase of RLP-C and RLP-TG (33). These data suggested the possibility that increased RLP in the postprandial state may be mainly composed of CM remnants. However, unexpectedly, we found no significant differences of apoB-48 levels in plasma or RLP apoB-48, but found significant differences of RLP aoB-100 levels between SCD and control death cases (14). As previously reported by Schneeman et al. (34), postprandial responses (after fat load) of apoB-48 and apoB-100 were highly correlated with those of TRL triglycerides. Although the increase in apoB-48 represented a 3.5-fold difference in concentration as compared with a 1.6-fold increase in apoB-100, apoB-100 accounted for about 80% of the increase in lipoprotein particles in TRL. Our results on plasma evaluation in SCD cases were very similar to the results reported by Schneeman et al (34). RLP apoB-100 levels were significantly elevated in SCD cases in the postprandial state (when RLP-C and RLP-TG were significantly elevated), however, plasma apoB-48 or RLP apoB-48 was not significantly elevated (14). These results strongly suggested that the major subset of RLP associated with fatal clinical events was apoB-100 carrying particles, but not apoB-48 particles.

The absolute amount of apoB-100 in RLP is much greater than that of apoB-48 in RLP. Hence, VLDL remnants, endogenous lipoprotein remnants, generated in the liver, may be more closely associated with the risk of sudden cardiac death than exogenous CM remnants, irrespective of the severity of coronary atherosclerosis. Furthermore, we often found SCD cases that had consumed alcohol on a full stomach. It is known that alcohol increases fatty acids in the liver and enhances VLDL production, and inhibit LPL activity (35). Alcohol intake with a fatty meal is known to greatly enhance TG increase in the postprandial state. The intake of alcohol together with a fatty meal may easily enhance the production of apoB-100 carrying VLDL in the liver, and increase VLDL remnants by inhibiting LPL activity and increase the potential risk of coronary artery in SCD cases.

4. Comparative reactivity of LDL and remnant lipoproteins to LDL receptor in liver

Clinical trials have shown that improvements in plasma LDL-C levels are associated with retardation of atherosclerosis and reduction in coronary artery morbidity and mortality [2, 36]. The major mechanism of statin therapeutic effect has been recognized as the increase of LDL receptor in liver to remove an elevated LDL-C in plasma. However, remnant lipoproteins have been also implicated in progression of atherosclerosis [37-40], with elevated remnant lipoprotein levels shown to independently predict clinical events in coronary artery disease (CAD) patients (4]. The direct comparison of reactivity between remnant lipoproteins and LDL to LDL receptor in liver has not been studied enough until recently.

Major target for remnant lipoprotein research has been focused on postprandial dyslipidemia. Postprandial dyslipidemia has been found to be associated with endothelial dysfunction [42, 43] an early indicator of atherogenesis. Previous studies have shown that normolipidemic patients with coronary disease have elevated postprandial levels of triglyceride-rich lipoproteins (TRLs) and their remnants compared with healthy control subjects [44-49]. Elevated remnant lipoprotein levels have also been associated with coronary endothelial dysfunction [50], with remnants shown to stimulate expression of proatherothrombotic molecules in endothelial cells [51]. Therefore, the prevention and treatment of atherosclerosis merits pharmacotherapy targeted at regulating postprandial dyslipidemia, namely remnant lipoproteins beyond LDL-C [52]. Postprandial remnant lipoproteins are the atherogenic lipoproteins which appear and increase postprandially into plasma at the initial step of lipoprotein metabolism after food intake and then change to further metabolized lipoproteins, such as LDL particles (Figure 1). The postprandial state with increased remnant lipoproteins in plasma continues almost whole day except in the early morning (6), while not the case in LDL. Therefore, if postprandial lipoproteins are atherogenic risks as Zilversmit proposed (53), those should be the primary therapeutic target to prevent cardiovascular disease. Increased LDL is not directly associated with the daily food intake as remnant lipoproteins.

Possible mechanisms suggested for abnormal accumulation of lipoproteins postprandially in plasma are defective clearance in liver via receptor-mediated pathways and/or increased competition for high-affinity processes because of increased numbers of intestinally and hepatically derived particles in the postprandial state [32]. HMG-CoA reductase inhibitors decrease cellular cholesterol synthesis and consequently reduce the hepatic production of very-low-density lipoproteins (VLDL) and increase the expression of LDL-receptors in liver [54]. These properties of statins suggest that they are potential agents for regulating the plasma levels of remnant lipoproteins as well as LDL-C.

Atorvastatin is an HMG-CoA reductase inhibitor found to be effective in lowering fasting LDL-C and triglyceride levels [55]. Favorable effects of atorvastatin on postprandial lipoprotein metabolism have been reported in healthy normolipidemic human subjects [56-58]. Recently, atorvastatin and rozuvastatin are reported to decrease small dense LDL-C significantly, which is highly correlated with remnant lipoproteins in plasma, possibly as a precursor of sdLDL (59).

We investigated whether RLP bound to LDL receptor more efficiently than LDL itself via apoE-ligand which is rich in RLP (6). RLP competed more efficiently with β-VLDL than LDL in LDL receptor transfected cells (to be published in Clin Chim Acta 2012 by Takahashi et al). These results suggested that RLP which is mainly apoE-rich VLDL more efficiently binds and internalizes into LDL receptor transfected cells than LDL. Similar results were observed in VLDL receptor transfected cells, although VLDL receptor is not present in liver (60). Takahashi et al found that pitabastatin (NK-104) induced VLDL receptor in skeletal muscle cells with significantly higher concentration (more than 10 folds) compared to HepG2, in which NK-104 enabled to induce LDL receptor.

In FH of a LDL receptor deficiency, statins have a dual mechanism of action involving an increase in the catabolism of LDL via up-regulation of LDL-receptors and a decrease in the hepatic secretion of apolipoprotein (apo) B-100. The net effect is a decrease in the concentration of apoB-containing lipoproteins. As CM remnants are also apo E-rich and mainly cleared via the LDL-receptor [61, 62], an increase in receptor activity and reduced competition from apoB-100-containing lipoproteins was hypothesized to increase the removal rate of remnant lipoproteins from circulation. A recent study investigating the effects of high-dose, long-term statin treatment on the metabolism of postprandial lipoproteins in heterozygous FH, reported a decrease in the fasting and postprandial RLP-C as well as LDL-C [63]. Statins can induce LDL receptor in heterozygous FH which enhance the removal of RLP and LDL simultaneously.

However, it has not been known which, RLP or LDL, is removed earlier or primarily from plasma by increased LDL receptor with statin treatment. Takahashi et al suggested the possibility that remnant lipoproteins are removed more primarily from plasma by statins and prevent cardiovascular disease, while LDL are more likely reduced as a consequence of reduction of the precursor lipoproteins (to be published in Clin Chim Acta 2012 by Takahashi et al).

Moreover, VLDL receptor which does not affect the removal of remnant lipoproteins in liver may affect on rhabdomyolysis in skeletal muscle cells, in case when VLDL receptors are significantly induced by statins in those cells. When plasma concentration of statins increased abnormally high, VLDL receptor could be induced in the skeletal muscle cells. Then, RLP binds and internalizes into skeletal muscle cells with significantly increased concentration and may cause the rhabdomyolysis in skeletal muscle cells by the cytotoxic effect of remnant lipoproteins (6, 64, 65).

The direct comparison between LDL and RLP has shown that RLP with its apoE-rich ligand has superior binding and internalization reactivity to LDL receptor than LDL in liver, which is a similar reactivity with VLDL receptor. These results suggest that RLP may be more primarily and efficiently metabolized in liver than LDL through increased LDL receptor when treated with statins.

5. Possible molecular mechanism of remnant lipoproteins associated with coronary artery vasospasm

Followings are the hypothesis of molecular mechanism on the initiation and progression of atherosclerosis associated with fatal cardiovascular events we have proposed from our studies on sudden cardiac death during last two decades (Figure 2).

Elevated plasma RLP first cause the initiation of vascular dysfunction at endothelial cell and smooth muscle cells through LOX-1 receptor and activate Rho-kinase pathway in vascular smooth muscle cells to induce coronary artery spasm as vascular smooth muscle hyperconstriction. However, LDL has no such biological properties to initiate the vascular dysfunction. Although Ox-LDL, derived from LDL modified, has very similar biological properties with remnant lipoproteins, the plasma concentration of Ox-LDL is significantly low and can not influence to the following phenomenon like remnant lipoproteins shown by in vitro studies (6).

5.1 Remnant lipoproteins and impaired endothelialium-dependent vasorelaxation

Endothelial activation or dysfunction is known to be an early event in the development of atherosclerosis which is not necessarily associated with strong morphological changes. Kugiyama et al (66) and Inoue et al (67) first found that plasma RLP-C levels, but not LDL-C levels, showed significant and independent correlation with impaired endothelial function reflected as impaired endothelium-dependent vasomotor function (vasorelaxation) in large and resistance coronary arteries in humans. These observations indicated the possibility that high plasma concentration of remnant lipoproteins impair endothelial cell function in human coronary arteries.

Flow-mediated vasodilation (FMD) of the brachial artery during reactive hyperemia has been used as a noninvasive method to assess endothelial function. Kugiyama et al (68) and Funada et al (69) examined FMD by high resolution ultrasound technique before and at the

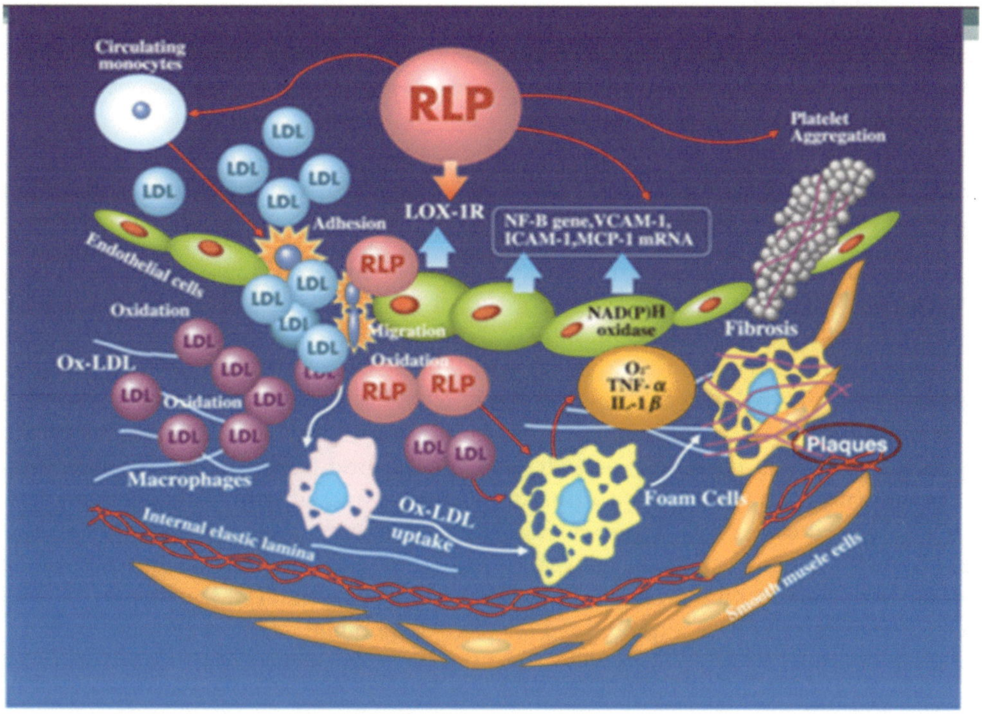

Fig. 2. Effect of RLP and Ox-LDL on athegenesis. The endothelial cell dysfunction is initiated by RLP in plasma followed by the induction of LOX-1 receptor and the associated pathway of various cytokines and enzymes. Ox-LDL promotes the progression of atherosclerosis in subendothelial space after a large efflux of LDL from plasma and form atherosclerotic plaques.

end of a 4 week treatment with oral administration of alpha-tocopherol acetate (300 IU/day). Alpha-tocopherol improved the impairment of endothelium-dependent vasodilation in patients with high RLP-C, but not in patients with low RLP-C. Similarly, RLP and their extracted lipids impaired endothelium-dependent vasorelaxation (EDR) of isolated rabbit aorta at the same concentration of serum RLP-C as found in patients with coronary artery disease (70). In contrast, non-RLP in the VLDL fraction had no effect on EDR. This in vitro study further showed that co-incubation of N-acetylcysteine and reduced glutathione (GSH), antioxidants, that were added to incubation mixture in isolated rabbit aorta containing RLP, almost completely reversed the impaired EDR, suggesting that reactive oxygen species contained in RLP or those generated by RLP played a significant role in the impairment of EDR. Further, Doi et al (51) showed that RLP isolated from patients undergoing treatment with alpha-tocopherol lost their inhibitory action on vasorelaxation of isolated rabbit aorta in response to Ach, whereas RLP from patients receiving placebo had inhibitory action on vasorelaxation. These results suggested that high RLP-C level being oxidized in plasma increased the oxidative stress and contribute to endothelial vasomotor dysfunction in patients with high plasma concentration of RLP-C. Ohara et al (17) reported that remnant lipoproteins isolated from SCD cases suppressed nitric oxide (NO) synthetase activity and attenuate endothelium-dependent vasorelaxation.

Probucol is known to inhibit the oxidative modification of LDL (71), lowering serum cholesterol levels. Ox-LDL has been shown to impair endothelium-dependent vasorelaxation and antioxidants, including probucol, suppressing the impaired EDR (72) as RLP described above.

5.2 Both Ox-LDL and remnant lipoproteins activate LOX-1 receptor in endothelial cells

A scavenger receptor independent pathway for acetyl LDL and oxidized LDL in cultured endothelial cells, has long been known; however, it has been difficult to isolate. Recently, Sawamura and his colleagues (73-76) discovered and characterized lectin-like oxidized LDL receptor-1 (LOX-1) as a vascular endothelial receptor for Ox-LDL. Endothelial dysfunction or activation invoked by oxidatively modified LDL has been implicated in the pathogenesis of atherosclerosis by enhanced intimal thickening and lipid deposition in the arteries. Ox-LDL and its lipid constituents, mainly composed of oxidized products of phospholipids such as lysophosphatidylcholine, impair endothelial production of NO, and induce the endothelial expression of leukocyte adhesion molecules and smooth muscle growth factors, which can contribute to atherogenesis via LOX-1 receptor. Vascular endothelial cells in culture and in vivo internalize and degrade Ox-LDL through a putative receptor-mediated pathway that does not involve macrophage scavenger receptor. The treatment of HUVECs with RLP increased LOX-1 expression in a dose dependent manner (Figure 3) and was completely inhibited by LOX-1- antisense, but not by LOX-1-sence. Monoclonal antibody to LOX-1 reported by Shin et al (77) and antisence LOX-1 oligodeoxynucleotide reported by Park et al (78) significantly reduced RLP-mediated production of superoxide (NADPH oxidase dependent), TNF-alpha, and interleukin-beta, NF-κB activation, DNA fragmentation (cell death: apoptosis). Further Shin et al (77) have emphasized the importance of RLP in increasing the expression of LOX-1 receptor protein in NADPH oxidase dependent superoxide production; the expression of adhesion molecules such as ICAM-1, VCAM -1 and MCP-1 stimulated by RLP is dependent on the activation of LOX-1 receptors. These findings strongly suggest that LOX-1 may play the role of a receptor of RLP as well as Ox-LDL in endothelial cells. Endothelial cell injury caused by RLP via LOX-1 receptor activation evidently can initiate atherosclerosis. Cilostazol, a platelet aggregation inhibitor and vasodilator (79), is known to reduce plasma RLP-C levels in patients with peripheral artery disease (80) and has showed significant protective effect against RLP-induced endothelial dysfunction by suppressing these variables both in-vitro and in-vivo with its antioxidative activity (81).

5.3 Remnant lipoproteins activate LOX-1 receptor in smooth muscle cell

Coronary vasospasm has been considered to occur at vascular smooth muscle cells (VSMCs) and the migration of VSMCs from media to intima and subsequent proliferation play key roles in atherogenesis. A previous report has demonstrated that RLPs induce VSMC proliferation [82]; however, receptors for RLPs in VSMCs have not yet been well characterized until recently reported by Aramaki et al (83), although LRP in the liver, apoB-48-R in macrophages, and VLDL receptor in heart, skeletal muscle, adipose tissue, brain and macrophages [84, 85] have been shown to act as a receptor for RLPs. LOX-1 expression is dynamically inducible by various proatherogenic stimuli, including tumor necrosis factor-α(TNF-α), heparin-binding epidermal growth factor-like growth factor (HB-EGF), and Ox-

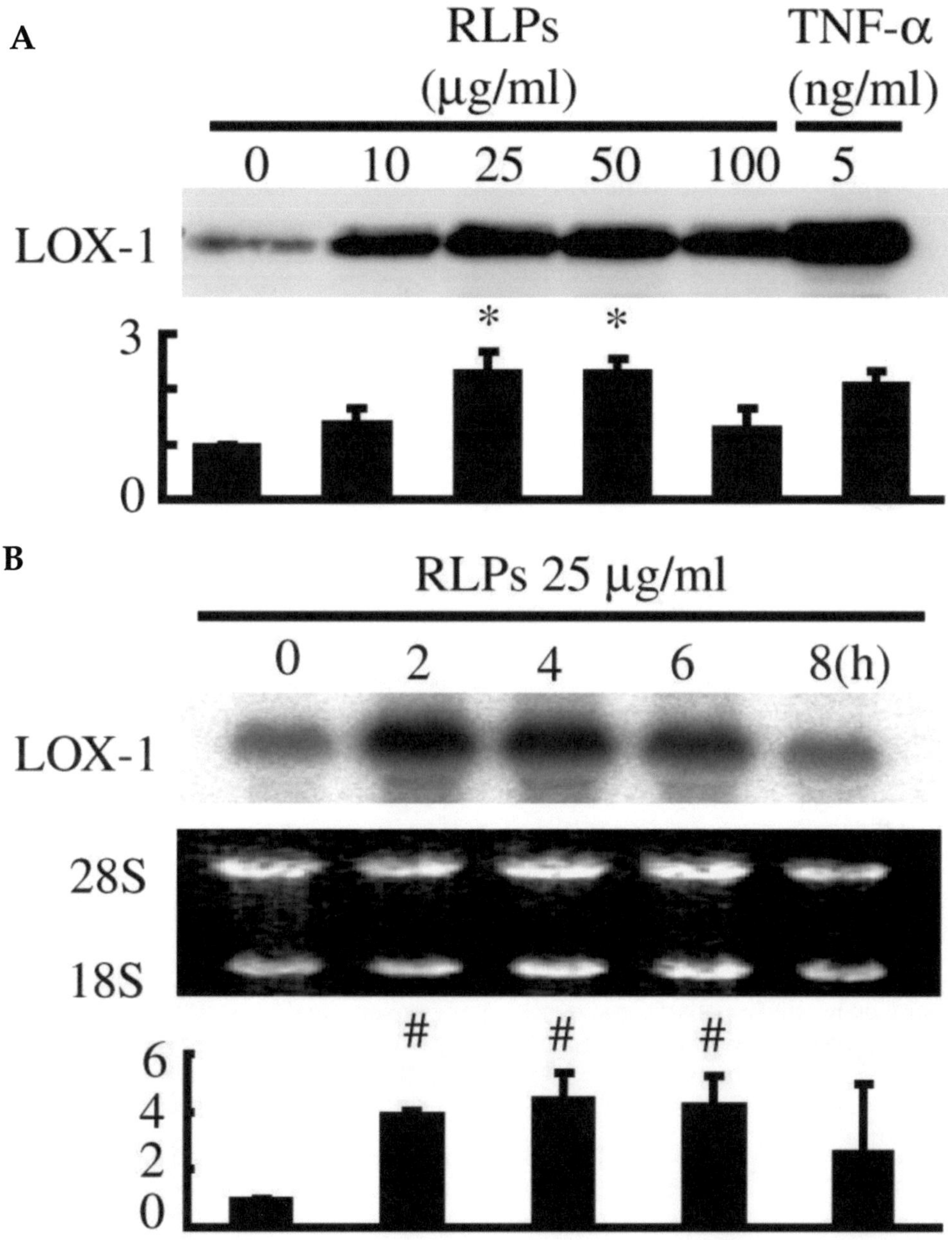

Fig. 3. RLPs, but not nascent VLDL (n-VLDL), induce LOX-1 expression in BVSMCs. (A) After BVSMCs were treated with the indicated concentrations of RLPs for 16 h, total cell lysates were subjected to immunoblotting for LOX-1. TNF-α served as a positive control. (B) After treatment with 25μg/ml of RLPs for the indicated time periods, total cellular RNA was subjected to Northern blot analyses. Bands for 28S and 18S ribosomal RNAs were visualized by ethidium bromide staining to control the amount of RNA loaded. (*) $p < 0.001$ vs. 0g/ml of RLPs, (#) $p < 0.05$ vs. 0 h incubation (cited from Ref 83).

LDL. Furthermore, LOX-1 is highly expressed by macrophages and VSMCs accumulate in the intima of advanced atherosclerotic lesions, as well as endothelial cells covering early atherosclerotic lesions in vivo, indicating that LOX-1 appears to play important roles at various stages of atherogenesis.. Aramaki et al (83) recently provided direct evidence, by cDNA and short interference RNAs (siRNAs) transfection, that LOX-1 acts as a receptor for RLP (Figure 1) and whereby induce VSMC migration, depending upon HB-EGF shedding and the downstream signal transduction cascades. The direct evidences that LOX-1 serves as a receptor for RLPs in vascular smooth muscle cells (VSMCs) were shown by use of two cell lines which stably express human or bovine LOX-1 and siRNA directed to LOX-1. In addition, involvement of metalloproteinase activation, HB-EGF shedding, EGFR transactivation, and activation of ERK, p38 MAPK and PI3K were also observed in RLP induced migration of BVSMCs. Competition studies in cells stably expressing LOX-1 indicated binding site(s) on the LOX-1 molecule for RLPs and oxidized LDL appear to be identical or overlapped, suggesting the C-terminal cysteine-rich C-type lectin-like domain was shown to be the responsible binding site(s) for RLPs [86]. These studies suggested the importance of LOX-1 in RLP-induced atherogenesis, as well as that induced by oxidized LDL. RLPs induced cell migration and LOX-1 expression by RLP-LOX-1 interactions, thus making a positive-feed back loop to further enhance the RLP-induced vascular dysfunction, as already showed in oxidized LDL-induced vascular dysfunction. In accordance with a previous report [77, 78], RLP-induced LOX-1 expression and cell migration depend upon HB-EGF shedding and subsequent EGFR transactivation demonstrated. Furthermore, the involvement of ERK, p38 MAPK and Akt as signal transducrion cascades located downstream to the EGFR transactivation were shown. JNK was not activated by RLPs or not involved in RLP-induced LOX-1 expression or cell migration (84).

These results suggested that RLP induced LOX-1 expression and enhance the activation of smooth muscle cells.

5.4 Remnant lipoproteins activate Rho-kinase in smooth muscle cells and induce vasospasm

Coronary vasospasm has been postulated to play an important role in SCD, although a direct demonstration for the hypothesis is still lacking. Shimokawa and his colleagues demonstrated the close relation between RLP and coronary vasospasm that is mediated by upregulated Rho-kinase pathway (18). The expression and the activity of Rho-kinase are enhanced at the inflammatory coronary lesions in the porcine model with interleukin-1 (19, 88).

RLP isolated from the plasma of SCD cases exert a potent upregulating effect on Rho-kinase in hcVSMC (18). In organ chamber experiments, serotonin caused hyperconstriction of vascular smooth muscle cells (VSMC) from RLP-treated segment, which was significantly inhibited by hydoxyfasudil (a selective Rho-kinase inhibitor). In cultured human coronary VSMC, the treatment with RLP significantly enhanced the expression and the activity of Rho-kinase. These results indicated that RLP isolated from the plasma of sudden cardiac death cases upregulated Rho-kinase in coronary VSMC (promoted inflammation) and markedly enhanced coronary vasospasmic activity.

Further, Oi et al (18) performed in vivo study on the formation of coronary vascular lesion by RLP, using healthy pigs in which they treated pig coronary arteries with RLP (an equivalent concentration of plasma RLP) isolated from the plasma of SCD cases. After 1 week, intracoronary serotonin caused hyperconstriction in the segment treated with RLP but not in the non-RLP VLDL treated segment (Figure 4). Likewise, RLP treated with hydroxyfasudil, a selective Rho-kinase inhibitor, dose dependently inhibited the coronary spasm in pigs.

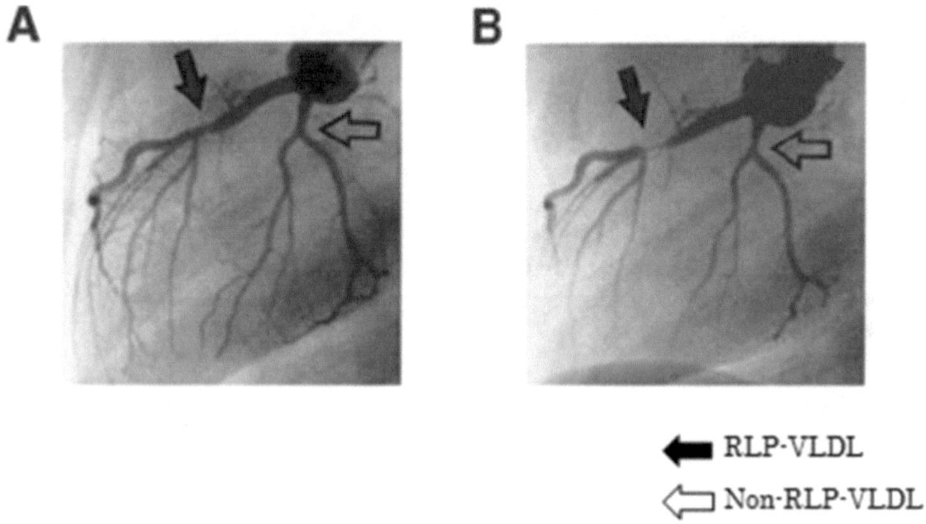

Fig. 4. RLP (RLP in VLDL fraction; RLP-VLDL) from patients with SCD markedly enhance coronary vasospastic activity in pigs. Coronary angiograms before (A) and after intracoronary serotonin (B). Black arrows indicate RLP site at coronary artery; white arrows, non-RLP site. RLP induced significant hyperconstriction at treated coronary site after 1 week, while hydroxyfasudil completely inhibited serotonin (5HT)-induced coronary hyperconstriction at RLP site (cited from Ref 18). These results were explained by the induction of Rho-kinase α and Rho-kinase β, of which mRNA expression was enhanced by the treatment with RLP but not that with non-RLP.

It has been recently reported that sphingosine 1-phosphate (S1P) and sphingosylphosphorylcholine, present in serum lipoproteins, behave as a lipid mediator and cause vasoconstriction through upregulation of Rho/Rho-kinase pathway (89). The possible role of S1P and sphingosylphosphorylcholine in the RLP fraction remains to be elucidated.

These results suggested the importance of intervention to suppress the cardiovascular events more aggressively by such as inhibiting Rho-kinase activation than to slow down the progression of atherosclerosis.

6. Conclusion remarks

Sudden and unexplained cardiac death has been known for many years in Southeast Asian countries, including Japan. These deaths were named differently in each country such as Pokkuri Death Syndrome in Japan, "Lai Tai" in Thailand, "Bangungut " in the Philippines, "Dream Disease" in Hawaii, and "Sudden Unexpected Nocturnal Death Syndrome" among South Asian immigrants in the USA. However, the clinical and pathological features of these sudden death cases are surprisingly similar with no coronary atherosclerosis and mainly occur among young males during sleep in the midnight, together with an excessive food and alcohol intake.

We have proposed a hypothesis that could explain a possible cause of PDS based on the postprandial increase of remnant lipoproteins in plasma and narrowed circumferences of coronary arteries in PDS cases. The elevated plasma RLP initiates the vascular dysfunction at endothelial cells in narrowed coronary arteries as an early event in the development of atherosclerosis and induces severe coronary spasm under stress or genetic disorder, possibly for example, through activating LOX-1 receptor and Rho-kinase pathway, at smooth muscle cells to cause cardiac arrest. LDL or low concentration of Ox-LDL could not explain these phenomena as RLP. Taken together, we have proposed that the severity of coronary atherosclerosis and the occurrence of cardiovascular events in CHD cases could be considered as separate factors, judging from the physiological role of LDL and RLP in plasma. Therefore, the intervention should be more targeted to suppress the plasma remnant lipoproteins to prevent cardiovascular events more aggressively rather than to slow down the progression of atherosclerosis by LDL.

7. Acknowledgment

This work is supported in part by Grant-in-Aid from Japan Society for the Promotion of Science (JSPS), No. 20406020. The authors deeply thank Dr. Richard Havel, University of California San Francisco and Dr. Ernest Schaefer, Tufts University for their long term collaboration on remnant lipoprotein research. Also we greatly thank Dr. Sanae Takeichi, Director of Takeichi Medical Research Laboratory (former professor of Tokai University School of Medicine, Department of Forensic Medicine) for her extensive research collaboration on sudden cardiac death.

8. References

[1] The Expert Panel. Report of the National Cholesterol Education Program Expert Panel on Detection, Evaluation and Treatment of High Blood Cholesterol in Adults. Arch Intern Med 1988;148:36-69

[2] The Scandinavian Sinvastatin Survival Study Group: Randomized trial of cholesterol lowering in 4444 patients with coronary heart disease: the Scandinavian Sinvastatin Survival Study (4S). Lancet 344:1383-1389,1994

[3] Steinberg D, Parthasarathy S, Crew TE, Khoo JC, and Witztum JL. Beyond cholesterol: modification of low-density lipoprotein that increase its atherogenecity. N Engl J Med 1989; 320: 915-924

[4] McNamara JR, Shah PK, Nakajima K,et al. Remnant-like particle (RLP) cholesterol is an independent cardiovascular disease risk factor in women: results from the Framingham Heart Study. *Atherosclerosis* 2001; 154:229-36.

[5] Twickler TB, Dallinga-Thie GM, Cohn JS, Chapman MJ. Elevated remnant-like particle cholesterol concentration: a characteristic feature of the atherogenic lipoprotein phenotype. Circulation 2004; 109:1918-25

[6] Nakajima K, Nakano T, Tanaka A. The oxidative modification hypothesis of atherosclerosis: The comparison of atherogenic effects on oxidized LDL and remnant lipoproteins in plasma. Clin Chim Acta 2006; 367: 36-47
[7] Sakata K, Miho N, Shirotani M, Yoshida H, Takada A. Remnant-like particles cholesterol is a major risk factor for myocardial infarction in vasospastic angina with nearly normal coronary artery. Atherosclerosis 1998; 136: 225-231.
[8] Miwa K, Makita T, Ihsii K, Okuda N,Taniguchi A. High remnant lipoprotein levels in patients with variant angina. Clin Cradiol 2004; 27:338-425.
[9] Kasteline JJ, Jukema IW , Zwinderman AH, et al. Lipoprotein lipase activity is associated with severity of angina pectoris. Circulation 2000; 102:1629-33
[10] Igarashi Y, Tamura Y, Suzuki K, et al. Coronary artery spasm is a major cause of sudden cardiac arrest in surviors without underlying heart disease. Coron Artery Dis 1993; 4: 177-185.
[11] Takeichi S, Nakajima Y, Yukawa N, et al. Association of plasma triglyceride-rich lipoprotein remnants with "Pokkuri disease". Legal Med 2001; 3: 84- 94.
[12] Takeichi S, Nakajima Y, Osawa M, et al. The possible role of remnant-like particles as a risk factor for sudden cardiac death. Int J Legal Med 1997;110:213-219.
[13] Takeichi S, Yukawa N, Nakajima Y, et al. Association of plasma triglyceride-rich lipoprotein remnants with coronary artery atherosclerosis in cases of sudden cardiac death. Atherosclerosis 1999;142:309-315.
[14] Nakajima K, Nakajima Y, Takeichi S, Fujita MQ. ApoB-100 carrying lipoprotein, but not apoB-48, is the major subset of proatherogenic remnant-like lipoprotein particles detected in plasma of sudden cardiac death cases. Atherosclerosis 2007, in press
[15] Nakajima K, Saito T, Tamura A, et al. Cholesterol in remnant-like lipoproteins in human serum using monoclonal anti apo B-100 and anti A-1 immunoaffinity mixed gels. Clin Chim Acta 1993; 223: 53-71
[16] Saniabadi AR, Takeichi S, Yukawa N, Nakajima Y, Umemura K, Nakashima M. Apo E4/3-rich remnant lipoproteins and platelet aggregation: A case report. Thromb Haemost 1998; 79: 878-879.
[17] Ohara N, Takeichi S, Naito Y, et al. Remnant-like particles from subjects who died of coronary artery disease suppress NO synthetase activity and attenuate endothelium-dependent vasorelaxation. Clin Chim Acta 2003; 338: 151-156.
[18] Oi K, Shimokawa H, Hiroki J, et al. Remnant lipoproteins from patients with sudden cardiac death enhance coronary vasospastic avtivity through upregulation of Rho-kinase. Arterioscler Thromb Vasc Biol 2004; 24:918-92211.
[19] Miyata K, Shimokawa H, Kandabashi T, et al. Rho-Kinase is involved in macrophage-mediated formation of coronary vascular lesions in pigs in vivo. Arterioscler Thromb Vasc Biol. 2000; 20: 2351-2358.
[20] Fuster V, Badimon J, CFallon JT et al. Plaque rupture, thrombosis, and therapeutic implications. Haemostasis 1996 ;26 (Suppl 4): 269-284
[21] Takeichi S, Nakajima Y, Yukawa N, et al. Validity of plasma remnant lipoproteins as surrogate markers of antemortem level in cases of sudden coronary death. *Clin Chim Acta* 2004;343:93-103.
[22] Nakajima, K, Nakajima,Y, Takeichi S, Fujita MQ. Plasma Remnant-Like Lipoprotein Particles or LDL-C as Major Pathologic Factors in Sudden Cardiac Death Cases. Atherosclerosis 2008; 198:237-46.

[23] Nakajima K, Takeichi S, Nakajima Y, Fujita MQ. Pokkuri Death Syndrome; Sudden Cardiac Death Cases without Coronary Atherosclerosis in South Asian Young Males. Forensic Sci Int 2010; 207:6-13.

[24] Takeichi S, Fujita MQ. Unveiling the cause of Pokkuri Disease—proposal of the concept for "Pokkuri Death" Syndrome (in Japanese). Igaku no Ayumi 2006; 217(4):347.

[25] Doi H, Kugiyama K, Ohgushi M, et al. Membrane active lipids in remnant lipoproteins cause impairment of endothelium-dependent vasorelaxation. Arterioscl Thromb Vasc Biol 1999;19:1918-2

[26] Fontbonne A, Eschwege E, Cambien F, et al. Hypertriglyceridemia as a risk factor of coronary heart disease mortality in subjects with impaired glucose tolerance or diabetes. Results from the 11-year follow-up of the Paris Prospective Study. Diabetologia 1989; 32: 300-4

[27] Walldius G, Junger I kolar W, Holme I , steiner E. High cholesterol and triglyceride values in Swedish male s and females: In creased risk of fatal myocardial infarction. Blood Press Suppl 1992;4:35-42

[28] Iso H, Naito Y, Sato S, et al. Serum triglycerides and risk of coronary heart disease among Japanese men and women. Am J Epidemiol 2001; 153:490-9

[29] Nordestrgaad BG, Benn M, Schnohr P, Tybjaerg-Hansen A. Nonfasting triglycerides and risk of myocardial infarction, ischemic heart disease, and death in men and women. JAMA 2007; 298:299-308

[30] Bansal S, Buring JE, Rifai N, Mora S, Sacks FM, Ridker PM. Fasting compared with nonfasting truglycerides and risk of cardiovascular events in women, JAMA 2007; 298; 309-16

[31] Imke C, Rodriguez BL, Grove JS, et al. Are remnant-like particles independent predictors of coronary heart disease incidence? The Honolulu heart study. Arterioscler Thromb Vasc Biol 2005; 25:1718-22.

[32] Karpe F, Steiner G, Olivecrona T, Carison LA, Hamsten A. Metabolism of triglyceride-rich lipoproteins during alimentary lipemia. J Clin Invest 1993;91: 748–58.

[33] Ooi TC, Cousins M, Ooi DS, et al. Postprandial remnant- like lipoproteins in hypertriglyceridemia. J Clin Endocrinol Metab 2001; 86:3134-42.

[34] Schneeman BO, Kotite L, Todd KM, Havel RJ. Relationships between the responses of triglyceride-rich lipoproteins in blood plasma containing apolipoprotein B-48 and B-100 to a fat-containing meal in normolipidemic humans. Proc Natl Acad Sci USA 1993; 90: 2069-73.

[35] Schneider J, Liesenfeld A, Mordasini R, et al. Lipoprotein fractions, lipoprotein lipase and hepatic triglyceride lipase during short-term and long term uptake of ethanol in healthy subjects. Atherosclerosis 1985; 57: 281–91.

[36] F.M. Sacks, M.A. Pfeffer, L.A. Moyle *et al.*, The effect of pravastatin on coronary events after myocardial infarction in patients with average cholesterol levels. *N Engl J Med* 1996; 335 : 1001–1009.

[37] F. Karpe, G. Steiner, K. Uffelman *et al.*, Postprandial lipoproteins and progression of coronary atherosclerosis. *Atherosclerosis* 1994; 106: 83–97.

[38] S.D. Proctor and J.C.L. Mamo, Arterial fatty lesions have increased uptake of chylomicron remnants but not low-density lipoproteins. *Coron Artery Dis* 1996; 7: 239–245.

[39] J.C.L. Mamo, Atherosclerosis as a post-prandial disease. *Endocrinol Metab* 1995; 2: 229–244.

[40] K. Kugiyama, H. Doi, K. Takazoe *et al.*, Remnant lipoprotein levels in fasting serum predict coronary events in patients with coronary artery disease. *Circulation* 1999; 99: 2858–2860.

[41] P. Lundman, M. Eriksson, K. Schenck-Gustafsson *et al.*, Transient triglyceridemia decreases vascular reactivity in young, healthy men without risk factors for coronary heart disease. *Circulation* 1997; 96: 3266–3268.

[42] R.A. Vogel, M.C. Corretti and G.D. Plotnick, Effect of a single high-fat meal on endothelial function in healthy subjects. *Am J Cardiol* 1997; 79: 1682–1686.

[43] D.S. Celermajer, K.E. Sorensen, V.M. Gooch *et al.*, Non-invasive detection of endothelial dysfunction in children and adults at risk of atherosclerosis. *Lancet* 1992; 340: 1111–1115.

[44] L.A. Simons, T. Dwyer, J. Simons *et al.*, Chylomicrons and chylomicron remnants in coronary artery disease: A case control study. *Atherosclerosis* 1987; 65: 181–189.

[45] P.H. Groot, W.A.H.J. van Stiphout, X.H. Krauss *et al.*, Postprandial lipoprotein metabolism in normolipidaemic men with and without coronary disease. *Arterioscler Thromb Vasc Biol* 1991; 11: 653–662.

[46] M.S. Weintraub, I. Grosskopf, T. Rassin *et al.*, Clearance of chylomicron remnants in normolipidaemic patients with coronary artery disease: Case control study over three years. *BMJ* 1996; 312: 935–939.

[47] E. Meyer, H.T. Westerveld, F.C. de Ruyter-Meijstek *et al.*, Abnormal postprandial apolipoprotein B_{48} and triglyceride responses in normolipidaemic women with greater than 70% stenotic coronary artery disease: A case-control study. *Atherosclerosis* 1996; 124: 221–235.

[48] D. Braun, A. Gramlich, U. Brehme *et al.*, Postprandial lipaemia after a moderate fat challenge in normolipidaemic men with and without coronary artery disease. *J Cardiol Risk* 1997; 4 : 143–149.

[49] K. Przybycień , Z. Kornacewicz-Jach, B. Torbus-Lisiecka *et al.*, Is abnormal postprandial lipaemia a familial risk factor for coronary artery disease in individuals with normal fasting concentrations of triglycerides and cholesterol?. *Coron Artery Dis* 2000; 11: 377–381.

[50] K. Kugiyama, H. Doi, T. Motoyama *et al.*, Association of remnant lipoprotein levels with impairment of endothelium-dependant vasomotor function in human coronary arteries. *Circulation* 1998; 97: 2519–2526.

[51] H. Doi, K. Kugiyama, K. Oka *et al.*, Remnant lipoproteins induce proatherothrombogenic molecules in endothelial cells through a redox-sensitive mechanism. *Circulation* 2000; 102: 670–676.

[52] J.S. Cohn, Postprandial lipemia: Emerging evidence for atherogenicity of remnant lipoproteins. *Can J Cardiol* 1998; 14: 18B–27B.

[53] Zilversmit DB. Atherogenesis: a postprandial phenomenon. Circulation 1979; 60:473-85.

[54] C.A. Aguilar-Salinas, H. Barrett and G. Schonfeld, Metabolic modes of action of the statins in hyperlipoproteinemias. *Atherosclerosis* 1998; 141: 203–207.

[55] A. Dart, G. Jerums, G. Nicholson *et al.*, A multicenter, double-blind, one-year study comparing safety and efficacy of atorvastatin versus simvastatin in patients with hypercholesterolaemia. *Am J Cardiol* 1997; 80: 39–44.

[56] H.N. Ginsberg, Hypertriglyceridemia: New insights and new approaches to pharmacologic therapy. *Am J Cardiol* 2001; 87: 1174–1180.

[57] J.R. Burnett, P.H.R. Barrett and P. Vicini, The HMG-CoA reductase inhibitor atorvastatin increases the fractional clearance of postprandial triglyceride-rich liporpoteins in miniature pigs. *Arterioscler Thromb Vasc Biol* 18 (1998), pp. 1906–1914.

[58] K.G. Parhofer, P.H.R. Barrett and P. Schwandt, Atorvastatin improves postprandial lipoprotein metabolism in normolipdaemic subjects. *J Clin Endocrinol Metab* 85 (2000), pp. 4224–4230.

[59] Ai M, Otokozawa S, Asztalos BF, et al. Effects of maximal doses of atorvastatin versus rosuvastatin on small dense low-density . Am J Cardiol. 2008; 101:315-8.

[60] Takahashi S, Sakai J, Fujino T, et al. The very low-density lipoprotein (VLDL) receptor: characterization and functions as a peripheral lipoprotein receptor. J Atheroscler Thromb 2004;11: 200–8lipoprotein cholesterol levels. Am J Cardiol. 2008; 101:315-8.

[61] Bowler A, Redgrave TG, Mamo JCL. Chylomicron-remnant clearance in homozygote and heterozygote Watanabe-heritable-hyperlipidaemic rabbits is defective. *Biochem J* 1991; 276:381–6.

[62] Cooper AD. Hepatic uptake of chylomicron remnants. *J Lipid Res* 1997; 38:2173–92.

[63] Twickler ThB, Dallinga-Thie de Valk HW, Schreuder PCNJ, Jansen H, Castro Cabezas M, Erkelens DW. High dose of simvastatin normalises postprandial remnant-like particle response in patients with heterozygous familial hypercholesterolaemia. *Arterioscler Thromb Vasc Biol* 2000;20:2422–7.

[64] Holbrook A, Wright M, Sung M, Ribic C, Baker S.Statin-associated rhabdomyolysis: is there a dose-response relationship? Can J Cardiol. 2011; 27:146-51.

[65] McAdams M, Staffa J, Dal Pan G. Estimating the extent of reporting to FDA: a case study of statin-associated rhabdomyolysis. Pharmacoepidemiol Drug Saf. 2008 Mar;17(3):229-39.

[66] Kugiyama K, Doi H, Motoyama T, et al. Association of remnant lipoprotein levels with impairment of endothelium-depedent vasomotor function in human coronary arteries. Circulation 1998; 97: 2519-26.

[67] Inoue T, Saniabadi AR, Matsunaga R, Hoshi K, Yaguchi I, Morooka S. Impaired endothelium-dependent acetylcholine-induced coronary artery relaxation in patients with high serum remnant lipoprotein particles. Atherosclerosis 1998; 139: 363-7.

[68] Kugiyama K, Motoyama T, Doi H, et al. Improvement of endothelial vasomotor dysfunction by treatment with alpha-tocopherol in patients with high remnant lipoprotein levels. J Am Colleg Cardiol. 1999; 33: 1512-18.

[69] Funada J, Sekiya M, Hamada M, Hiwada K. Postprandial elevation of remnant lipoproteins lead to endothelial dysfunction. Circ J. 2002 ; 66:127-32

[70] Doi H, Kugiyama K, Ohgushi M,et al. Remnants of chylomicron and very low density lipoprotein impair endothelium-dependent vasorelaxation. Atherosclerosis 1998; 137: 341-349.

[71] Parthasarathy S, Young SG, Witztum JL, Pittman RC, Steinberg D. Probucol inhibits oxidative modification of low density lipoprotein. J Clin Invest 1986; 77: 641-44.

[72] Keary JF, Xu A, Cunnibgham D, Jackson T, Frei B, Vita JA. Dietary probucol preserve endothelial function in cholestrol-fed rabbits by limiting vascular oxidative stress and superoxide generation. J Clin Invest. 1995; 95:2520-9

[73] Sawamura T, Kume N, Aoyama T, et al. An endothelial receptor for oxidized low-density lipoprotein. Nature 1997; 386: 73-7.

[74] Moriwaki H, Kume N, Sawamura T, et al. Ligand specificity of LOX-1, a novel endothelial receptor for oxidized low density lipoprotein. Arterioscler Thromb Vasc Biol 1998; 18: 1541-7.

[75] Kume N, Murase T, Morikawa H, et al. inducible expression of lectin-like oxidized LDL receptor-1 in vascular endothelial cells. Circ Res 1998; 83: 322-7.

[76] Kume N and Kita T. Roles of lectin-like oxidized LDL receptor –1 and its soluble forms in atherogenesis. Curr Opin Lipidol. 2001; 12: 419-423.

[77] Shin HK, Kim YK, Kim KY, Lee JH, Hong KW. Remnant lipoprotein particles induce apoptosis in endothelial cells by NAD(P)H oxidase-mediated production of superoxide and cytokines via lectin-like oxidized low-density lipoprotein receptor-1 activation: prevention by cilostazol. Circulation 2004; 109: 1022-8.

[78] Park SY, Lee JH, Kim YK, et al. Cilostazol prevents remnant lipoproteinparticle-induced monocyte adhesion to endothelial cells by suppression of adhesion molecules and monocyte chemoattractant protein-1 expression via lectin-like receptor for oxidized low-density lipoprotein receptor activation. J Pharmacol Exp Ther 2005; 312: 1241-48.

[79] Kimura Y, Tani T, Kanbe T, and Watanbe K. Effect of cilostazol on platelet aggregation and experimental thrombosis. Arzneimittelforshung 1985; 35: 1144-49.

[80] Wang T, Elam MB, Forbes WP, Zhong J, Nakajima K. Reduction of remnant lipoprotein cholesterol concentrations by cilostazol in patients with intermittent claudication. Atherosclerosis 2003; 171: 337-42.

[81] Lee JH, Oh GT, Park SY, et al. Cilostazol reduces atherosclerosis by inhibition of superoxide and tumor necrosis factor-alpha formation in low-density lipoprotein receptor- null mice fed high cholesterol. J Pharmacol Exp Ther 2005; 313: 502-509.

[82] Kawakami A, Tanaka A, Chiba T, et al. Remnant lipoprotein-induced smooth muscle cell proliferation involves epidermal growth factor receptor transactivation. Circulation 2003; 108: 2679–88.

[83] Aramaki Y, Mitsuoka H, Toyohara M, et al. Lectin-like oxidized LDL receptor-1 (LOX-1) acts as a receptor for remnant-like lipoprotein particles (RLPs) and mediates RLP-induced migration of vascular smooth muscle cells. Atherosclerosis. 2008 ; 198: 272-9.

[84] Hussain MM, Maxfield FR, Mas-Oliva J, et al. Clearance of chylomicron remnants by the low density lipoprotein receptor-related protein/alpha 2-macroglobulin receptor. J Biol Chem 1991; 266:13936–40.

[85] Gianturco SH, Ramprasad MP, Song R, et al. Apolipoprotein B- 48 or its apolipoprotein B-100 equivalent mediates the binding of triglyceride-rich lipoproteins to their unique human monocyte- macrophage receptor. Arterioscler Thromb Vasc Biol 1998;18: 968–76.

[86] Chen M, Narumiya S, Masaki T, Sawamura T. Conserved C-terminal residues within the lectin-like domain of LOX-1 are essential for oxidized low-density-lipoprotein binding. Biochem J 2001;355: 289–96.

[87] Shimokawa H, Ito A, Fukumoto Y, et al. Chronic treatment with interleukin-1 beta induces coronary intimal lesions and vasospastic responses in pigs in vivo. The role of platelet-derived growth factor. J Clin Invest. 1996; 97:769–776.
[88] Tosaka M, Okajima F, Hashiba Y,et al. Sphingosine 1-phosphate contracts canine basilar arteries in vitro and in vivo: possible role in pathogenesis of cerebral vasospasm. *Stroke.* 2001; 32: 2913–19.

3

Cardiovascular Risk Factors and Liver Transplantation

Anna Rossetto, Umberto Baccarani and Vittorio Bresadola
University of Udine,
Italy

1. Introduction

In the last decades, the survival of liver transplanted patients and grafts have had a great improvement due to many factors. Careful preoperative evaluation in transplant recipients, experience and a multidisciplinary approach have, without any doubt, a major role in the selection of candidates and in the diagnosis and treatment of preoperative complications. Moreover, with the introduction of new generation immunosuppressive drugs and careful pharmacological monitoring, both the episodes of acute rejection and toxic effects have been minimized (1)

In consequence, since the graft and the patient post-transplant survival have been improved, the transplanted population has started showing long term medical complications.

Besides the risk correlated with graft rejection, the transplanted population has an increased risk of developing many malignancies. A number of hematologic diseases, skin cancer, gastrointestinal tumors seems to recognize a possible trigger factor in immunosuppressive drugs and the patient's immunological status but also in serological status and viral infections quite common in immunosuppressed patients. As for frequency, after these two groups of complications, cardiovascular diseases are the third cause of death in the transplanted population (1)

Eligibility to liver transplant, once based on Child Pugh system, has been regulated, since a few years, by MELD score, an index of survival probability of the end stage liver disease (2). This score is obtained on three variables, INR, creatinine and bilirubine. Due to the well known inadequate number of available grafts, if compared to patients requiring liver transplantation and to the risk of mortality while in the waiting list, this score supplies a priority system, based on the severity of the disease, for the organ allocation. The cut off value normally considered for eligibility to liver transplantation is a MELD score ≥15. Since the evaluation of the MELD score is obtained with this mathematical formula:

$$10\{0.957\mathrm{Ln(Scr)}+0.378\mathrm{Ln(Tbil)}+1.12\ \mathrm{Ln\ (INR)}+0.643\}$$

eligibility to transplantation undergoes the parameter of severity of the disease, selecting the population of patients with generally worse clinical conditions. Moreover, the median age of the patients waiting for transplantation seems to be higher, essentially due to the improvement in the antiviral therapies and the better medical treatment in the hepatological patient; for these reasons, the impairment of the liver function resulting in an eligible score can be delayed, with a longer conservative treatment and an older age of the patients who undergo liver transplantation.

Like in general population, the risk of developing cardiovascular disease increases with age, but liver disease by itself is often related to cardiovascular disease or higher cardiovascular risk factors (2, 3). Therefore, an accurate cardiovascular risk assessment of these patients, besides the whole pretransplant evaluation, is essential, both for the increased risk of cardiovascular diseases after liver transplant and for the cardiovascular risk assessment of the pre-transplant condition.

2. Pretransplant cardiovascular risk

Advanced hepatic liver disease is responsible for many changes in the physiology and biochemistry of the cardiovascular system, affecting contractility, heart rate, conduction and repolarization (4, 5, 6).

Cirrhotic cardiomyopathy is a pathological condition characterized by an increased cardiac output, impaired ventricular response to stress, decreased beta-agonist transduction, increased circulating inflammatory mediators with cardio depressant effect, alteration in repolarization, low systemic vascular resistance and bradycardia, altered function of muscarinic function and beta adrenergic stimulatory system, heart cell membrane abnormalities due to altered membrane fluidity and a modified calcium concentration, overproduction of nitric oxide, cardio depressant effects of an increased level of carbon monoxide (7).

Both the systolic and diastolic functions seem to be damages: the former, even if in cirrhotic cardiomyopathy the cardiac output is high, can be revealed by stress test, and can be caused by a reduced cardiovascular reactivity during exercise; the latter determined by fibrosis, myocardial hypertrophy and sub endothelial edema results in the impairment of compliance and relaxation. (4, 5, 6)

Abnormalities at the ECG, such electromechanical dissociation, which results in a prolongation of the QT interval , and chronotropic incompetence given by an impaired response to beta stimulation, are very common in cirrhosis and seem to be mainly related to portal hypertension and portosystemic shunting, but also to alterations of the heart rate with a central hypovolemia, loss of renal excretion of water and sodium and an altered baroreflex sensitivity which contribute to impair the cardiovascular system.(4, 5, 6, 8)

These conditions can lead to a higher risk of torsade de pointes, rhythm disturbances but also to the inability to develop physiologic tachycardia when required.

Some liver diseases seem to show a correlation also on the coronary blood flow. Diffuse but undetectable coronary atherosclerosis, reduced coronary micro vascular bed and impaired endothelium function are reported in NAFLD (9, 10).

Pre-transplant diabetes is another cardiovascular risk factor, and, in liver diseases the possibility to find an insulin resistance can be related to the pathogenesis of liver disease (non alcoholic fatty liver disease), where the deregulation of fat metabolism causes an overproduction of very low density proteins involved in the metabolic syndrome, and, after the initial over activity with hyperinsulinemia, there is an impairment of islet beta cells; on the other hand, the liver glycogenogenesis and glycogenolysis pathways for the regulation of carbohydrate metabolism can be impaired due to the hepatic disease itself (10, 11, 12, 13, 14, 15, 16, 17).

Renal dysfunction is not uncommon (microalbuminuria, hepato-renal syndrome), and also pulmonary heart disease has to be considered such as Hepatopulmonary Syndrome where a mismatch between ventilation and perfusion is involved with hypoxemia due to an excess of perfusion because of abnormal intrapulmonary vascular dilation. (5, 9, 11, 16)

Portopulmonary Hypertension, is a condition where pulmonary arterial hypertension is associated with liver disease or portal hypertension due to many factors such as hyperdinamic circulation, release of mediators from the congested bowel because of splancnic overload, vasoconstriction and remodeling of the lung vascular endothelium.(16)

The American Association for the Study of Liver Diseases (2) recommends a rigorous pre-operative Assessment

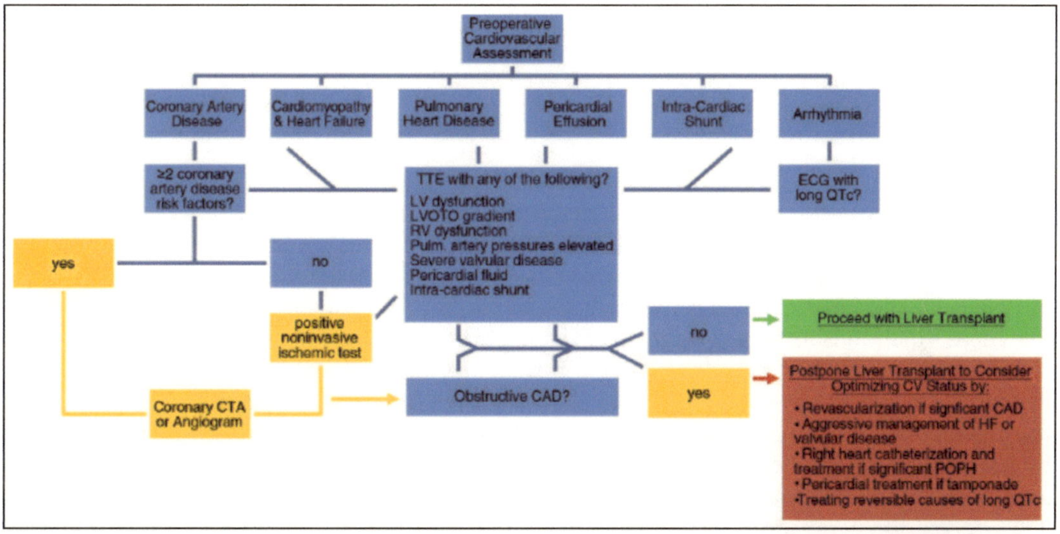

CAD= coronary artery disease; CTA= computed tomography angiogram; ECG= electrocardiogram; H= heart failure; LV= left ventricular; LVOTO= left ventricular outflow tract obstruction; POPH= portopulmonary hypertension; Pulm.= pulmonary; QTc= corrected QT interval; RV= right ventricular; TTE= transthoracic

Fig. 1. Suggested strategy for pre-operative cardiac assessment of liver transplant candidates

3. Post transplant cardiovascular risk

Patients who undergo liver transplantation have an around doubled risk of developing cardiovascular disease if compared to non transplanted population. To investigate the risk of such complications, multiple risk factors have to be added up. On one hand, there are all the risk factors of the general population such as advanced age, male gender, smoking history, high body mass index, pre-transplant diabetes mellitus, marital status. On the other hand, some peculiar risk related to the etiology of the underlying liver cirrhosis have to be considered, since liver disease caused by criptogenetic, alcohol and hepatitis C seems to be related to an increased cardiovascular risk. Moreover, after transplantation, a new physiological condition arises from the hemodynamic, biochemical and drug related standpoint. The vasodilatation existing in the cirrhotic patient has been solved and a systemic vasoconstriction is quite often present in the transplanted patient. Many factors seem to be involved in such systemic resistance modification but a definite pathogenesis is still under debate. The renin-angiotensin system seems to be involved but also the effect of endothelin, which seems to be higher then normal after LT, with its vasoconstrictor effect and which could determine the arterial pressure increase as well as the arterial stiffness which are clearly related to high pressure. Anyway a high arterial blood pressure before transplant seems to be a factor contributing the post transplant development of arterial hypertension (1, 18, 19)

The metabolic syndrome is apparently another risk factor, quite common in transplanted patient. In liver cirrhosis the patient generally suffers from a hypermetabolic condition and insulin resistance is very common. The normalization of the metabolic status, and the change induced in the metabolism of lipoproteins, in absence or combined with insulin resistance or diabetes due to the pancreas cells function impairment, can explain some effects of the post-transplant status while the underlying liver disease itself (HCV infection and relapse) seems to be related to diabetes affecting the insulin pathway and directly affecting the pancreatic beta cells (20, 21, 22, 23)

A major role in the cardiovascular risk factors lies in the irreplaceable use of immunosuppressive drugs (1, 18, 24)

Immunosuppressive drugs are related to arterial hypertension, and especially calcineurin inhibitors, have turned out to affect the vascular bed causing endothelial dysfunction. Besides their direct effect on the vascular endothelium, they also affect the vascular smooth muscle cells and have effects on the release and production of nitric oxide and endotheline. The renal function is impaired because of the nephrotoxic effects of many of these drugs that cause an impairment of the glomerular filtration rate and side effects on arterial pressure. Immunosuppressive drugs have also a pancreatic beta cells toxicity leading to a decrease in the production and secretion of insulin and an increased risk of diabetes (18). This condition by itself impairs the micro vascular bed and renal function. These drugs, especially M-tor inhibitors, affect the lipid metabolism, with the development of high levels of cholesterol and triglyceride concentration requiring lipid-lowering drugs. This side effect seems to be due to a decreased drug related bile acid synthesis but also to the agonist effects of some immunosuppressive drugs with low density lipoprotein cholesterol receptors, with a higher quantity of circulating low density lipoprotein. These side effects cause a further impairing in the vascular beds status, with effects of stiffness on the vascular walls. Also the steroids, frequently used in combination with immunosuppressive drugs or as treatment of acute rejection, have their well known effects on the vascular system, causing vasoconstriction, arterial hypertension, truncal fat deposition, and on the glucydic metabolism, causing a decreased insulin production, and impairing the peripheral glucose utilization, resulting in an insulin resistance or diabetes (1, 18, 25, 26).

4. Immunosuppression and cardiovascular risk factors

Transplantation soared in the 1980s thanks to the introduction of a new immunosuppressive drug: Cyclosporine. Before that, survival after liver transplantation was strongly impaired by the common onset of rejection and graft loss, when the immunosuppressive strategies were poor and crude such as the whole-body x-radiation at the very beginning (1960s) and azathioprine, prendisolone and anti-lymphocytes antibodies about ten years later. (27)

The experience in liver transplant shows that liver transplant recipients develop a lower rate of rejection if compared to other organs (heart, kidney) possibly because a form of microchimerism due to a large number of donor's cells within the allograft. Also the production by the liver of soluble donor MHC class 1 molecules has been mentioned to explain this resistance to rejection in liver transplantation. The size and regenerative properties of liver can also play a role.(27, 28)

Nevertheless, although the liver is less prone to rejection then other organs, the immunosuppressive regimen remains mandatory after liver transplantation. The selection of immunosuppressive drugs is not universal but has to be done considering the pretransplant history and the medical conditions, considering for example pretransplant poor renal function, diabetes or hepatocellular carcinoma. Therefore a careful balance between pros and cons is essential.

At present, calcineurin inhibitors are the most large used immunosuppressive drugs for liver transplantation, with well known side effects such as neurotoxicity, nephrotoxicity, hypertension, increased risk of death due to cardiovascular risk factors, gingival hyperplasia, hirsutism and diabetes.

Cyclosporine, the oldest one, is derived from the fungus Tolypocladium inflatum and is a polypeptide of 11 amino acids. Tacrolimus, the most recent one, is derived from Streptomyces tsukabaensis and is a macrolide compound.

Cyclosporine inhibits interleukin 2 gene transcription, binding cyclophilin, inhibiting the calcium/calmodulin phosphatase dependent calcineurin complex. It causes a dephosphorilation of activated T cell which is important for the transcription of cytokines for the activation of T cells, while Tacrolimus, from the same group of immunosuppressive drugs and with a similar mechanism of action, inhibits calcineurin binding to another specific immunophilin, FK binding protein 12. (27, 28, 29)

These drugs seem to have complex activities besides immunosuppression, causing endothelial dysfunction and more specifically a decrease in the production of the vasodilator nitric oxide (NO) by endothelial NO synthase (eNOS), affecting the vasodilator function by negatively altering endothelial intracellular Ca2+ and eNOS phosphorylation. Ca2+ concentration is altered by intracellular Ca2+ leak and decreased agonist-induced intracellular Ca2+ release which negatively affects eNOS phosphorylation, NO production, and endothelium-dependent dilatation. The precise mechanisms leading to hyperlipidemia are not completely known. There are contributing factors such as corticosteroids use and obesity. Anyway cyclosporine is related to an increase of VLDL and LDL while Tacrolimus seems to be characterized by VLDL increase alone. The mechanisms which underlie these side effects seem to be the increase in free intracellular cholesterol levels due to an impaired cholesterol esterification, but also the activation of the transcription factor responsible for the expression of lipid related genes. Oxidative processes may also underlie the atherosclerotic effect.

The nephrotoxic effects are well known, and they can by themselves be related to the development of arterial hypertension. The mechanism, beside a possible involvement of the tubular epithelium, seems to be more strongly related to vascular alteration of the afferent arterioles, with consequent ions alteration and hyperkaliemia. (28, 29, 30)

The arteriolar vasoconstriction and renal ischemia are related to an imbalance between the vasoactive messengers (endothelin-1 and tromboxane A2), the dysregulation of nitric-oxide formation and the renin-angiotensin system. Besides these vascular effects altering the renal control of arterial pressure, the nephrotoxic direct effects should also be mentioned, with tubular cell apoptosis and necrosis, but also the effects on the cell cycle compromising the proliferation capacity and accelerating cell aging possibly mediated by an oxidative stress caused by reactive oxygen species (ROS) and lipid peroxides. This effect has been demonstrated as an abnormality in permeability of the mitochondria causing an isometric vacuolization resulting in the presence of giant mitochondria. Thus, the endoplasmic reticulum undergoes enlargement and the proteic syntesis is affected. Cyclosporine can act as an endoplasmic reticulum stress inducer causing epithelial phenotypic changes leading to nephrotoxicity (30, 31, 32, 33, 34).

Endoplasmic reticulum stress seems to play a major role in many diseases such as atherosclerosis, Alzheimer, diabetes and inflammatory bowel diseases, leading the unfolded protein response to an adaptative response. (35, 36)

The above mentioned stress is involved in post transplant diabetes, promoting insulin resistance and cells death. Insulin secerning cells undergo proteins synthesis stress and are very sensitive to any status causing accumulation of anomalous proteins. The pathophisiology of pancreatic beta cells damage during treatment with Tacrolimus and Cyclosporine is still matter of debate, but it seems related to the endoplasmic reticulum stress which modify cells vitality, since in animal models treated with calcineurin inhibitors, nuclear inclusions, dilatation in cistern of the granulous endoplasmic reticulum with degranulation and degeneration of pancreatic beta islets have been shown (35, 36)

Steroids are often used in immunosuppressive therapeutic schemes in the perioperative period, both intraoperatively, and after transplantation for a period ranging from 3 to 6 months for liver transplantation. Moreover, at the possible onset of acute rejection, bolus of steroids are administered. The steroid immunosuppressive function derives from the inactivation of the response of lymphocytes and macrophages by inhibiting the production of cytokines, but also suppressing antigens and stimulating the migration of T cells to the lymphoid tissue.(30)

A large body of evidence supports the theory that steroids induce an imbalance between vasoconstriction and vasodilatation, favoring vasoconstriction, resulting in arterial hypertension.

The increased vasoconstriction is mediated by several mechanisms. In large part vasoconstriction is mediated by the increased endothelin-1 synthesis and secretion, increased erythropoietin levels by the increased level of cytosolic calcium, increased sympathetic activity that is mediated by the increase of Beta1-adrenergic receptor expression and increased synthesis of catecholamines, by the increased expression of various enzymes involved in the catecholamines biosynthesis including tyrosine hydroxilase and phenyl ethanolamine N-methyltransferase and altered availability of Alfa1-adrenergic receptors in vascular smooth muscles, leading to an increased vascular reactivity, pressure responsiveness and hypertension. The vasoconstriction and hypertension induced by steroids are also mediated through enhanced synthesis and action of vasoactive substances and their receptors, including neuro peptide Y (NPY), arginine vasopressin (AVP) and atrial natriuretic peptide (ANP).

Another interesting issue is the role of the renin-angiotensin system activation in the development of steroids induced hypertension. Steroids act directly at the liver site, enhancing the synthesis of angiotensinogen. (29, 37)

On the other hand, steroids negatively affect various vasodilatory systems causing nitric oxide (NO) deficiency through a range of a negative influences on the NO biosynthetic pathways involving alteration in the activity and expression of NO synthase, decreased availability of tetrahydrobiopterin (BH4) and decreased NO precursor L-arginine. Moreover steroids affect the production of other vasodilatatory substances as prostacyclin, prostaglandin E2 and kallikrein.

Steroids induce insulin resistance in skeletal muscle by directly interfering with the insulin signaling cascade. The same effect is produced also in hepatic cells and thus endogenous glucose production is increased. (28, 29, 37)

Steroids appear to have a direct causal effect relationship with cardiovascular disease depending on dose, duration, cumulative dose of exposure and route of administration. The increased risk is mediated through the induction of several risk factors for cardiovascular disease.

Since the late 1990s other immunosuppressive drugs have been introduced into the world of transplantation: the group of m-Tor inhibitors (Sirolimus and Everolimus) (27, 28, 29).

Sirolimus is derived from actinomycete Streptomyces hygroscopicus. It has a homologous structure if compared to Cyclosporine and Tacrolimus and it also binds to FK bindig proteins family (FKBP-12) which binds to mammalian targets of rapamycin (MTOR) which has a kinase activity. Sirolimus plays its action on the signal transduction pathway, blocking the IL-2 and IL-5 induction of B and T cell proliferation. It inhibits the normal cell proliferation in response to IL-2. Everolimus, is a macrolide derived from Sirolimus, with a similar mechanism of action, inhibiting the activation of immunophyllin FKBP-12. Unlike Sirolimus it has pharmacokinetics properties which make it easier to handle.

These drugs are particularly interesting and under debate. Based on their anti proliferative effects, they also seem to have anti-neoplastic effects based on the fact that they inhibit angiogenesis, inhibit cancer cells survival and also cancer stem cells survival (27, 28, 29).

They seem to have less nephrotoxic effects than calcineurin-inhibitors provided there is no pre-existing renal disease, basing their action on m-Tor contrasting the renal fibrosis caused by TGF-beta. There's anyway a risk of proteinuria or of renal damage amplification in an already compromised renal function.

They show interesting properties in promoting tolerance but Sirolimus is considered an unsafe drug for the 1st month after transplantation for a higher risk of developing hepatic artery thrombosis and for a slower and more difficult wounds healing. Mouth ulcers and leg edema are common. It's strongly related to high risk of developing of hyperlipidemia which seems to be caused by an increased hepatic secretion of VLDL, increased hepatic synthesis of apoB100 and a reduction in the hepatic catabolism of LDL. The action of lipoprotein lipase is decreased and the expression of apoCIII and lipase in adipose tissue are increased. Anyway these drugs have effects on macrophages and antiproliferative effects which could protect from the cardiovascular risk of atherosclerosis (27, 28, 29, 38, 39).

Antimetabolites such as mycophenolate mofetil and mycophenolate sodium have immunosuppressive properties which were recognized in the 1990s although these drugs are older. Their action derive from the blockage of inosine-5^{1}-monophosphate deydrogenase (IMPDH) resulting in the selective lymphocyte proliferation blockage. They have probably less cardiovascular side effects, mainly gastrointestinal disorders, bone marrow depression, some infections. Their exclusive use is hardly ever considered due to their insufficient protection from acute rejection if not combined to m-Tor or CNI. Yet their use anyway often allows a lower CNI or m-Tor dosage with side effects sparing properties. (27, 28, 29, 40)

Both polyclonal and monoclonal antibodies [anti- thymocites globilin (ATG), anti-lymphocyte globulin (ALG), monoclonal antibodies (OKT3, Campath, Basiliximab)] are also largely used in combination with CNI or m-Tor delayed introduction as induction therapies, minimizing the side effects of CNI and m-Tor inhibitors.

Other immunosuppressive drugs are currently undergoing trials such as Belatacept, which inhibits T cell activation binding CD80 and CD86, and looks promising, with less renal toxicity, and Efalizumab which inhibits T cell-APC stabilization and blocks lymphocyte adhesion to endothelial cells, with good results as for immunosuppressive properties but with an increased risk of onset of post-transplant lymphoproliferative disorders (27, 28, 29).

5. Risk of new onset of diabetes (36)

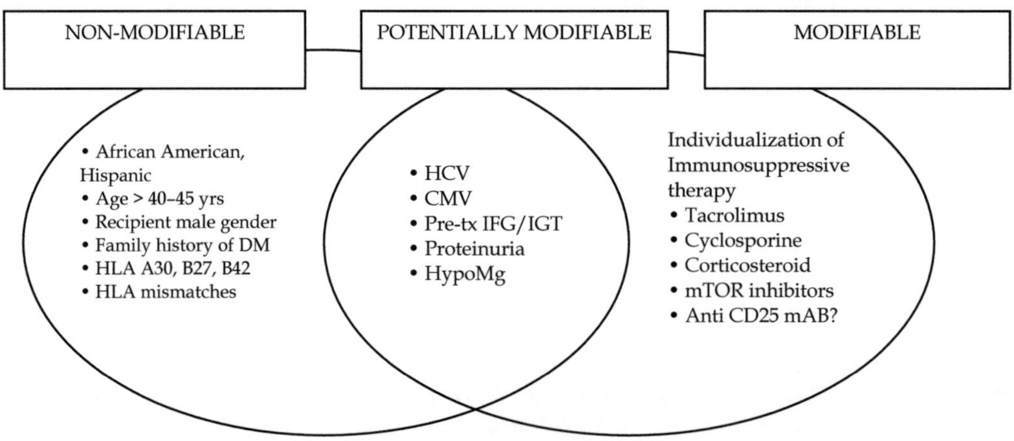

LEGEND:
IGT: impaired glucose tolerance, IFG: impaired fasting glucose, Anti CD25 mAb, Anti CD25 monoclonal antibody, CMV:cytomegalovirus, HCV: hepatitis C, HypoMg: hypomagnesemia, Pre-Tx: pre-transplant

IMMUNOSUPPRESSIVE AGENT	MECHANISM OF ACTION
CALINEURINE INHIBITORS	Inhibit signal 2 trasduction via T cell receptor
MAMMALIAN TARGET OF RAPAMYCIN INHIBITORS	Inhibit Signal 3 trasduction via IL-2 receptor
MYCOPHENOLIC ACID	Inhibit purine and DNA synthesis
CORTICOSTEROIDS	Inhibit cytokine transcription by antigen presenting cell; Selective lysis of immature cortical thymocytes
AntiCD3 monoclonal antibodies	Depletion and receptor modulation in T cell Interferes with Signal 1
Antithymocyte globuline	Depletion and receptor modulation in T cells Interferes with Signal 1, 2, 3 Inhibits lymphocytes trafficking
Anti IL-2 alpha chain receptor antibodies	Inhibit T cell proliferation to IL-2
Anti –CD52 monoclonal antibodies	Cause depletion of thymocytes, T cells, B cells and monocytes

IMMUNOSUPPRESSIVE AGENT	SIDE EFFECTS
CALINEURINE INHIBITORS	Hypertension, Renal toxicity, neurotoxicity, diabetes, dislipidemia, gingival hyperplasia, hirsutism.
MAMMALIAN TARGET OF RAPAMYCIN INHIBITORS	Dislipidemia, anemia, leucopenia, thrombocytopenia, HAT, wound dehiscence, aphtous ulcers, arthralgia, proteinuria
MYCOPHENOLIC ACID	Anorexia, abdominal pain, gastritis, diarrhea, neutropenia

CORTICOSTEROIDS	Hypertension, pancreatitis, peptic ulcer, osteoporosis, aseptic necrosis of femoral head, diabetes, hyperlipidemia, risk of infections, difficult wound healing
AntiCD3 monoclonal antibodies	Fever, hypotension, headache, aseptic meningitis, dyspnea, vomiting, diarrhea
Antithymocyte globuline	Leucopenia, thrombocytopenia
Anti IL-2 alpha chain receptor antibodies	Risk of acute rejection
Anti -CD52 monoclonal antibodies	Risk of acute rejection

6. Conclusions

Besides the cardiovascular risk factors related to age, family disease and life habits, the transplant candidate has a particular hemodynamic, biochemical, cardiac and systemic condition depending on the hepatic disease. After transplantation, these paraphysiologic modifications suddenly change, with the onset of a new systemic condition, the appearance of organ damages not evident before, a new risk factors profile related to the new situation and to unavoidable life-saving drugs treatment.

For these reasons the pre-transplant cardiovascular evaluation and the post-transplant accurate monitoring followed by a careful choice of the immunosuppressive therapeutic regimen, drug level monitoring, educational efforts to ameliorate life style and risk factors are mandatory for a satisfactory outcome.

7. References

[1] Rossetto A, Bitetto D, Bresadola V, Lorenzin D, Baccarani U, De Anna D, Bresadola F, Adani GL. Cardiovascular risk factors and immunosuppressive regimen after liver transplantation. Transplant Proc. 2010 Sep;42(7):2576-8.

[2] Raval Z, Harinstein ME, Skaro AI, Erdogan A, DeWolf AM, Shah SJ, Fix OK, Kay N, Abecassis MI, Gheorghiade M, Flaherty JD. Cardiovascular risk assessment of the liver transplant candidate. J Am Coll Cardiol. 2011 Jul 12;58(3):223-31.

[3] Aberg F, Jula A, Höckerstedt K, Isoniemi H. Cardiovascular risk profile of patients with acute liver failure after liver transplantation when compared with the general population. Transplantation. 2010 Jan 15;89(1):61-8.

[4] Zardi EM, Abbate A, Zardi DM, Dobrina A, Margiotta D, Van Tassell BW, Afeltra A, Sanyal AJ. Cirrhotic cardiomyopathy. J Am Coll Cardiol. 2010 Aug 10;56(7):539-49. Review. Erratum in: J Am Coll Cardiol. 2010 Sep 14;56(12):1000.

[5] Lee RF, Van Tassel,Glenn TK, Lee SS. Cardiac dysfunction in cirrhosis. Best Pract Res Clin Gastroenterol. 2007;21(1):125-40.
[6] Møller S, Henriksen JH. Cirrhotic cardiomyopathy. J Hepatol. 2010 Jul;53(1):179-90. Epub 2010 Mar 31. Review.
[7] Rockey DC.Vascular mediators in the injured liver. Hepatology. 2003 Jan;37(1):4-12. Review.
[8] Yilmaz Y, Kurt R, Yonal O, Polat N, Celikel CA, Gurdal A, Oflaz H, Ozdogan O, Imeryuz N, Kalayci C, Avsar E. Coronary flow reserve is impaired in patients with nonalcoholic fatty liver disease: association with liver fibrosis. Atherosclerosis. 2010 Jul;211(1):182-6. Epub 2010 Feb 7.
[9] Mandell MS, Lindenfeld J, Tsou MY, Zimmerman M. Cardiac evaluation of liver transplant candidates.World J Gastroenterol. 2008 Jun 14;14(22):3445-51. Review.
[10] Fon Tacer K, Rozman D.Nonalcoholic Fatty liver disease: focus on lipoprotein and lipid deregulation J Lipids. 2011;2011:783976. Epub 2011 Jul 2.
[11] Garcia-Compean D, Jaquez-Quintana JO, Gonzalez-Gonzalez JA, Maldonado-Garza H.Liver cirrhosis and diabetes: risk factors, pathophysiology, clinical implications and management. World J Gastroenterol. 2009 Jan 21;15(3):280-8. Review.
[12] Parekh S, Anania FA. Abnormal lipid and glucose metabolism in obesity: implications for nonalcoholic fatty liver disease. Gastroenterology. 2007 May;132(6):2191-207. Review.
[13] Alexander S. Petrides, Leif C. Groop, Caroline A. Riely, and Ralph A. DeFronzo. Effect on physiologic hyperinsulinemia on glucose and lipid metabolism in cirrhosis. J. Clin. Invest. Volume 88, August 1991, 561-570
[14] Krok KL, Milwalla F, Maheshwari A, Rankin R, Thuluvath PJ.Insulin resistance and microalbuminuria are associated with microvascular disease in patients with cirrhosis.Liver Transpl. 2009 Sep;15(9):1036-42.
[15] García-Compean D, Jaquez-Quintana JO, Maldonado-Garza H.Hepatogenous diabetes. Current views of an ancient problem. Ann Hepatol. 2009 Jan-Mar;8(1):13-20.
[16] Hoeper MM, Krowka MJ, Strassburg CP. Portopulmonary hypertension and hepatopulmonary syndrome. Lancet. 2004 May 1;363(9419):1461-8. Review.
[17] Laish I, Braun M, Mor E, Sulkes J, Harif Y, Ben Ari Z. Metabolic syndrome in liver transplant recipients: prevalence, risk factors, and association with cardiovascular events. Liver Transpl. 2011 Jan;17(1):15-22. doi: 10.1002/lt.22198.
[18] Tepperman E, Ramzy D, Prodger J, Sheshgiri R, Badiwala M, Ross H, Raoa V. Surgical biology for the clinician: vascular effects of immunosuppression. Can J Surg. 2010 Feb;53(1):57-63.
[19] Neal DA, Brown MJ, Wilkinson IB, Alexander GJ. Mechanisms of hypertension after liver transplantation. Transplantation. 2005 Apr 27;79(8):935-40.
[20] Watt KD, Charlton MR.Metabolic syndrome and liver transplantation: a review and guide to management. J Hepatol. 2010 Jul;53(1):199-206. Epub 2010 Mar 31. Review.
[21] Sorice GP, Muscogiuri G, Mezza T, Prioletta A, Giaccari A. Metabolic syndrome in transplant patients: an academic or a health burden? Transplant Proc. 2011 Jan-Feb;43(1):313-7.
[22] Pagadala M, Dasarathy S, Eghtesad B, McCullough AJ. Posttransplant metabolic syndrome: an epidemic waiting to happen. Liver Transpl. 2009 Dec;15(12):1662-70. Review.

[23] Ruiz-Rebollo ML, Sánchez-Antolín G, García-Pajares F, Fernández-Orcajo P, González-Sagrado M, Cítores-Pascual MA, Velicia-Llames R, Caro-Patón A.Risk of development of the metabolic syndrome after orthotopic liver transplantation. Transplant Proc. 2010 Mar;42(2):663-5.
[24] Pérez MJ, García DM, Taybi BJ, Daga JA, Rey JM, Grande RG, Lombardo JD, López JM. Cardiovascular risk factors after liver transplantation: analysis of related factors. Transplant Proc. 2011 Apr;43(3):739-41.
[25] Farge D, Julien J.Effects of transplantation on the renin angiotensin system (RAS). J Hum Hypertens. 1998 Dec;12(12):827-32. Review.
[26] Bahirwani R, Reddy KR.Outcomes after liver transplantation: chronic kidney disease. Liver Transpl. 2009 Nov;15 Suppl 2:S70-4.
[27] Geissler E.K., Schlitt H.J. Immunosuppression for liver transplantation. Gut 2009; 58:452-463
[28] Pillai A. A., Levitsky J. Overview of immunosuppression in liver transplantation. Worl J Gastroentol 2009 September 14; 15(34): 4225-4233.
[29] Mukherjee S., Mukherjee U. A comprehensive revies of immunosuppression used for liver transplantation. Journal of transplantation
[30] Kockx M., Jessup W., Kritharides L. Cyclosporin A and atherosclerosis- Cellular pathways in atherogenesis. Pharmacology & Therapeutics 128 (2010) 106-118
[31] Halloran P.F. Mechanism of action of the calcineurin inhibitors. Transplant Proc. 2001; 33: 3067-3069
[32] J. R. Chapman. Chronic Calcineurin Inhibitor Nephrotoxicity—Lest We Forget American Journal of Transplantation 2011; 11: 693–697
[33] F. Lamoureux, E. Mestre, M. Essig, F.L. Sauvage, P. Marquet, L.N. Gastinel. Quantitative proteomic analysis of cyclosporine-induced toxicity in a human kidney cell line and comparison with tacrolimus. Journal of Proteomics (2011) article in press
[34] Nicolas Pallet, Sophie Fougeray,Philippe Beaune,Christophe Legendre,Eric Thervet, and Dany Anglicheau. Endoplasmic Reticulum Stress: An Unrecognized Actor in Solid Organ Transplantation. Transplantation 2009;88: 605–613
[35] Nicolas Pallet, Nicolas Bouvier, Philippe Beaune, Christophe Legendre, Dany Anglicheau, Éric Thervet. Implication du stress du reticulum endoplasmique en transplantation d'organe solide MEDECINE/SCIENCES 2010 ; 26 : 397-403
[36] Phuong-Thu T Pham, Phuong-Mai T Pham, Son V Pham, Phuong-Anh T Pham, Phuong-Chi T Pham. New onset diabetes after transplantation (NODAT): an overview Diabetes, Metabolic Syndrome and Obesity: Targets and Therapy Dovepress DOI: 10.2147/DMSO.S19027
[37] Gabardi S., Pharm D., Baroletti S., Pharm D. Everolimus: A proliferation signal inhibitor with clinical applications in organ transplantation, oncology and cardiology. Phramacotherapy 2010; 30(10): 1044-1056
[38] Webster A. C., Lee V.W.S., Chapman J. R., Craig J.C. Target of rapamycin inhibitors (Sirolimus and Everolimus) for primary immunosuppression of kidney transplant recipients: a systematic review and meta-analysis of randomized trials. Transplantation 2006; 9 (15): 1234-1248
[39] Allison A. C., Eugui E.M. Mycophenolate mofetil and its mechanism of action. Immunopharmacology 2000; 47:85-118

4

Pathogenesis of Renovascular Hypertension: Challenges and Controversies

Blake Fechtel, Stella Hartono and Joseph P. Grande
Mayo Clinic,
USA

1. Introduction

With an aging population, renovascular hypertension has become a major public health problem (Safian & Textor, 2001). Although various forms of fibromuscular disease of the renal arteries and/or traumatic disruption of renal vessels are the most common cause of RVH among the younger individuals, atherosclerotic renal artery disease (ARAD) is the most common lesion producing hypertension by far (Garovic & Textor, 2005). ARAD is present in over 6.8% of individuals over 65 years of age and is found in up to 49.1% of patients with coronary artery disease or aortoiliac disease (Iglesias et al. 2000; Valabhji et al. 2000; Hansen et al. 2002; Rihal et al. 2002; Weber-Mzell et al. 2002; Textor 2003). Although many patients with asymptomatic renovascular disease do not develop progressive renal dysfunction, overall morbidity and mortality is significantly increased (Chabova et al. 2000; Textor 2002; Textor 2003; Textor 2003; Foley et al. 2005; Foley et al. 2005). On the other hand, some studies suggest that from 10% to 40% of elderly hypertensive patients with newly discovered end stage renal disease and no identifiable parenchymal renal disease have significant RAS (Textor and Wilcox 2001). As in other forms of renal disease, the severity of interstitial fibrosis, tubular atrophy, interstitial inflammation, and glomerular sclerosis are important predictors of renal outcome (Wright et al. 2001). It has been postulated that this acquired tubulointerstitial injury may contribute to at least some forms of essential hypertension (Raghow 1994). Mechanisms underlying vascular and renal dysfunction in RAS have not been well delineated, despite intense study (Textor 2004). This information is essential for the development of therapies - surgical or medical - to treat RAS.

The hallmark of RVH arising from unilateral RAS is atrophy of the stenotic kidney and compensatory hyperplasia/hypertrophy of the contralateral kidney. Although this compensatory hypertrophy serves an adaptive function, this process may render the contralateral kidney more susceptible to other injuries (due to diabetes, glomerulonephritis, etc.) (Wenzel et al. 2002). Although the corresponding histologic, hemodynamic, and tubular alterations in the stenotic and contralateral kidneys have been superficially described in experimental animals, mechanisms underlying these alterations and the identification of markers that predict response to therapy have not been well defined. In particular, the stage in evolution of RAS at which the atrophic changes in the stenotic kidney preclude recovery of renal function after revascularization is not known. This lack of basic mechanistic knowledge is underscored by the variable response of RAS to surgical revascularization; significant improvement in blood pressure control and recovery of renal function is achieved in only about half of patients, with approximately one-quarter showing no significant changes, and up to one-quarter of patients developing progressive deterioration of renal function (Textor and Wilcox 2001; Textor 2003; Textor 2004). Furthermore, angiotensin-converting enzyme (ACE) inhibitors or angiotensin receptor blockers potentiate hypoperfusion of the stenotic kidney, but have been advocated to prevent deterioration of function in the contralateral kidney (Mann et al. 2001; Schoolwerth et al. 2001). The stage during development of RVH and circumstances in which this treatment should be initiated are not known. This lack of understanding of basic mechanisms underlying the development of human RVH has prompted the development of animal models to address this issue.

1.1 Animal model of renovascular disease

The classic "Goldblatt" 2K1C rat model of RAS has been extensively used to model human RVH (Goldblatt et al. 1934). In the stenotic kidney, reduced renal perfusion stimulates renin secretion through the renal baroreceptor system, leading to increased plasma levels of angiotensin II (A-II), provoking systemic hypertension (Martinez-Maldonado 1991). A-II may increase blood pressure directly or through elaboration of other vasoconstrictors (such as endothelin, thromboxanes, etc.); aldosterone promotes sodium and water retention and secondarily suppresses renin release. Over time, secondary structural damage occurs to the kidneys, vessels, and other end organs. In this chronic phase, the role of A-II in maintaining elevated blood pressure is not clear, as this phase no longer completely responds to ACE inhibitor therapy. In this chronic phase, the renal damage and endothelial dysfunction may be associated with near-normal renin and A-II levels (Okamura et al. 1986; Carretero and Scicli 1991). Indeed, lack of response to A-II inhibition in experimental animals with sustained RVH may predict lack of response to surgical intervention to remove the RAS (Pipinos et al. 1998).

In the 2K1C model, the weight of the stenotic kidney tends to be lower than that of normal or sham-treated controls, indicating that the kidney has undergone atrophy. The weight of the contralateral kidney is higher than that of normal controls, indicative of a hypertrophic/hyperplastic response. Histopathologic alterations in this model are variable, and probably depend upon the extent of blood pressure elevation. As originally described, the "Goldblatt" 2K1C is a model of accelerated, or "malignant" hypertension, with mean systolic blood pressures >200 mmHg (Goldblatt et al. 1934; Wilson and Byrom 1939; Wilson and Byrom 1940). Under these conditions, the contralateral kidney, despite low renin expression, develops interstitial fibrosis, tubular atrophy, interstitial inflammation, glomerulosclerosis, and hyalinosis (Mai et al. 1993; Sebekova et al. 1998; Kobayashi et al. 1999; Gauer et al. 2003). These chronic tubulointerstitial alterations are associated with increased TGF-β expression (Wenzel et al. 2003). Reported histopathologic alterations in the stenotic kidney are variable, and range from minimal alterations (Eng et al. 1994) to focal interstitial fibrosis and tubular atrophy without significant glomerulosclerosis (Wenzel et al. 2002).

In a rat 2K1C model that develops moderate hypertension (mean arterial pressure 158 mmHg), atrophy of the stenotic kidney and hypertrophy of the contralateral kidney is observed. The stenotic kidney shows increased staining for renin associated with interstitial fibrosis and tubular atrophy, with minimal alterations observed in the contralateral kidney (Richter et al. 2004). In this model, COX-2 inhibitors significantly reduce interstitial fibrosis in the stenotic kidney (Richter et al. 2004).

The 2K1C model has been established in mice using a clip of 0.12 mm (Wiesel et al. 1997). Four weeks after clipping, these investigators reported that 2K1C hypertensive mice exhibited blood pressure approximately 20 mm Hg higher than their sham operated controls. We have recently defined the histopathologic alterations connected with renal artery stenosis in animal model (Figure 1) (Cheng et al., 2009) and human (Keddis et al., 2010). In a murine model of 2K1C of RVH, we found that both the clipped and the contralateral kidney underwent minimal histopathological alterations during the first two weeks following surgery. Subsequently, the clipped kidney underwent atrophy, with generalized tubular atrophy, interstitial fibrosis and focal mononuclear infiltrates, whereas the contralateral kidney underwent hypertrophy/hyperplasia with minimal histopathologic alterations (figure 2). We propose that the murine 2K1C model is a good model of renovascular disease in humans with moderate hypertension. These animal models have helped to elucidate and suggest which cytokines and pathways are involved in RVH. Of these, the renin-angiotensin-aldosterone system, long known to have effects on the hemodynamics of RAS, is becoming more interesting for the inflammatory effects it causes as well.

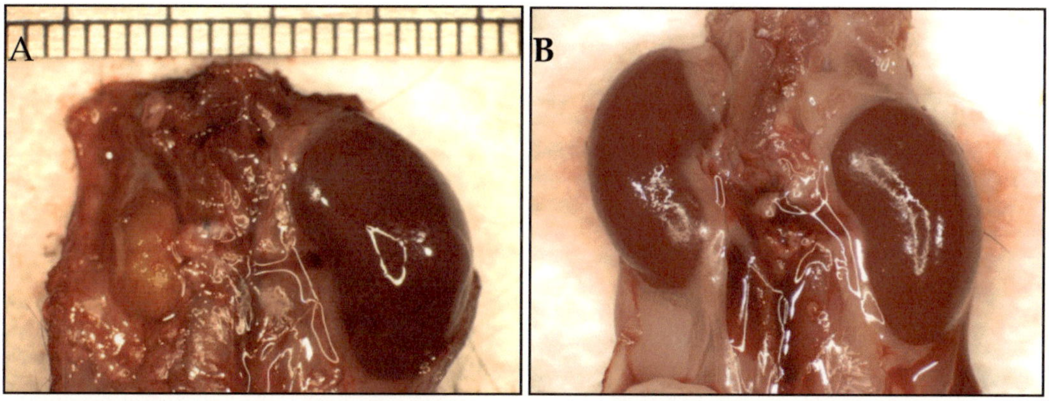

Fig. 1. Gross picture of the stenotic and contralateral kidney of mice (A) after placement of renal artery clip, the 2K1C model, compared to (B) sham procedure.

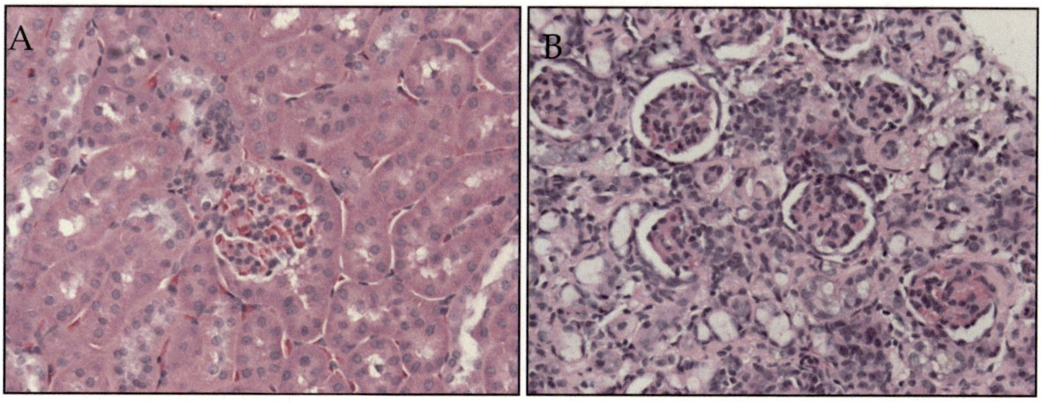

Fig. 2. Glomerular appearance of the (A) contralateral and (B) stenotic kidney with H&E staining.

1.2 The Renin-Angiotensin System and renovascular disease

Though its normal function is to preserve organ perfusion by regulating sodium and water balance, extracellular fluid volume and cardiac activity, the Renin-Angiotensin-Aldosterone System (RAAS) also plays an integral part in RVH. The RAAS has been found to be significantly activated in the presence of RAS. It is known that the increase in blood pressure caused by the RAAS has significant detrimental effects on the body, but it may also play a number of other roles in the development and progress of RVH.

Renin is made primarily by the juxtaglomerular cells in the Juxtaglomerular apparatus in response to 1) low pressure in the afferent renal artery, 2) sympathetic nervous system activity 3) A-II levels and 4) low sodium delivered to the macular densa in the distal convoluted tubule of the nephron. Other signals, such as potassium concentration, atrial natruretic peptide and endothelin also modulate renin synthesis. Renin enzymatically converts angiotensinogen, made in the liver, to angiotensin I. ACE, synthesized primarily in the lungs (though also in other tissues), then converts angiotensin I to A-II, a significantly biologically active molecule. A-II, in addition to its numerous tissue effects, induces the synthesis of aldosterone in the zona glomerulosa of the adrenal medulla, which then acts on mineralocorticoid receptors throughout the body, though when considering RAS, their most notable function is in the kidney (Laragh et al., 1992). This pathway is also located completely within other organs, including, the kidney. The proximal tubule, interstitium and medulla of the kidney have higher-than-systemic concentrations of A-II, because of local synthesis, which allows it to act in a paracrine function (Johnston et al., 1992). A-II and aldosterone can also be synthesized through an ACE-independent pathway, which is what allows for the return to normal A-II levels in the presence of ACE inhibition. This effect is also particularly prominent in the kidneys, where an estimated 40% of renally-synthesized A-II does not rely on ACE (Hollenberg, 1999).

A-II acts on 2 different receptors (angiotensin receptor type 1, or AT-1, and angiotensin receptor type 2, or AT-2) producing very different biological responses. Of these, AT-1 appears to play the most significant role in renal vascular disease (AT-2 is mostly known for its role in fetal organ development). Stimulation of the AT-1 receptor is best known for its systemic vasoconstrictive effects, and its vasoconstrictive effects on the efferent renal arteriole. The former causes general rises in systolic blood pressure, while the later decreases renal plasma flow, but increases glomerular filtration fraction. AT-1 stimulation also causes salt-retention through a number of mechanisms, increasing blood pressure even further (Dzau & Re, 1994; Liu & Cogan, 1989; Brewster & Perazella, 2004). A-II also mediates non-hemodynamic effects. A-II has the ability to promote fibrosis through a number of mechanisms, including induction of collagen synthesis, inhibition of collagen-cleaving proteases, stimulation of the secretion of platelet-derived growth factor, and, most interestingly, direct stimulation of TGF-β receptor type II(Luft, 2003; Wolf, 2000). AT-1 stimulation also has the ability to promote fibrosis by up-regulating expression and synthesis of NF-κB and thus TGF-β, as well as a number of other cytokines (Tsuzuki, 1996). Downstream, aldosterone, in addition to its hypertensive effects mediated through the mineralocorticoid receptor, also up-regulates the expression of TGF-β (Juknevicius et al., 2000). These studies have supported a widespread use of RAAS inhibitors (ACE-inhibitors, AT-1 inhibitors and aldosterone receptor inhibitors) to prevent renal disease progression. However, there is concern with the often-seen deleterious effects on renal function of the stenotic kidney caused by these anti-hypertensive agents. With already compromised blood flow, concern about increased damage to the ischemic kidney must be weighed with the benefits to the contralateral kidney (Jackson et al., 1986). With substanstial arterial obstruction, simply reducing perfusion pressure can reduce post-stenotic blood flow beyond that required for metabolic demands in the kidney. Early experimental studies in rats emphasized the potential for irreversible damage to the clipped kidney in animals treated with ACE inhibitors, resulting in "medical nephrectomy" (Jackson, 1990). However, it is important to note that this adverse reaction can develop with any forms of antihypertensive therapy (Textor et al., 1983). The risk factors for this adverse event include older age groups, pre-existing renal dysfunction, and episodes of acute illness leading to volume depletion (such as diarrhea or reduced intake during diuretic administration) (Speirs, et al., 1988).

With the increasing evidence of the involvement of TGF-β in RAS induced damage, the role of the RAAS in RAS, especially with respect to its induction of an inflammatory response, is being re-thought. There should be careful consideration and evaluation of the role of the immunologic and cytokine-associated effects of RAAS in the pathological process and initiation of RAS induced kidney damage. Such research may shed new light on whether the benefits of RAAS inhibition outweigh the costs in patients with RAS.

1.3 TGF-β and renovascular disease

Mechanisms underlying the differential response of the stenotic and contralateral kidney during the development and progression of RVH have not been adequately defined, despite numerous studies (Goldblatt et al., 1934; Martinez-Maldonado, 1991; Carretero, 1991). TGF-β is involved in a number of processes relevant to the development of RVH, including cell cycle regulation leading to hypertrophy and/or apoptosis, MAPK activation, inflammation, and extracellular matrix synthesis (Cheng & Grande, 2002).

It is well recognized that TGF-β plays a central role in fibrotic diseases (Cheng & Grande, 2002; Border et al., 1990; Border & Noble, 1994, 1997; Border & Ruoslahti, 1992). All aspects of fibrogenesis have been shown to be regulated by TGF-β, including the initial inflammatory phase in which infiltrating inflammatory cells and macrophages set the stage for the subsequent fibrotic phase in which activated fibroblasts and myofibroblasts contribute to the pathogenic accumulation of matrix (Cheng et al., 2005). In the past few years, receptors and signal transduction pathways mediating the effects of TGF-β on cells have been identified, enabling the identification of specific pathways involved in pathogenic events dependent on this cytokine. TGF-β signals through a set of transmembrane receptor serine/threonine kinases unique to the larger superfamily of TGF-β-related proteins. The active heteromeric receptor complex is formed by binding of ligand to a type II receptor, recruitment and activation of the type I receptor kinase, and phosphorylation of intracellular mediating target proteins (Massague, 1992, 1998; Attisano et al., 1994). Increased TGF-β receptor expression is observed in experimental glomerulonephritis (Shankland et al., 1996; Tamaki et al., 1994). In experimental renal disease associated with epithelial to mesenchymal transformation, TGF-β type 1 receptor expression is increased in tubular epithelial cells (Yang & Liu, 2002). Downstream mediators are the Smad family of proteins (Piek et al., 1999). Smad2 and 3 are phosphorylated directly by the type I receptor kinase, after which they partner with Smad4 and translocate to the nucleus where they act as transcriptional regulators of target genes, including those essential for apoptosis, inflammation, differentiation, and growth inhibition (Massague & Wotton, 2000; Derynck et al., 1998; Attisano et al., 2001). TGF-β plays a critical role in chronic inflammatory changes of the interstitium and extracellular matrix accumulation during fibrogenesis (Cheng & Grande, 2002; Grande et al., 1997, 2002). TGF-β initiates the transition of renal tubular epithelial cells to myofibroblasts, the cellular source for extracellular matrix deposition, leading to irreversible renal failure (Yang & Liu, 2001; Iwano et al., 2002; Li et al., 2002).

A predominant role of TGF-β1 in regulation of extracellular matrix deposition is highlighted in our published studies employing renal tubular epithelial cells derived from animals bearing a homozygous deletion of the TGF-β1 gene (Grande et al, 2002). Although the most direct means to test the hypothesis that T TGF-β1 plays a central role in the development of RVH would be to perform these studies in mice bearing homozygous deletion of the TGF-β1 gene, the phenotype of these animals precludes such studies. TGF-β1 KO animals have an extremely high rate of embryonic lethality, and the few surviving mice develop a systemic inflammatory syndrome, leading to their death within 2-4 weeks of age (Letterio et al, 1994; Martin et al., 1995; Kulkarni & Karlsson, 1993; Boivin et al., 1995). For this reason, more recent studies have employed mice with genetic manipulation of the Smad proteins to define potential mechanisms by which the TGF-β signaling pathway is involved in chronic tissue injury. Smad3 KO mice show accelerated healing of wounds, in association with decreased local inflammation (Ashcroft et al., 1999). Smad3-null mice have been used in several chronic injury models, including ureteric obstruction (Sato et al., 2003). In WT mice, unilateral ureteric obstruction (UUO) produces extensive interstitial fibrosis and tubular atrophy, with TGF-β1-driven epithelial to mesenchymal transformation of tubular epithelial cells, as evidenced by reduction in E-cadherin staining and de novo induction of α-smooth muscle actin (α-SMA) staining. This is associated with extensive influx of monocytes. In Smad3 KO animals subjected to UUO, there was a marked reduction in interstitial fibrosis, and epithelial to mesenchymal transformation, indicating that the Smad pathway is necessary for epithelial to mesenchymal transformation by TGF-β (Itoh et al., 2003; Yu et al., 2002).

1.4 MAPK pathways and renovascular disease

It is well recognized that cellular adaptive responses to environmental stimuli, including hypertrophy, hyperplasia, and atrophy associated with increased apoptotic activity, are transduced through the MAPK pathway(s) (Kyriakis 2000; Kyriakis and Avruch 2001). Cardiac hypertrophy in A-II dependent hypertension is associated with activation of p38, whereas ERK and JNK are preferentially stimulated in an A-II independent model of RVH (Pellieux et al. 2000). The development of hypertension is associated with persistent ERK activation in the aorta of Dahl salt-sensitive rats and stroke-prone spontaneously hypertensive rats (Kim et al. 1997; Hamaguchi et al. 2000). In human diabetic nephropathy, there is increased immunohistochemical staining for p-ERK in glomeruli which correlates with the severity of glomerular lesions and increased p-p38 staining which correlates with severity of tubulointerstitial lesions and number of CD68-positive macrophages (Adhikary et al. 2004; Toyoda et al. 2004; Sakai et al. 2005). Hypertension accelerates the development of diabetic nephropathy in a rat model of type 2 diabetes through induction of ERK and p38, as well as TGF-β (Imai et al. 2003). Similarly, the p38 and JNK pathways are activated in the early stages of experimental proliferative glomerulonephritis, whereas the ERK pathway is persistently activated (Bokemeyer et al. 1998). Both p38 and JNK are activated in experimental anti-glomerular basement membrane antibody mediated glomerulonephritis (Stambe et al. 2003). In a variety of other human renal diseases, p-ERK expression is observed in regions of tubulointerstitial damage, within α-SMA positive myofibroblasts (Masaki et al. 2004). In cultured cells, ERK is involved in epithelial to mesenchymal transformation (Li et al. 2004; Xie et al. 2004; Yang et al. 2004). We have previously identified ERK, p38, and JNK as essential intermediates for MC mitogenesis, and ERK and p38 as essential intermediates for TGF-β stimulated collagen IV mRNA expression and MCP-1 production (Cheng et al. 2002; Cheng et al. 2004). We have also shown that ERK is significantly upregulated in a rat model of salt sensitive hypertension (Diaz et al., 2008). Others have shown that p38 activation is necessary for TGF-β stimulation of fibronectin production (Suzuki et al. 2004).

The MAPK pathways are involved in regulation of cell cycle arrest and apoptosis, which is of direct relevance to the renal atrophy which occurs in the stenotic kidney of the 2K1C RAS model. Activation of ERK is necessary for TGF-β-mediated induction of p21 and cell cycle arrest (Hu et al. 1999). High glucose promotes hypertrophy of MC through ERK mediated phosphorylation of p27 (Wolf et al. 2003). Activation of p38 or JNK is frequently associated with cell cycle arrest or apoptosis (Cardone et al. 1997; Frasch et al. 1998). Induction of apoptosis in MC requires sustained activation of JNK (Guo et al. 1998). Apoptosis and other cellular responses may be directed by a balance between ERK and JNK activation (Xia et al. 1995).

Based on these considerations, there has been intense interest in developing low molecular weight pathway specific MAPK inhibitors as therapeutic agents to treat cancer and fibroproliferative inflammatory conditions (Duncia et al. 1998; Sebolt-Leopold et al. 1999; Clemons et al. 2002; Duan et al. 2004; Sebolt-Leopold and Herrera 2004; Jo et al. 2005; McDaid et al. 2005). These agents have been employed in experimental renovascular disease, with mixed results. The ERK inhibitor U0126 was effective in reducing acute renal injury in an experimental mesangial proliferative glomerulonephritis model (Bokemeyer et al. 2002). In human renal diseases associated with injury to podocytes, p38 is induced. The p38 inhibitor FR167653 prevents renal dysfunction and glomerulosclerosis in chronic adriamycin nephropathy (Koshikawa et al. 2005) and in experimental crescenteric glomerulonephritis (Wada et al. 2001). Similarly, the p38 inhibitor NPC31145 reduced acute inflammatory injury in an experimental anti-glomerular basement membrane glomerulonephritis model (Stambe et al. 2003). On the other hand, the p38 inhibitor FR167653 increased proteinuria in a passive Heymann nephritis model of podocyte injury (Aoudjit et al. 2003), suggesting that activation of p38 protects podocytes from complement mediated injury. Furthermore, the p38 inhibitor NPC31169 exacerbated renal damage in a remnant kidney model due to in vivo induction of ERK (Ohashi et al. 2004).

1.5 The role of inflammation in renovascular disease

RVH initiates activation of the renin–angiotensin system and structural remodeling, evidenced by fibrosis and vascular deterioration in the affected kidney. Although the renin-angiotensin system tends to resolve once a stable blood pressure (BP) is reached, it has been suggested that transient elevation of plasma A-II could precipitate macrophage infiltration, thereby initiating an inflammatory response within the kidney (Ozawa et al., 2007). This inflammatory cascade may well underlie the degenerative processes within the kidney as its renal artery begins to narrow.

We performed PCR array studies of renal homogenates obtained from mice subjected to RAS or sham surgery. The results of our PCR Array studies (Table 1) implicate monocyte chemoattractant protein-1 (MCP-1) as a key chemokine in this inflammatory response. In addition to infiltrating inflammatory cells, tubular epithelial cells of the stenotic kidney of mice exposed to RAS express high level of MCP-1 (figure 3). Our findings are in accord with those of other investigators who have studied renovascular hypertension. High salt diet in DSS rats caused expression of NADPH oxidase and MCP-1 in the dilated renal tubules and resulting in interstitial inflammation and migration of mononuclear cells (Shigemoto et al., 2007). Increased MCP-1 levels also seem to stimulate TGF-β formation in glomerular cells despite the absence of infiltrating inflammatory cells (Wolf et al., 2002). Studies in the swine model of renovascular hypertension using bindarit, a selective MCP-1 blocker, show that inhibition of MCP-1 confers renal protective effects by blunting renal inflammation and reducing the level of collagen deposition, thereby preserving the kidney in chronic RAS (Zoja et al., 1998; Zhu et al., 2009). It was further indicated that MCP-1 contributes to functional and structural impairment in the RAS kidney, specifically in the tubulo-interstitial compartment.

Gene function	Gene symbol	Gene name	Fold change
Inflammation	Ccl2	MCP-1 (monocyte chemoattractant protein 2)	+43
	Ccl3	MIP-1α (macrophage inflammatory protein 1α)	+22
	Ccl4	MIP-1β (macrophage inflammatory protein 1β)	+8
	Ccl5	RANTES (regulated upon activation, normal T-cell expressed and secreted cytokine)	
	Ccl7	MCP-3 (monocyte chemoattractant protein 3)	+153
	Ccl8	MCP-2 (monocyte chemoattractant protein 2)	+149
	Ccl12	MCP-5 (monocyte chemoattractant protein 5)	+56
	Ccl20	MIP-3α (macrophage inflammatory protein 3α)	+105
	Ccl22	MDC (macrophage derived chemokine)	+41
	Ccr2	Chemokine (C-C motif) receptor 2	+30
	Ccr3	Chemokine (C-C motif) receptor 3	+35
	Ccr4	Chemokine (C-C motif) receptor 4	+6
	Cxcl2	MIP-2α (macrophage inflammatory protein 2α)	+208
	Cxcl3	MIP-2β (macrophage inflammatory protein 2β)	+7
	Cxcl5	AMCF-II (alveolar macrophage chemotactic factor)	+653
	Cxcl9	Mig (monokine induced by γ-interferon)	+5
	IL1α	Interleukin-1α	+18
	IL1β	Interleukin-1β	+11

Table 1. PCR array results of proinflammatory cytokine expression in stenotic kidneys of RAS mouse

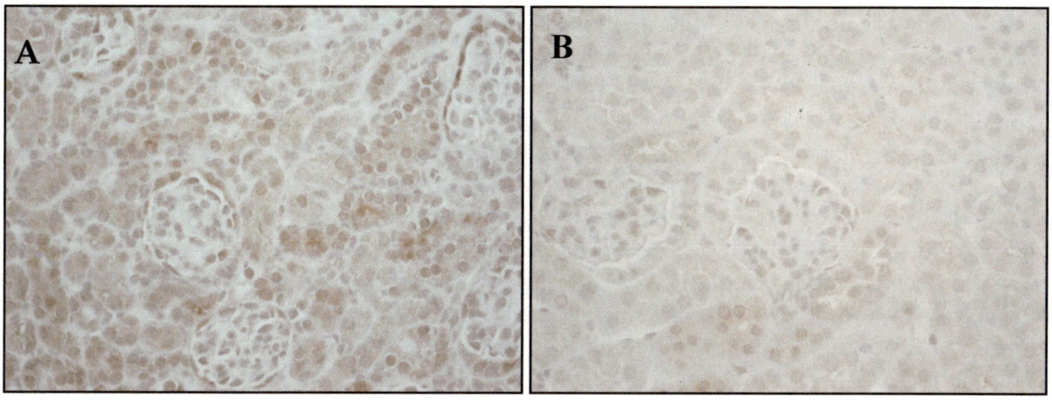

Fig. 3. MCP-1 staining in the (A) contralateral kidney and (B) stenotic kidney of C57BLKS mouse 4 weeks after placement of renal artery clip.

At a cellular level, it is apparent that the renal artery stenosis did elicit an inflammatory cascade in the kidney as evidenced by macrophage infiltration, the rise in MCP-1 and its receptor chemokine (C-C motif) receptor 2 (CCR2), NFκB, protein kinase C (PKC) and TGF-β. Remarkably, we also saw transient increase in MCP-1 and TGF-β in the contralateral kidney which indicates some inflammatory process taking place despite lack of inflammatory cells and/or tissue damage. It is apparent that blockade of the MCP-1 receptor does offer renal protection and prevents the progressive fibrosis development in renovascular hypertension. Elucidating the underlying mechanisms of this protection will allow us to develop preventive measures and novel therapeutic interventions that could possibly be applied to other renal diseases.

1.6 Therapeutic implication

Hypertension is one of the most common reasons for a visit to a physician. There are several key issues that need to be addressed during evaluation of a patient with hypertension: accurate blood pressure reading, determination of target organ damage due to hypertension, screening for other cardiovascular risk factor, stratification of cardiovascular disease, and assessment for the cause of hypertension (primary vs. secondary hypertension). Thorough assessment of the cause of hypertension is essential for determining the correct treatment approach, especially in children where atherosclerosis is not common. For children with hypertension, it is necessary to consider genetic diseases (i.e. coarctation of the aorta, primary aldosteronism) and auto-immune diseases (i.e. post-infectious-glomerulonephritis). When initiating treatment, it is important to maintain low systolic pressure as systolic pressure is a stronger predictor of cardiovascular event (Mancia et al. 2009; Cherubini et al. 2010). Maintenance of blood pressure goal should ideally be achieved within 6 to 9 months of therapeutic initiation.

2. Conclusion

Optimal management of renovascular hypertension requires an understanding of the disease process and remains an important challenge for clinicians caring for patients with hypertension. Although the pathophysiology and the consequence to human health caused by RVH are well understood, the exact mechanism by which the stenosis of the renal artery induces the damage is not. Revascularization studies have demonstrated highly variable results, with significant improvement in a small subset of patients, but an overall lack of justification of the risks, when applied to large groups of patients (Textor et al., 2009). While parsing out why some patients benefit while others do not will be an important task in the years to come, the more significant benefit will be from determining the reasons for the continued renal damage in the majority of revascularized patients. Developing novel therapies to address these yet-unknown pathological processes will yield benefit for all RAS patients. Recent studies implicate the non-hemodynamic effects of the renin-angiotensin-aldosterone system and the inflammatory chemokines as possible initiating signals for the atrophic, inflammatory and fibrotic changes seen. Elucidating, more thoroughly, the role these pathways play in renal damage due to RAS could identify new targets for therapeutic intervention and the first biomarkers to aid in diagnosis, limiting the need for costly and damaging imaging studies. Many questions remain to understand how these pathways are initiated, how they interact and how they ultimately lead to renal damage. What cells first sense the stenosis, and how do they sense it? Which of the pathways contribute to damage and which are necessary to preserve kidney function? The answer to these and other such questions hold the possibility to further the science, diagnostics and treatment of renovascular hypertension, and to improve the lives of the millions it affects.

3. References

Adhikary L, Chow F, Nikolic-Paterson DJ, Stambe C, Dowling J, Atkins RC, et al. (2004). Abnormal p38 mitogen-activated protein kinase signalling in human and experimental diabetic nephropathy. *Diabetologia,* 47(7):1210-22.

Aoudjit L, Stanciu M, Li H, Lemay S, Takano T. (2003). p38 mitogen-activated protein kinase protects glomerular epithelial cells from complement-mediated cell injury. *Am J Physiol Renal Physiol,* 285(4):F765-74.

Ashcroft G, Yang X, Glick A, Weinstein M, Letterio J, Mizel D, et al. (1999). Mice lacking Smad3 show accelerated wound healing and an impaired local inflammatory response. *Nature Cell Biology,* 1:260-266.

Attisano L, Tuen Lee-Hoeflich S. (2001). The Smads. *Genome Biololgy,* 2(8).

Attisano L, Wrana JL, Lopez-Casillas F, Massague J. (1994). TGF-β receptors and actions. *Biochemica et Biophysica Acta,*1222:71-80.

B Jackson, BP McGrath, PG Matthews, C Wong and CI Johnston. (1986). Differential renal function during angiotensin converting enzyme inhibition in renovascular hypertension. *Hypertension.* 8:650-654

Boivin GP, O'Toole BA, Orsmby IE, Diebold RJ, Eis MJ, Doetschman T, et al. (1995). Onset and progression of pathological lesions in transforming growth factor-β1-deficient mice. *Am J Pathol,* 146(1):276-88.

Bokemeyer D, Guglielmi KE, McGinty A, Sorokin A, Lianos EA, Dunn MJ. (1998). Different activation of mitogen-activated protein kinases in experimental proliferative glomerulonephritis. *Kidney Int Suppl,* 67(5):S189-91.

Bokemeyer D, Panek D, Kramer HJ, Lindemann M, Kitahara M, Boor P, et al. (2002). In vivo identification of the mitogen-activated protein kinase cascade as a central pathogenic pathway in experimental mesangioproliferative glomerulonephritis. *J Am Soc Nephrol;*13(6):1473-80.

Border WA, Noble NA. (1997). TGF-β in kidney fibrosis: A target for gene therapy. *Kidney Int*;51(5):1388-1396.

Border WA, Noble NA. (1994). Transforming growth factor β in tissue fibrosis. *N Engl J Med*, 331:1286-1292.

Border WA, Okuda S, Languino LR, Sporn MB, Ruoslahti E. (1990). Suppression of experimental glomerulonephritis by antiserum against transforming growth factor β-1. *Nature*;346:371-374.

Border WA, Ruoslahti E. (1992). Transforming growth factor β in disease: The dark side of tissue repair. *J Clin Invest*, ;90:1-7.

Brewster UC, Perazella MA. (2004). The reninangiotensin-aldosterone system and the kidney: effects on kidney disease. *Am J Med*, 116:263-72

Cardone MH, Salvesen GS, Widmann C, Johnson G, Frisch SM. (1997). The regulation of anoikis: MEKK-1 activation requires cleavage by caspases. *Cell*, 90(2):315-23.

Carretero OA, Scicli AG. (1991). Local hormonal factors (intracrine, autocrine, and paracrine) in hypertension. *Hypertension*, 18(3 Suppl):I58-69.

Chabova V, Schirger A, Stanson AW, McKusick MA, Textor SC. (2000). Outcomes of atherosclerotic renal artery stenosis managed without revascularization. *Mayo Clin Proc*, 75(5):437-44.

Cheng, J., Zhou, W., Warner, GM., Knudsen, BE., Garovic, VD., Gray, CE., Lerman, LO., Platt, JL., Romero, JC., Textor, SC., Nath, KA. & Grande, JP. (2009). Temporal analysis of signaling pathways activated in a murine model of two-kidney, one-clip hypertension. *Am J Physiol Renal Physiol.* 297:(4) F1055-F1068

Cheng J, Diaz Encarnacion MM, Warner GM, Gray CE, Nath KA, Grande JP. (2005). TGF-beta1 stimulates monocyte chemoattractant protein-1 expression in mesangial cells through a phosphodiesterase isoenzyme 4-dependent process. Am J Physiol Cell Physiol;289(4):C959-70.

Cheng J, Grande JP. (2002). Transforming growth factor-beta signal transduction and progressive renal disease. Exp Biol Med;227:943-956.

Cheng J, Gray C, Warner G, Grande J. (2002). Regulation of monocyte chemoattractant protein-1 (MCP-1) by MAPK inhibitors in rat mesangial cells. J Am Soc Nephrol, 13:136A.

Cheng J, Thompson MA, Walker HJ, Gray CE, Diaz Encarnacion MM, Warner GM, et al. (2004). Differential Regulation of Mesangial Cell Mitogenesis by cAMP Phosphodiesterase Isozymes 3 and 4. Am J Physiol Renal Physiol, 287(5):F940-53.

Cherubini, A., D. T. Lowenthal, et al. (2010). "Hypertension and cognitive function in the elderly." Disease-a-month : DM 56(3): 106-147.

Clemons AP, Holstein DM, Galli A, Saunders C. (2002). Cerulein-induced acute pancreatitis in the rat is significantly ameliorated by treatment with MEK1/2 inhibitors U0126 and PD98059. Pancreas, 25(3):251-9.

Derynck R, Zhang Y, Feng X. (1998). Smads: transcriptional activators of TGF-β responses. Cell, 95:737-740.

Diaz Encarnacion MM, Warner GM, Gray CE, Cheng J, Keryakos HK, Nath KA, and Grande JP (2008) Signaling pathways modulated by fish oil in salt-sensitive hypertension. Am J Physiol Renal Physiol 294:F1323–F1335

Duan W, Chan JH, Wong CH, Leung BP, Wong WS. (2004). Anti-inflammatory effects of mitogen-activated protein kinase kinase inhibitor U0126 in an asthma mouse model. J Immunol, 172(11):7053-9.

Duncia JV, Santella JB, 3rd, Higley CA, Pitts WJ, Wityak J, Frietze WE, et al. (1998). MEK inhibitors: the chemistry and biological activity of U0126, its analogs, and cyclization products. Bioorg Med Chem Lett, 8(20):2839-44.

Dzau VJ, Re R. (1994). Tissue angiotensin system in cardiovascular medicine: a paradigm shift? Circulation. 89:493–498.

Eng E, Veniant M, Floege J, Fingerle J, Alpers CE, Menard J, et al. (1994). Renal proliferative and phenotypic changes in rats with two-kidney, one-clip Goldblatt hypertension. Am J Hypertens;7(2):177-85.

Foley R, Wang C, AJ C. (2005). Cardiovascular risk factor profiles and kidney function stage in the US general population: The NHANES III Study. Mayo Clin Proc, 80(10):1270-1277.

Foley RN, Murray AM, Li S, Herzog CA, McBean AM, Eggers PW, et al. (2005). Chronic kidney disease and the risk for cardiovascular disease, renal replacement, and death in the United States Medicare population, 1998 to 1999. J Am Soc Nephrol, 16(2):489-95.

Frasch SC, Nick JA, Fadok VA, Bratton DL, Worthen GS, Henson PM. (1998). p38 mitogen-activated protein kinase-dependent and -independent intracellular signal transduction pathways leading to apoptosis in human neutrophils. *J Biol Chem*, 273(14):8389-97.

Garovic V, Textor SC. (2005). Renovascular hypertension: current concepts. *Semin Nephrol*, 25:261-271.

Garty H. (1992). Regulation of sodium permeability by aldosterone. Semin Nephrol.;12:24–29

Gauer S, Hartner A, Hauser IA, Fierlbeck W, Eberhardt W, Geiger H. (2003). Differential regulation of osteopontin expression in the clipped and nonclipped kidney of two-kidney, one-clip hypertensive rats. Am J Hypertens;16(3):214-22.

Goldblatt H, Lynch J, Hanzal R, Summerville W. (1934). Studies on experimental hypertension; I: The production of persistent elevation of systolic blood pressure by means of renal ischemia. J Exp Med, 59:347-79.

Grande J, Warner G, Walker H, Yusufi A, Gray C, Kopp J, et al. (2002). TGF-β1 is an autocrine mediator of renal tubular epithelial cell growth and collagen IV production. Exp Biol Med ,227:171-181.

Grande JP, Melder DC, Zinsmeister AR. (1997). Modulation of collagen gene expression by cytokines: Stimulatory effect of transforming growth factor-β1, with divergent effects of epidermal growth factor and tumor necrosis factor-α on collagen type I and collagen type IV. J Lab Clin Med ,130:476-486.

Guo YL, Baysal K, Kang B, Yang LJ, Williamson JR. (1998). Correlation between sustained c-Jun N-terminal protein kinase activation and apoptosis induced by tumor necrosis factor- in rat mesangial cells. J Biol Chem , 273(7):4027-34.

Hamaguchi A, Kim S, Izumi Y, Iwao H. (2000). Chronic activation of glomerular mitogen-activated protein kinases in Dahl salt-sensitive rats. J Am Soc Nephrol, 11(1):39-46.

Hansen KJ, Edwards MS, Craven TE, Cherr GS, Jackson SA, Appel RG, et al. (2002). Prevalence of renovascular disease in the elderly: a population-based study. J Vasc Surg, 36(3):443-51.

Hollenberg NK. (1999). Pharmacologic interruption of the renin-angiotensin system and the kidney: differential responses to angiotensinconverting enzyme and renin inhibition. J Am Soc Nephrol, 10(suppl):S239–S242

Hu PP, Shen X, Huang D, Liu Y, Counter C, Wang XF. (1999). The MEK pathway is required for stimulation of p21(WAF1/CIP1) by transforming growth factor-beta. J Biol Chem, 274(50):35381-7.

Iglesias JI, Hamburger RJ, Feldman L, Kaufman JS. (2000). The natural history of incidental renal artery stenosis in patients with aortoiliac vascular disease. Am J Med, 109(8):642-7.

Imai G, Satoh T, Kumai T, Murao M, Tsuchida H, Shima Y, et al. (2003). Hypertension accelerates diabetic nephropathy in Wistar fatty rats, a model of type 2 diabetes mellitus, via mitogen-activated protein kinase cascades and transforming growth factor-beta1. Hypertens Re, 26(4):339-47.

Itoh S, Thorikay M, Kowanetz M, Moustakas A, Itoh F, Heldin CH, et al. (2003). Elucidation of Smad requirement in transforming growth factor-beta type I receptor-induced responses. J Biol Che, 278(6):3751-61.

Iwano M, Plieth D, Danoff TM, Xue C, Okada H, Neilson EG. (2002). Evidence that fibroblasts derive from epithelium during tissue fibrosis. J Clin Invest, 110(3):341-50.

Jackson B, Franze L, Sumithran E, Johnston CI. (1990). Pharmacologic nephrectomy with chronic angiotensin converting enzyme inhibitor treatment in renovascular hypertension in the rat. J Lab Clin Med., 115:21–27

Jo SK, Cho WY, Sung SA, Kim HK, Won NH. (2005). MEK inhibitor, U0126, attenuates cisplatin-induced renal injury by decreasing inflammation and apoptosis. Kidney Int;67(2):458-66.

Johnston CI. (1992). Renin-angiotensin system: a dual tissue and hormonal system for cardiovascular control. *J Hypertens Suppl.*, 10(suppl):S13–S26

Juknevicius I, Segal Y, Kren S, et al. (2000). Aldosterone causes TGF-β expression. J Am Soc Nephrol.;11:59-66

Keddis, MT., Garovic, VD., Bailey, KR., Wood, CM., Raissian, Y. & Grande, JP. (2010). Ischaemic nephropathy secondary to atherosclerotic renal artery stenosis: clinical and histopathological correlates. *Nephrol. Dial. Transplant.* 25: 3615-3622

Kim S, Murakami T, Izumi Y, Yano M, Miura K, Yamanaka S, et al. (1997). Extracellular signal-regulated kinase and c-Jun NH2-terminal kinase activities are continuously and differentially increased in aorta of hypertensive rats. *Biochem Biophys Res Commun*, 236(1):199-204.

Kobayashi S, Ishida A, Moriya H, Mori N, Fukuda T, Takamura T. (1999). Angiotensin II receptor blockade limits kidney injury in two-kidney, one-clip Goldblatt hypertensive rats with special reference to phenotypic changes. J Lab Clin Med;133(2):134-43.

Koshikawa M, Mukoyama M, Mori K, Suganami T, Sawai K, Yoshioka T, et al. (2005). Role of p38 Mitogen-Activated Protein Kinase Activation in Podocyte Injury and

Proteinuria in Experimental Nephrotic Syndrome. J Am Soc Nephrol;16(9):2690-701.

Kulkarni AB, Huh C-G, Becker D, Geiser A, Lyght M, Flanders KC, et al. (1993). Transforming growth factor -1 null mutation in mice causes excessive inflammatory response and early death. Proceedings of the National Academy of Sciences;90:770-774.

Kulkarni AB, Karlsson S. (1993). Transforming growth factor β-1 knockout mice. A mutation in one cytokine gene causes a dramatic inflammatory disease. American Journal of Pathology;143:3-9.

Kyriakis JM, Avruch J. (2001). Mammalian mitogen-activated protein kinase signal transduction pathways activated by stress and inflammation. Physiol Rev;81(2):807-69.

Kyriakis JM. (2000). MAP kinases and the regulation of nuclear receptors. Sci STKE;2000(48):E1.

Laragh JH, Angers M, Kelly WG, Lieberman S. (1960). Hypotensive agents and pressor substances: the effect of epinephrine, norepinephrine, A-II, and others on the secretory rate of aldosterone in man. JAMA. 1960;174:234–240

Letterio JJ, Geiser AG, Kulkarni AB, Roche NS, Sporn MB, Roberts AB. (1994). Maternal rescue of transforming growth factor-β1 null mice. Science 1994;264:1936-1938.

Li J, Zhu H, Huang X, Lai K, RJ J, Lan H. (2002). Smad7 inhibits fibrotic effect of TGF-β on renal tubular epithelial cells by blocking Smad2 activation. J Am Soc Nephrol;13:1464-1472.

Li JH, Wang W, Huang XR, Oldfield M, Schmidt AM, Cooper ME, et al. (2004). Advanced glycation end products induce tubular epithelial-myofibroblast transition through the RAGE-ERK1/2 MAP kinase signaling pathway. Am J Pathol;164(4):1389-97.

Liu FY, Cogan MG. (1989). A-II stimulates early proximal bicarbonate absorption in the rat by decreasing cyclic adenosine monophosphate. J Clin Invest.;84:83–91.

Luft FC. (2002). Proinflammatory effects of A-II and endothelin: targets for progression of cardiovascular and renal disease. Curr Opin Nephrol Hypertens.;11:59–66.

Mai M, Geiger H, Hilgers KF, Veelken R, Mann JF, Dammrich J, et al. (1993). Early interstitial changes in hypertension-induced renal injury. Hypertension;22(5):754-65.

Mancia, G., S. Laurent, et al. (2009). "Reappraisal of European guidelines on hypertension management: a European Society of Hypertension Task Force document." Journal of hypertension 27(11): 2121-2158.

Mann JF, Gerstein HC, Pogue J, Bosch J, Yusuf S. Renal insufficiency as a predictor of cardiovascular outcomes and the impact of ramipril: the HOPE randomized trial. Ann Intern Med 2001;134(8):629-36.

Martin JS, Dickson MC, Cousins FM, Kulkarni AB, Karlsson S, Akhurst RJ. (1995). Analysis of homozygous TGF-β1 null mouse embryos demonstrates defects in yolk sac vasculogenesis and hematopoiesis. Annals of the New York Academy of Sciences 1995;752:300-308.

Martinez-Maldonado M. (1991). Pathophysiology of renovascular hypertension. Hypertension 1991;17(5):707-19.

Masaki T, Stambe C, Hill PA, Dowling J, Atkins RC, Nikolic-Paterson DJ. (2004). Activation of the extracellular-signal regulated protein kinase pathway in human glomerulopathies. J Am Soc Nephrol 2004;15(7):1835-43.

Massague J, Wotton D. (2000). Transcriptional control by the TGF-beta/Smad signaling system. Embo J;19(8):1745-54.

Massague J. (1992). Receptors for the TGF-beta family. Cell 1992;69:1067-1070.

Massague J. (1998). TGF-β signal transduction. Annu Rev Biochem;67:753-791.

McDaid HM, Lopez-Barcons L, Grossman A, Lia M, Keller S, Perez-Soler R, et al. (2005). Enhancement of the therapeutic efficacy of taxol by the mitogen-activated protein kinase kinase inhibitor CI-1040 in nude mice bearing human heterotransplants. Cancer Res;65(7):2854-60.

Ohashi R, Nakagawa T, Watanabe S, Kanellis J, Almirez RG, Schreiner GF, et al. (2004). Inhibition of p38 mitogen-activated protein kinase augments progression of remnant kidney model by activating the ERK pathway. Am J Pathol;164(2):477-85.

Okamura T, Miyazaki M, Inagami T, Toda N. (1986). Vascular renin-angiotensin system in two-kidney, one clip hypertensive rats. Hypertension;8(7):560-5.

Ozawa Y, Kobori H, Suzaki Y, Navar LG. (2007). Sustained renal interstitial macrophage infiltration following chronic angiotensin II infusions. Am J Physiol Renal Physiol 2007; 292:F330–F339

Pellieux C, Sauthier T, Aubert JF, Brunner HR, Pedrazzini T. (2000). Angiotensin II-induced cardiac hypertrophy is associated with different mitogen-activated protein kinase activation in normotensive and hypertensive mice. J Hypertens;18(9):1307-17.

Piek E, Heldin C-H, Ten Dijke P. Specificity, diversity, and regulation in TGF-β superfamily signaling. FASEB J 1999;13:2105-2124.

Pipinos, II, Nypaver TJ, Moshin SK, Careterro OA, Beierwaltes WH. Response to angiotensin inhibition in rats with sustained renovascular hypertension correlates with response to removing renal artery stenosis. J Vasc Surg 1998;28(1):167-77.

Raghow R. The role of extracellular matrix in postinflammatory wound healing and fibrosis. Federation of American Societies for Experimental Biology 1994;8:823-831.

Richter CM, Godes M, Wagner C, Maser-Gluth C, Herzfeld S, Dorn M, et al. Chronic cyclooxygenase-2 inhibition does not alter blood pressure and kidney function in renovascular hypertensive rats. J Hypertens 2004;22(1):191-8.

Rihal CS, Textor SC, Breen JF, McKusick MA, Grill DE, Hallett JW, et al. Incidental renal artery stenosis among a prospective cohort of hypertensive patients undergoing coronary angiography. Mayo Clin Proc 2002;77(4):309-16.

Safian RD, Textor SC. Renal-artery stenosis. N Engl J Med 2001;344(6):431-42.

Sakai N, Wada T, Furuichi K, Iwata Y, Yoshimoto K, Kitagawa K, et al. Involvement of extracellular signal-regulated kinase and p38 in human diabetic nephropathy. Am J Kidney Dis 2005;45(1):54-65.

Sato M, Muragaki Y, Saika S, Roberts AB, Ooshima A. Targeted disruption of TGF-beta1/Smad3 signaling protects against renal tubulointerstitial fibrosis induced by unilateral ureteral obstruction. J Clin Invest 2003;112(10):1486-94.

Schoolwerth AC, Sica DA, Ballermann BJ, Wilcox CS. Renal considerations in angiotensin converting enzyme inhibitor therapy: a statement for healthcare professionals from the Council on the Kidney in Cardiovascular Disease and the Council for High

Blood Pressure Research of the American Heart Association. Circulation 2001;104(16):1985-91.

Sebekova K, Dammrich J, Fierlbeck W, Krivosikova Z, Paczek L, Heidland A. Effect of chronic therapy with proteolytic enzymes on hypertension-induced renal injury in the rat model of Goldblatt hypertension. Am J Nephrol 1998;18(6):570-6.

Sebolt-Leopold JS, Dudley DT, Herrera R, Van Becelaere K, Wiland A, Gowan RC, et al. Blockade of the MAP kinase pathway suppresses growth of colon tumors in vivo. Nat Med 1999;5(7):810-6.

Sebolt-Leopold JS, Herrera R. Targeting the mitogen-activated protein kinase cascade to treat cancer. Nat Rev Cancer 2004;4(12):937-47.

Shankland SJ, Pippin J, Pichler RH, Gordon KL, Friedman S, Gold LI, et al. Differential expression of transforming growth factor- isoforms and receptors in experimental membranous nephropathy. Kidney Int 1996;50(1):116-124.

Shigemoto Fujii, Ling Zhang and Hiroaki Kosaka. Albuminuria, Expression of Nicotinamide Adenine Dinucleotide Phosphate Oxidase and Monocyte Chemoattractant Protein-1 in the Renal Tubules of Hypertensive Dahl Salt-Sensitive Rats. Hypertension Research 30, 991-998 (October 2007)

Speirs CJ, Dollery CT, Inman WHW, et al. Postmarketing surveillance of enalapril II: investigation of the potential role of enalapril in deaths with renal failure. Br Med J. 1988;297:830–832

Stambe C, Atkins RC, Hill PA, Nikolic-Paterson DJ. Activation and cellular localization of the p38 and JNK MAPK pathways in rat crescentic glomerulonephritis. Kidney Int 2003;64(6):2121-32.

Stambe C, Atkins RC, Tesch GH, Kapoun AM, Hill PA, Schreiner GF, et al. Blockade of p38alpha MAPK ameliorates acute inflammatory renal injury in rat anti-GBM glomerulonephritis. J Am Soc Nephrol 2003;14(2):338-51.

Suzuki H, Uchida K, Nitta K, Nihei H. Role of mitogen-activated protein kinase in the regulation of transforming growth factor-beta-induced fibronectin accumulation in cultured renal interstitial fibroblasts. Clin Exp Nephrol 2004;8(3):188-95.

Swartbol P, Thorvinger BO, Parsson H, et al. Renal Artery Stenosis in patients with peripheral vascular disease and its correlation to hypertension. A retrospective study. Int Angiol 1992; 11:195-199.

Tamaki K, Okuda S, Ando T, Iwamoto T, Nakayama M, Fujishima M. TGF-β1 in glomerulosclerosis and interstitial fibrosis of adriamycin nephropathy. Kidney Int 1994;45:525-536.

Textor SC, Novick AC, Steinmuller DR, Streem SB. Renal failure limiting antihypertensive therapy as an indication for renal revascularization. Arch Int Med. 1983;143:2208–2211

Textor SC, Wilcox CS. Renal artery stenosis: a common, treatable cause of renal failure? Annu Rev Med 2001;52:421-42.

Textor SC. Ischemic nephropathy: where are we now? J Am Soc Nephrol 2004;15(8):1974-82.

Textor SC. Managing renal arterial disease and hypertension. Curr Opin Cardiol 2003;18(4):260-7.

Textor SC. Progressive hypertension in a patient with "incidental" renal artery stenosis. Hypertension 2002;40(5):595-600.

Textor SC. Stable patients with atherosclerotic renal artery stenosis should be treated first with medical management. Am J Kidney Dis 2003;42(5):858-63.

Textor S, Lehrman L, and McKusick M. The Uncertain Value of Renal Artery Interventions: Where Are We Now? J. Am. Coll. Cardiol. Intv. 2009;2;175-182

Toyoda M, Suzuki D, Honma M, Uehara G, Sakai T, Umezono T, et al. High expression of PKC-MAPK pathway mRNAs correlates with glomerular lesions in human diabetic nephropathy. Kidney Int 2004;66(3):1107-14.

Tsuzuki S, Matoba T, Eguchi s, aalnagami T. A-II type 2 receptor inhibits cell proliferation and activates tyrosine phosphatase. Hypertension. 1996;28:916-918

Valabhji J, Robinson S, Poulter C, Robinson AC, Kong C, Henzen C, et al. Prevalence of renal artery stenosis in subjects with type 2 diabetes and coexistent hypertension. Diabetes Care 2000;23(4):539-43.

Wada T, Furuichi K, Sakai N, Hisada Y, Kobayashi K, Mukaida N, et al. Involvement of p38 mitogen-activated protein kinase followed by chemokine expression in crescentic glomerulonephritis. Am J Kidney Dis 2001;38(6):1169-77.

Weber-Mzell D, Kotanko P, Schumacher M, Klein W, Skrabal F. Coronary anatomy predicts presence or absence of renal artery stenosis. A prospective study in patients undergoing cardiac catheterization for suspected coronary artery disease. Eur Heart J 2002;23(21):1684-91.

Wenzel UO, Wolf G, Jacob I, Schwegler C, Qasqas A, Amann K, et al. Beneficial and adverse renal and vascular effects of the vasopeptidase inhibitor omapatrilat in renovascular hypertensive rats. Nephrol Dial Transplant 2003;18(10):2005-13.

Wenzel UO, Wolf G, Jacob I, Thaiss F, Helmchen U, Stahl RA. Chronic anti-Thy-1 nephritis is aggravated in the nonclipped but not in the clipped kidney of Goldblatt hypertensive rats. Kidney Int 2002;61(6):2119-31.

Wiesel P, Mazzolai L, Nussberger J, Pedrazzini T. Two-kidney, one clip and one-kidney, one clip hypertension in mice. Hypertension 1997;29(4):1025-30.

Wilson C, Byrom F. Renal changes in malignant hypertension. Lancet 1939;1:136-39.

Wilson C, Byrom F. The vicious circle in chronic Bright's disease: experimental evidence from the hypertensive rat. QJ Med 1940;10:65-96.

Wolf G, Reinking R, Zahner G, Stahl RA, Shankland SJ. Erk 1,2 phosphorylates p27(Kip1): Functional evidence for a role in high glucose-induced hypertrophy of mesangial cells. Diabetologia 2003;46(8):1090-9.

Wolf G. A-II as a mediator of tubulointerstitial injury. Nephrol Dial Transplant. 2000;15:61–63

Wolf, Gunter, Thomas Jocks, Gunther Zahner, Ulf Panzer, and Rolf A. K. Stahl. Existence of a regulatory loop between MCP-1 and TGF- β in glomerular immune injury. Am J Physiol Renal Physiol 283: F1075–F1084, 2002

Wright JR, Duggal A, Thomas R, Reeve R, Roberts IS, Kalra PA. Clinicopathological correlation in biopsy-proven atherosclerotic nephropathy: implications for renal functional outcome in atherosclerotic renovascular disease. Nephrol Dial Transplant 2001;16(4):765-70.

Xia Z, Dickens M, Raingeaud J, Davis RJ, Greenberg ME. Opposing effects of ERK and JNK-p38 MAP kinases on apoptosis. Science 1995;270(5240):1326-1331.

Xie L, Law BK, Chytil AM, Brown KA, Aakre ME, Moses HL. Activation of the Erk pathway is required for TGF-beta1-induced EMT in vitro. Neoplasia 2004;6(5):603-10.

Yang J, Liu Y. Blockage of tubular epithelial to myofibroblast transition by hepatocyte growth factor prevents renal interstitial fibrosis. J Am Soc Nephrol 2002;13(1):96-107.

Yang J, Liu Y. Dissection of key events in tubular epithelial to myofibroblast transition and its implications in renal interstitial fibrosis. Am J Pathol 2001;159(4):1465-75.

Yang M, Huang H, Li J, Li D, Wang H. Tyrosine phosphorylation of the LDL receptor-related protein (LRP) and activation of the ERK pathway are required for connective tissue growth factor to potentiate myofibroblast differentiation. Faseb J 2004;18(15):1920-1.

Yu L, Hebert MC, Zhang YE. TGF-beta receptor-activated p38 MAP kinase mediates Smad-independent TGF-beta responses. Embo J 2002;21(14):3749-59.

Zhu X-Y, Chade AR, Krier J, Daghini E, Lavi R, Guglielmotti A, Lerman A, Lerman LO. The chemokine monocyte chemoattractant protein-1 contributes to renal dysfunction in swine renovascular hypertension. J Hypertens 2009; 27:2063–2073

Zoja C, Corna D, Benedetti G, Morigi M, Donadelli R, Guglielmotti A, et al. Bindarit retards renal disease and prolongs survival in murine lupus autoimmune disease. Kidney Int 1998; 53:726–734

5

Cardiovascular Disease in Inflammatory Disorders – Psoriasis and Psoriatic Arthritis

Aizuri Murad and Anne-Marie Tobin
Department of Dermatology, Adelaide and Meath Hospital and Trinity College Dublin, Ireland

1. Introduction

Psoriasis, a papulosquamous skin disease, was originally thought to be a disorder primarily of epidermal keratinocytes, but is now recognised as one of the commonest immune-mediated disorders. It is a chronic skin disorder that causes areas of thickened, inflamed, red skin, often covered with silvery scales. Worldwide psoriasis prevalence rates range from 0.6 percent to 4.8 percent. Children and adolescents can develop psoriasis, but it occurs primarily in adults. There seem to be two peaks in onset: one between ages 20 and 30 and another between 50 and 60. Women and men are equally affected. The immune system is involved and appears to be overactive in a way that causes inflammation. Specifically, there is excessive production of T-Helper 1 cytokines, particularly TNFα. These have many effects, including growth of extra blood vessels within the skin and increased turnover of the skin cells. Like most diseases, psoriasis is influenced by inherited characteristics. Up to 50% of people with psoriasis will know of another affected family member. Patients with a family history of psoriasis tend to develop psoriasis earlier in life than those without a family history.

It is associated with comorbidities that include metabolic syndrome and increased cardiovascular risk. These conditions share etiologic features and health consequences that directly correlate with the severity of psoriatic disease. Up to thirty percent of patients with psoriasis develop psoriatic arthritis, this is an erosive, seronegative arthritis, which is associated with inflammation of tendon insertion points (enthesitis). An increased risk of cardiovascular disease was first noted in patients with rheumatoid arthritis and it became apparent that chronic inflammation was associated with increased risk of cardiovascular or cerebrovascular disease.

While heart disease remains a quiet killer, psoriasis is a visible disease whose impact on social interaction and quality of life usually prompt earlier physician consultation. Psoriasis patients are at increased risk of being obese and therefore are at greater risk than the general population to develop myocardial infarction, metabolic syndrome and other comorbidities. It has become evident that patients with psoriasis and psoriatic arthritis have an increased incidence of cardiovascular disease and also certain cardiovascular risk factors such as smoking, hypertension and metabolic syndrome compared to the normal population. They also have increased non-conventional risk factors such as raised levels of homocysteine and excessive alcohol consumption.

2. Psoriasis, psoriatic arthritis and cardiovascular disease

An association between psoriasis and cardiovascular risk was first described in 1978. Patients with psoriasis in an outpatient clinic had 2.2 times higher incidence of venous and arterial vascular disease in a clinic-based control study (McDonald & Calabresi, 1978). Gelfand and colleagues published a large cross -sectional study of the UK General Practice Database reporting a higher death rate from cardiovascular disease in those with severe psoriasis compared to the general population (Gelfand et al.,2006). The investigators controlled for diabetes, hyperlipidaemia, hypertension, body mass index, age, sex and smoking and found that psoriasis appeared to confer an independent risk for myocardial infarction. This risk is greater in younger patients (Gelfand et al.,2006). A second group utilising the same data found an increased incidence of risk factors for cardiovascular disease, as well as increased rates of myocardial infarction, angina, stroke and peripheral vascular disease (Henseler & Christophers, 1995). Patients were also found to have an increased risk of cardiovascular mortality that is independent of traditional cardiovascular risk factors (Mehta et al., 2010). More recently, a study has shown that psoriasis conferred an additional 6.2% absolute risk of 10 year major adverse cardiac events after adjusting for age, gender, diabetes, hypertension, tobacco use and hyperlipidaemia (Mehta et al., 2011).

A hospital based study from Sweden, Germany and Finland previously documented increased rates of risk factors such as hypertension, diabetes and obesity in patients with psoriasis. Poikolainen and Mallbris found that patients with severe psoriasis who required hospitalisation for treatment of their psoriasis had increased mortality from cardiovascular disease (Mallbris et al, 2004; Poikolainen et al., 1999). Patients managed as out-patients however did not have excess risk, suggesting that more severe disease was associated with a higher risk of cardiovascular disease. In a Danish nationwide cohort study, psoriasis was shown to be associated with increased risk of adverse cardiovascular events and all cause of mortality especially in young patients with severe disease (Ahlehoff et al., 2011). Furthermore, a separate Danish study showed that psoriasis significantly impaired prognosis in patients after myocardial infarction (Ahlehoff et al., 2011).

An observational study by Prodanovich and colleagues examined the cardiovascular risk factors in psoriasis and found psoriasis to be associated with atherosclerosis and this association applies to coronary artery, cerebrovascular and peripheral vascular diseases (Prodanovich et al., 2009). A cross sectional prevalence-based study from 2 American healthcare databases showed an increase prevalence of cardiovascular diseases and risk factors in patients with psoriasis compared with general population (Kimball et al., 2008). In Israel, Shapiro and colleagues showed a strong association between psoriasis, atherosclerosis, heart failure and diabetes (Shapiro et al., 2007). In addition to large clinical studies, several studies have documented subclinical cardiovascular disease.

A Chinese study showed that young patients with psoriasis have increased arterial stiffness compared with healthy controls. More importantly, CRP positively correlated with, and independently predicted, arterial stiffness. This suggests that systemic inflammation in patients with psoriasis is associated with premature atherosclerosis (Yiu et al., 2011). In another Asian study, Mazlan and colleagues also showed that there was a significant association between cardiovascular risk and intima-media thickness in psoriatic arthritis patients. However, it was not associated with disease activity, disease severity and DMARDS therapy (Mazlan et al., 2009). Karadag and colleagues demonstrated a significant endothelial dysfunction and increased insulin resistance in patients with psoriasis (Karadag et al., 2010). In a separate Turkish study, aortic elasticity in patients with psoriasis was found to be significantly lower than the control group. In psoriatic patients without cardiac involvement, aortic elasticity was decreased and this decrease was correlated with the duration and severity of the disease (Bicer et al., 2009). A study by El-Mongey and colleague showed an increase in carotid artery intima-media thickness in patients with chronic psoriasis suggesting that chronic psoriasis is associated with subclinical atherosclerosis with increased risk of cardiovascular disease (El-Mongy et al., 2010). Patients with psoriatic arthritis also had a higher prevalence of subclinical atherosclerosis as measured by intima-media wall thickness (Eder et al., 2008; Kimhi et al., 2007) and endothelial dysfunction even without any overt cardiovascular disease (Gonzalez-Juanatey et al., 2007). More recently, subclinical left ventricular dysfunction has also been shown in psoriatic arthritis patients who had no established cardiovascular disease or risk factors (Shang et al., 2011). Risk factors for cardiovascular disease as well as other vascular diseases were shown by Kaye and colleagues to occur with higher incidence in patients with psoriasis than in the general population (Kaye et al., 2008). The study by Jamnitski and colleague showed the prevelance of cardiovascular diseases in psoriatic arthritis resembles that of rheumatoid arthritis (Jamnitski et al., 2011).

There are several theories to explain the association between psoriasis and increased cardiovascular risk. Both psoriasis and atherosclerosis involve Th-1 lymphocytes and cytokines and it is suggested that the excess inflammatory cells and mediators produced in psoriasis may contribute to the development of atherosclerotic plaques. A recent case-control study in 2011 on inpatients with psoriasis and dermatitis by Shapiro and colleagues supports previous reports of an association between psoriasis and CVD risk factors, suggesting that the inflammatory process in psoriasis, but not in dermatitis which is a T helper-2 mediated condition is involved in athersclerosis (Shapiro et al., 2011). Subsequently, Armstrong and colleagues have investigated the different inflammatory pathways which are common in psoriasis and atherosclerosis. They have found that psoriasis and atherosclerosis are diseases in which effector T lymphocytes such as Helper T cells type 1 (Th1) and 17 (Th17) play integral roles in disease pathogenesis and progression. Regulatory T cells (Treg) also exert clinically important anti-inflammatory effects that are pathologically altered in psoriasis and atherosclerosis. These shared pathways provide the basis for mechanisms that may explain the epidemiologic observation that patients with psoriasis have an increased risk of heart disease (Armstrong et al., 2011).

In patients with psoriatic arthritis, it was shown recently that better control of inflammation with TNF-alpha blockers may inhibit the cascade that causes raised vascular risks in this cohort of patients. They were found to have thinner carotid intima-media thickness compared to those who were treated with DMARDs (Di Minno et al., 2011). With these findings, it is possible that control of chronic inflammation in these patients may have a significant role in preventing vasculopathy. Apart from this, screening and modification other cardiovascular risk factors in these patients should form part of their assessment.

Cardiovascular risk factors found with increased frequency in patients with psoriasis include conventional cardiovascular risk factors such as obesity, diabetes mellitus, hypertension, dyslipidaemia and smoking. Oxidative stress, endothelial cell dysfunction, abnormal platelet adhesion and hyperhomocysteinemia which may also increase cardiovascular risk have all been reported to occur with greater prevalence in psoriasis.

3. Conventional risk factors in psoriasis

3.1 Smoking and psoriasis

Smoking and psoriasis have been associated by several studies and from the disease perspective, it appeared to have an adverse effect with treatment response and patients in this cohort seem to have more severe disease. There is an increased rate of smoking in patients with psoriasis compared to controls (Christophers, 2001; Griffiths & Barker, 2007; McDonald & Calabresi, 1978; Stern et al., 2004; Veale & Fitzgerald, 2002). Poikolainen and colleagues found that smoking is a risk factor for psoriasis in women. Negative life events and smoking were more common among psoriasis patients than among controls (Poikolainen et al., 2004). Furthermore, the risk for psoriasis was higher in ex-smokers and current smokers compared to individuals who had never smoked (Mills et al., 1992; Naldi et al., 1999,2005; Poikolainen et al., 2004; Williams, 1994).

Behnam and colleagues found that women who are smokers have an up to 3.3-fold increased risk of developing plaque-type psoriasis. Men who are smokers do not exhibit such an increased risk, but studies have shown that smoking more than 10 cigarettes per day by men who are psoriasis patients may be associated with a more severe expression of disease in their extremities. In addition, smoking among both men and women who are psoriasis patients has been shown to reduce improvement rates (Behnam et al., 2005). Smoking also adversely affects the natural history of psoriasis in both genders especially in those who smoked more than 20 cigarettes a day. An Italian hospital-based cross-sectional study by Fortes and colleagues showed high intensity of smoking (>20 cigarettes daily) vs a lower level of consumption (< or =10 cigarettes daily) was associated with a more than 2-fold increased risk of clinically more severe. Separate analyses for men and women showed that the effect of cigarette-years was stronger for women (Fortes et al., 2005). Therefore, patients with psoriasis who smoke tend to have a less favourable outcome and disease that is more difficult to control.

Some researchers have found that heavier smokers have a greater risk of developing psoriasis and this only falls back to normal 20 years after quitting. There are good reasons for these patients to cease smoking to improve their psoriasis and more importantly, for their general health (Behnam et al., 2005; Fortes et al., 2005; Setty et al., 2007).

3.2 Hypertension and psoriasis

The association between elevated blood pressure and psoriasis was first described in 1977 and further studies showed an increased prevalence of essential hypertension in patients with psoriasis (Gisondi et al., 2007). In these patients, their hypertension is likely to be more severe and requires more medication to control it.

Enhanced activity of the renin-angiotensin system (Cohen et al., 2008) and increased levels of endothelin-1 released from vascular endothelium (Binazzi et al., 1975) were factors that contribute to the increased incidence of hypertension in patients with psoriasis. More recently, a hospital-based case-controlled study by Armesto and colleague evaluated the prevalence of hypertension in psoriasis based on a sample of Spanish population. The prevalence of hypertension was significantly higher in psoriasis patients than controls (Armesto et al., 2011). Armstrong and colleague showed that compared to hypertensive patients without psoriasis, psoriasis patients with hypertension were 5 times more likely to be on a monotherapy antihypertensive regimen, 9.5 times more likely to be on dual antihypertensive therapy, 16.5 times more likely to be on triple antihypertensive regimen, and 19.9 times more likely to be on quadruple therapy or centrally-acting agent (Armstrong et al., 2011).

3.3 Dyslipidaemia and psoriasis

Several mechanisms including unhealthy lifestyle, activation of T Helper-1 lymphocytes and autoantibodies recognizing oxidized low-density lipoprotein may induce dyslipidaemia in psoriatic patients. Moreover, the levels of antibodies against oxidized low-density lipoprotein correlate with the disease activity. A large study on lipid profile at the onset of psoriasis showed significantly higher very low-density lipoprotein and high density lipoprotein fractions (Mallbris et al., 2006). This study was controlled for gender, blood pressure, BMI, physical activity, smoking and alcohol consumption. Later, a large cross-sectional study using a population-based database by Dreiher and colleagues found that psoriatic patients had higher triglyceride and lower high-density lipoprotein cholesterol levels compared to control (Dreiher et al., 2008).

In a separate study, children with psoriasis were found to have elevated total plasma cholesterol and HDL cholesterol and a decrease in the ratio of HDL to LDL cholesterol (Ferretti et al.,1993,1994). Dyslipidaemia observed in patients with psoriasis is compounded by increased oxidative stress and decreased anti-oxidant capacity. Autoantibodies recognizing oxidized LDL have been found in psoriasis, with their levels correlating with disease activity as measured by PASI (Offidani et al., 1994).

More recently, it has been suggested that statin therapy may have beneficial effects by downregulating lymphocyte function-associated antigen-1, inhibiting leukocyte endothelial adhesion, extravasation and natural killer cell activity, all of which are key to the development of psoriasis lesions. They also reduce levels of proinflammatory cytokines such as tumour necrosis factor-alpha, interleukin 1 and 6, lowering C-reactive protein promote T (H) 1 cytokine receptors on T cell, leading to inhibition of activation of lymphocytes and infiltration into inflammatory sites.

Overall, statin therapy for associated dyslipidaemia in patients with psoriasis has shown clinical improvement due to its immunomodulatory and anti-inflammatory effects (Ghazizadeh et al., 2011).

3.4 Diabetes mellitus and psoriasis

The association between psoriasis and hyperglycaemia was documented as early as 1967 (Lynch, 1967). Since then, numerous studies have confirmed the association between psoriasis, hyperglycaemia and relative insulin resistance (Fratino et al., 1979; Neimann et al., 2006; Pelfini et al., 1979; Reynoso-von Drateln et al., 2003; Sommer et al., 2006). A cross-sectional study by Ucak and colleagues found that psoriatic patients were more insulin resistant than healthy subjects and type II psoriatics(late onset) were more susceptible than type I psoriatics(onset before 35 years of age) to develop impaired glucose tolerance (Ucak et al., 2006). Qureshi and colleagues found that women with psoriasis were 63% more likely to develop diabetes and around 17% more likely to develop hypertension, than women without psoriasis (Qureshi et al., 2009). Genetic analysis of two non-major histocompatibility complex (MHC) in patients with psoriasis found the strongest phenotypic marker for a loci mapping to chromosome 6p22. This marker maps to CDKAL1, a gene associated to type 2 diabetes, suggesting a possible role for pleiotropic susceptibility loci for both conditions (Wol et al., 2008).

Boehncke and colleagues found a significant correlation between the Psoriasis Area and Severity Index (PASI) score and insulin secretion. The PASI score was significantly correlated with serum resistin levels, a cytokine known to be increased in insulin resistance (Boehncke et al., 2007). Patients with psoriasis demonstrate hyperinsulinaemia which correlates with disease severity (Boehncke et al., 2007;Ucak et al., 2006) and increased levels of insulin results in excessive levels if insulin-like growth factors (IGF) which appear to have a role in epidermal hyperproliferation in psoriasis (Hodak et al., 1996; Wraight et al., 2000; Xu et al, 1996). Induction of interleukin-6 and vascular endothelial growth factor has been postulated as underpinning IGF's role in the development of psoriatic plaques (Kwon et al., 2000, 2004).

More recently, a cohort analysis by Solomon and colleagues on patients with psoriasis showed a reduced risk of diabetes mellitus (DM) with the use of a tumor necrosis factor α (TNF-α)inhibitor or hydroxychloroquine, but not with methotrexate, compared with other nonbiologic disease-modifying antirheumatic drugs (DMARDs). Evidence suggests a possible role for DMARDs and immunosuppression in DM prevention (*Solomon* et al., 2011) along with adopting a healthy lifestyle, regular physical activity and good nutrition.

3.5 Obesity and metabolic syndrome in psoriasis.

In a case control study, we found that patients with psoriasis had higher Body Mass Index (BMI) compared to controls (Tobin et al., 2011). Individuals with psoriasis were more likely than controls to be obese. An increased adiposity and weight gain were strong risk factors for the development of psoriasis. A case-controlled study by Chen and colleagues found high levels of leptin more often in females, the obese and those with high blood pressure, metabolic syndrome and psoriasis. Hyperleptinemia in psoriasis is associated with higher risk of developing metabolic syndrome, which may be defined as the concurrence of hypertension, dyslipidaemia, diabetes and central adiposity. This finding links the chronic inflammation of psoriasis with metabolic disturbances. The high circulating leptin levels in individuals with psoriasis may derive not only from fat tissue but also from inflammation (Chen et al., 2008). Body weight loss has been reported to significantly decrease leptin levels and improve insulin sensitivity and may reduce the likelihood of developing metabolic syndrome and adverse cardiovascular diseases. Psoriasis and obesity are linked through a common pathophysiological mechanism of chronic low grade inflammation. Not only is obesity associated with a higher incidence of psoriasis and greater severity, it also affects response to treatment. Weight loss could potentially become part of the general treatment of psoriasis, especially in patients with obesity.

Furthermore, when age, smoking and alcohol intake were all controlled for, there was a strong association between BMI and psoriasis (Setty et al., 2007).

Metabolic syndrome has been reported to be strongly associated with psoriasis. A hospital-based case-control study by Gisondi and colleagues showed a higher prevalence of metabolic syndrome in patients with psoriasis. These patients were found to be older and had longer disease duration compared with those without metabolic syndrome. However, there was no correlation between disease severity and prevalence of this syndrome (Gisondi et al., 2007). Another case-control study by Cohen and colleagues showed metabolic syndrome was more common in male psoriatic patients who are above 50 years of age (Cohen et al., 2008). Management of these patients should also target these metabolic conditions associated with psoriasis which are significant predictors of a cardiovascular event. Therefore, healthy diet and lifestyle should be emphasized.

4. Conventional risk factors in psoriatic arthritis

There is less research on cardiovascular disease and risk factors in psoriatic arthritis compared to psoriasis but it has been shown that patients with psoriatic arthritis have an increased prevalence of cardiovascular risk factors, type 2 diabetes, hyperlipidaemia and hypertension.

A slightly different pattern of dyslipidaemia was found in these patients. They had higher HDL cholesterol and apolipoprotein A1 levels, lower total cholesterol and low density lipoprotein cholesterol levels and lower total cholesterol to HDL cholesterol ratio (Tam et al., 2008). Older studies have shown that psoriatic arthritis patients with synovitis had lower total cholesterol, low density lipoprotein (LDL) and high density lipoprotein (HDL) (Lazarevic et al., 1992; Skoczynska et al., 2003).

Individual components of metabolic syndrome such as hypertension, obesity, insulin resistance and dyslipidaemia (Jones et al., 2000; Tam et al., 2008) have been reported in psoriatic arthritis patients but the full spectrum of metabolic syndrome has not been studied in these patients.

5. Non-conventional risk factors in psoriasis and psoriatic arthritis

5.1 Inflammation

Chronic inflammation is known to play a role in the development of atherosclerosis involving the innate immune system and T helper-1 lymphocytes (Hansson et al., 2002, 2006). This is similar to the pattern of immune mediated inflammation seen in psoriasis and with chronic low grade circulating inflammatory cells and cytokines which invoke endothelial inflammation, could ultimately lead to plaque formation (Wakkee et al., 2007). The increase prevalence of obesity in psoriasis and psoriatic arthritis may also increase the burden of inflammation (Hammings et al., 2006).

C - reactive protein is a moderate predictor for cardiovascular disease (Danesh et al., 2004) and a marker that correlates well with joint inflammation. However, a large Italian study showed that it is more valuable in severe joint disease (Cervini et al., 2005). In another study, raised plasma fibrinogen levels are shown to be associated with an increased risk of vascular events. This may be mediated by adverse effects of fibrinogen on plasma viscosity, coagulation, platelet activity, inflammation and atherogenesis (Dziedzic, 2008; Kakfika et al., 2007). It is also known to be elevated in psoriasis and psoriatic arthritis (Marongiu et al.,

1994; Rocha - Pereira et al., 2004; Vanizor Kural et al., 2003). This would indicate chronic inflammation and a possible role in increasing cardiovascular risk.

5.2 Endothelial dysfunction

Patients with psoriasis were found to have increased calcification in their coronary arteries compared to controls. Ludwig and colleagues found a significantly increased prevalence and severity of coronary artery calcification in patients with psoriasis and is likely to be an independent risk factor (Ludwig et al., 2007). Chronic inflammation causes endothelial dysfunction which leads to formation of atherosclerotic plaques in association with raised plasma lipids. Increased levels of oxidized low density lipoprotein in psoriatic plaques have been reported compared to controls (Rocha - Pereira et al., 2004; Vanizor Kural et al., 2003). Oxidized low-density lipoprotein is thought to promote atherosclerosis through complex inflammatory and immunologic mechanisms that lead to lipid dysregulation and foam cell formation. Recent findings suggested that oxidized LDL forms complexes with beta2-glycoprotein I (beta2GPI) and/or C-reactive protein (CRP) in the intima of atherosclerotic lesions. Oxidative stress has a critical role in causing damage to endothelial cells (Matsuura et al., 2006).

5.3 Fibronectin and platelets: Atherothrombotic markers

Atherothrombosis results in myocardial infarction, stroke and peripheral vascular disease. Low levels of fibronectin have been suggested as a marker of atherothrombosis and this has been shown in patients with psoriasis with active disease and in remission (De Pita et al., 1996). Increased platelet aggregation has also been found in these patients compared to controls. Hayashi and colleagues found platelet aggregation was significantly increased in psoriatics compared with normal controls. An additive effect was observed when diabetes was associated with psoriasis, with platelet aggregation being further increased by ADP. The increased platelet aggregation with ADP and epinephrine was significantly reduced when the skin lesions had cleared (Hayashi et al., 1985).

5.4 Homocysteine

Homocysteine causes endothelial dysfunction and is an independent risk factor for development of cardiovascular disease (Graham et al., 1997). In a case controlled study we showed that psoriatic patients have a relative risk 7.1 times greater than controls of having significantly raised levels of homocysteine (Tobin et al., 2011). This was also found in 2 uncontrolled studies and one in the context of patients who are taking methotrexate (Vanizor Kural et al., 2003). Refsum and colleagues investigated the effect of low-dose methotrexate on plasma homocysteine in patients who had psoriasis. Psoriasis patients had significantly higher basal plasma homocysteine levels (Refsum et al., 1989). High levels of homocysteine have been documented in small number of patients with psoriatic arthritis (Segal et al., 2004).

5.5 Increased alcohol consumption

Excessive alcohol consumption has been widely documented in patient with psoriasis (Higgins, 2000) and some researchers believe that drinking large amounts of alcohol predisposes to psoriasis (Segal et al., 2004). There is a high prevalence of psoriasis in patients with alcoholic liver disease (Tobin et al., 2009). Patients undergoing phototherapy for psoriasis also had an increased prevalence of excessive alcohol intake (Kirby et al., 2011). Treatment outcome is adversely affected in patients who consume excess alcohol (Gupta et al., 1993).

Overall, alcohol misuse is common in patients with moderate to severe psoriasis. Proper screening allows identification of these patients who would benefit from appropriate intervention. There are limited studies about alcohol consumption in patients with psoriatic arthritis.

Sporadic heavy drinking (binge drinking) increases the risk of developing coronary heart disease, the most common form of heart disease. Men nearly double their chances of developing coronary heart disease by drinking more than eight units of alcohol a day. Women have a 1.3 times greater risk of developing coronary heart disease when they drink more than six units a day. Women who persistently drink more than three units of alcohol a day and men, who drink more than four, are more likely to suffer from the risk factors associated with cardiovascular disorders such as high blood pressure. Alcohol can increase levels of homocysteine. High homocysteine levels increase the risk of thrombosis. Long-term drinking and heavy alcohol consumption is linked with weakness of the heart muscle, known as cardiomyopathy.

There is evidence to suggest that a regular pattern of drinking relatively small amounts of alcohol (one or two drinks a few times a week) reduces the risk of heart disease in men over the age of 40 and post-menopausal women. Therefore, excess amount of alcohol appear to be harmful whereas small amounts seem to be cardioprotective.

6. Does treatment of inflammation ameliorate cardiovascular risk?

Much has been said about the effects of chronic inflammation on cardiovascular risk factors and cardiac events. Researchers have tried to investigate if systemic therapy may improve cardiac biomarkers in patients with severe psoriasis. A German study by Boehncke and colleagues investigated the effects of continuous systemic therapy on the cardiovascular risk of patients with severe psoriasis. There was a trend towards reduced serum levels of vascular endothelial growth factor (VEGF) and resistin, while the potentially cardio-protective adiponectin showed a trend toward increased serum levels under therapy. This was parallel to improvement in C-reactive protein, PASI and insulin responsiveness (Boehncke et al., 2011). The impact on the metabolic state was found to be better if the psoriatic inflammation was controlled for longer (Boehncke et al., 2011). However, Abuabara and colleagues investigated on the effect of systemic treatment on the incidence of myocardial infarction in a control group treated with UVB therapy that has limited systemic anti-inflammatory effects. The risk of developing myocardial infarction in patients with severe psoriasis receiving systemic therapy was not reduced compared to a group undergoing phototherapy (Abuabara et al., 2011).

7. Conclusion

The increased cardiovascular risks in patients with psoriasis and psoriatic arthritis may be due to higher prevalence of multiple risk factors in these patient cohorts. It is very unlikely that all patients with psoriasis and psoriatic arthritis have increased cardiovascular risks. However, steps should be taken to identify those who are at risk early for intervention. With the evidence indicating a higher incidence of metabolic syndrome and cardiovascular disease, it is important for physicians to identify at risk patients and initiate an interdisciplinary approach for the screening and management of their co - morbidities.

8. References

Abuabara K, Lee H & Kimball AB. (2011) The Effect of Systemic Psoriasis Therapies on the Incidence of Myocardial Infarction: A Cohort Study. Br J Dermatol. July 20. doi: 10.1111/j.1365-2133.2011.10525.x.

Ahlehoff O, Gislason GH, Charlot M, Jørgensen CH, Lindhardsen J, Olesen JB, Abildstrøm SZ, Skov L, Torp- Pedersen C & Hansen PR. (2011) Psoriasis is associated with clinically significant cardiovascular risk: a Danish nationwide cohort study. J Intern Med. August; 270(2):147-57.

Ahlehoff, Gislason GH, Lindhardsen J, Olesen JB, Charlot M, Skov L, Torp-Pedersen C & Hansen PR (2011) Prognosis following first-time myocardial infarction in patients with psoriasis: a Danish nationwide cohort study. J Intern Med. September; 270(3):237-44.

Armesto S, Coto-Segura P, Osuna CG, Camblor PM, Santos-Juanes J. (2011) Psoriasis and hypertension: a case- control study. J Eur Acad Dermatol Venereol. May. doi: 10.1111/j.1468-3083.2011.04108.x

Armstrong AW, Voyles SV, Armstrong EJ, Fuller EN & Rutledge JC. (2011) A tale of two plaques: convergent mechanisms of T-cell-mediated inflammation in psoriasis and atherosclerosis. Exp Derm. July; 20(7):544-9.

Armstrong AW, Lin SW, Chambers CJ, Sockolov ME & Chin DL. (2011) Psoriasis and hypertension severity: results from a case-control study. PLoS One. March 29;6(3):

Behnam SM, Behnam SE & Koo JY. (2005) Smoking and psoriasis. Skinmed. May-June;4(3):174-6

Bicer A, Acikel S, Kilic H, Ulukaradag Z, Karasu BB, Cemil BC, Dogan M, Baser K, Cagirci G, Eskioglu F & Akdemir R. (2009) Impaired aortic elasticity in patients with psoriasis. Acta Cardiol. October; 64(5):597-602.

Binazzi M, Calandra P, Lisi P. (1975) Statistical association between psoriasis and diabetes: further results. Arch Dermatol Res. November; 254(1): 43-8

Boehncke S, Thaci D, Beschmann H, Ludwig RJ, Ackermann H, Badenhoop K, Boehncke WH. (2007) Psoriasis patients show signs of insulin resistance. Br J Dermatol. December; 157(6): 1249-51

Boehncke S, Fichtlscherer S, Salgo R, Garbaraviciene J, Beschmann H, Diehl S, Hardt K, Thaçi D & Boehncke WH. (2011) Systemic therapy of plaque-type psoriasis ameliorates endothelial cell function: results of a prospective longitudinal pilot trial. Arch Dermatol Res. August; 303(6):381-8.

Boehncke S, Salgo R, Garbaraviciene J, Beschmann H, Hardt K, Diehl S, Fichtlscherer S, Thaçi D & Boehncke WH. (2011) Effective continuous systemic therapy of severe plaque-type psoriasis is accompanied by amelioration of Biomarkers of cardiovascular risk: results of a prospective longitudinal observational study. J Eur Acad Dermatol Venereol. January. doi: 10.1111/j.1468-3083.2010.03947.x

Cervini C, Leardini G, Mathieu A, Punzi L & Scarpa R. (2005) Psoriatic arthritis: epidemiological and clinical aspects in a cohort of 1,306 Italian patients. Reumatismo. December; 57(4): 283-90.

Christophers E. (2001) Psoriasis - epidemiology and clinical spectrum. Clin Exper Dermatol. June; 26(4): 314-320

Chen YJ, Wu CY, Shen JL, Chu SY, Chen CK, Chang YT & Chen CM. (2008)Psoriasis independently associated with hyperleptinemia contributing to Metabolic Syndrome Arch Dermatol. December; 144(12):1571-1575

Cohen AD, Sherf M, Vidavsky L, Vardy DA, Shapiro J & Meyerovitch J. (2008) Association between psoriasis and the metabolic syndrome. A cross-sectional study. Dermatology. January; 216(2): 152-2

Danesh J, Wheleler JG, Hirschfield GM, Eda S, Eiriksdottir G, Rumley A, Lowe GD, Pepys MB & Gudnason V.(2004) C-reactive protein and other circulating markers of inflammation in the prediction of coronary artery disease. N Engl J Med. April; 350(14): 1387-97.

De Pita O, Ruffelli M, Cadoni S, Frezzolini A, Biava GF, Simom R, Bottari V, De Sanctis G. (1996) Psoriasis: comparison of immunological markers in patients with acute and remission phase. J Dermatol. Sci. November; 13(2): 118-24

Di Minno MN, Iervolino S, Peluso R, Scarpa R & Di Minno G. (2011) Carotid intima-media thickness in psoriatic arthritis: differences between tumor necrosis factor-α blockers and traditional disease- modifying antirheumatic drugs. Arterioscler Thromb Vasc Biol. March; 31(3):705-12.

Dreiher J, Weitzman D, Davidovici B, Shapiro J & Cohen AD. (2008) Psoriasis and dyslipidaemia: a population-based study. Acta Derm Venereol. 88(6):561-5.

Dziedzic T. (2008) Clinical significance of acute phase reaction in stroke patients. Front Bisoci. January; 13: 2922-7.

Eder L, Zisman D, Barzilai M, Laor A, Rahat M, Rozenbaum M, Bitterman H, Feld J, Rimar D & Rosner I. (2008) Subclinical atherosclerosis in psoriatic arthritis: a case-control study. J Rheumatol. May; 35(5): 877-82.

El-Mongy S, Fathy H, Abdelaziz A, Omran E, George S, Neseem N & El-Nour N. (2010) Subclinical atherosclerosis in patients with chronic psoriasis: a potential association. J Eur Acad Dermatol Venereol. June; 24(6):661-6.

Ferretti G, Simonett O, Oftidani AM, Messini L, Cinti B, Marshiseppe I, Bossi G & Curatola G. (1993) Changes of plasma lipids and erythrocyte membrane fluidity in psoriatic children. Pediatr Res. May; 33(5): 506-9.

Ferretti G, Alleva R, Taus M, Simonette O, Cinti B, Oftidani AM, Bossi G & Curatola G. (1994) Abnormalities of plasma lipoprotein composition and fluidity in psoriasis. Acta Derm Venerol. May; 74(3): 171-5.

Fortes C, Mastroeni S, Leffondre K, Sampogna F, Melchi F, Mazzotti E, Pasquini P & Abeni D. (2005) Relationship between smoking and the clinical severity of psoriasis. Arch Dermatol. December; 141(12):1580-4;

Fratino P, Pelfine C, Jucci A & Bellazi R. (1979) Glucose and insulin in psoriasis: the role of obesity and diabetic genetic history. Panminerva Med. 21: 167-72.

Gelfand, Neimann AL, Shin DB, Wang X, Margolis DJ & Troxel AB. (2006) Risk of myocardial infarction in patients with psoriasis. JAMA October; 296(14): 1735-41

Ghazizadeh R, Tosa M & Ghazizadeh M. (2011) Clinical improvement in psoriasis with treatment of associated hyperlipidemia. Am J Med Sci. May; 341(5):394-8

Gisondi P, Tessari G, Conti A, Piaserico S, Schianchi S, Peserico A, Giannetti A & Girolomoni G. (2007) Prevalence of metabolic syndrome in patients with psoriasis: a hospital-based case-control study. Br J Dermatol. July;157(1):68-73

Gonzalez-Juanatey C, Llorca J, Miranda-Filloy JA, Amigo-Diaz E, Testa A, Garcia-Porrua C, Martin J & Gonzalez-Gay MA. (2007). Endothelial dysfunction in psoriatic arthritis patients without clinically evident cardiovascular disease or classis atherosclerosis risk factors. Arthritis Rheum. March; 57(2): 287-93.

Graham IM, Daly LE, Refsum Hm, Robinson K, Brattström LE, Ueland PM, Palma-Reis RJ, Boers GH, Sheahan RG, Israelsson B, Uiterwaal CS, Meleady R, McMaster D, Verhoef P, Witteman J, Rubba P, Bellet H, Wautrecht JC, de Valk HW, Sales Lúis AC, Parrot-Rouland FM, Tan KS, Higgins I, Garcon D, Andria G, et al. (1997)Plasma homocysteine as a risk factor for vascular disease: The European Concerted Action Project. JAMA June; 277(22): 1775-81.

Griffiths CE & BarkerJN. (2007) Pathogenesis and clinical features of Psoriasis. Lancet July; 370(9583): 263-71

Gupta MA, Schork NJ, Gupta AK & Ellis CN. (1993)Alcohol intake and treatment responsiveness of psoriasis: a prospective study. J Am Acad Dermatol. May; 28(5 Pt 1):730-2.

Hammings EA, van der Lely AJ, Neumann HA & Thio HB. (2006) Chronic inflammation in psoriasis and obesity: implications for therapy. Med Hypotheses June; 67(4): 768-773.

Hansson GK, Libby P, Schonbeck U & Yan ZQ. (2002) Innate and adaptive immunity in the pathogenesis of atherosclerosis. Circ Res. August; 91(4): 281-9.

Hansson GK & Libby P. (2006) The immune response in atherosclerosis: a double-edged sword. Nat Rev Immunol. July; 6(7): 508-19.

Hayashi S, Shimizu I, Miyauchi H & Watanabe S. (1985) Increased platelet aggregation in psoriasis. Acta Derm Venereol. 65(3): 258-62

Henseler & Christophers. (1995) Disease concomitance in psoriasis.J Am Acad Dermatol. June; 32(6): 982-6.

Higgins E. (2000) Alcohol, smoking and psoriasis. Clin Exp Dermatol. March; 25(2): 10.

Hodak E, Gottlieb AB, Anzilotti M & Krueger JG. (1996) The insulin-like growth factor 1 receptors is expressed by epithelial cells with proliferative potential in human epidermis and skin appendages: correlation of increased expression with epidermal hyperplasia. J Invest Derm. March; 106(3): 564-70

Jamnitski A, Visman IM, Peters MJ, Boers M, Dijkmans BA & Nurmohamed MT. (2011) Prevalence of cardiovascular diseases in psoriatic arthritis resembles that of rheumatoid arthritis. Ann Rheum Dis. May; 70(5):875-6

Jones SM, Harris CP, Lloyd J, Stirling CA, Reckless JP & McHugh NJ. (2000) Lipoproteins and their subfractions In psoriatic arthritis: identification of an atherogenic profile with active joint disease. Ann Rheum Dis. November; 59(11): 904-9.

Kakafika, Liberopoulos EN & Mikhailidis DP. (2007) Fibrinogen: a predictor of vascular disease. Curr Pharm Des. 13(16): 1647-59

Karadag AS, Yavuz B, Ertugrul DT, Akin KO, Yalcin AA, Deveci OS, Ata N, Kucukazman M & Dal K. (2010) Is psoriasis a pre-atherosclerotic disease? Increased insulin

resistance and impaired endothelial function in patients with psoriasis. Int J Dermatol. June; 49(6):642-6.
Kaye JA, Li L & Jick SS. (2008) Incidence of risk factors for myocardial infarction and other vascular diseases in patients with psoriasis. Br J Dermatol. September; 159(4):895-902.
Kimball AB, Robinson D Jr, Wu Y, Guzzo C, Yeilding N, Paramore C, Fraeman K & Bala M. (2008) Cardiovascular disease and risk factors among psoriasis patients in two US healthcare databases, 2001-2002. Dermatology. March; 217(1):27-37.
Kimhi O, Caspi D, Bornstein NM, Maharshak N, Gur A, Arbel Y, Comaneshter D, Paran D, Wigler I, Levartovsky, Berliner S & Elkayam O. (2007) Prevalence and risk factors of atherosclerosis in patients with psoriatic arthritis. Semin Arthritis Rheum. February; 36(4): 203-9.
Kirby B, Dudley J, Tobin AM et al. Psychological distress but not alcohol intake affects the time to clearance of psoriasis patients treated with narrow-band UVB. In press Clin Exp Derm
Kwon YW, Jang ER, Lee YM, Kim YS, Kwon KS, Jang HS, Oh CK & Kim KW. (2000) Insulin-like growth factor II induces interleukin-6 expression via NF kappa B activation in psoriasis. Biochem Biophys Res Commun. November; 278(2): 312-7.
Kwon YW, Kwon KS, Moon HE, Park JA, Choi KS, Kim YS, Jang HS, Oh CK, Lee YM, Kwon YG, Lee YS, Kim KW. (2004) Insulin-like growth factor -II regulates the expression of vascular endothelial growth factor by the human keratinocye cell line HaCaT. J Invest Dermatol. July; 123(1): 152-8
Lazarevic MB, Vitic J, Mladenovic V. Moynes BL, Skosey JL & Swedler WI. (1992) Dyslipoproteinemia in the course of active rheumatoid arthritis. Semin Arthritis Rheum. December; 22(3): 172-8.
Ludwig RJ, Herzog C, Rostock A, Ochsendorf FR, Zollner TM, Thaci D, Kaufmann R, Vogl TJ & Boehncke WH. (2007) Psoriasis: a possible risk factor for development of coronary artery calcification. Br J Dermatol. February; 156(2): 271-276.
Lynch PJ. (1967) Psoriasis and blood sugar levels. Arch Dermatol. March; 95(3): 255-8.
Mallbris, Akre O, Granath F, Yin L, Lindelöf B, Ekbom A & Ståhle-Bäckdahl M. (2004) Increased risk for cardiovascular mortality in psoriasis inpatients but not in outpatients. Eur J Epidemiol March; 19(3): 225-30.
Mallbris L, Granath F, Hamsetn A & Stahle M. (2006) Psoriasis is associated with lipid abnormalities at the onset of skin disease. J Am Acad Dermatol. April; 54(4): 614-21.
Marongiu F, Sorano GG, Bibbo C, Pistis MP, Conti M, Mulas P, Balestrieri A & Biggio P. (1994) Abnormlaities of blood coagulation and fibrinolysis in psoriasis. Dermatology. 189(1): 32-7
Mazlan SA, bin Mohamed Said MS, Hussein H, binti Shamsuddin K, Shah SA & Basri H. (2009) A study of intima media thickness and their cardiovascular risk factors in patients with psoriatic arthritis. Acta Medica. 52(3):107-16
Matsuura E, Kobayashi K, Tabuchi M, Lopez LR. (2006) Oxidative modification of low-density lipoprotein and immune regulation of athersclerosis. Prog Lipid Res. November; 45(6): 466-86.
McDonald & Calabresi. (1978) Psoriasis and occlusive vascular disease. BrJ Dermatol. November; 99(5): 469-75.

McDonald CJ & Calabresi P. (1978) Psoriasis and occlusive vascular disease. BrJ Dermatol. November; 99(5): 469-75

Mehta, Azfar RS, Shin DB, Neimann AL, Troxel AB & Gelfand JM. (2010) Patients with severe psoriasis are at increased risk of cardiovascular mortality: cohort study using the General Practice Research Database Eur Heart J. April; 31(8):1000-6.

Mehta, Yu Y, Pinnelas R, Krishnamoorthy P, Shin DB, Troxel AB & Gelfand JM. (2011) Attributable Risk Estimate of Severe Psoriasis on Major Cardiovascular Events. Am J Med. August;124(8): 775

Mills CM, Srivastava ED, Harvey IM, Swift GL, Newcombe RG, Holt PJ & Rhodes J. (1992) Smoking habits in psoriasis: a case control study. Br J Dermatol. July; 127(1): 18-21.

Naldi L, Chatenoud L, Linder D, Belloni Fortina A, Peserico A, Virgili AR, Bruni PL, Ingordo V, Lo Scocco G, Solaroli C, Schena D, Barba A, Di Landro A, Pezzarossa E, Arcangeli F, Gianni C, Betti R, Carli P, Farris A, Barabino GF & La Vecchia C. (2005) Cigarette smoking, body mass index, and stressful life events as risk factors for psoriasis: results form an Italian case-control study. J Invest Dermatol. July; 125(1): 61-7

Naldi L, Peli L & Parazzini F. (1999) Association of early-stage psoriasis with smoking and male alcohol consumption: evidence from an Italian case-control study. Arch Dermatol. December; 135(12): 1479-84.

Neimann AL, Shin DB, Wang X, Margolis DJ, Troxel AB & Gelfand JM. (2006) Prevalence of cardiovascular risk factors in patients with psoriasis. J Am Acad Dermatol. November; 55(5): 829-35

Offidani AM, Ferretti G, Taus M, Simonetti O, Dousset N, Valdiguie P, Curatola G & Bossi G. (1994) Lipoprotein peroxidation in adult psoriatic patients. Acta Derm Venerol Suppl (Stockh) 186: 38-40.

Pelfini C, Jucci A, Fratino P, De Marco R & Serri F. (1979) Insulinogenic indexes in psoriasis: Acta Derm Venereol Suppl (Stoch); 87: 48-50

Poikolainen, K, Karvonen J & Pukkala E (1999) Excess mortality related to alcohol and smoking among hospital treated patients with psoriasis Arch Dermatol. December; 135(12): 1490-3.

Poikolainen K, Renula T & Karvonen J. (1994) Smoking, alcohol and life events related to psoriasis among women, Br J Dermatol. April; 130(4): 473-7

Poikolainen K, Reunala T, Karvonen J, Lauharanta J & Kärkkäinen P. (1990)Alcohol intake: a risk factor for psoriasis in young and middle-aged men. BMJ. March; 300(6727): 780-3

Proanovich, Kirsner RS, Kravetz JD, Ma F, Martinez L & Federman DG. (2009) Association of psoriasis with coronary artery, cerebrovascular, and peripheral vascular diseases and mortality. Arch Dermatol. June; 145(6):700-3.

Qureshi AA, Choi HK, Setty AR & Curhan GC. (2009) Psoriasis and the risk of diabetes and hypertension: a prospective study of US female nurses. Arch Dermatol April; 145(4):379-82.

Refsum H, Helland S & Ueland PM. (1989) Fasting plasma homocysteine as a sensitive parameter of antifolate Effect: a study of psoriasis patients receiving low-dose methotrexate treatment. Clin Pharmacol Ther November; 46(5): 510-20

Reynoso-von Drateln C, Matrinez-Abundis E, Balcazar - Munoz BR, Bustos-Saldana R & Gonzalez-Ortiz M. (2003) Lipid profile, insulin secretion, and insulin sensitivity in psoriasis. J AM Acad Dermatol. June; 48(6): 882-5.

Rocha - Pereira P, Santos-Silva A, Rebelo I, Figuiredo A, Quintanilha A & Teixera F. (2004) The inflammatory response in mild and in severe psoriasis. Br J Dermatol. May; 150(5): 917-28.

Segal R, Baumoehl Y, Elkayam O, Levartovsky D, Litinsky I, Paran D, Wigler I, Habot B, Leibovitz A, Sela BA & Caspi D (2004) Anemia, serum vitamin B12, and folic acid in patients with rheumatoid arthritis, psoriatic arthritis, and systemic lupus erythematosus. Rheumatol Int. January; 24(1): 14-9.

Setty AR, Curhan G & Choi HK. (2007.) Obesity, Waist Circumference, Weight Change, and the Risk of Psoriasis in Women. Nurses' Health Study II. Arch Intern Med. August; 167(15): 1670-5

Setty AR, Curhan G & Choi HK. (2007) Smoking and the risk of psoriasis in women: Nurses' Health study II. Am J Med. November;120(11):953-9

Shang Q, Tam LS, Yip GW, Sanderson JE, Zhang Q, Li EK, Yu CM. (2011) High prevalence of subclinical left ventricular dysfunction in patients with psoriatic arthritis. J Rheum July; 38(7):1363-70.

Shapiro J, Cohen AD, Weitzman D, Tal R & David M. (2011) Psoriasis and cardiovascular risk factors: A case-control study on inpatients comparing psoriasis to dermatitis. J Am Acad Dermatol. July 8. [Epub ahead of print]

Shapiro J, Cohen AD, David M, Hodak E, Chodik G, Viner A, Kremer E & Heymann A. (2007) The association Between psoriasis, diabetes mellitus, and atherosclerosis in Israel: a case-control study. J Am Acad Dermatol April; 56(4):629-34.

Skoczynska AH, Turczyn B, Brancewicz-Losek M, Martynowicz H. (2003) High-density lipoprotein cholesterol in patients with psoriatic arthritis. J Eur Acad Dermatol Venereol. May; 17(3): 362-3.

Solomon DH, Massarotti E, Garg R, Liu J, Canning C & Schneeweiss S. (2011)DMARDs Reduce Diabetes Risk in RA and Psoriasis. JAMA June;305(24):2525-2531.

Sommer DM, Jenisch S, Suchan M, Christophers E, Weichenthal M. (2006) Increased prevalence of the metabolic syndrome in patients with moderate to severe psoriasis. Arch Dermatol Res. December; 298(7): 321-8.

Stern R, Nijsten T, Feldman S, Margolis J & Rolstad T. (2004) Psoriasis is common, carries a substantial burden even when not extensive, and is associated with wide-spread treatment dissatisfaction. J Invest Dermatol. March; 9(2):136-9

Tam LS, Tomlinson B, Chu TT, Li M, Leung YY, Kwok LW, Li TK, Yu T, Zhu YE, Wong KC, Kun EW & Li EK. (2008)Cardiovascular risk profile of patients with psoriatic arthritis compared to controls- the role of inflammation. Rheumatology. May; 47(5): 718-23.

Tobin AM, Hughes R, Hand E, Leong T, Graham IM & Kirby B. Homocysteine status and cardiovascular risk factors in patients with psoriasis: a case control study. In press Clin Exper Dermatol

Tobin AM, Higgins EM, Norris S & Kirby B. (2009) The prevalence of psoriasis in patients with alcoholic liver disease. Clin Exp Derm. August; 34(6):698-701

Ucak S, Ekmekci TR, Basat O, Koslu A & Altuntas Y. (2006) Comparison of various insulin sensitivity indices in psoriatic patients and their relationship with type of psoriasis. J Eur Acad Dermatol Venereol. May; 20(5): 517-22

Vanizor Kural B, Orem A, Cimsit G, Yandi YE & Calapoglu M. (2003) Plasma homocysteine and its relationship with atherothrombotic markers in psoriatic patients. Clin Chim Acta June; 332(1-2): 23-30

Veale DJ & Fitzgerald O. (2002) Psoriatic arthritis - pathogenesis and epidemiology. Clin Exp Rheumatol. Nov-Dec; 20(6 Suppl 28):S27-33

Wakkee M, Thio HB, Prens EP, Sijbrands EJ & Neumann HA. (2007) Unfavourable cardiovascular risk profiles in untreated and treated psoriasis patients. Atherosclerosis. January; 190(1): 1-9.

Williams HC. (1994)Smoking and psoriasis. BMJ February; 308(6926): 428-9

Wolf N, Quaranta M, Prescott NJ, Allen M, Smith R, Burden AD, Worthington J, Griffiths CE, Mathew CG, Barker JN, Capon F & Trembath RC. (2008) Psoriasis is associated with pleiotropic susceptibility loci identified in type II diabetes and Crohn's disease. J Med genet. February; 45(2): 114-116.

Wraight CJ, White PJ, McKean SC, Fogarty RD, Venables DJ, Liepe IJ, Edmondson SR & Werther GA. (2000) Reversal of epidermal hyperproliferation in psoriasis by insulin-like growth factor 1 receptor antisense oligonucleotides. Nat Biotechnol. May; 18(5): 521-6

Xu S, Cwyfan-Hughes SC, van der Stappen JW, Sansom J, Burton JL, Donnelly M & Holly JM. (1996)Altered insulin-like growth factor-II(IGF-II) level and IGF-binding protein-3 (IGFBP-3) protease activity in interstitial fluid taken from the skin lesion of psoriasis. J Invest Dermatol. January; 106(1): 109-12.

Yiu KH, Yeung CK, Chan HT, Wong RM, Tam S, Lam KF, Yan GH, Yue WS, Chan HH & Tse HF. (2011) Increased arterial stiffness in patients with psoriasis is associated with active systemic inflammation. Br J Dermatol. March; 164(3):514-20.

6

Cardiovascular Risk Factors in Elderly Normolipidaemic Acute Myocardial Infarct Patients

Arun Kumar
Department Of Biochemistry, International Medical School, Management and Science University, Malaysia

1. Introduction

Cardiovascular diseases (CVD) are a group of disorders of the heart and blood vessels, and include coronary heart disease (CHD), cerebrovascular disease (stroke), raised blood pressure (hypertension), peripheral artery disease, rheumatic heart disease, congenital heart disease and heart failure. According to the World Health Organization, CVD are the number one cause of death globally and claim 17 million lives each year. By 2030, almost 24 million people will die from CVD, mainly from heart disease and stroke. These are projected to remain the single leading causes of death (World Health Organization. Cardiovascular diseases (CVDs). Available from: http://www.who.int/mediacentre/factsheets/fs 317/en/index.html). In the United States, CVD account for more than one-third (34.3%) of deaths annually, and responsible for nearly 3 million Americans reporting disability. The costs of CVD are also staggering. In 2010, the total cost including health care services, medications and lost productivity, is estimated to be over $503 billion in the United States (Centers for Disease Control and Prevention. Heart Disease and Stroke Prevention. Addressing the nation's leading killers: at a glance 2010. Available from: http://www.cdc.gov/chronicdisease/resources/publications/AAG/dhdsp.htm). Similarly, the National Heart Foundation of Australia reported that CVD are the leading cause of mortality and morbidity in Australia, killing one person nearly every 10 minutes (National Heart Foundation of Australia. Data and statistics. Available from: http:// www.heartfoundation.org.au/information-for-professionals/data-and-statistics). Despite improvements over the last few decades, CVD remain as the second largest disease burden to our society after cancers. As the population ages, the economic impact of CVD on the health care system will become even greater. Tobacco smoking, an unhealthy diet, physical inactivity and high alcohol consumption increase the risk of CVD. Indeed, behavioral and dietary risk factors are responsible for about 80% of coronary heart disease and cerebrovascular disease (World Health Organization. Cardiovascular diseases (CVDs). Available from: http://www.who.int/mediacentre/factsheets/fs317/en/index.html).

Interestingly, both the incidence and mortality rate of CVD are much lower in Japan than other countries (Mozaffarian D) which may be attributed to the high consumption of fish/seafood by the Japanese population (Meyer BJ). The fact that fish is abundant in omega-3 polyunsaturated fatty acids has opened an effective venue to the prevention and treatment of this disease by either dietary modifications or pharmacological supplementation.

Cardiovascular disease is multi-factorial which is associated with factors like hereditary, hyperlipidemia, obesity, hypertension, environmental and life style variables like stress, smoking, alcohol consumption, etc (Chopra and Wasir 1998). Lipoprotein profile has been investigated extensively in recent years, which is deranged in large proportion of coronary artery disease (CAD) patients; especially Asians showing a mixed picture of dyslipidemia (Vasisht *et al*, 1990). Literature survey reveals dyslipidaemic subjects are more prone to myocardial infarction, due to increased free radical generation and ischemia as it is a conventional risk factor. (Malhotra *et al*, 2003; Mishra *et al*, 2005; Ghosh *et al*, 2006; Patil *et al*, 2007; Rajasekhar *et al*, 2004; Rani *et al*, 2005; Gomez *et al*,1996). Lowering of high density lipoprotein- cholesterol (HDL-C) is a common phenomenon observed in MI patients supported by previous studies (Malhotra *et al*, 2003; Mishra *et al*, 2005; Ghosh *et al*, 2006; Patil *et al*, 2007; Rajasekhar *et al*, 2004; Rani *et al*, 2005). High density lipoprotein- cholesterol (HDL-c) is the most important independent protective factor for arteriosclerosis which underlies coronary heart disease (CHD). High density lipoprotein- cholesterol (HDL-c) associated paraoxonase-1 (PON1) enzyme is protective against lipid peroxidation (Singh *et al*, 2007). Numerous cohort studies and clinical trials have confirmed the association between a low high density lipoprotein- cholesterol (HDL-c) and increased risk of coronary heart disease (CHD). Low density lipoprotein-cholesterol (LDL-C) is considered as the most important risk factor of coronary artery disease (CAD). Its oxidized form promotes foam cells formation which initiates the process of atherosclerosis by accumulating in sub-endothelium cells leading to fatty streaks and complex fibro fatty or atheromatous plaques formation (Berliner *et al*, 1995). The oxidation of low-density lipoprotein (LDL) can be limited by antioxidant enzyme system, including superoxide dismutase, catalase, glutathione peroxidase and antioxidant vitamins C, A, E and other carotenoids. Among the endogenous antioxidant system, includes albumin, uric acid, and total bilirubin. Imbalance of this reaction either due to excess free radical formation or insufficient removal by antioxidants leads to oxidative stress (Frei *et al*, 1998; Shrinivas *et al*, 2000; Maritim *et al*, 2003).

Various other risk factors have been identified apart from dyslipidemia are caeruloplasmin, C-reactive proteins, Lipoprotein (a), plasma fibrinogen, etc. Since we have encountered myocardial infarct patients with normal serum lipid concentration, we conducted a prospective case-control study to evaluate the concentration of antioxidant enzymes, degree of lipid peroxidation and other risk factors associated with acute myocardial infarction.

2. Materials and methods

The prospective case-control study consisted of 165 patients (123 men and 42 women) with AMI, admitted to the Intensive Cardiac Care Unit (ICCU), Sharda Hospital, India. The diagnosis of AMI was established according to diagnostic criteria: chest pain lasting for ≤3 hours, electrocardiographic (ECG) changes (ST elevation ≥ 2 mm in at least two leads) and elevation in enzymatic activities of serum creatine phosphokinase (CPK) and aspartate aminotransferase (AST). The control group consisted of 165 age/sex-matched healthy volunteers (123 men and 42 women). The design of this study was pre-approved by the institutional ethical committee board and informed consent was obtained from the patients and controls. Inclusion criteria were patients with a diagnosis of acute myocardial infarction (AMI) with normal lipid profile. Patients with diabetes mellitus, renal insufficiency, current and past smokers, hepatic disease or taking lipid lowering drugs or antioxidant vitamin supplements were excluded from the study. Normolipidemic status was judged by the following criteria: LDL≤160 mg/dl; HDL, ≥35 mg/dl; total cholesterol (TC), <200 mg/dl; and triglycerides (TG), <150 mg/dl (NCEP, ATP-III, 2001). Ten milliliters of blood was collected after overnight fasting for lipid profile assay. For ischemia-modified albumin (IscMA) analysis, 2 ml of blood was collected from the patients immediately after admission to intensive care unit.

Lipid Profile Total cholesterol (TC), triglyceride (TG) and high density lipoprotein-cholesterol (HDL-c) were analyzed enzymatically using kit obtained from Randox Laboratories Limited, Crumlin, UK. Plasma low density lipoprotein -cholesterol was determined from the values of total cholesterol and high density lipoprotein-cholesterol using the following formula:

$$\text{LDL-cholesterol} = \text{TC} - \frac{\text{TG}}{5} - \text{HDL-cholesterol}\,(\text{mg/dl})$$

Other assays - Serum albumin was measured by Bromocresol green binding method (Perry *et al*, 1979). Serum uric acid was estimated by the method of Brown based on the development of a blue color due to tungsten blue as phosphotungstic acid is reduced by uric acid in alkaline medium (Brown ,1945). Serum total bilirubin was estimated by the method of Jendrassik and Grof (Jendrassik and Grof, 1938).

The glutathione peroxidase (GPx) activity was determined by the procedure of Paglia and Valentine (Paglia and Valentine,1967). Superoxide dismutase (SOD) enzyme activity was measured by SOD assay kit using rate of inhibition of 2-(4-indophenyl)-(4-Nitrophenol)-5-phenyltetrazolium chloride (I.N.T) reduction method modified by Sun et al (Sun *et al*, 1988). Catalase activity was measured spectrophotometrically as described by Beutler (Beutler, 1984). MDA levels were estimated by thiobarbituric acid (TBA) reaction (Bernheim *et al*, 1948).Conjugated diene (CD) levels were measured by Recknagel and Glende method (Recknagel and Glende, 1984) with little modification. Caeruloplasmin assay was done by *p*-phenylene diamine method (Ravin, 1961). Ischemia-modified albumin (IscMA) concentration was determined by addition of a known amount of cobalt (II) to a serum sample and measurement of the unbound cobalt (II) by the intensity of colored complex formed after reacting with dithiothreitol (DTT) by colorimeter (Libby ,2003). Lipoprotein (a), levels were determined by Latex- Enhanced turbidimetric method. Serum paraoxonase was estimated using Zeptometrix Assay Kit obtained from Zeptometrix Corp, New York, 14202 based on the cleavage of phenyl acetate resulting in phenol formation. The rate of formation of phenol is measured by monitoring the increase in absorbance at 270 nm at 25°C.

Estimation of ascorbic acid was carried out by Roe and Kuether method (Roe and Kuether, 1943). The C-reactive protein were determined using high sensitivity enzyme Immunoassay kit manufactured by Life Diagnostics,inc., Catalog Number: 2210. The principle of the assay was based on a solid phase enzyme-linked immunosorbent assay (Kumar and Sivakanesan,

2008). The plasma fibrinogen was determined using kit which was obtained from TEClot Fib Kit 10 Catalog No: 050-500, manufactured by TECO GmbH, Dieselstr. 1, 84088 Neufahrn NB Germany (Kumar and Sivakanesan, 2008).

All chemicals of analytical grade were obtained from Sigma-Aldrich Company, New Delhi.

3. Results

Anthropometric parameters in acute myocardial infarction (AMI) patients and control are shown in Table 1. Total cholesterol, its ratio to high density lipoprotein -cholesterol (TC/HDL-C) and triglyceride were significantly higher in both sexes of patients compared with control (Table 2 and 3). The low density lipoprotein –cholesterol (LDL-c) and its ratio to high density lipoprotein –cholesterol (LDL-c) (LDL-C/HDL-C) were higher in acute myocardial infarction (AMI) subjects than in control (Table-3). The behavioral pattern and familial history of cardiovascular disease is presented in Table 4. The distribution of risk factors and relative risk according to potential risk factors among cases and controls are presented in Table 5 and Table 6. The status of antioxidants and lipid peroxidation are shown in Tables 7. All antioxidants were significantly decreased in patients compared with controls. In agreement with this serum malondialdehyde (MDA) and conjugated diene (CD) were more abundant in patients compared with controls. Ischemia-modified albumin (IscMA) levels were also greater in both male and female patients compared with control (Table 7).Serum fibrinogen, caeruloplasmin, ischemia- modified albumin and C-reactive protein were significantly higher where as arylesterase activity were significantly lowered in cases compared with controls (Table 8).

	Control *(n=165)*	MI patients *(n=165)*	P- value (95%CI)
Age (years) Range (years)	60.5 ± 3.4 *(48-69)*	61.8 ± 3.8 *(48-69)*	0.0037 (61.26- 62.33)
Height (m)	1.63 ± 0.04	1.64 ± 0.59	0.2919 (1.55-1.72)
Weight (kg)	68.34 ± 3.97	72.01 ± 5.37	<0.01 (71.25-72.76)
BMI (kg/m^2)	25.40 ± 1.20	26.16 ± 1.45	<0.01 (25.95-26.36)
Waist Circumference (cm)	93.70 ± 3.63	100.77 ± 6.06	<0.01 (99.91-101.62)
Hip Circumference (cm)	100.01 ± 3.16	105.72 ± 5.23	<0.01 (104.82-106.45)
Waist-Hip ratio	0.93 ± 0.01	0.95 ± 0.01	<0.001 (0.94-0.95)
Mid Arm Circumference (cm)	29.70 ± 1.47	30.63 ± 1.87	<0.01 (30.36-30.89)
Biceps skin fold thickness (mm)	6.95 ± 1.05	7.5 ± 1.38	<0.001 (7.30-7.69)
Triceps skin fold thickness (mm)	11.97 ± 1.27	12.89 ± 1.69	<0.001 (12.65-13.12)
Systolic blood pressure (mmHg)	121.06 ± 4.19	134.32 ± 11.65	<0.05 (132.67-135.96)
Diastolic blood pressure (mmHg)	79.90 ± 3.64	86.04 ± 4.25	<0.05 (85.44-86.63)

Table 1. Anthropometric data of control and patients (mean ± SD)

Variables	*Controls (n=165)*	*Patients (n=165)*	*P-value (95%CI)*
Age	60.55 ± 3.98	61.84 ± 3.80	0.0037(61.26-62.42)
Total Cholesterol (mg/dl)	168.58 ± 12.16	186.44 ± 13.95	<0.001(184.31-188.56)
HDL-Cholesterol (mg/dl)	50.51 ± 6.78	41.27 ± 4.62	<0.001(40.56-41.97)
Triglycerides (mg/dl)	107.84 ± 11.51	128.96 ± 12.19	<0.001(127.10-130.82)
LDL-Cholesterol (mg/dl)	83.59 ± 11.95	119.37 ± 14.05	<0.001(17.22-21.51)
TC: HDL-C	3.39 ± 0.36	4.57 ± 0.58	<0.001(4.48-4.65)
LDL:HDL-C	1.90 ± 0.31	2.93 ± 0.51	<0.001(2.85-3.00)
TG: HDL-C	2.17 ± 0.35	3.16 ± 0.49	0.3149(3.086-3.234)

Table 2. Lipid profile in patients and healthy controls (mean ± SD)

Ratio	Controls (n=165)	Patients (n=165)
TC/HDL-C		
2-3	2.90 ± 0.09 (n=28)	-
3-4	3.44 ± 0.25 (n=129)	3.70 ± 0.20 (n=31)
4-5	4.19 ± 0.22 (n=8)	4.53 ± 0.27 (n=90)
5-6	-	5.26 ± 0.23 (n=44)
TG/HDL-C		
1-2	1.77 ± 0.13 (n=56)	-
2-3	2.38 ± 0.23 (n=109)	2.65 ± 0.27 (n=59)
3-4	-	3.42 ± 0.26 (n=99)
4-5	-	4.22 ± 0.19 (n=7)
LDL-C/HDL-C		
1-2	1.71 ± 0.17 (n=106)	1.86 ± 0.15 (n=5)
2-3	2.23 ± 0.21 (n=59)	2.57 ± 0.27 (n=81)
3-4	-	3.32 ± 0.21 (n=74)
4-5	-	4.11 ± 0.12 (n=5)

Table 3. Distribution of Lipid ratios in patients and healthy controls (mean ± SD)

		Control Group	Study Group
Hyperactive	*Yes*	39 *(23.63)*	68 *(41.21)*
	no	126 *(76.36)*	97 *(58.78)*
Triffle thinker *	*yes*	30 *(18.18)*	99 *(60.00)*
	no	135 *(81.81)*	66 *(40.00)*
Irrelevant thinker	*yes*	50 *(30.30)*	106 *(64.24)*
	No	115 *(69.69)*	59 *(35.75)*

Numbers in parentheses are percent unless mentioned otherwise
*Triffle thinker: subjects who thinks and worries on unnecessary small things

Table 4. Behavioral Pattern in AMI patients and control

	AMI Cases (*n=165)*	Controls (*n= 165)*
Age (y)	61.84 ± 3.80	60.55 ± 3.98
BMI (kg/m^2)	26.16 ± 1.45	25.40 ± 1.20
Waist-to-hip ratio	0.95 ± 0.11	0.93 ± 0.08[a]
Alcohol intake (servings/d)	0.36 ± 0.68	0.15 ± 0.34[a]
Physical activity (MET-min/d)	56.23 ± 123.8	97.83 ± 174.8[a]
Current cigarette smokers (%)	14.45	3.6[b]
Current bidi smokers (%)	23.67	12.31[c]
Family history of MI (%)	37.57	8.48[d]
Hypertension (%)	49.09	1.8[e]
Alcoholics (%)	47.87	20.60[f]

Values are in Mean ± SD
[a,b,c,d,e,f] Significantly different from cases (*t* test for matched data): [a,b,c] $P \leq 0.001$, [d,e] $P \leq 0.0001$, [f] $P \leq 0.003$

Table 5. Distribution of risk factors among AMI patients and control

	No. of cases *N*	No. of controls *N*	Age- and sex-adjusted RR (95% CI)[b]	Multivariate RR (95% CI)[c]
Cigarette smoking				
Never smoker	120	136	1.0	1.0
>10 cigarettes/d	36	6	7.8 (4.9, 13.5)	7.4 (4.3, 15.2)
Bidi smoking*				
Never smoker	120	136	1.0	1.0
> 10 bidis/d	49	8	8.2 (5.2, 14.2)	6.5 (3.9, 12.9)

BMI (kg/m²)				
20-24.9	30	51	1.0	1.0
≥ 25	135	114	2.7 (1.8,4.1)	2.9 (1.6, 5.1)
Waist -to-hip ratio				
≤ 0.95	52	137	1.0	1.0
> 1.0	113	28	3.9 (2.1, 6.3)	2.8 (1.6, 5.7)
Family history of MI				
No	97	151	1.0	1.0
Yes	62	14	2.1(1.6, 2.7)	2.7 (1.8, 3.8)
History of Hypertension				
No	136	142	1.0	1.0
Yes	29	23	2.1 (1.7, 3.2)	1.9 (1.4, 2.9)
Education level				
Highest level of education	25	27	1.0	1.0
None	101	132	3.1 (1.3, 5.1)	3.6 (1.0, 6.2)
Type of Family				
Split	20	64	1.0	1.0
Joint	145	101	4.5 (1.5- 2.9)	3.9(1.2-2.6)
Civil Status				
Lower Class	10	19	1.0	1.0
Middle Class	119	131	3.4 (4.3, 6.7)	2.8 (3.7, 5.9)
Higher Class	36	15	4.7 (4.9, 7.2)	3.8 (3.1, 4.7)
Leisure -time exercise				
Non-exerciser	82	58	1.0	1.0
≥ 145 MET-min/d	83	107	0.76 (0.4, 0.8)	0.68 (0.4, 0.7)
Household income				
>10 000 rupees/month	155	146	1.0	1.0
<5000 rupees/month	10	19	1.8 (1.2, 2.7)	1.7 (1.0, 3.1)
Hindu religion				
No	33	12	1.0	1.0
Yes	132	153	0.8 (0.6, 1.1)	0.9 (0.7, 1.3)

[a] MET, metabolic equivalent. RR estimates were obtained by using conditional logistic regression analysis controlled for the matching factors (age, sex, and hospital) and then additional potential risk factors.

[b] Also adjusted for hospital.

[c] Covariates controlled for in the multivariate model were as follows: age; sex; hospital; cigarette smoking never, current (≤10 cigarettes/d, >10 cigarettes/d)]; bidi smoking [never, current (≤10 bidis/d, >10 bidis/d)]; BMI, in kg/m² (20-24.9, ≥25); waist-to-hip ratio (≤0.95, >1.0); leisure time physical exercise (none, < 145 MET-min/d, ≤145 MET-min/d); history of hypertension (no, yes); history of diabetes (no, yes); history of high cholesterol (no, yes); family history of IHD (no, yes); education (none, primary school, middle, secondary, higher secondary, college, graduate or professional); household income (<5000, 5000-10000, 10000-15000,>10000 rupees/mo); and Hindu religion (no, yes).

[*] Bidis (pronounced bee-dees) are small hand-rolled cigarettes manufactured in India and other southeast Asian countries. They are exported to as many as 122 countries, according to one bidi manufacturer. Bidi cigarettes are made of tobacco wrapped in tendu or temburni leaf *(Diospyros melanxylon)*.

Table 6. Relative risk (RR) of Acute Myocardial Infarction (AMI) according to potential risk factors[a]

	Control *(n=165)*	AMI patients *(n=165)*	P value (95%CI)
Serum albumin (mg/dl)	4.4 ± 0.3	4.2 ± 0.3	<0.001(4.17-4.28)
Serum uric acid (mg/dl)	5.8 ± 1.2	4.3 ± 0.9	<0.01(4.18-4.45)
Serum ascorbic acid (mg/dl)	5.3 ± 1.2	2.8 ± 0.7	<0.0001(2.70-2.89)
Serum Total bilirubin (mg/dl)	0.8 ± 0.2	0.7 ± 0.2	<0.001(0.62-0.69)
Serum superoxide dismutase (U/gHb)	1826.5 ± 31.9	813.9 ± 208.9	<0.02 (784.42-843.37)
Serum glutathione peroxidase (U/gHb)	61.3 ± 3.9	42.6 ± 6.3	<0.001(41.71- 43.48)
Serum catalase (k/gHb)	256.2 ± 26.7	193.1 ± 35.9	<0.001(188.03-198.16)
Serum Lipoprotein (a) (mg/dl)	3.0 ± 1.1	10.9 ± 2.2	<0.0001 (10.58-11.21)
Serum malondialdehyde (nmol/L)	5.7 ± 1.0	14.8 ± 1.7	<0.02(11.55-15.06)
Serum conjugated dienes (μmol/L)	31.0 ± 2.7	48.3 ± 5.5	<0.001(47.44-49.11)

Table 7. Antioxidant status and Lipid Peroxidation in Control and AMI patients (mean ± SD)

	Control *(n=165)*	AMI patients *(n=165)*	*P* value (95% CI)
Plasma fibrinogen (mg/dl)	237.5 ± 17.4	357.8 ± 23.2	<0.0001 (354.52 -361.07
Serum caeruloplasmin (mg/dl)	20.4 ± 2.3	51.5 ± 2.4	<0.0001 (51.16-51.83)
Serum Arylesterase activity (kU/L)	98.4 ± 6.2	69.7 ± 10.0	<0.0001(68.28-71.11)
Serum Ischemia modified albumin (U/ml)	81.9 ± 3.9	97.5 ± 11.7	<0.001(95.84-99.15)
Serum C-reactive protein (mg/dl)	1.1 ± 0.3	3.0 ± 1.1	<0.0001(2.84-3.15)

Table 8. Other Biochemical parameters in Control and AMI patients (mean ± SD)

4. Dicussion

Coronary artery disease (CAD) remains the major cause of morbidity and mortality in all developed and developing countries in the world including India (Reddy and Yusuf, 1998). Dyslipidemia is one of the major modifiable risk factors for CAD (Chopra *et al*, 1998; Vasisht *et al*, 2000; Malhotra *et al*, 2003).

The coronary artery disease (CAD) risk factors do not predict the occurrence of acute myocardial infarction (AMI) as variation in risk factors is observed in South Asian population due to varied dietary habits and life style (Mishra *et al*, 2005). The search for various conventional risk factors among Asians could be helpful in recognizing the future events of stroke. These curiosities prompted us to identify the newer risk factors, with respect to Indian population.

The search for the newer risk factors continues and researchers are investigating the role of inflammatory markers and other potential risks factors which could link with acute myocardial infarction (AMI).

In this prospective case-control study in India, only normolipidaemic acute myocardial infarction (AMI) patients were selected. The study was designed to identify and evaluate potential risk factors in normolipidaemic acute myocardial infarction (AMI) patients. The subjects selected for the study comprised of 165 controls, 48-69 y and 165 acute MI patients, 48-69 y.

Anthropometric variables in acute myocardial infarction (AMI) patients showed highly significant differences in waist/hip ratio and biceps skin fold thickness. Study reported (Heitman *et al*, 2004) that waist /hip ratio is a dominant, independent and predictive variable of cardiovascular disease and coronary heart disease deaths in Australian men and women. Megnien *et al*, 1999 also reported high hip circumference relative to weight and waist circumference is a better predictor of low incidence of cardiovascular disease and coronary heart disease. The present study is in good agreement with the observations of the above studies. Among Indians the cardiovascular risk is high even the prevalence of obesity is minimal (Megnien *et al*, 1999). In the present study the mean body mass index and waist /hip ratio in all subjects was 26.56 and 0.96 respectively, showing a significantly higher body mass index and weight /hip ratio in patients compared with control.

Based on the observations of the aforementioned studies and further supported by the present study it could be concluded that weight/hip ratio is a better predictor of cardiovascular disease (CVD) than body mass index. So it is better tool for indentifying the future risk of acute myocardial infarction (AMI) in subjects by non-invasive procedures.

Observations of lipid profile

The mean total cholesterol level of the controls compared with acute myocardial infarction patients (186.44 ± 13.95 mg/dl) was significantly ($p<0.001$) higher compared with controls (168.58 ± 12.16 mg/dl). The mean high density lipoprotein-cholesterol level in the patients was significantly lower ($p<0.001$) compared with controls. Triglyceride (TG) values observed in acute myocardial infarction (AMI) patients was (129mg/dl) significantly higher than controls (107.8mg/dl). The mean low density lipoprotein-cholesterol (LDL-c) levels in patients was (119.4mg/dl) significantly higher than controls (83.6 mg/dl). The total cholesterol / high density lipoprotein - cholesterol ratio in acute myocardial infarct patients (4.6) was significantly ($p<0.001$) higher compared with controls (3.4). The present study observed significantly higher ratio (2.9) in acute myocardial infarction patients compared with control (1.9).

Earlier studies in lipid profile analysis conducted on acute myocardial infarction patients (Mishra *et al*, 2001; Das *et al*, 2002; Goswami *et al*, 2003; Kharb *et al*, 2003; Malhotra *et al*, 2003; Burman *et al*, 2004; Rajashekhar *et al*, 2004; Sivaraman *et al*, 2004; Rani *et al*, 2005; Shindhe, *et al*, 2005; Yadhav *et al*, 2006; Patil *et al*, 2007) observed higher total cholesterol, triglyceride, low-density lipoprotein –cholesterol and lower levels of high-density lipoprotein-cholesterol in patients compared to controls.

Also higher ratio of total cholesterol to high density lipoprotein-cholesterol, low-density lipoprotein-cholesterol to high-density cholesterol-lipoprotein and higher triglyceride to high-density cholesterol-lipoprotein was observed in the present study. The present study concludes the importance of assessing the lipid ratios even in normolipidaemic subjects as it is one of the atherogenic factors for development of myocardial infarction and other coronary complications. The practice of computing the ratio should be implemented even in a normal health check up packages. In the final analysis it appears that myocardial infarction and coronary artery disease are not always associated with an elevated serum total cholesterol concentration. The major concern of this observation is that subjects who maintain desirable total cholesterol concentration also are targets for myocardial infarction (MI) and coronary artery disease (CAD) and therefore analysis of other risk factors that are non-conventional and newly emerging will be of immense important in the eventual assessment of the risk status. The existing literature and the results of the present study all point out that acute myocardial infarction and coronary artery disease patients have significantly higher total cholesterol concentration whether the values are in the desirable range or elevated.

Antioxidant status

The serum endogenous antioxidants were decreased in acute myocardial infarction compared to controls. Similarly the enzyme antioxidants were also significantly lowered in patients.

Study conducted (Olusi *et al*, 1999; Djousse *et al* 2003) in acute myocardial infarction patients, reported significantly lower ($p<0.0001$) albumin and bilirubin ($p<0.0001$), where as lower levels of uric acid (Jing *et al*, 2000; Brand *et al*, 1985; Niskanen *et al*, 2004) and ascorbic acid (Nyossen *et al*, 1997; Bhakuni *et al*, 2006; Das *et al*, 2002; Kurl *et al*, 2002) in acute myocardial infarct patients were reported.

The aforementioned studies suggested the expected risk of acute myocardial infarction is increased where these endogenous antioxidants are lowered due to enhanced utilization during oxidative stress in patients. Though, uric acid is well established antioxidant, but at times it can also act as a pro-oxidant, which might increase the risk of myocardial infarction. Aulinskas *et al*, (1983) established the role of ascorbic acid as up regulator of low density -lipoprotein (LDL) receptors, facilitating the clearance of low density - lipoprotein (LDL). The low levels of ascorbic acid in acute myocardial infarction (AMI) patients in the present study might be due to enhanced utilization of ascorbic acid during oxidative stress in patients.

The enzymatic antioxidants namely superoxide dismutase, catalase and glutathione peroxidase are also lowered in patients compared with controls. The findings of the present study concurs to earlier studies (Senthil *et al*, 2004; Bhakuni *et al*, 2006; Jain *et al*, 2000; Rajashekhar *et al*, 2004; Das *et al*, 2002; Gupta *et al*, 2006; Patil *et al*, 2007) where lower activities of superoxide dismutase, catalase and glutathione peroxidase. Studies conducted (Senthil *et al*, 2004; Shindhe *et al*, 2005; Rajasekhar *et al*, 2004; El-Badry *et al*, 1995; Gupta *et al*, 2006 and Kharb 2003) also reported reduced activities of glutathione peroxidase in patients compared with controls. These studies are based on the hypothesis of decreased antioxidants due to oxidative insult in myocardial infarct patients. Thus it is indicative that low levels of both endogenous and enzyme antioxidants in circulation may be due to its increased utilization to scavenge toxic lipid peroxides.

Lipoprotein (a) and lipid peroxidation

The mean serum Lipoprotein (a) malondialdehyde (MDA) and conjugated diene (CD) levels in MI patients were higher compared with controls. Earlier studies conducted (Burman *et al*, 2004; Guha *et al*, 2001; Bal *et al*, 2001; Rajashekhar *et al*, 2004) also observed higher Lipoprotein (a) in AMI patients where as Nascetti *et al*, (1996) did not observed any change in Lipoprotein (a) levels in cardiovascular disease (CVD) patients and concluded lipoprotein (a) not to be considered as an independent risk factor in cardiovascular disease (CVD) patients.

Studies conducted (Senthil *et al*, 2004; Das *et al*, 2002; Kharb 2003; Bhakuni *et al*, 2006; Shindhe *et al*, 2005; Gupta *et al*, 2006) reported higher levels of malondialdehyde (MDA) in myocardial infarct patients.

Other biochemical parameters

The levels of caeruloplasmin, C-reactive protein, fibrinogen, ischemia-modified albumin were higher and arylesterase activities were lowered in patients. Studies conducted (Grobusch *et al*, 1999; El-Badry *et al*, 1995; Giurgie, 2005; Awadallah *et al*, 2006) observed significantly higher ($p<0.001$) levels of caeruloplasmin where as (Berton *et al*, 2003; Bhagat *et al*, 2003; Sivaraman *et al*, 2004; Kulsoom *et al*, 2006; Boncler *et al*, 2006) observed higher levels of C-reactive protein in patients. Shukla *et al*, (2006) stated elevated levels of caeruloplasmin as a risk factor for acute myocardial infarct patients. The reactive oxygen species disrupts copper binding to caeruloplasmin thus impairing its antioxidant property and further promoting oxidative pathology. Studies conducted on plasma fibrinogen levels in acute myocardial infarct patients (Harkut *et al*, 2004; Coppola *et al*, 2005; Beg *et al*, 2007; Sivaraman *et al*, 2004) reported rise in plasma fibrinogen as the present study. Earlier study conducted (Chawla *et al*, 2006; Auxter, 2003; Bar-Or *et al*, 2001) in acute myocardial infarct patients also reported higher levels in patients as observed by the present study. Studies on arylesterase activities in acute myocardial infarct patients (Aviram *et al*, 1999; Ayub *et al*, 1999; Richard *et al*, 2000; Jarvik *et al*, 2002; Azizi *et al*, 2002; Singh *et al*, 2007; Sarkar *et al*, 2006) also observed lower activities as concurrent to the current study. Increased C-reactive protein (CRP) concentrations in patients with unstable angina and acute myocardial infarct might induce the production by the monocytes of the tissue factor which initiates the coagulation process. C-reactive protein together with fibrinogen acts as a chemotactic factor. Fibrinogen is responsible for the adhesion of macrophages to the endothelial surface for their migration into the intima. The elevated c-reactive protein levels have been found to be related to the occurrence of cardiovascular complications such as sudden cardiac death or AMI (Pepys and Hirschfield, 2003).

Our study concluded apart from lipid profile, other variables which could be a probable risk for the future myocardial events have to be equally monitored. It is also recommended to increase dietary antioxidant intake in persons who already have known risk factors so that to some extent the myocardial infarction could be delayed. It is also important to check inflammatory markers like c-reactive protein and ischemia-modified albumin in a regular period of time after stepping early forties as they could be a cost effective mode of diagnosis and the subjects can be efficiently monitored and complications of myocardial infarction can be prolonged.

5. References

Auxter S. Cardiac Ischemia testing: a new era in chest pain evaluation. *Clin Lab News* 2003; 29, 1-3.

Aulinskas TH, Vander Westhuyzen DR. Coetzee GA. Ascorbate increases the number of low density lipoprotein receptors in cultured arterial smooth muscle cells. *Atherosclerosis* 1983; 47: 159-71.

Aviram M, Rosenblat M, Billecke S, Eroul J, Sovenson R, Bisaier CL. Human serum paraoxonase (PON1) is in activated by oxidized low density lipoprotein and preserved by antioxidants. *Free Radic Biol Med* 1999; 26:892-904.

Awadallah SM, Hamad M, Jbarah I, Salem NM, Mubarak MS. Autoantibodies against oxidized LDL correlate with serum concentrations of caeruloplasmin in patients with cardiovascular disease. *Clin Chim Acta* 2006; 365: 330-336.

Ayub A, Mackness MI, Sharon A, Mackness B, Patel J, Durrington PN. Serum Paraoxonase After Myocardial Infarction. *Arteriosclerosis, Thrombosis, and Vascular Biology* 1999; 19:330-335.

Azizi F, Rahmani M, Raiszadeh F, Solati M, Navab M. Associations of lipids, lipoproteins, apolipoproteins and paraoxonase enzyme activity with premature coronary artery disease. *Coronary Artery Dis* 2002; 13(1): 9-16.

Balarajan R. Ethnicity and variations in mortality from coronary heart disease. *Health Trends* 1996; 28:45–51.

Bar-Or,D, Lau E, Rao N, Bampos N, Winkler JV, Curtis CG. Reduction in the cobalt binding capacity of human albumin with myocardial ischemia. *Ann. Emerg. Med* 1999; 34: 556.

Berliner JA, Navab M, Fogelman AM, Frank JS, Demer LL, Edwards PA, et al. Atherosclerosis: basic mechanisms. Oxidation. Inflammarion, and genetics. *Circulation* 1995; 91:2488-96.

Bernheim S, Bernheim MLC, Wilbur KM. The reaction between thiobarbituric acid and the oxidant product of certain lipids. *J Biol Chem* 1948; 174: 257-264.

Berton G, Cordiano R, Palmieri R, Pianca S, Pagliara V, Palatini P. C-Reactive Protein in Acute Myocardial Infarction: Association With Heart Failure. *Am Heart J* 2003; 145(6):1094-1101.

Beutler E. Red Cell Metabolism: *A Manual of Biochemical Methods, 3rd edition. New York, Grune and Stratton* 1984; 105.

Beg M, Nizami A, Singhal KC, Mohammed J, Gupta A, Azfar SF. Role of serum fibrinogen in patients of ischemic cerebrovascular disease. *Nepal Med Coll J* 2007; 9: 88-92.

Bhagat S, Gaiha M, Sharma VK, Anuradha S A. Comparative Evaluation of C - reactive protein as a Short-Term Prognostic Marker in Severe Unstable Angina- A Preliminary Study. *Journal of Assoc Physicians* 2003; 51:349-354.

Bhakuni P, Chandra M, Misra MK. Levels of free radical scavengers and antioxidants in post perfused patients of myocardial infarction. *Current Science* 2005; 89: 168-170.

Bhakuni P, Chandra M, Misra MK. Oxidative stress parameters in erythrocytes of post-reperfused patients with myocardial infarction. *J Enzyme Inhib Med Chem* 2005; 20(4):337-81.

Boncler M, Luzak B, Watala C. Role of C-reactive protein in atherogenesis. *Postepy Hig Med Dosw* 2006; 60:538-46.

Brand FN, Mcgee DL, Kannel WB, Stokes J, Castelli W P. Hyperuricemia as a rsik factor of coronary heart disease: The Framingham Study. *American Journal of Epidemiology* 1985; 121: 11-18.

Brown H. *J Clin Chem* 1945; 158:601.

Bulatao RAO, Stephens PW. Demographic estimates and projections, by region, 1970-2015. In: Jamison DT, Mosley WH, eds. Disease control priorities in developing countries. *Washington, DC: World Bank,* 1990. (Health sector priorities review no. 13.)

Burman A, Jain K, Gulati R, Chopra V, Agrawal DP, Vaisisht S. Lipoprotein (a) as a marker of Coronary Artery Disease and its Association with Dietary Fat. J Assoc Physicians India 2004; 52:99-102.

Centers for Disease Control and Prevention. Heart Disease and Stroke Prevention. Addressing the nation's leading killers: at a glance 2010. Available from: http://www.cdc.gov/chronicdisease/resources/publications/AAG/dhdsp.htm

Chawla R, Goyal N, Calton R, Goyal S. Ischemia modified albumin: A novel marker for acute coronary syndrome. *Indian Journal of Clinical Biochemistry* 2006; 21(1):77-82.

Chopra V, Wasir H. Implications of lipoprotein abnormalities in Indian patients. *Journal Assoc Physicians of India* 1998; 46:814-8.

Coppola G, Rizzo M, Maurizio GA, Corrado E, Alberto DG, Braschi A, Braschi G, Novo S. Fibrinogen as a predictor of mortality after acute myocardial infarction: a forty-two-month follow up study. *Ital Heart J* 2005; 6:315-322.

Das S, Yadav D, Narang R, Das N. Interrelationship between lipid peroxidation, ascorbic acid and superoxide dismutase in coronary artery disease. *Current Science* 2002; 83:488-491.

Djousse L, Rothman KJ, Cupples LA, Levy D, Ellison RC. Effect of serum albumin and bilirubin as a risk factor for Myocardial infarction. *Am J Cardiol* 2003; 91: 485- 488.

El- Badry I, Abon El N, Yehia T K, Zakhari MM. Free radicals activity in Acute Myocardial Infarction. *The Egyptian Heart Journal* 1995; 47: 71-78.

Executive Summary of The Third Report of The National Cholesterol Education Program (NCEP) Expert panel on Detection, Evaluation, and treatment of high Blood Cholesterol in Adults (Adult Treatment Panel III). Expert Panel of Detection, Evaluation, and Treatment of High Blood Cholesterol in Adults. *JAMA* 2001; 285(19):2486-97.

Frei B, Stocker R, Ames BN. Antioxidant defenses and lipid peroxidation in human blood plasma. *Proc Natl Acad Sci USA* 1988; 85: 9748-9752.

Friedewalds, WT, Levy RI, Fredrickson DS. Estimation of the concentration of low density lipoprotein cholesterol in plasma without the use of preparative ultracentrifuge. *Clin. Chem* 1972; 18, 499-502.

Ghosh J, Mishra TK, Rao YN, Aggarwal SK. Oxidised LDL, HDL Cholesterol, LDL Cholesterol levels in patients of Coronary Artery Disease. *Indian Journal of Clinical Biochemistry* 2006; 21(1):181-184.

Giurgea N, Constantinescu MI, Stanciu R, Suciu S, Muresan A. Caeruloplasmin- acute – phase reactant or endogenous antioxidant? The case of cardiovascular disease. *Med Sci Monit* 2005; 11: RA 48-51.

Gomez MA, Anderson JL, Karagounis LA, Muhlestein JB, Mooers FB. An emergency medicine based protocol for rapidly ruling out myocardial ischemia reduces hospital time and expense. Results of randomized study (ROMO). *J. Am. coll. Cardiol* 1996; 28:25-33.

Goswami K Bandyopadhyay. Lipid profile in middle class Bengali population of Kolkata. *Ind J of Clin Biochem* 2003; 18:127-130.

Gupta M, Chari S. Proxidant and Antioxidant status in patients of type II Diabetes Mellitus with IHD. *Indian Journal of Clinical Biochemistry* 2006; 21(2):118-122.

Harkut PV, Sahashrabhojney VS, Salkar RG. Plasma fibrinogen as a marker of major adverse cardiac events in patients of type 2 Diabetes with unstable angina. *Int J Diab Dev Countries* 2004; 24: 69-74.

Heitman BL, Frederickson P, Lissner L. Hip Circumference and Cardiovascular Morbidity and Mortality in Men and Women. *Obesity Research* 2004; 12:482-487.

Jarvik GP, Tsai NT, Mckinstry LA, Wani R, Victoria HB, Richter RJ, Schellenberg GD, Heagerty PJ, Hatsukami TS, Furlong CE. Vitamin C and E Intake Is Associated With Increased Paraoxonase Activity. *Arteriosclerosis, Thrombosis, and Vascular Biology* 2002; 22:1329.

Jendrassik L, Grof B. *Biochem Zeit* 1938; 297:81 9.

Jing F, Alderman M H. Serum uric acid and cardiovascular mortality. *JAMA* 2000; 283: 2404-2410.

Kharb S. Low Glutathione levels in acute myocardial infarction. *Ind J Med Sci* 2003; 57; Issue8: 335-7.

Kurl S, Tuomainen TP, Laukkanen JA, Nyyssonen K, Lakka T, Sivenius J, Salonen JT. Plasma Vitamin C Modifies the Association Between Hypertension and Risk of Stroke. *Stroke* 2002; 33:1568.

Kulsoom B, Nazrul SH. Association of serum C - reactive protein and LDL: HDL with myocardial infarction. *J Pak Med Assoc* 2006; 56 (7):318-22.

Kumar A, Sivakanesan R. Does plasma fibrinogens and C-reactive protein predict the incidence of myocardial infarction in patients with normal lipids profile? *Pak J Med Sci* 2008; 24:336-339.

Libby P. Vascular biology of atherosclerosis: Overview and state of art. *Am J Cardiol* 2003; 91(suppl): 3A-6A.

Malhotra P, Kumari S, Singh S, Verma S. Isolated Lipid Abnormalities in Rural and Urban Normotensive and Hypertensive North-West Indians. *Journal of Assoc Physicians of India* 2003; 51:459-463.

Maritim AC, Sanders RA, Watkins JB. Diabetes, oxidative stress, and antioxidants: a review. *J Biochem Mol Toxicol* 2003; 17: 24-38.

Megnien JL, Denarie N, Cocaul M. Predicitve value of Waist-to-hip ratio on Cardiovascular Risk Events. *Int J Obes Relat Metab Disord* 1999; 23:90-97.

Meyer BJ. Are we consuming enough long chain omega-3 polyunsaturated fatty acids for optimal health? *Prostaglandins Leukot Essent Fatty Acids.* 2011;DOI: 10.1016/j.plefa.2011.04.010

Mishra A, Luthra K, Vikram NK. Dyspipidemia in Asian Indians: Determminants and Significance. *Journal Assoc Physicians India* 2005; 52:137-142.

Mishra TK, Routray SN, Patnaik UK, Padhi PK, Satapathy C, Behera M. Lipoprotein (a) and Lipid Profile in Young Patients with Angiographically Proven Coronary Artery Disease. *Indian Heart Journal* 2001; 53 :(5) Article No. 60.

Mozaffarian D. JELIS, fish oil and cardiac events. *Lancet*. 2007; 369(9567):1062-1063.

Nascetti S, D' Addato S, Pascarelli N, Sangiorgi Z, Grippo MC, Gaddi A. Cardiovascular disease and Lp(a) in the adult population and in the elderly: the Brisighella study. *Riv Eur Sci Med Farmacol* 1996; 18(5-6):205-12.

National Heart Foundation of Australia. Data and statistics. Available from: http://www.heartfoundation.org.au/information-for-professionals/data-and-statistics

Niskanen LK, Laaksonen DE, Nyyssonen K, Alfthan G, Lakka H M, Lakka TA, Salonene JT. Uric acid level as a risk factor for cardiovascular and all- cause moratlity in middle-aged men: a prospective study. *Arch Intern Med* 2004; 164:1546-51.

Nyyssonen K, Markku TP, Salonen R, Tuomilehto J, Salonen JT. Vitamin C deficiency and risk of myocardial infarction: prospective population study of men from eastern Finland. *BMJ* 1997; 314:634.

Olusi SO, Prabha K, Sugathan TN. Biochemical Risk factors for Myocardial Infarction Among South Asian Immigrants and Arabs. *Annals of Saudi Medicine* 1999; 19: 147-149.

Paglia DE, Valentine WN. Studies on quantitative and qualitative characterization of erythrocyte glutathione peroxidase. *J Lab Clin Med* 1967; 70: 158-69.

Patil N, Chavan V, Karnik ND. Antioxidant Status in Patients with Acute Myocardial Infarction. *Indian Journal of Clinical Biochemistry* 2007; 22(1):45-51.

Pepys MB and Hirschfield G M. C-reactive protein: a critical update. *J Clin Invest* 2003; 111(12): 1805-1812. doi: 10.1172/JCI200318921.

Perry BW, Doumas BT. Effect of heparin on albumin determination by use of bromocresol green and bromocresol purple. *Clin Chem* 1979; 25:1520-1522.

Rajasekhar D, Srinivasa Rao PV, Latheef SA, Saibaba KS, Subramanyam G. Association of serum antioxidants and risk of coronary heart disease in South Indian population. *Indian J Med Sci* 2004; 58(11):465-71.

Rani SH, Madhavi G, Ramachandra RV, Sahay BK, Jyothy A. Risk factors for coronary heart disease in type II diabetes. *Indian Journal of Clinical Biochemistry* 2005; 20(2):75-80.

Ravin HA. An improved colorimetric enzymatic assay of caeruloplasmin. *J. Lab. Med* 1961; 58, 161-168.

Recknagel RO, Glende EA. Spectrophotometric detection of lipid conjugated dienes. *Methods Enzymol* 1984; 105:331-337.

Reddy KS. Cardiovascular disease in India. *World Health Stat Q* 1993; 46:101-7.

Reddy KS, Yusuf S. Emerging epidemic of cardiovascular disease in developing countries. *Circulation* 1998; 97:596–601.

Richard JW, Leview I, Righetti A. Smoking Is Associated With Reduced Serum Paraoxonase Activity and Concentration in Patients With Coronary Artery Disease. *Circulation* 2000; 101:2252.

Roe JH, Kuether CA. *J. Biol Chem* 1943; 147:399.

Sarkar PD, TMS Madhusudhan B. Association between paraoxonase activity and lipid levels in patients with premature coronary artery disease. *Clin Chim Acta* 2006; 373:77-81.

Senthil S, Veerappan RM, Ramakrishna RM, Pugalendi KV. Oxidative stress and antioxidants in patients with cardiogenic shock complicating acute myocardial infarction. *Clin Chim Acta* 2004; 348 (1-2):131-7.

Shrinivas K, Vijaya Bhaskar M, Aruna Kumari M, Nagaraj K, Reddy KK. Antioxidants, lipid peroxidation and lipoproteins in primary hypertension. *Indian Heart J* 2000; 52:285-88.

Shinde S, Kumar P, Patil N. Decreased Levels Of Erythrocyte Glutathione In Patients With Myocardial Infarction. *The Internet Journal of Alternative Medicine* 2005; 2:1.

Singh S, Venketesh S, Verma JS, Verma M, Lellamma CO, Goel RC. Paraoxonase (PON11) activity in northwest Indian Punjabis with coronary artery disease & type II diabetes mellitus. *Indian J Med Res* 2007; 125:783-7.

Sivaraman S K, Zachariah G, Annamalai PT. Evaluation of C - reactive protein and other Inflammatory Markers in Acute Coronary Syndromes. *Kuwait Medical Journal* 2004; 36(1):35-37.

Sun Y, Oberly LW, Li Y. A simple method for clinical assay of superoxide dismutase. *Clin Chem* 1988; 34: 497-500.

Vasisht S, Narula J, Awtade A, Tandon R, Srivastava LM. Lipids and lipoproteins in normal controls and clinically documented coronary heart disease patients. *Ann Natl Acad Med Sci (India)* 1990; 26:57-66.

World Health Organization. Cardiovascular diseases (CVDs). Available from: http://www.who.int/mediacentre/factsheets/fs317/en/index.html

Yadhav AS, Bhagwat VR, Rathod IM. Relationship of Plasma homocysteine with lipid profile parameters in Ischemic Heart disease. *Indian Journal of Clinical Biochemistry* 2006; 21(1):106-110.

7

Erectile Dysfunction Complicating Cardiovascular Risk Factors and Disease

Irekpita Eshiobo, Emeka Kesieme and Taofik Salami
Ambrose Alli University, Ekpoma, Nigeria

1. Introduction

Erectile Dysfunction (ED) is the persistent inability to achieve and or maintain penile erection sufficient for satisfactory sexual Intercourse. [1] *In 1995 it was estimated that 152 million men world-wide experienced ED and it was projected that by 2025, the prevalence worldwide would be 320 million.*[2] In the United states alone, 34 million men suffer from ED[3] while in China, according to Yang et al, [4] prevalence is reported to be 73.1% in the general population. Shaeer et al [5] in their study of the prevalence of ED in diverse nationalities representing a wide range of cultural, religious, racial and socio-economic backgrounds concluded that prevalence rates from various countries are difficult to compare because of variable definition and age range. So far, the most comprehensive epidemiological study of ED has been the Massachusetts male aging study[6] which reported ED to be present in 10% of men aged between forty and fifty years and almost 70% in Men aged 70% years and above.

	COUNTRIES	PREVALENCE
1.	Malaysia	17.0%
2.	Germany	19.0%
3.	Japan	34.0%
4.	United States of America	52.0%
5.	Morocco	53.6%
6.	Nigeria	57.4%
7.	Egypt	63.6%
8.	Turkey	64.3%
9.	China	73.1%
10.	Pakistan	80.8%

Table 1. Reported Prevalence of ED in selected Countries.

In the early 1980s, issues of quality of life (Qol) were brought into the fore of medical practice prompting the rise of ED into prominence as a diagnostic entity. According to Pomerville [7] '20 years ago, ED did not exist as a diagnostic term. Its former name 'Impotence' carried a heavy connotation - an impotent man was powerless, worthless, less than a man. Impotence was seldom discussed in the locker rooms or bed rooms of nations" Impotence was relegated and considered to be due to the wears and tears of the aging process for which there is no treatment. This is strongly supported by the following statement by Wyne et al:[8] "for centuries, sexual medicine was a taboo subject practiced by quasiscientists, back alley charlatans and village shamans. Because of a paucity of basic knowledge about the anatomy, Physiology and Pharmacology of the erectile process, many myths on causation and therapy were promulgated through time."

This perception has changed remarkably due to research into ED in the last century which led to the discovery that certain factors are associated with ED with a cause- effect relationship.[9] [10] Currently, there is a better understanding of the incidence, prevalence, etiology and risk factors for ED.

ED is classified as psychogenic, neurological and vasculogenic. Vasculogenic erectile dysfunction, similar to coronary artery disease, is usually due to atherosclerosis, in the case of ED, arthrosclerosis of the branches of the pudendal artery. Cardiovascular risk factors are so classified because of their propensity for causing artherosclersis[12] which may involve the coronary artery thereby predisposing the heart to myocardial hypoperfussion disease. The common denominator in ED and CAD therefore, is arthrosclerosis whose main causes are these life style abnormities referred to as cardiovascular risk factors. The implication of this is that the risk factors for ED and CAD are similar or are in fact the same.[13 14 15]

Hypertension, Diabetes mellitus, dyslipidemia and cigarette smoking have been well documented as predisposing to atherosclerosis of the coronary artery which has earned them the term 'cardiovascular risk factors". Currently, reduced androgen level, particularly testosterone, is under intense research as another risk factor because of the vascular changes associated with it.[16] Several epidemiological studies have demonstrated that ED is more prevalent in men with atherosclerotic disease than the general population. [17] It is now generally accepted that ED, like CAD, results from the endothelial dysfunction which usually co-exist with or predates true atherosclerotic vascular changes.[18]

Documented Risk Factors	**CVS RISK FACTOR BEING EVALUATED**
Cigarette smoking **Dyslipidemia** **Diabetes Mellitus** **Hypertension**	**Low testosterone level**

Table 2. CVS risk factors.

In spite of the adverse effects of ED on quality of life of the affected men, the disease is generally under-reported and under-treated[19] due to poor self reporting as a result of cultural taboos, fear of stigmatization, ignorance on the part of the patient or physician and unavailability of specialists in the area. Erectile dysfunction is a treatable disease and many men have been treated and have returned to normal life especially with the advent of the phosphodiesterase 5 inhibitors. [20] This chapter focuses on erectile dysfunction and its cardiovascular system correlates.

2. Neuroanatomy and physiology of penile erection

The human penis is made up of two dorsally located corpora cavernosa and one ventrally placed corpus spongiosum.[21] The corpus spongiosum expands proximally to form the bulb of the penis while distally it expands to form the glans penis, the most sensitive part of the organ. Proximally, the two corpora cavernrnosa diverge laterally and are attached, one on each side, to the inferior surface of the ischio pubic rami.[22] The erectile tissue proper is located in the corpora cavernosa and surrounded by a tough fibrous tissue called the tunica albuginea.

The corpora cavernosa consist of sinusoids with smooth muscle lined internally by endothelium similar to that of blood vessels. The helicine arteries, the terminal branches of the cavernosal arteries, open directly into the sinusoids. The blood is drained by veins which course beneath the tunica albuginea before piercing it. These join the dorsal vein complex.

The penis is innervated by both autonomic and somatic nerves; the latter supplies the skin while the former sub serves the erectile tissue proper.[23] Somatic supply consist of free nerve endings (receptors) in the skin of the penis, usually up to ten times as numerous in the penile skin and the glans particularly. These receptors coalescence to form the dorsal nerve of the penis, a branch of the pudendal nerve which originates from the dorsal rami of S2 -4. [24] The nerve fibres are mainly unmyelinated C and A delta fibres which sub serve the sensation of pain, pressure and touch (tactile stimulus), the stimulus responsible for reflexogenic erection.The para sympathetic pathway which serves the cavernosa arises from neurons in the S2- 4[25] and follow the ventral rami. This group of cells constitutes the Onuf nucleus and their preganglionic fibres join the sympathetic fibers from the hypogastric plexus to form the pelvic plexus (pelvic splachnic nerves). The post ganglonic fibres (nervi erigentis) arise from the pelvic plexus and passing anterior to the rectum and posteriolateral to the prostate, they pierce the pelvic membrane to reach the corpora cavernosa. They are often damaged during surgical procedures which involve total removal of the prostate and the rectum because of which these procedures are often complicated by erectile dysfunction.[26]

The sympathetic pathway whose fibres are mainly inhibitory originate from T11 - L2 spinal segment. The fibres pass through the white rami to the sympathetic ganglion. Some of these fibres reach the inferior mesenteric and superior hypogastric plexus through the lumbar splanchnic nerves. From the hypogastric plexus, some fibres reach the pelvis and join the parasympathetic fibres to form the pelvic plexus. The fibres from the pelvic plexus which reach the carvenosa along with those from S2-4 are mainly from T10 -12. [27] These fibres also carry impulses which control ejaculation and may be damaged during radical retro peritoneal dissection as they course behind the peritoneum. [28]

The central control of penile erection depends on the input from somatic and autonomic pathways and environmental factors, which include smell, sight and thought of Sex. Tactile impulses from the dorsal nerve of the penis travel via the spino thalamic and spino reticular pathways to the thalamus and sensory cortex for sensory interpretation. Studies have shown that the medial pre-optic area and the para ventricular nucleus of the hypothalamus are the integration centre for erection and sexual activity.[29] It is currently suggested that there may be projections from the hypothalamic nuclei to the sacral erection centre, S2 – 4, as is found in animals. Other centres which contribute to control of sexual activity also abound in the mid brain and medulla.[30]

Several neuro transmitters are involved in penile erection and control of sexual activity. The neuro transmitter traditionally associated with the parasympathetic (parasympathetic finally control erection) is acetylcholine while nor– adrenaline and adrenaline are involved in sympathetic transmission. Other neuro-transmitters secreted at the level of the autonomic nervous system in the genito-urinary tract are vaso- active intestinal peptide (VIP) and several prostaglandins. These neurotransmitters do not however, completely account for the events that lead to penile erection. Currently, the substance which is considered to act as the neurotransmitter involved in penile erection is a non adrenergic, non cholinergic (NANC) and it is now known to be nitric oxide (NO). [31]

Nitric oxide is a ubiquitous neuro-transmitter in the lower urinary tract [32] and its role in penile erection process is presently well documented. It is formed from L-arginine under the control of Nitric oxide synthase. [33] There are three isoforms of Nitric oxide synthase; eNos, nNos and iNos depending on the cell in which it is synthesized. Neural stimulation causes release of Nitric oxide from neurons while its release from endothelium is in response to sheer stress. [34] The neurotransmitters involved in the central control of penile erection and sexual activity include oxytocin, gama amminobutyric acid and serotonin.

In the flaccid state, the smooth muscle of the cavernosa is semi contracted under the tonic influence of the sympathetic system, its intrinsic myogenic activity and endothelium derived factors such as prostaglandin $_{F2}$ alpha. [37] In this state, the blood flow to the penis is kept at the barest minimum required to meet its nutritional needs at a pCo2 of 35mmHg.[38] Following sexual stimulation, the non adrenergic non cholinergic fibres which accompany the parasympathetic to the cavernosa, release nitric oxide which triggers the erectile process [39].

- Central (smell, thought) and tactile (penile skin) stimulus
- Processing of resulting impulses by the Onuf nucleus.
- Activation of the effector pathway (nervi-erigentes).
- Release of neuronal NO following neuronal NO Synthase activation.
- Activation of the NO-cGMP pathway.
- Increase blood flow into the cavernous sinus-penile erection.
- Increase flow stimulates release of endothelial NO- sustained erection

Table 3. Summary of physiology of penile erection.

Nitric oxide is a potent vasodilator which readily diffuses into the cell to initiate a series of bio-chemical events. Nitric oxide modulates the activities of guanylate cyclase, [40] an action which leads to the conversion of guanosine triphosphate (GTP) to cyclic guanosine monophosphate (cGMP). The latter, acting as a second messenger, regulates calcium channel activities including those of intracellular contractile proteins that lead to the relaxation of corpus cavernosal smooth muscle.[41] Specifically, cGMP activates protein

Kinase G leading to a decrease in calcium influx into the cell which in turn causes activation of myokinase and finally, relaxation of corpora smooth muscle, a sine qua non in the erectile process [42].

Penile erection is classified as: Central, reflexogenic and Nocturnal. [43] In central erection, the stimulus is from thought, site and smell related to Sexual intercourse which activates the spinal centres, the impulses of which travel through the parasympathetic to the corpora. Reflexogenic erection results from tactile stimulation of the dorsal nerve of the penis. The afferent pathway reaches the onuf nucleus which then activates the erectile parasympathetic pathway via the same process as in central erection. Nocturnal Penile tumescence (NPT) is currently poorly understood. It occurs during rapid eye movement sleep and it is presently thought to play a key role in keeping the erectile tissue per fussed. [3]

Following central or reflexogenic stimulus, there is activation of the parasympathetic erectile pathway with the release of nitric oxide and the consequent cascade of events which lead to relaxation of cavernous smooth muscle and the helicine arteries. The ensuing rapid influx of blood into the sinusoids leads to increased intra cavernosal pressure and compression of the sub tunical venous system against the tunica abulginea. There is reduced outflow in the presence of markedly increased inflow and the penis becomes firm and increased in size - phase of full erection. Through the pudendal nerve, sexual impulses also reach the ischio carveranosus and bulbospongiosus muscles which contract vigorously, further impeding venous drainage - phase of rigid erection.

Penile detumescense is a consequence of the intense, diffuse sympathetic discharge which herald orgasm, emission and ejaculation. The catecholamines released in the process cause smooth muscle contraction, thereby terminating erection. The smooth muscle contraction leads to reduced blood flow into the sinusoids, reduced intra cavernosa pressure and the opening of the venous channels. There is therefore increased venous outflow in the presence of reduced arterial inflow. The trapped blood in the sinusoids is expelled and the penis becomes flaccid[23].

Parasympathetic NANC system

↓

Guanylate Cyclase

↓ ↓

Smooth muscle←GTP **CGMP→SMC relax**

Contraction

and detumescense **and penis erect**

↑

PDES5

↑

Sympathetic System

Fig. 1. Penile tumescence and detumescence

3. Atherosclerosis

Arteries vary in wall thickness and size and based on these, they are classified as[45] (A) Elastic or large arteries. A typical example is the aorta, Innorminate, subclavian and illiac arteries (b) Medium sized arteries typical of which are coronary arteries (c) Small arteries. These are usually less than 2mm in diameter, coursing for most of their path through the substance of the issue or organ. A good example is the pudendal and cavernosa arteries which supply the penile erectile tissue and upon which erection depends. The arterial wall, independent of class, is made up of three layers namely;

1. Adventitia. This is a fibrous tissue which covers the artery externally and separates it from the surrounding structures or tissues.
2. The media. This is responsible for most of the wall thickness and consists mostly of smooth muscle cells (SMC) which are under the tonic control of the endothelium.[46] It is from this layer that SMC are recruited in the formation of atheroma.
3. The intima. This consists of a single layer of endothelium which rests on a basement membraine. The endothelial cells are joined together by tight junctions which are normally impermeable to most substances in the blood.

The endothelium is physiologically endowed to control the vessel in order to vary blood flow according to tissue, organ and regional requirements. It is in most part, responsible for the smooth flow of blood and therefore has profound effect on vascular reactivity and thrombogenesis. It inhibits platelet aggregation, reduces the recruitment of inflammatory cells into the intima and the entry of lipids into the arterial wall.

The endothelium secretes a wide variety of substances with paracrine effect while also expressing receptors for various substances in the blood stream, the latter including hormones, local mediators and vasoactive substances. Based on these, the endothelium is capable of sensing and responding to local changes either by causing vasodilatation or constriction. The overall effect of endothelial reactivity is however vasodilatation or a tendency to vasodilatation reaching up to 80% in the penile arterial bed as against 15% in other tissues.[47 48]

Nitric oxide (NO) is a major neurotransmitter produced by the endothelium and is responsible for the endothelium derived vasodilatation. It is produced, as a neurotransmitter, in most parts of the lower urinary tract either normally or pathologically.[49] It inhibits cytochrome C oxidase, reduces oxygen consumption by the vasculature and inhibits or modifies the endothelial cells for circulating white blood cells. Its release is stimulated by acetyl choline, brandykin, substance P and sheer stress on the arterial wall.

- Endothelial dysfunction is defined as a state of altered phenotype which leads to impairment of vascular reactivity or an induced surface which is thrombogenic or abnormally adhesive for inflammatory cells.[45] This change may predate or co-exist with atherosclerosis and is characterized by loss of vascular reactivity. The initial phase is characterized by decreased bioavailability of nitric oxide either due to reduced production or increased breakdown. There is therefore loss of the endothelium derived smooth muscle relaxation with a tendency to vasoconstriction and increased peripheral resistance. These effects have been implicated in hypertension, diabetes mellitus, cigarette smoking and hyperlipidemia, all of which are risk factors for ED and CAD.

Endothelial dysfunction is a systemic disease and it is usually as a result of diverse injury including sheer stress, trauma and inflammation. It occurs in the initial and subsequent phases of atherosclerosis. Though all arterial beds are affected, the effects manifests earlier in the smaller vessel beds[50] such as the pudendal artery which supply the erectile tissue of the penis. In the presence of endothelial dysfunction, the endothelium becomes unduly permeable, allowing substances such as lipids, proteins and macrophages into the intima, a sin-qua non for atherosclerotic changes.

- Atherosclerosis is characterized by intimal lesion called atheroma or atheromatous plagues or fibrofatty plagues which project into the lumen of the vessel. It forms the common pathway through which the well documented cardiovascular risk factors cause their deleterious effects on the heart, cerebrum and the erectile tissues. Endothelial dysfunction results from inhibition of dimethyl arginine dimethyl amino hydrolase which catalyses the hydrolysis of asymmetric dimethyl arginine, an inhibitor of endothelial nitric oxide synthase. The subsequent uncoupling of eNos leads to endothelial oxidative stress and formation of peroxy nitrates, oxidation of pro-inflammatory nuclear factor Kappa B and hence cellular inflammation.[51]

Endothelial inflammation causes increase permeability of the endothelial cells and the tight junctions. The subsequent increased movement of lipids, protein and inflammatory cells, particularly macrophages into the intima, initiates the process of atherosclerosis which affects all the arterial bed. Timing of clinical appearance however depends on the severity and size of the affected vessel as up to 75% of the vessel lumen maybe occluded before effects become obvious.[52] Smaller vessels such as the pudendal artery may be occluded up to ten years before bigger vessels like the coronary arteries are affected. This explains why erectile dysfunction usually precedes the occurrence of coronary artery diseases or stroke.

Cvs Risk Factors
↓
Endothelial dysfunction → activation of hydrolase
↓ ↓
Increase permeability to lipids/others
↓
Atheroma formation → ED &CAD ← Inhibition of eNos

Fig. 2. Mechnisms by which CVS risk factors cause ED and CAD

4. Cardiovascular risk factors and erectile dysfunction

4.1 Diabetes mellitus

Diabetes mellitus(DM) is defined as persistent hyperglycemia secondary to relative or absolute insulin deficiency. This has a profound effect on protein, lipid and carbohydrate metabolism with a myriad of complications of which ED is one. These complications can broadly be classified as vascular or neurologic and ED has been documented in both classes. In DM, neurologic damage which may predispose to ED usually result from peripheral neuropathy and ED is well known to be associated with both somatic and autonomic neuropathies. [53] Both types of autonomic neuropathies ie, axonal and demyelinating, occur in DM and are responsible for the 'failure to initiate' type of ED.

Vascular damage from DM causes the 'failure to fill' type of erectile dysfunction. This results from endothelial dysfunction and or atherosclerosis both of which are companions of diabetes mellitus. Diabetes mellitus is associated with low grade inflammation, dyslipidemia, hypertension and the metabolic syndrome all of which, as independent entities, are risk factors for ED. This low grade inflammatory state in DM has been well documented by many authors who have demonstrated elevated c-Reactive protein, Tumor Necrosis Factor alpha (TNF) and interleukin 6 (IL-6) in diabetic patients with ED who have no other risk factors. [54 55 56]

The low grade inflammation in DM causes endothelial dysfunction which leads to an endothelium that is more thrombogenic and permeable to lipids, inflammatory cells such as macrophages. This initiates the process of atherosclerosis which is usually diffuse and occurs earlier in diabetic patients. (The reader is referred to standard vascular texts for the pathology of atherosclerosis) The ensuing diffuse atherosclerosis and micro-angiopathy is responsible for the nephropathy, retinopathy, stroke, coronary artery disease and ED that accompany DM. According to Meng et al, [57] higher glucose levels induces apoptosis in endothelial cells while Di Filippo et al [58] conclude that DM is associated with increased cardiovasular disease due to established risk factors such as dyslipdemia , hypertension and atherosclerosis as a result of increased inflammation. This leads to the production of free oxygen radicals, impaired NO metabolism and increased movement of lipids into the intima leading to early and diffuse atherosclerosis. Through this atherosclerotic damage, cerebral, cardiac, renal and erectile function maybe impaired.

The pathophysiologic relationship between diabetes mellitus and erectile dysfunction, according to Moore et al, [59] is multifactorial. They proposed the mechanism of ED in DM to include elevated advance glycation end products, increased level of free oxygen radicals, impaired NO synthesis, increased endothelin B binding sites and ultrastructural changes, up regulated Rhoa/ Rho-Kinase pathway, NO dependent selective nitregic nerve degeneration and impaired c-GMP dependent kinase. Overall, there is impaired flow mediated dilatation in DM patients which is in part secondary to increased inflammation and endothelial and platelet activation[60]

- Other associated CVS risk factors e.g. hypertension, dyslipidemia.
- Low grade inflammation causing endothelial dysfunction.
- Production of free O2 radicals, impaired NO metabolism.
- Elevated advance glycation end products.
- Increased endothelin B receptor binding sites.
- Up regulation of RhOA/Rho-Kinase Pathway.
- Nitric oxide dependent selective nitregic nerve degeneration.

Table 4. Summary of Causes of ED in DM.

ED is highly common in type 2 DM (T2DM) patients and the duration of DM is usually longer in ED patients. The atherosclerotic process is usually ongoing, dynamic and progressive [61]making the clinical course of ED in DM gradual and ED may be the only sign[62]. As DM, especially type 2, maybe present for years before diagnosis, many patients already have complications before or at presentation and this may include ED. Based on these, it has been proposed that ED should be regarded as an observable marker of DM. In a study of ED In diabetics, Sun et al [63] concluded that men with ED are more than twice likely to have DM, strongly so for men 45 years and below but not for men older than 66 years. Twelve percent of men studied by Deutsch et al [64] were found to have unrecognized DM while the Massachusetts Male Aging Study (MMAS) [65] showed that the probability of ED is three times more common in men who reported being treated for DM and figures as high as three quarters of all diabetics have been documented. DM has other complications such as leg ulcers which impact negatively on psyche and quality of life and in such patients, ED may be partly psychogenic. This should not be underestimated in the course of evaluation.

4.2 Hypertension

Essential hypertension is the leading risk factor for mortality worldwide accounting for 13% of all deaths globally.[66] It is the most common non communicable disease in Nigeria[67] and according to Essien et al,[68] the mean venous blood glucose level of hypertensive adult Nigerians is higher than their normotensive counterparts. According to recent studies, approximately 67-68% of men with hypertension have some degree of erectile dysfunction.[69]

Erectile dysfunction in hypertension, similar to diabetes mellitus, results from endothelial dysfunction and or atherosclerosis. Endothelial dysfunction in hypertension is caused by the sheer stress of elevated blood pressure on the vessel wall.[70] This endothelial damage causes the impairment of endothelium derived relaxation. The inflammation which accompanies endothelial dysfunction leads to altered NO metabolism, formation of free oxygen radicals and an increased movement of lipids into the intima, a necessity for atheromatous vascular damage. Hypertension is associated with structural and functional changes in the arterial wall and this is responsible for the mortality and morbidity associated with it.[71]

In a number of cardiovascular pathologies, such as hypertension and heart failure, according to Boulauger et al,[72] the balance in the endothelial production of vasodialating mediators is altered. The underlying dysfunction is likely to be the consequence of the high blood pressure and could facilitate the maintenance of elevated peripheral resistance with subsequent development of atherosclerosis. The ensuing arterial stiffness is an independent cardiovascular risk factor.[73] From this perspective, it can be deduced that hypertension is an independent risk factor for coronary heart disease and vasculogenic erectile dysfunction. In the work of Modebe[74] in Nigeria, 8% of the untreated hypertension population had erectile dysfunction while this was 61% in the treated group. Treatment, rather than the hypertension therefore, may be responsible for the ED and may account for the non compliance with treatment frequently seen in this group of patients who may want to maintain their potency. This agrees with the of opinion of Shiri et al[75] who in their study concluded that the risk of ED is higher in men suffering from treated hypertension and heart disease than in those with the untreated condition

Erectile function and neuromuscular transmission are calcium dependent phenomena, which to a large extent, depends on the general physical well being of the man. Erectile dysfunction is associated with the use of calcium channel blockers, angiotensin II antagonist, non selective alpha blockers and diuretics. The continuous use of diuretics, particularly thiazide diuretics, is often accompanied by dehydration, electrolyte imbalance and elevated blood sugar all of which may lead to ED or aggravate an already existing mild disease. ED is however not currently known to be associated with the use of organic nitrates, angiotensin converting enzymes (ACE) inhibitors, selective alpha blockers and drugs that lower serum lipid levels.

• Ultrastructural changes in the vessel wall. • Endothelial dysfunction and atherosclerosis. • Medication side effect e.g. diuretics. • Target organ damage e.g. stroke and heart failure.

Table 5. Summary of causes of ED in hypertension

The preliminary report of the telmisartan alone, and in combination with ramipril global end point trial/telmisartan randomized assessment study in ACE – intolerant subjects with cardiovascular disease (ONTARGET/TRACEND) study[76] has shown that on the contrary, calcium channel blockers tend to have a significant adverse effect on erectile function whereas diuretics, beta blockers, ACE inhibitors, ATI antagonist and alpha blockers do not. Treatment with ACE inhibitors and ATI antagonist or a combination of both is suggested to improve erectile function in cardiovascular high risk patients.

On the overall, hypertension is complicated by numerous vascular conditions which impact negatively on the quality of life of the affected men. Apart from coronary heart disease and erectile dysfunction, conditions such as hypertensive renal damage, intermittent claudication, retinal damage and heart failure often complicate hypertension and lower the quality of life of these men, with severe effect on their psyche. Like DM therefore, the contribution of psychogenic erectile dysfunction in hypertensives should not be underestimated in the course of treatment.

5. Cigarrette smoking/dylipidemia

Cigarette smoking is currently a major health concern and in spite of the vigorous campaign against it, more people continue to take to smoking in many countries of the world. The most well mentioned and documented toxin of cigarette smoke is nicotine but others exist. Cigarette smoke is directly toxic to vascular endothelium[77] and this culminates in vascular endothelial dysfunction, functional and architectural changes in the vessel wall.[78] The cascade of events which follow this endothelial dysfunction is similar to that in DM and hypertension. The end result is atherosclerosis and its deleterious effect on penile erectile, cardiac and cerebral function.

According to Chen et al, [79] an increased ED prevalence has been reported in patients with chronic obstructive airway diseases and sustained inflammation seem to play a central role in this linkage. Cigarette smoking has traditionally been associated to chronic obstructive airway disease (chronic bronchitis, emphysema) and through this mechanism, it may contribute significantly to the burden of ED. These conditions, similar to DM, are accompanied by low level chronic inflammation, elevated c-Reactive protein and may be followed by diffuse endothelial dysfunction and atherosclerosis.[80] This low grade inflammatory state allow increase in low density lipoprotein transport across the endothelium into the intima, thereby initiating the process of atherosclerosis.

• Direct toxicity to vascular endothelium. • Functional and structural changes in vessel wall. • Chronic obstructive airway disease. • Endothelial dysfunction and atherosclerosis. • Reduction in concentration of NO synthase.

Table 6. Summary of causes of ED in cigarette smoking and Dyslipidemia

Dyslipidemia and obesity are major components of the metabolic syndrome (MS) which is currently well documented as being accompanied by a low systemic inflammatory state which predisposes to vascular endothelial dysfunction.[81]This is the underlying mechanism of ED in men who have the metabolic syndrome and concomitant ED. This is evidenced by the presence of raised level of inflammatory markers in the affected men. MS and obesity are linked to lowered serum testosterone[82] in a double edge manner and low serum testosterone as an independent cardiovascular risk factor, is presently being examined. It is considered to be due to the reduced level of sex hormone binding globulin. Additionally, in obesity which is often present in MS, there is increased level of low density lipoprotein as a result of abnormal insulin metabolism.[82]

A third of citizens of the United States are presently considered, by current definition, to be obese[83] and the prevalence of MS in ED population is 45% compared with 24% in matched control.[84] Conversely, the prevalence of ED in MS population is 34 - 43% and this depends on the number of independent risk factors-[85] dyslipidemia, hypertension and diabetes mellitus. Dyshpidemia is also often an accompaniment of DM and hypertension in different combinations. However, dyslipidemia is an independent risk factor for ED and CAD.[86] Hypercholesterolemia has a well established link with endothelial dysfunction with oxidized low density lipoprotein being a key mediator.[87] According to Brunner et al, [77] in familial hypercholesterolemia, endothelial dysfunction is present prior to clinical arterial disease. Endothelial dysfunction is related to particle size and concentration, [88] transport across the endothelium being inversely related to the particle size and directly to the concentration. This explains why low density lipoprotein, and not high density lipoproteins, [89] is incriminated in endothelial dysfunction. Low density lipoprotein leads to reduction in endogenous NO synthase[90] which in turn causes a reduced bioavailability of the endothelium derived relaxation factor, NO, probably by enhancing super oxide anion. Lipoproteins are transported across the endothelium by the process of transcytosis and in the presence of endothelial dysfunction, reduced NO bioavailability and increased concentration of LDL, this process is enhanced leading to atherosclerotic vascular changes. In contrast, HDLs are presently considered to enhance endothelial function and a low concentration may predispose to endothelial dysfunction.[91]

6. Coronary Artery Disease (CAD)

In Britain, approximately a quarter of all deaths among men and one-fifth of all deaths among women are due to ischemic heart diseases.[92] In England and Wales, 30% of all deaths among men and 22% among women are as a result of ischemic heart diseases. [93] Through atherosclerotic narrowing, cardiac ischemia precipitates cardiac malfunction and sometimes infarction of the myocardium. The major risk factors for endothelial dysfunction and atherosclerosis, which are also the cause of CAD and ED, are hypertension DM, dyslipidemia and cigarette smoking and these life style abnormalities have been traditionally documented as cardiovascular risk factors.

ED is related to CAD in a double edged manner. ED represents an independent risk factor for feature CVS event independent of classic risk factors such as hypertension, DM and dyslipidema [94]. The common denominator for ED, CAD and these cardiovascular risk factors is endothelial dysfunction which is usually diffuse, affecting several arterial beds such as the pudendal and coronary arteries and thereafter culminating in atherosclerosis. In 2003 Montorsi et al [95] proposed the small artery theory to explain the earlier occurrence of ED than CAD. Coronary arteries, being larger than the pudendal arteries, take a longer period for occlusion from endothelial dysfunction and atherosclerotic vacscular narrowing to occur. Eventually, as the atherosclerosis progresses, larger vessels such as the cerebral, coronary and renal arteries become involved and this precipitates target organ damage.

Several studies have documented this with clear evidence. In the study by Pritzter, [96] of 20 men, out of a study group of 50 who were investigated angiographically following self reported ED without any other complaints, all have demonstrable disease. They compared sexual function to the penile stress test as a window to the hearts of men. Vlachopoulos et al [97] investigated men whose only complaint was ED and found angiographically silent CAD in 19%. Bensal et al [98] also in their work documented 56% asymptomatic CAD in an ED population. Ultimately, in some of these men, CAD become overt, and as documented by Rodriguez et al [99] in DM, taking an average period of 38.8 months. According to their study, 100% of DM men experienced ED prior to onset of CAD. Based on this premise, ED is currently considered a sentinel event for CAD as both have their origin from endothelial dysfunction and atherosclerosis.[100] These are mounting evidence therefore, that ED is an early predictor of CAD and that there is need for physicians to evaluate men who present with ED, with no other cardiovascular symptom, for CAD and its risk factors. [101]

CAD is an independent risk factor for ED and the prevalence of ED in CAD population is remarkable. James et al[102] studied the relation between ED and CAD in men referred for stress myocardial perfusion single-photon emission computed tomography (MPS). They concluded that men sent for MPS have a higher prevalence of ED. Also, men with ED exhibited a higher prevalence of severe CAD and left ventricular dysfunction than those without ED. In the work of Bensal, [98] 75% of men with CAD have symptoms of ED and 91% of their ED populations have cardiovascular risks. This has implication for men who have CAD and who intend to engage in sexual activity. Herschorn[100] in his work on cardiovascular safety of phosphodiestares 5 inhibitors said that "in general, sexual activity has an effect similar to mild-moderate exercise in increasing heart rate, blood pressure, cardiac output and respiratory rate. The degree of change in these physiologic parameters however, is greater than expected because of disproportionate increase in sympathetic activation. The absolute risk of sexual activity triggering a myocardial infarction (MI) is low. Men with CAD or previous MI have a 10-fold higher risk, which means that during sexual inter-course, the probability of such a man having MI is 20/Million/hour".

7. Heart failture (HF)

Several cardiovascular disorders cause heart failure which may be left or right sided failure. These include hypertension, congenital and acquired heart defects and cardiomyophathies. Left side failure usually results from hypertension, mitral and aortic valvular abnormalities which may be acquired or congenital. Eventually, left sided failure leads to pulmonary hypertension and with continued back pressure, right sided failure which is referred to as congestive cardiac failure (CCF). Heart failure may occur independent of traditional cardiovascular risk factors or in association with one or more of them. For instance, Ukoh[103] et al in their study observed hyperlipidemia in three groups of patients. (1) Hypertensive's with or without heart disease (2) patients with ischemic heart disease and (3) those with hypertensive cardiomyopathy. ED may therefore occur in men with heart failure not because of the failure itself, but because of the background cardiovascular risk factors present.

The prevalence of heart failure (HF) in the United States, according to the American Heart Association, is estimated at 5.3 million.[104] ED is present, estimatedly, in 60.8% of heart failure patients and prevalence ranging from 81 to 91% has been documented in this group.[105] In CCF, there is peripheral venous stasis, decreased venous return, reduced stroke volume and cardiac output, a must situation for physical in-activity or under-activity. Most patients with chronic cardiovascular disease experience decreased libido and frequency of sexual activity as well as ED.

- Endothelial dysfunction.
- Reduced cardiac output.
- Exercise in tolerance from PH.
- Associated CVS Risk factors.
- Drug side effect.

Table 7. Causes of ED in Heart Failure

The ED in HF patients is multifactorial in origin. Anxiety or depression may lead to performance fears and therefore psychogenic ED. The reduced pulmonary and cardiac reserve in CCF patients makes exercise intolerable, bearing in mind that sexual activity involve mild to moderate exercise and that most of erectile function is CVS event. Treatment of heart failure may lead to ED as a side effect of the drugs used. Diuretics, particular thiazides,[106]are associated with ED through unknown mechanism which may not be unconnected with the accompanying electrolyte imbalance. Beta blockers, Digoxin and aldosterone are also documented as causing ED. Heart failure is accompanied by endothelial dysfunction which as an independent factor, may cause ED in these men.[107]

8. Treatment of ED complicating CVS risk factors and disease

Following the evaluation of these men (this is beyond the scope of this chapter), there is need for treatment in order to improve their quality of life. Gerald et al[108] evaluated the sexual attitudes and beliefs of middle aged and older adults in non-European 'Westernized' countries in their work. Approximately 85% of men and women felt that satisfactory sexual intercourse is essential for the maintenance of a relationship. Most respondents felt that it is acceptable for older men to use medication to enable them to continue to enjoy sexual activity. By extension, this is necessary if they are to continue to maintain spousal relationship which at this age has profound effect on quality of life and longevity.

ED is multifactorial in terms of etiology, the implication of which is that treatment should be holistic. It is based on this premise that David et al[109] proposed a multifaceted approach with the argument that no single agent has proven to be highly efficacious. He supported this with the work of Goldstein et al[110] in which though, 84% of men had improved function following treatment with sildenafil, they achieved a fully rigid erection only four times per month. This is limiting for a couple and may therefore not be enough to maintain a satisfactory relationship.

9. Life style modification

9.1 Smoking and alcohol

According to Feldman et al, [6] smoking doubles the risk of developing ED. Cigarette smoking increases the risk of death from CAD and according to Derling et al,[111] also the incidence of ED. Traditionally, alcohol has been associated with the capacity to lower serum cholesterol and therefore improve erectile function. Alcohol has a central sedating effect which may be over powering. It is also associated with lowered NO production.[112] Men who smoke and drink alcohol should be advised to cease smoking and alcohol consumption. The later may be restricted to a single daily drink, preferably, red wine which has been documented to improve NO production.

9.2 Regular exercise

Regular exercise is beneficial to all body tissues and organs particularly in healthy individuals. During exercise, the cardiac output, the chronotropic and inotropic activity of the heart increase and the circulation therefore becomes more rapid. The blood supply to different organs and tissues, particularly the heart and muscles, increase with remarkable improvement in tissue perfusion. A sedentary life style is three times as likely to lead to ED where as moderate physical activity reduces the risk of ED by two-thirds.[113] The sheer stress of increase blood flow stimulates the production of NO, an effect which lasts for up to 2-7days with a magnitude in the order of fourfold.[114] During penile erection, the increase in flow is more than this, implying a more increased production of NO. On this premise, some studies have shown improved erectile function in men with regular and frequent sexual activity.

Regular exercise also may help control weight gain, obesity, dyslipidimia and the metabolic syndrome. Reduction in weight in the already obese men may lead to regularization of testosterone concentration and correct the loss of libido often associated with ED in the obese. Men with ED should therefore be advised on regular physical exercise and sexual activity.

9.3 Modification of diet

Diet has a profound effect on the general well being and it is part of general healthy living that men should be mindful of what they eat. Diet modification can help control weight gain, glucose level in diabetes and cholesterol level in dyslipidemic men. When combined with regular exercise, the effect may be synergistic with remarkable weight loss and it has been documented that about one-third of obese men with ED are able to improve sexual function through life style changes.[115] Dietary modification should involve the services of a trained dietician who should set a target from the beginning, bearing in mind existing co-morbidities and the age of the patients.

9.4 Principles of medical treatment

The medical treatment for erectile dysfunction complicating CVS risk factors and disease should necessarily include treating for the underlying risk factors[107]. These include the control of hypertension, diabetes mellitus, dyslipidemia, heart failure and coronary artery disease. Although this therapeutic approach, according to Tikkanen et al[116], appears justified, relatively few intervention studies have investigated the effect of risk factor reduction on established ED. However, in the work by Saltzman et al[117], artovastatin treatment of men with hyperlipidemia as the only risk factor, for instance, led to an improvement in erectile function. The medical treatment of these risk factors is beyond this chapter but a few guiding principles need to be explained.

Route of Administration	Drugs Used
1. Oral	a. Phosphodiesterase 5 inhibitors 1. Sildenafil 2. Vardanefil 3. Tadalafil b. Peripheral alpha 1 blockers 1. Phentolamine Mesylate c. Central Alpha2 antagonist 1. Yohimbine d. Dopamine agonists 1. Apomorpine
2. Intra-Urethral	a. Direct smooth muscle relaxant 1. Aprostodil (PGEI)
3. Intra-cavernosal (injectable)	a. Phosphodiesterase Inhibitor 1. Papaverine b. Peripheral alpha 1 blocker 1. Phentolamine c. Direct smooth muscle relaxant 1. Aprostodil (PGEI) 2. Vaso-active intestinal peptide (VIP).

Table 8. Summary of Drugs used in Pharmacotherapy for ED

There are conflicting reports on the effects of the drugs used for specific therapy of these risk factors and disease on ED. Statins have been reported to improve erectile function due to their positive effect on endothelial function.[118] There are however observational reports associating statin use with ED.[119] Diuretics, calcium channel blockers and beta blockers used for the treatment of hypertension and digoxin used for heart-failure have all been reportedly linked with ED. The preliminary report of the telmisartan alone, and in combination with ramipril global end point trial/telmisartan randomized assessment study in ACE-intolerant subjects with cardiovascular Disease (CONTARGET/TRANCEND) study[76] shows that calcium channel blockers tend to have a significant adverse effect on erectile function while treatment with beta blockers, diuretics, ACE inhibitors, ATI antagonist and alpha antagonist do not. Treatment with ACE inhibitors, ATI antagonist or a combination of both is suggested to improve erectile function in cardiovascular high risk patients. Based on this premise, the treating physician is advised to document the base-line erectile function at the commencement of treatment as subsequent development of ED is often quoted as responsible for non compliance by the affected men who may wish to maintain their potency. In the course of treatment, these men should be questioned directly about erectile function, and if this wanes or the patients complain, the drugs should be withdrawn. If erectile function returns, the drug/drugs can then be documented as the culprit and permanently withdrawn. This emphasizes the need for individualization of the management of these men.

Erectile dysfunction has social implications for the couple and any treatment regimen should necessarily take the female partner into consideration[114]. Some modalities of treatment may require the co-operation of the female partner due to their psychosocial and medical side effects which may be distressful to the couple. For instance, apormorphine may cause nausea and or vomiting sometimes necessitating the use of anti-emetics. Table 8 shows some of the drugs for the treatment of ED, their mode of administration and some of their side effects. Also, the use of phosphodiesterase 5 inhibitors is associated with diverse reaction which may threaten life.

9.5 Treatment of ED in CAD and HF patients; Use of PDE 5 inhibitors

The development and approval for use of the phosphodiesterase 5 inhibitors has revolutionized the treatment of erectile dysfunction, but this is not without short-comings especially in men with HF and CAD. The main stay of the treatment of CAD is the use of nitrates which dilate the coronary arterial bed. The active factor in the nitrates is the nitric-oxide which it releases and which is also the endothelium dependent vasodilator and neurotransmitter mostly responsible for penile erection in man. The phosphodiesterase 5 inhibitors inhibit the breakdown of nitric oxide, an action which potentiates that of the nitrates used for the treatment of CAD.

Patients with heart disease have a reduced exercise tolerance because of which there is need to assess and advise them on fitness to undergo sexual activity. They should be stratified into low risk, intermediate risk and high risk based on the presence and number of risk factors, angina, previous MI and their New York Heart Association classification status[121]. The amount of energy required for sexual activity has been shown to be about 20-40 metabolic equivalent of the tasks which is equivalent to doing easy house hood work or climbing a flight of stairs. This should guide the physician in advising patients with heart failure provided that aortic stenosis and obstructive valvular cardiomyophathy have been excluded.

Opinions are varied as to whether the phosphodiesterase 5 inhibitors should be used in patients who have coronary artery disease and concomitant erectile dysfunction. According to George et al[121], on the basis of the pharmacokinetic profile of sildenafil for instance, the co-administration of a nitrate within the first 24 hours is likely to produce a severe, potentially, life threatening hypotensive response and it is therefore contradicted. However, Parker et al[122] insist in their work that though contradicted, there are occasions when a patient who has recently taken a phosphodiesterase 5 inhibitor might need intravenous nitroglycerin treatment with the proviso that such patients should be closely monitored and should have stable CAD. In the work by Webb et al,[123] when sublingual nitroglycerin was administered, there was a fourfold decrease in systolic blood pressure In patients with sildenafil treatment. Their conclusion was that sildenafil potentiated the hypotensive effect of nitrates and their concomitant use was absolutely contra indicated. According to Velasquez et al[124] adverse cardiac event associated to sildenafil use, for instance, include MI, angina, ventricular tachycardia and death. Therefore, the use of phosphodiesterase 5 inhibitors and nitrates in men with ED and concomitant CAD should be done with caution, individualized and in consultation between the physician and Urologist in order to optimize care.

10. Surgical treatment

Surgical treatment of ED has been relegated to the background as the last option with the advent of effective medical therapy. The main-stay of surgical treatment includes the use of penile implants and penile arterial revascularization procedures.[125] Infection is a major setback in the use of penile implants particularly in DM.Penile revascularization procedures may be complicated by numbness of the glans and penile skin, defeating the aim of the surgery. Penile venous surgery is presently considered historical.

11. Use of vacuum erection devices

These devices induce erection by increasing corporal perfusion and or impeding venous return.[126] Their efficacy profile is good but non compliance by patients is high due to difficulty with operating them and the associated ejaculatory problems. In truth, vacuum erection devices cause a hinged erection and the penis is rather truly not rigid.

12. Conclusion

Endothelial dysfunction and atherosclerosis are the pathways through which cardiovascular risk factors predispose to coronary artery disease, stroke and erectile dysfunction, the ED occurring earlier because of the small size of the pudendal artery which supplies the cavernous bed. As atherosclerosis is a progressive and dynamic disease, larger vessels are eventually involved and this often includes the coronary artery with the development of CAD. ED is presently regarded as a sentinel event for CAD and patients who present with ED with no other risk factors should be evaluated for silent CAD. The drugs used for the treatment of CVS risk factors may have ED as side effect and patients should therefore be questioned directly for the occurrence of ED. The concomitant use of nitrates and phosphodiesterase 5 inhibitors calls for caution.

13. References

[1] National Institute of Health Consensus Development Panel on Impotence. Proceeding of a conference held December 7/9, 1992, Bethesda (Maryland), USA. *JAMA* 1993:270:83-90

[2] Ayta 1A, Mckinlay JB, Krane RJ. The likely world-wide increase in erectile dysfunction between 1995 and 2005 and some possible policy consequences. *BJU Int.* 1999,84:50-56

[3] Hoffman BM, Sherwood A, Smith PJ, Babyak MA, Doraiswamy PM, Hinderliter A. Cardiovascular disease risk, vascular Health and erectile dysfunction among middle-aged clinically depressed men. *Inter J Impot Res* 2010; 22:30-35.

[4] Yang G, Pan C, Lu J. Prevalence of erectile dysfunction among Chinese men with type 2 diabetes mellitus. *Inter J Impot Res*2010; 22:310-317.

[5] Shaeer KZM, Osegbe DN, Siddiqui SH, Razzaque A, Glasser DB, Jaguste R. Prevalence of erectile dysfunction and its correlates among men attending primary care clinic in three countries: Pakistan, Egypt and Nigeria. *Int J Imp Res* 2003; 5:8-14.

[6] Fedman HA, Goltstein I, Hatzichristo DG, Krane RJ, Mcklinlay JB. Impotence and its medical and Psychosocial correlates. Results of the Massachusetts male aging study. *J Urol* 1994; 15:54-61.

[7] Pomerville P. Erectile dysfunction, an over-view. *Can J Urol* 2003; 10(1): 2-6.

[8] Wyne. JG Hellstrom. The Molecular basis of erectile physiology: from bench to bedside. *Journal of Andrology* 2002; 23 (5):83-4.

[9] Miner M, Billups KL. Erectile dysfunction and dyslipidemia: Relevance and role of phosphodiesterase types 5 inhibitors and statins. *J sex med.* 2005; 5 (5):1066-78.

[10] Conti CR, Pepine CJ, Sweeney M. Efficacy and safety of sildenafil citrate in the treatment of erectile dysfunction in patients with ischemic heart disease. *Am J Cardiol* 1999; 83 (5A):29c-34c.

[11] Ross R. Atherosclerosis-an inflammatory disease. *N Engl. J med.* 1999; 340:115-126.

[12] Ponholzer A, Gutjahr G, Temml V, Madersbacher. Is erectile dysfunction a predictor of cardiovascular event or stroke? A prospective study using a validated questionnaire. *Int J Impot Res* 2010; 22:25-29.

[13] Chang ST, Chu CM, Hsu JT, Hsiao JF, Chung CM, Ho C et al. Independent determinants of coronary artery disease in erectile dysfunction patients. *J sex med.* 2010;7 (4pt1): 1478-87.

[14] George G, Fluchter S, Kirsteir M, Kunze T. [sex, erectile dysfunction and the heart a growing problem]. *Herz* 2003; 28 (4):284-290.

[15] Nehra A. Erectile dysfunction and cardiovascular disease; efficacy and safety of phosphodiesterase type 5 inhibitors in men with both conditions. *Mayo Clin Proc.* 3009; 84(2):139-148.

[16] Maggio M, Basaria S. Welcoming testosterone as a cardiovascular risk factor. *Int J Impot Res* 2009; 21161-164.

[17] Munhall JP, Kaminestsky JC, Althof S, Goldstein 1, Creanga D, Marfatia A. Correlation with satisfaction measures in men treated with phosphodiestrase inhibitors for erectile dysfunction. *Am J Mens Health* 2011;

[18] Shindel AW, Kishore S, Lue TF. Drugs designed to improve endothelial function: effects on erectile function. *Curr Pharm. Des* 2008; 14(35):58-67.

[19] Kloner RA, Mullin SH, Shook T, Mathews R, Mayeda G, Bursteins S. Erectile dysfunction in the cardiac patients: how common and should we treat? *J Urol* 2003; 170(2N1):546-50.
[20] Dhir RR Lin HC, Confield SE, Wang R. Combination therapy for erectile dysfunction: an update review. *Asian J. Androl* 2011.
[21] Gillenwater JY, Howards SS, Mitchell ME, Grayhack T. Adult and pediatric urology. 4th ed. Philadelphia (PA): Lippincott Williams and Wilkins; 2001 p. 1956-1983
[22] Richard L Drake, Wayne A Vogl, Adam W M Mitchell. Grays Anatomy for Students.2nd ed. Philadelphia(PA) Churchill Livingstone;2010 p 484.
[23] Alastair JJ, Wood MD. Erectile dysfunction. *The New England Journal of Medicine* 2000; 342(24):1802-1812.
[24] John R, Brewster S, Biers S. Oxford Hand book of Urology. New York (NY): Oxford University Press; 2006.P.476.
[25] Ahmed 1. El-Sakka, Tom F. Lue. Physiology of penile erectile. *The world scientific Journal* 2004; 4(51):128-134.
[26] Walsh PC, Donker PS, Impotence following radical prostatectomy: insight into a etiology and prevention. *J Urol* 1998; 12:694.
[27] Simerly RB, Swanson LW. Projections of the medial pre-optic nucleus; a phaseolus vulgaries leucoagglutronation anterograde tract-tracing in the rat. *J Comp Neurol* 1988; 270:209.
[28] Degroat WC, Booth AM. Neural control of penile erection. In Magi CA, ed. The automatic nervous system, nervous control of the genito-urinary system. Chap 12. London: Harwood. Pp 465-513.
[29] Donohue JP, Einhorn LH, Williams SD, Cytoreduction surgery for metastatic testes cancer. Consideration of time and extent. *J Urol* 1980; 123:876.
[30] Robert C, Dean F Lue. Physiology of penile erection and pathophysiology of penile erection. *Urol Clin North Am* 2005; 32(4):379.
[31] Davis MG, Fulton GJ, Hager PO. Clinical biology of Nitric oxide. *British Journal of Surg* 1995; 82:1598-1610.
[32] Koshland DE Jr. Nitric Oxide: the molecules of the year. *Science* 1992; 258:186 (Editorial).
[33] Palmer RMJ, Astib DS, Moncada S. Vascular endothehal cells synthesize nitric oxide from L-arginine. Nature 1988; 333:664
[34] Ghabayiri IF. Nitric Oxide-Cyclic GMP pathways with some emphasis on cavernosal contractility. *Int J Impot Res.* 2004; 16(6):459-69.
[35] Saenz de Tejada 1, Kim N, Lagan 1, Krane RJ, Goldstein1. Regulation of adrenergic activity in penile corpus cavernosa. *J Urol* 1989;1117-21
[36] Anderson KE, Wanger G. physiology of penile erection. *Physiol Rev.* 1995; 75:191-236.
[37] Italiano G. Calabro A, Spini S, Ragazzi E, Pagano I. Functional response of Cavernosal tissue to dissection. *Urol Res* 1998; 26:39-44.
[38] Sattar AA, Salpigides G, Vanderhaegken JJ. Cavernous oxygen tension and smooth muscle fibres: relation and function. *J Urol* 1995; 154:1736.
[39] Basu A, Ryder RE. New treatment options for erectile dysfunction in patients with diabetes mellitus. *Drugs* 2004;(23):2667-88
[40] Zusman RM, Morales A, Glasser DB, Osterioh LH. Overall cardiovascular profile of sildenafil citrate. *Am J Cardiol* 1999; 83(5A) 35c-44c.

[41] Burnett AL. The role of nitric oxide in erectile dysfunction; implication for medical therapy. *J Clin hypertens* (GreenWich) 2006; 8(12):53-62.

[42] Montorisi F, Briganti A, Salonia A, Deho F, Zanni G, Cestari A et al. The aging male and erectile dysfunction. *Br J Urol* 2003; 92:516-520.

[43] Christ GJ, Richard S, Winkler A integrative erectile biology: the role of signal transduction and cell to cell communication in co-coordinating corporal smooth muscle tone and penile erection". *Int J. Impot Res.* 1997;9:69-84,

[44] Davis MG, Tulton GJ, Hagen PO. Clinical biology of Nitric oxide. *Br. J Surg* 1995; 82:1598-1610.

[45] Fredrick JS, Ramzi SC. Blood Vessels. In Ramzi RS, Vinay K, Ticker C, editors. Robins Pathological basis of diseases 6th ed. Philadelphia (PA): WB Sauders Company: 1999 P8-10.

[46] Furchgott RE, Zawadzki JV. The obligatory role of endothelial cells in the relaxation of arterial smooth muscle by acetyl choline. *Nature* 1980; 288:373-376.

[47] Kaiser DR, Billups K, Mason C, Wetterling R, Lundberg JL, Bank AJ. Impaired Branchial artery endothelium-dependent and independent vasodilatation in men with erectile dysfunction and no other clinical cardiovascular disease. *J Am Coll cordiol* 2004; 43:279-184.

[48] Henderson AH. St Cyres lecture. Endothelium in control. *Br Heart J* 1991; 65:116-125.

[49] Mumtax FH, Khan MA, Thompson CS, Mosgan RJ. Nutric oxide in the urinary tract: Physiological and pathological implicatipons. *BJU* 2000; 35:567-578

[50] Hodges LD, Kirby M, O, Donnell J, Brodie DA. The temporal relationship between erectile dysfunction and cardiovascular disease. *Int J. Clin Pract.* 2007; 61:2019-2025.

[51] Ahmad AH, Hemant S, Ryan JL, Verghese M, Abhiram P,Geralyn P. Coronary endothelial dysfunction is associated with erectile dysfunction and elevated asymmetric dimethylarginine in patients with early atherosclerosis. *Eur Heart J* 2006;27:824-31

[52] Schwartz BG, Economides C, Mayeda GS, Burstern S, Kloner RA. The endothelial cell in health and disease: its function, dysfunction measurement and therapy. *Int J Impot Res* 2010; 22:77-90.

[53] Boulton AJM, Malik AR, Arezzo JC, Sosenko JM. Diabetic Somatic neuropathies. *Diabetes Care* 2004; 27(6)1458-1486.

[54] Nystrom T, Nygren A, Sjoholm A, Economides C. Increased levels of tumor necrosis factor alpha (TNF-alpha) in patients with type II diabetes mellitus after myocardial infarction are related to endothelial dysfunction. *Clin Sci.* (London) 2006; 110(6)673-81.

[55] Yu. H1, Sheu WH, Song YM, Liu HC, Chen YT. C-reative protein and risk factors for peripheral vascular disease in subjects with type 2 diabetes mellitus. *Diabetic Med.* 2004; 21(4):336-41.

[56] Arena Rasainz MD, Ojede MO, Acosta JR, Ellias_Calles LC, Gonzalez NO Honera OT. Imbalanced low-grade Inflammation and Endothelial Activation in Patients with type 2 Diabetes Mellitus and erectile dysfunction. *J Sex Med.* 2011'

[57] Meng X, Li ZM, Zhou YJ, Cao Yl, Zhaag J. Effect of anti oxidant alphalipolic acid on apoptosis in human endothelial cells induced by higher glucose. *Clin Exp Med.* 2008; 8:34-49.

[58] Di Filippo C, Verza M, Coppola L, Rossi F, D Amico M, Marfella R. Insulin resistance and post prandial hyperglycemia the bad Companion in natural history of diabetes: effects on health of vascular tree. *Curr diabetes review* 2007; 3:268-273.

[59] Moore CR, Wang R. Pathophysiology and treatment of diabetes erectile dysfunction. *Asian J Androl* 2006; 8(6)675-84.

[60] Woodman RJ, Watts GF, Puddey 1B, Burke V, Mori TA, Hodgson JM et al. Lenkocyte count and vascular function in type 2 diabetes subjects with treated hypertension. *Atherosclerosis* 2002; 163(1):175-81.

[61] Nystrom T, Nygren A, Sjoholm A Persistent endothelial dysfunction is related to elevated C-reative protein (CRP) levels in type 2 diabetes patients after acute myocardial infarction. *Clin Sci.* (London) 2005; 108(2):121-8.

[62] Sun P, Cameroon A, Seftel A, Shabsigh R, Niederberger C, Guay A. Erectile dysfunction. An observable marker of diabetes mellitus? A large national epidemiology study. *J Urol* 2006; 176(3):1081-5.

[63] Colagiuri S, Cull CA, Holman RR. Are lower fasting plasma glucose levels at diagnosis of type 2 diabetis associated with improved outcomes? UK prospective diabetic study 67. Diabetes Care 2002; 25: 1410 - 1417

[64] Deutsch S, Sherman l. Previously unrecognized diabetes mellitus in sexually impotent men. *JAMA* 1980; 224-243.

[65] Feldman HA, Golosterin 1, Hatzichristou DG, Kraine RJ, Mckinlay JB. Impotence and its medical and psychosocial correlates: results of the Massachusetts male aging study. *J Urol* 1994; 151:54-61.

[66] Michell DL, Andrews KL, Chin-Dustong JP. Endothelial dysfunction in hypertension: the role of arginase. Pront Biosai (Schol Ed) 2011; 3:946-960.

[67] Ayodele AE, Alebiosu CO, Salako BL Awoden OG, Abigun AD. Target organ damage and associated clinical conditions among Nigerians with treated hypertension. *Cardiovasc J S Afr* 2005; 16:89-93.

[68] Essien OE, Peters ET, Udoh AE, Ekot JU, Odigwe CD. Prevalence and pattern of abnormal glucose tolerance in adult Nigerians with primary hypertension. *Niger J Med.* 2007; 16:50-56.

[69] Kloner R. Erectile dysfunction and hypertension. *Int. j impot Res.* 2007; 19:296-302.

[70] Irekpita E, Salami TAT. Erectile dysfunction:its relationship with cardiovascular risk factors and disease. *Saudi med J* 2009; 30(2)1296-1302.

[71] Asmar R. Effects of anti hypertensive agents on arterial stiffness as evaluated by pulse wave velocity: clinical implications- *Am J Cardiovasc Drugs* 2001; 1(5):387-97.

[72] Boulauger CM. Secondary endothelial dysfunction: Hypertension and heart failure. *J Mol Cell Cardiol* 1999; 31(1):39-49.

[73] Petri P,Vyssoulis G,Vlachopoulos C,Zervodaki A, Gialerivos T, Aznaouridis K, et al. Relationship between low grade inflammation and arterial stiffness in patients with essential hypertension. *J Hypertens* 2006; (11):2231-8.

[74] Modebe O. Erectile failure among clinical medical patients. *Afr J Med. Sci* 1990; 19:259-364.

[75] Shiri R, koskimaki J, Hakkinen J, Tamadela TL Auvinen A,Tamela TL, Hakama M. Cardiovascular drug use and the incidence of erectile dysfunction. *Int. j Impot. Res* 2007; 19:208-212.

[76] Bolm M, Baumhakel M, Probstfield JL, Schimieder R, Yusuf S, Zhao F et al. Sexual function, satisfaction and association of erectile dysfunction with cardiovascular disease and risk factor in cardiovascular high risk patients: sub-study of the on-going telmisartrain alone, and combination with Ramipril Global End-point Trial/Telmisartran Randomized Assessment study in ACE-INtolerant subjects with cardiovascular Disease (ONTARGET/TRANCEND). *Am Heart J* 2007; 154:94-101.

[77] Brunner H. Endothelial function and dysfunction. Part 2: Association with cardiovascular risk factors and disease. A statement by the working group on Endothelins and Endothelial factors of the European Society of hypertension. *J Hypertens* 2005; 23:233-246.

[78] Rodrigues JJ, Al Dashti R, Schwartz ER. Linking erectile dysfunction and coronary artery disease *Int J Import. Res.* 2005; 17; 512-518

[79] Chou KT, Hung CL, Chen YM, Perng DW, Chao HS, Chang WH, et al. Asthma and risk of erectile dysfunction. A nationwide population based study. *J Sex Med* 2011;

[80] WU C, Zhang H, Gao Y, Tan A, Yang X, LU z, et al. The association of smoking and erectile dysfunction: Results from the frangchenggang Area Male health and examination Survey (FAMHES). *J Androl* 2011

[81] Eiton EB, Liu YL Mittleman MA, Miner M, Glasser DB, Rimm EB. A retrospective study of the relationship between biomarkers of atherosclerosis and erectile dysfunction in 988 men. *Int J Res Impot* 2007; 19:218-225.

[82] Allen NE, Appleby PN, Davey GK, Key TT. Lifestyle and nutritional determinants of bio-available androgens and related hormones in British men. *Cancer Causes Control* 2002; 13:352-363.

[83] Ogden CL, Carroll MD, Gurtin LR, Mcdowell MA, Tabak CJ, Flegal KM. Prevalence of overweight and obesity in the United States, 1999-2004 *JAMA* 2006;295:1549-1555.

[84] Bensal TC, Guay AT, Jacobson J, Woods BO, Nesto RW. Incidence of metabolic syndrome and insulin resistance in a population with organic erectile dysfunction. *J Sex. Med.* 2005; 2:96-103.

[85] Roumeguere T, Wespes E, Carpentier Y, Hoffmann P, Schulman CC. Erectile dysfunction is associated with a high prevalence of hyperlipidemia and coronary heart disease risk. *Eur urol* 2003; 44:355-359.

[86] Bortolotti A, Parazzini F, Colli E, Ladoni M. The epidemiology of erectile dysfunction and its risk factors. Int. *J Androl* 1997; 20:323-334.

[87] Miner M, Billups K. Erectile dysfunction and dyslipidemia:relevance and role of phosphodiesterase 5 inhibitors and statins. *J Sex Med* 2008;5(5):1066-78

[88] Chang ST, Chu CM, Hsu JT, Hsiao JF, Chung CM, Ho C, et al. Independent determinants of coronary artery disease in erectile dysfunction patients .*J Sex Med* 2010;7(4pt1):1478-87.

[89] Quyyumi A et al. coronary vascular nitric oxide activity in hypertension and hypercholesterolemia. Comparism of acetyl choline and substance P. *Circulation* 1997; 95:104-110.

[90] Vallance P, Chan N. Endothelial function and nitric oxide: clinical relevance. *Heart* 2004; 85:342-350.

[91] Kuvin JJ et al. A Novel mechanism for the beneficial vascular effects of high density lipoprotein cholesterol: enhanced vaso-relaxation and increased endothelial Nitric oxide synthase expression. *Am Heart J* 2002; 144:165-172.

[92] Ness AR, Smith GD. The epidemiology of ischemic heart disease. In Warell DA, Cox JM, Firth JD, Edward J, Benz MD, editors Oxford Text Book of Medicine. 4th ed. Oxford (UK): Oxford University Press: 2003.P.315-607.

[93] Alkhayal S, Lehmaun V, Thomas P. A simple non invasive test to detect vascular disease in patients with erectile dysfunction: a novel method. *J Sex Med.* 2006; 3:331-336.

[94] Thompson 1M, Tangen CM, Goodman PJ, Probsfield JL, Moinpour CM, Cottman CA. Erectile dysfunction and subsequent cardiovascular disease. *JAMA* 2005; 294:2996-3002.

[95] Montorsi P, Montorsi F, Schulman CC. Is erectile dysfunction the tip of the iceberg of a systemic vascular disorder? *Eur Urol* 2003; 44:352-354.

[96] Pritzker MR. The Penile stress test: a window to the heart of men? *Circulation* 1999; 100(1):1-711.

[97] Vlachopoulos C, Rokkas K, Ioakeimidis N, Aggeli C, Michealides A,Roussakis G et al. Prevalence of asymptomatic coronary artery disease in men with vasculogenic erectile dysfunction: a prospective angiographic study. *Eur Urol* 2005; 48:996-1003.

[98] Bensal TC, Gnay AT, Jacobson J, Woods BO, Nesto RW. Incidence of metabolic syndrome and insulin resistance in a population with organic erectile dysfunction. *J Sex Med.* 2005; 2:96-103.

[99] Rodriguez JJ, AL Dashti R, Schwatz ER. Linking erectile dysfunction and coronary artery disease. *Int. J Impot Res* 2005; 17:12-18.

[100] Herschorn S. Cardiovascular safety of PDE 5 inhibitors. *Can J Urol* 2003; 10(1):S23-S25

[101] Harin P, Shabsigh R, Sildenafil citrate (viagra) (R): a review. *Am J Urol* 1999; 18:274-279.

[102] James KM, Kim AW, Tochi M, George WB, Michael SP, Parker R. Prediction of coronary Heart disease by erectile dysfunction in men referred for nuclear stress test. *Arch Inter Med.* 2006; 166:201-206.

[103] Ukoh VA, Okorofua IA. Plasma lipid profile in Nigerians with normal blood pressure, hypertension and other acquired cardiac conditions. *East Afr Med J* 2007; 84: 267 - 270

[104] Rosamond N, Flegal K, Furie K Go A, Greenland K, Haase N et al. Heart disease and stroke statistics - 2008 update: a report from American Heart Association statistics committee and stroke statistics Subcommittee. *Circulation* 2008; 117: e25 - 146

[105] Herbert K, Lopez B, Castellano J, Palacio A, Tamari L, Arcemen LM. The prevalence of erectile dysfunction in heart failure patients by race and ethnicity. *Int J Import Res* 2008; 20: 507 - 511

[106] Barsdale JD, Gardner SF. The impact of first line antihypertensive drugs on erectile function. *Pharmacotherapy* 1999: 19: 573 - 581

[107] Gupta S, Salinpour P, Seanz de Tajeda 1, Daley J, Gholamai S, Baller M ,et al. A possible mechanism for alteration human erectile function by digoxin: inhibition of corpus cavernosum sodium/potassium adenosin triphosphate activity. *J. Urol* 1998; 158: 1529 - 1536.

[108] Gerald B, Lauman EO, Glasser DB et al. Sexaual attitudes and beliefs of middle aged and older adults in non-European Westernised countries. The global study of sexual attitude and behavior. Can *J Urol* 2004; II (3): 2271

[109] David RM, Jospeh CG, Marge AM, Louis JI. Multifaced approach to maximize erectile function and cardiovascular health. *Fertility and sterility* 2010; 7 (94): 2514 - 2520

[110] Goldstein I, Lu TF, Padma-Nathan H, Rosen RC, Steers WD, Wicker PA. Oral sildenafil in the treatment of erectile dysfunction. *N Engl J Med* 1998; 338: 1397 - 404

[111] Derby CA, Mohr BA, Goldstein I, Feldman HA, Johanness CB, Mckinly JB. Modifiable risk factors and erectile dysfunction: Can lifestyle changes modify risk. *Urology* 2000; 58: 302 - 306.

[112] Aydinoglu F, Yilmaz SN, Coskun B, Daglioglu N, Ogulener N. Effect of ethanol treatment on the neurogenic and endothelium dependent relaxation of corpus cavernosum smooth muscle in the mouse. *Pharmacol Rep* 2008; 60: 725 - 34

[113] Selvin E, Burnett AL, Platz EA. Prevalence and risk factors for erectile dysfunction in the US. *Am J Med* 2007; 120: 151 - 157.

[114] Haram PM, Adams V, Kemi OJ, Brabakk AO, Hambrech LR, Ellingsen O, et al. Time course of endothelial adaptation following acute and regular exercise. *Eur J cardoivac. Prev rehabil* 2006; 13: 585 - 591

[115] Esposito K, Giughano F, Di Palo C, Giugliano G, Marfella RD, Andrea F, et al. Effect of life-style changes on erectile dysfunction in obese men: A randomized controlled study. *JAMA* 2004: 291: 2978 - 2984

[116] Tikkanen KM, Jackson G, Tammela T, Assmann G, Polamaki M, Kupari M, et al. Erectile dysfunction as a risk factor for coronany heart disease: Implications for prevention. *Int J Clin Pract* 2007; 61: 265 - 268

[117] Saltzman EA, Guay AT, Jacobson J. Improvement in erectile function in men with organic erectile dysfunction by correction of elevated cholesterol levels: a clinical observation. *J urol* 2004; 172: 255 - 8

[118] Grundy SM, Gleeman JI, Merz CN, Brewer Jnr HB, Clark LT, Huninghake DB, et al. Implications of recent clinical trial for the national cholesterol Adult Education Program Treatment III Panel guidelines . *Circulation* 2004; 110: 227 - 239

[119] Solomon H, Samarasinghe YP, Feher MD, Man J, Rivas - Toro H, Lumb PJ, et al. Erectile dysfunction and statin treatment in high cardiovascular risk patients. I*nt J Clin Pract.* 2006; 60: 141 - 145

[120] Glenn Matfin. New treatments of erectile dysfunction. *Sexuality Reproduction and Menopause* 2003; 1 (1): 40 - 45

[121] Gorge G, Fluchter S, Kirstein M, Kunz T. (Sex, erectile dysfunction, and the heart: a growing problem). *Herz* 2003; 28(4): 284-90

[122] Parker JD, Bart BA, Webb DJ, Koren MJ, Siegel RL, Wang H, et al. Safety of intravenous nitroglycerin after administration of sildanefil citrate to men with coronary artery disease: a double blind placebo controlled randomized crossover trial. *Crit Care Med* 2007; 35:1863-1868.

[123] Webb DJ, Freestone S, Allen MJ, Muirhead GJ. Sildenafil citrate and blood pressure lowering drugs: results of the drug interaction study with an organic nitrate and a calcium antagonist. *Am J Cardiol* 1999; 83 C21 - C28

[124] Velasquez Lopez JG, Agudelo Restrepo CA, Yapes Gomex D, Uribe Trufillo CA. (Acute myocardial infarction associated to the sildenafil consumption. A case report and review of the literature). *Actas Urol Esp* 2007; 31: 52 - 57

[125] Derouet A, Caspari D, Rohdi V, Rommel G, Ziegler M. Treatment of erectile dysfunction with external vacuum devices. *Andrologia* 1999; 31 (1) 89 - 94

[126] Goldstein 1, New man L, Baum N, et al. Safety and efficacy outcome of mentor alpha 1 inflatable penile prosthesis implantation for impotence treatment. *J Urol* 1997; 157: 833 - 839.

8

Vascular Dysfunction in Women with Recurrent Pregnancy Loss

Mikiya Nakastuka
Graduate School of Health Sciences, Okayama University
Department of Obstetrics and Gynecology, Okayama University Hospital
Japan

1. Introduction

Women have unique risk factors for cardiovascular diseases and cerebrovascular diseases such as pregnancy and hormone replacement therapy. Pregnancy provides an opportunity to reveal various cardiovascular disease risk factors and estimate a woman's lifetime risk because of its unique cardiovascular and metabolic stress.

The causes of recurrent pregnancy loss (RPL) are classified as genetic, anatomic, endocrinologic, immunologic, microbiologic, environmental, and further more (Kutteh, 1999; Christiansen et al., 2005). Several lines of study have suggested that certain coagulation abnormalities such as antiphospholipid antibodies or Factor V Leiden, the genetic defect underlying resistance to activated protein C, are causes of RPL (Kutteh, 1999).

New diagnostic methods have improved the clinical triage of RPL (Kutteh, 1999; Li, 1998). Transvaginal pulsed Doppler ultrasonography allows noninvasive evaluation of uterine circulation. The introduction of pulsed Doppler ultrasonography has provided noninvasive means for the evaluation of uterine impedance, and gives physiologic data, rather than anatomic information alone. It is known that resistance to uterine arterial blood flow is associated with poor obstetrical outcome such as preeclampsia and fetal growth restriction (Nakatsuka et al, 1999b; Nakatsuka et al, 2002; Takata et al, 200).

We have reported that impaired uterine perfusion is observed in a portion of women with RPL (Habara et al., 2002; Nakatsuka et al., 2003a, 2003b). Pulsed Doppler ultrasonography in the uterine artery may be useful in distinguishing women with RPL caused by vascular dysfunction from women with unexplained RPL (Habara et al., 2002). Furthermore, the plasma level of adrenomedullin, which is often associated with pathological processes of the vasculature (Hinson, 2000), is elevated in women with RPL (Nakatsuka et al., 2003a). However, vascular changes in women with RPL have not been fully elucidated.

Antiphospholipid antibody syndrome (APS), which is an autoimmune disease associated with coagulopathy, is a well-known cause of RPL (Nakatsuka et al., 2003b). Antiphospholipid antibodies refer to several groups of autoantibodies with specificity for a number of negatively-charged phospholipids such as cardiolipin, phosphatidylserine, and phosphatidylethanolamine, or phospholipid-binding glycoproteins such as β2 glycoprotein I (β2GPI) and prothrombin. There are currently data supporting an association between various types of antiphospholipid antibodies and vascular diseases (Nayak & Komatireddy et al., 2002). Previous studies suggest that predominantly IgG and to lesser extent IgM isotype of antiphospholipid antibodies and lupus anticoagulant (LAC) are associated with arterial and venous thrombosis, thrombocytopenia, and livedo reticularis (Nayak & Komatireddy et al., 2002). Anti-cardiolipin and anti-β2GPI antibodies are elevated in patients with coronary artery disease. Anti-cardiolipin antibodies are also associated with typical chest pain, significant coronary artery stenosis on angiography and prediction of myocardial infarction (Sherer &Shoenfeld, 2003).

Premature atherosclerosis is a clinical feature of thrombotic patients with primary APS (Ames et al., 2009). Early data from the Italian Antiphospholipid Registry calculated a 2.5% patient/year incidence of recurrent thrombosis often fatal; a prospective Spanish study demonstrated that 5.2% of primary APS patients died of recurrent arterial occlusions; Italian longitudinal study showed a 5.2% patient/year mortality rate for recurrent arterial thrombosis and a Russian group recently reported a 17% 8-year vascular mortality for primary APS (Ames et al., 2009).

Polycystic ovary syndrome (PCOS) is one of the most common endocrinological disorders among reproductive-age women (Franks, 1995; Dunaif, 1997, The Rotterdam ESHRE/ASRM-Sponsored PCOS consensus workshop group, 2004). Using a combination of clinical, ultrasonographic, and biochemical criteria, the diagnosis of PCOS is usually reserved for those women who display one or more clinical symptoms including chronic anovulation, an ultrasonographical morphology of polycystic ovaries, inappropriate gonadotropin secretion, and hyperandrogenism (Franks, 1995; Dunaif, 1997). It is reported that women with PCOS have adverse pregnancy outcome including miscarriage (Abbott et al., 2002; Doldi et al., 1998; Glueck et al., 1999; Wang et al., 2001; Diejomaoh et al., 2003).

We and the other researchers demonstrated an impaired uterine perfusion in women with PCOS (Ajossa et al., 2002; Chekir C et al., 2005). Abnormal sex steroid hormones have been suggested as the cause for the elevated blood flow resistance in the uterine artery of women with PCOS (Zaidi et al., 1998). Furthermore, risk factors for cardiovascular disease including central obesity, hyperandrogenism, hyperinsulinemia, and dyslipidemia, which are commonly observed in women with PCOS, may lead to impairment of uterine perfusion and vascular dysfunction (Slowinska-Srzednicka et al., 1991; Legro ,2003; Sabuncu et al., 2001; Fenkci et al., 2003; Setji & Brown, 2007).

In the light of these studies, vascular dysfunction may be the key to the pathophysiology of pregnancy loss. This chapter reviews association between RPL and vascular dysfunction.

2. Impaired uterine arterial blood flow in women with RPL

Pregnancy loss in LPS-treated rats is associated with coagulopathy, decreased placental blood flow, and placental and fetal hypoxia. This impairment in uteroplacental hemodynamics in LPS-treated rats is linked to increased uterine artery resistance (Graham et al., 2011). In Human, peripheral vascular resistance in normal pregnancy decreases as early as 5 weeks of gestation (Robson, 1989). Resistance in uterine arterial blood flow also exhibits a progressive decrease after implantation while it increases in women with preeclampsia or fetal growth restriction (Steel et al., 1990). Pulsed Doppler velocimetry of the uterine artery has been reported to predict preeclampsia, fetal growth restriction, or gestational diabetes (van den Elzen et al., 1995). However, predictive value of uterine arterial pulsed Doppler velocimetry in pregnancy loss is controversial (van den Elzen et al., 1993; Jauniaux, et al., 1994; Kurjak et al., 1994; Alcázar, 2000; Nakatsuka et al., 2003a)..

2.1 Pregnant women with RPL associated with antiphospholipid antibodies

We measured the resistance in the uterine arteries of 104 pregnant women with and without RPL at 4 to 5 weeks' gestation and evaluated association of autoantibodies including antiphospholipid antibodies (Nakatsuka et al., 2003a). In this study, uterine arterial pulsatility index (PI) in the RPL group was significantly higher than that in the control group (Figure 1). Women with antiphospholipid antibodies had an elevated PI in the uterine artery, which is prominent in women with RPL (Table 1). Coagulopathy and vascular dysfunction caused by antiphospholipid antibodies may impair uterine perfusion.

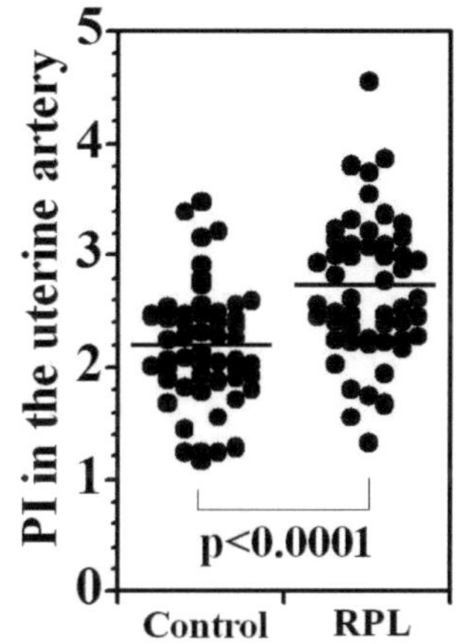

Fig. 1. Resistance in uterine arterial blood flow of women with recurrent pregnancy loss (Nakatsuka et al., 2003a).

	APA (-) (n=89)	APA (+) (n=15)	p value
Control (n=52)	2.19±0.54 * (52)	n.a. (0)	n.a.
Recurrent pregnancy loss (n=52)	2.51±0.52 * (37)	3.18±0.64 (15)	<0.0003
Total (n=104)	2.32±0.55	3.18±0.64	<0.0001

APA : Antiphospholipid antibodies,
n.a.: not available, Student's t-test* : p<0.007.
(Nakatsuka et al., 2003a).

Table 1. Antiphospholipid antibodies and pulsatility index in the uterine artery

Pregnancies complicated with hypertensive disorders and/or fetal growth restriction are known to be associated with a defective trophoblastic invasion. Antiphospholipid antibodies are known to interfere with syncytialization of the trophoblasts in early pregnancy and cause decidual vasculopathy, thrombosis, and placental infarction later in pregnancy. However, the elevation of uterine arterial PI that we observed is more likely to be associated with vascular dysfunction rather than impaired trophoblastic invasion. Trophoblastic invasion affects little on uterine arterial blood flow at 4-5 weeks of gestation because decrease in blood flow resistance in the uterine artery is very slow until 8 weeks of gestation (Dickey et al., 1995).

Pregnant women with antiphospholipid antibodies have vascular dysfunctions in the uterine artery although the prediction of adverse pregnancy outcome is not conclusive (Caruso et al, 1993; Venkat-Raman et al, 2001; Nakatsuka et al., 2003a).

Interestingly, the uterine arterial PI in RPL women without antiphospholipid antibodies is significantly higher than that in the control pregnant women even among women without antiphospholipid antibodies in our study (Nakatsuka et al., 2003a).

2.2 Non-pregnant women with unexplained RPL

Pulsed Doppler ultrasonography demonstrated blood flow changes in the uterus and ovaries during the menstrual cycle (Goswamy and Steptoe, 1988a; Chekir et al., 2005). The uterine arterial PI has been known to diminish progressively during the luteal phase, during which implantation occurs. Differences in uterine blood flow impedance between fertile and infertile women (Goswamy et al., 1988b; Steer et al., 1994). Based on studies from the IVF-ET programme, impedance of blood flow through the uterine arteries is a good indicator of the probability of subsequent pregnancy (Salle et al., 1998).

We investigated whether women with unexplained RPL have impaired uterine perfusion in the mid-luteal phase of non-conception cycles (Habara et al., 2002). The uterine arterial PI of 121 women including 49 women with unexplained RPL was measured by transvaginal pulsed Doppler ultrasonography. The uterine artery PI in RPL group (2.54±0.45, mean ±S.D.) was significantly higher than that in the control group (2.20±0.35). In the RPL group, the PI in the uterine artery of women with antinuclear antibodies (ANA) was significantly higher than that of women without ANA (Figure 2). There is no significant difference between the PI in the uterine artery of women with ANA and that of women without ANA in control group. Among women without ANA, the uterine artery PI in RPL group was also significantly higher than that in the control group.

Although ANA are not specific pathogens for pregnancy loss (Ogasawara, et al., 1996), women with positive ANA may have other autoimmune antibodies causing vasculopathy or coagulopathy. These pathological changes are likely to cause elevation of the uterine arterial blood flow resistance and lead to RPL, early onset preeclampsia, or fetal growth restriction. Although the apparent underlying pathophysiology of these cases was not elucidated, they may have subclinical vasculopathy, which was not diagnosed by routine screening tests for RPL.

2.3 Women with PCOS

Relatively high rate of pregnancy loss has been reported in women with PCOS. We performed a pulsed Doppler study on uterine arterial blood flow in 25 women with PCOS and 45 control women with regular menstrual cycles (Chekir et al.,2005). Among the control group, the uterine arterial PI in the luteal phase was significantly lower than that in the follicular phase (Figure 3). Among women with PCOS, the uterine arterial PI in the luteal phase tended to be lower than that in the follicular phase. The PI in the uterine artery in women with PCOS was significantly higher than that for the control group both in the follicular phase and in the luteal phase. Among women with PCOS, women with amenorrhea had a significantly higher uterine arterial PI than that of women with oligomenorrhea.

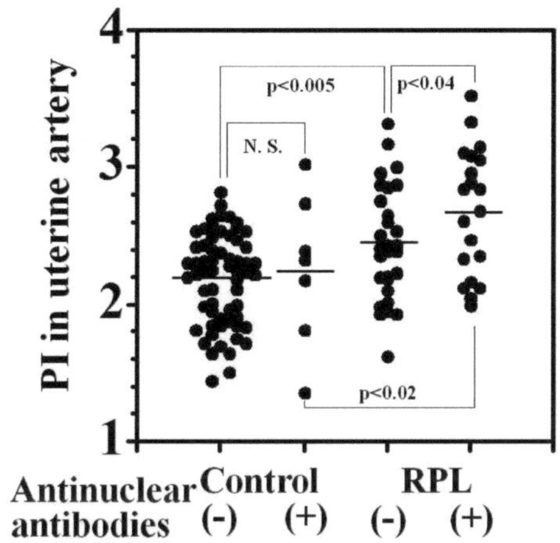

Fig. 2. Pulsatility index in the uterine artery of women with or without antinuclear antibodies in control or RPL group. Bars, Mean. Values are expressed as mean ±S.D. (Habara et al., 2002)

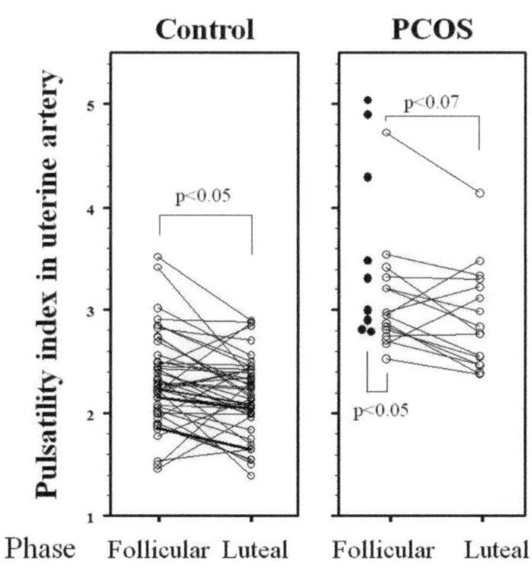

Fig. 3. Pulsatility index in the uterine artery in control women and women with PCOS. Left panel: Uterine arterial PI in control women. Data from control women during the follicular phase and the luteal phase are indicated by open circles. Right panel: Uterine arterial PI in women with PCOS. Data from women with amenorrhea during the follicular phase are indicated by closed circles. Data from women with oligomenorrhea during the follicular phase and the luteal phase are indicated by open circles (Chekir et al, 2005).

The uterine arterial PI was correlated with body mass index, luteinizing hormone /follicle-stimulating hormone ratio, or low-density lipoprotein-cholesterol (LDL-C)/high-density lipoprotein-cholesterol (HDL-C) ratio while it was inversely correlated with the HDL-C level.

3. Biomarkers for cardiovascular risk assessment in women with RPL

The introduction of pulsed Doppler ultrasonography has provided the means for the noninvasive evaluation of uterine impedance, thus providing physiologic data on hemodynamic abnormalities in early pregnancy failures. Are these vascular changes in women with PRL observed solely in the uterine artery? Biomarkers for cardiovascular risk assessment are substances that are released into the blood when the vasculature is damaged. Some biomarkers cause vascular dysfunction directly or indirectly. It may be worth measuring biomarkers for cardiovascular risk assessment in women with RPL.

3.1 Thrombomodulin

Thrombomodulin binds thrombin, changes thrombin conformation and allows thrombin to activate protein C, which inhibits coagulation and thrombin-activatable fibrinolysis inhibitor, which inhibits fibrinolysis. Increased serum thrombomodulin, cleaved products of cellular thrombomodulin, has been demonstrated previously in preeclampsia (Dusse et al., 2011). Endothelial thrombomodulin is known to be a major vasoprotective molecule. However, elevated serum thrombomodulin is also likely to be a response to vascular activation.

We measured serum levels of soluble thrombomodulin of 54 pregnant women at 4-8 weeks of gestation (Nakatsuka et al., 2004). Serum thrombomodulin was significantly elevated in women with antiphospholipid antibodies in RPL group compared with control women and with RPL women without antiphospholipid antibodies. Among women with APS, serum thrombomodulin in women who subsequently had a growth-restricted fetus had been significantly higher than that in women who subsequently had an appropriate-for-date fetus. Elevation of thrombomodulin is likely to indicate impaired uterine blood flow in women with RPL.

It is controversial whether the soluble thrombomodulin level is an independent risk factor for coronary heart disease (Wu, 2003; Huang et al., 2008; Karakas et al., 2011). However, anti-cardiolipin antibodies are reported to be important not only in the pathogenesis of mixed connective tissue disease (MCTD) but in the induction of endothelial cell causing elevation of soluble thrombomodulin, and may play crucial roles in the development of early atherosclerosis in MCTD (Soltesz, 2010). It is also known that development of atherosclerosis and elevation of soluble thrombomodulin in serum of systemic lupus erythematosus (SLE) patients with metabolic syndrome (Mok et al., 2010).

3.2 Adrenomedullin

Adrenomedullin, a 52-amino acids-ringed, structured peptide, mediates vasodilatory properties through the second messenger cyclic adenosine, 3,5-monophosphate (Jougasaki & Burnett, 2000). The main source of plasma adrenomedullin is considered to be vascular endothelial cells and vascular smooth muscle cells.

Adrenomedullin has interaction with various bioactive molecules including nitric oxide, prostaglandins, atrial natriuretic peptide, renin, aldosterone, norepinephrine, arginine vasopressin, endothelin-1, and adrenocorticotropic hormone (Jougasaki & Burnett, 2000). The plasma level of adrenomedullin is elevated in various diseases including hypertension, diabetes, cardiac failure, septic shock, or SLE, which are often associated with pathologic processes of the vasculature (Jougasaki & Burnett, 2000; Hinson et al., 2000).

We measured plasma levels of adrenomedullin of 100 pregnant women in the midluteal phase of a nonpregnant cycle (Nakatsuka et al., 2003b). We also measured the PI in the uterine arteries by transvaginal pulsed Doppler ultrasonography at the same time. The plasma level of adrenomedullin in women with RPL was significantly higher than that in control women. Uterine arterial PI of women with RPL was significantly higher than that in control women. Plasma level of adrenomedullin had a significant positive correlation with uterine arterial PI both in the control group ($r=0.58$, $p < 0.001$) and in the RPL group ($r=0.78$, $p < 0.001$) (Figure 4). Both plasma adrenomedullin concentration and uterine arterial PI were significantly high in women with antiphospholipid antibodies.

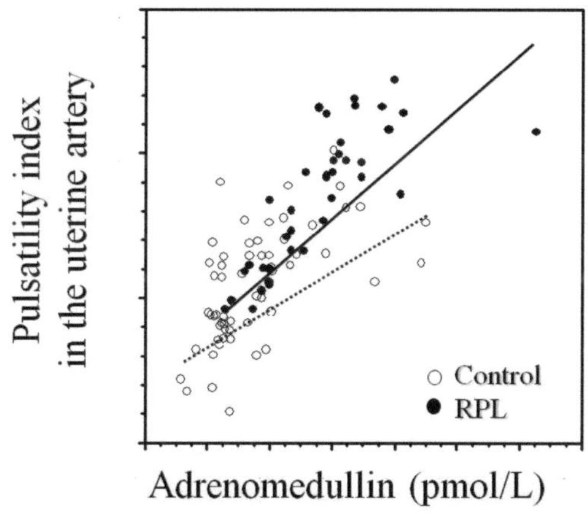

Fig. 4. Plasma adrenomedullin and uterine arterial pulsatility index.
A) Plasma adrenomedullin concentration and uterine arterial pulsatility index in control women. A significant positive correlation was determined by Pearson correlation coefficient ($r =0.58$, $p<0.001$). B) Plasma adrenomedullin concentration and uterine arterial pulsatility index in women with recurrent pregnancy loss. A significant positive correlation was determined by Pearson correlation coefficient ($r =0.78$, $p <0.001$). (Nakatsuka et al., 2003b)

Increased plasma adrenomedullin in women with RPL is likely to be a response to vascular damage and increased vascular tone. Plasma adrenomedullin levels observed in women with recurrent pregnancy loss were similar to the values reported in patients with hypertension, mitral stenosis, primary aldosteronism, or SLE (Nakatsuka et al., 2003b).

Although the pathophysiologic roles of adrenomedullin in RPL have not been fully elucidated, this peptide may serve as a biochemical marker to identify women with impaired uterine perfusion (Nakatsuka et al., 2003b; Ashraf et al., 2011) and also impaired systemic vasculatures.

3.3 The other markers associated with cardiovascular diseases

We have previously reported that there is no significant difference in serum nitric oxide metabolite level between control women and women with recurrent pregnancy loss (Habara et al., 2002). However, anti-cardiolipin antibodies induce nitric oxide and superoxide production from vascular vessels, resulting in enhanced local levels of plasma peroxynitrite (Alves & Grima, 2003), which is a powerful pro-oxidant molecule (Nakatsuka et al, 1999). These oxidative damages in the cardiovascular system may be involved in atherosclerosis.

PCOS has deserved major attention because it is linked to the same cluster of events that promote the metabolic syndrome. We have reported that women with PCOS had significantly higher total cholesterol, triglyceride, and β-lipoprotein levels than those of the control group. Significantly lower HDL-C, higher LDL-C, and consequently a higher LDL-C/HDL-C ratio were observed in women with PCOS as compared to those of the control women. Fasting serum insulin and homeostasis model assessment-R (HOMA-R), which are indexes of insulin resistance, in women with PCOS were significantly higher than those for the control group.

It has been reported that isolated adipocytes from women with PCOS express higher mRNA concentrations of some adipokines involved in cardiovascular risk and insulin resistance (Garruti et al., 2009). The actions of adipokines and adipocytokines on platelets and vascular smooth muscle cells, both of which are deeply involved in atherothrombosis, have been reported (Anfossi et al, 2010). Adipose tissue from individuals with central obesity synthesizes and releases increased amount of proinflammatory chemokines and cytokines, such as monocyte chemoattractant protein-1 (MCP-1), macrophage migration inhibitory factor (MIF), tumor necrosis factor-α (TNF-α), and interleukins, including interleukin-1β (IL-1β) and interleukin-6 (IL-6); procoagulant and proinflammatory mediators such as tissue factor (TF) and plasminogen activator inhibitor-1 (PAI-1); vasoactive substances such as angiotensinogen and endothelin-1 (ET-1); molecules involved in the pathogenesis of insulin resistance, such as TNF-α and resistin (Anfossi et al, 2010). Elevated levels of PAI-1, the major natural antifibrinolytic agent, are involved in atherothrombosis in women with PCOS (Ehrmann, 2005). Women with RPL, who are characterized as PCOS might be monitored by measuring these bioactive molecules to predict development of cardiovascular diseases.

4. Arterial stiffness in women with RPL

Impaired uterine arterial blood flow and elevated cardiovascular disease risk markers suggest that early changes of systemic vasculature may be progressing in women with RPL. These changes lead to athrosclerosis and atherothrombosis and may cause coronary heart disease and/or stroke.

4.1 Evaluation methods of arterial stiffness

Reductions in the elasticity of central arteries may act as a marker of early changes that predispose to the development of major vascular disease. Arterial stiffness has been known as a major contributory factor to cardiovascular morbidity and mortality in patients with hypertension. Independent studies have shown that central arterial stiffness is increased in older individuals and in those with coronary artery disease, myocardial infarction, heart failure, hypertension, stroke, diabetes mellitus, end-stage renal disease, hypercholesterolemia, and inflammation (Nichols, 2005).

There are various methods in evaluation of atherosclerosis. Intima media thickness (IMT) of carotid arteries is used to evaluate early atherosclerosis and the risk of associated cardiovascular disease (Burke, et al., 1995). The The ankle-brachial index (ABI) for each leg was calculated as the ratio of the systolic pressures in the leg and the systolic pressure of either the left or right arm. An ABI < 1.0 in either leg was considered abnormal, suggesting peripheral arterial disease; progressively lower ABI values indicate more severe obstruction (Sacks et al., 2002).

Pulse wave velocity (PWV) and the augmentation index (AI) are widely used as arterial stiffness indices. Recently, brachial-ankle PWV (baPWV) measurement can be performed easily by simultaneous oscillometric measurement of pulse waves in all four extremities. Brachial-ankle PWV was used as a substitute for aortic PWV because baPWV is known to be strongly correlated with aortic PWV (Matsui et al., 2004). PWV are known to be a marker of both the severity of vascular damage and the prognosis of atherosclerotic vascular diseases in patients with hypertension (Blacher et al., 1999), end-stage renal failure (London & Cohn, 2002), and diabetes (Yokoyama et al., 2003). Increased PWV is known to be an independent predictor of the prognosis in hypertension, including in subjects under anti-hypertensive medication (Laurent et al., 2001).

Carotid AI (cAI) was assessed by the proportion of the central pulse pressure resulting from peripheral arterial wave reflection. The AI is known to be an independent predictor of all-cause and cardiovascular mortality in end-stage renal failure patients (London et al., 2001). It has been also reported that increased AI is associated with the presence and severity of coronary artery disease, particularly in younger and middle-aged male patients (Weber et al., 2004). Although PWV and AI have been known to be useful indices of atherosclerotic vascular diseases, data in young females are scarce.

4.2 Women with PRL associated with antiphospholipid antibodies

Antiphospholipid antibodies is known to play a central role in both pregnancy loss and cardiovascular diseases (Mackworth-Young, 2004). Antiphospholipid antibodies is a risk factor for incident stroke, however, the evidence to support the role of antiphospholipid antibodies in recurrent stroke is conflicting (Brey, 2004). Neither anti-cardiolipin antibodies nor anti-β2GPI antibodies is reported to be associated with atherosclerosis in premenopausal women with APS and SLE, who have an increased prevalence of carotid and femoral plaque (Vlachoyiannopoulos et al., 2003). Furthermore, previous studies have paradoxically proposed a beneficial role for some antiphospholipid antibodies in atherosclerosis (Nicolo & Monestier, 2004).

We assessed arterial stiffness of 153 women with RPL and 66 healthy women with one or less pregnancy loss. It is reported that abnormal ABIs are more common in primary APS than in healthy controls (Baron et al., 2005). However, we did not observe significant difference in ABI value or incidence of abnormal ABI between RPL women with antiphospholipid antibodies and control women. More sensitive methods may be necessary to detect early changes of vascular system in younger patients with antiphospholipid antibodies.

Women with RPL had significantly higher baPWV than control women (Figure 5). Mean value of baPWV of RPL women with antiphospholipid antibodies is significantly higher than that in control women. None in control women or women with unexplained RPL showed abnormal baPWV while five in RPL women with antiphospholipid antibodies showed abnormal baPWV (baPWV > 1,400 m/sec, American Heart Association Medical/Scientific Statement, 1993). Women with RPL had significantly higher cAI (22.5 ± 171.2 %) than control women (-67.3 ± 151.7 %) ($p<0.0005$). Mean value of cAI of women with unexplained RPL or that of RPL women with antiphospholipid antibodies is significantly higher than that in control women (Figure 6).

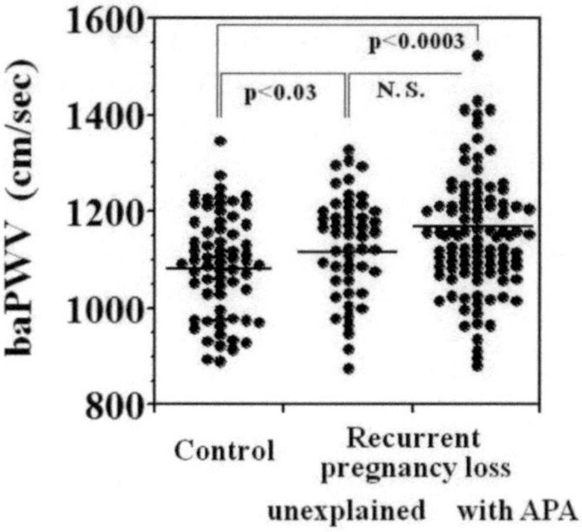

Fig. 5. baPWV of women with RPL

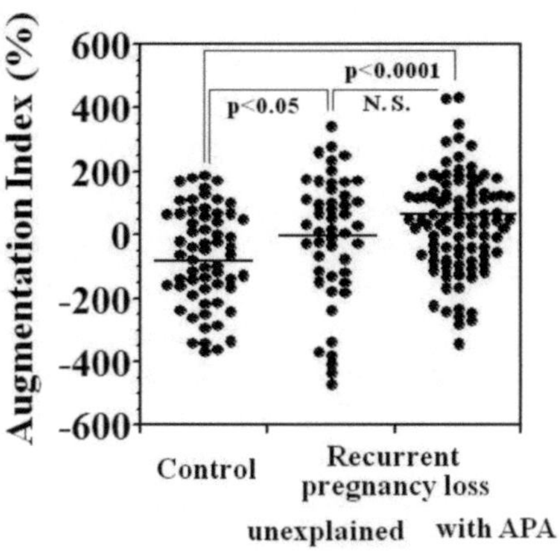

Fig. 6. cAI of women with RPL

4.3 Types of autoimmune antibodies and arterial stiffness in women with RPL

Antiphospholipid antibodies are a heterogeneous group of autoantibodies directed against phospholipid binding proteins, such as anti-cardiolipin antibodies, anti-β2GPI antibodies, and anti-phosphatidylserine/prothrombin antibodies, lupus anticoagulant, anti-phosphatidylserine antibodies and anti-phosphatidylethanolamine antibodies. Pathogenesis of antiphospholipid antibodies may vary depending on types and target phospholipid. There is an increasing interest in clinical significance of various types of antiphospholipid antibodies to define the patient's risk of arterial and venous thrombosis (Galli et al., 2005) although it is inconclusive.

Petri have reported that twenty years after diagnosis, SLE patients with lupus anticoagulant have a 50% chance of a venous thrombotic event and myocardial infarction occurs significantly more often (22%) in those with lupus anticoagulant (Petri, 2004). However, neither anti-cardiolipin nor lupus anticoagulant is associated with an increase of carotid IMT, carotid plaque, nor coronary calcium by helical CT, which are signs of subclinical atherosclerosis (Petri, 2004). In our study, we could not find any significant differences in baPWV or cAI between women with lupus anticoagulant and control women (Figure 7).

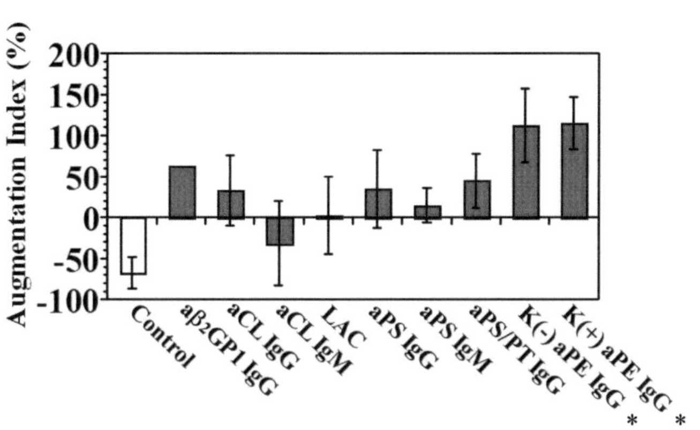

*:p<0.05 vs. Control, aβ2GPI: anti-β2GPI antibodies, aCL: anti-cardiolipin antibodies, LAC: lupus anticoagulant, aPS: anti-phosphatidylserine antibodies, aPS/PT: antibodies against phosphatidylserine/prothrombin complex, K(-)aPE: kininogen independent anti phosphatidylethanolamine antibodies, K(+)aPE: kininogen dependent anti-phosphatidylethanolamine antibodies

Fig. 7. cAI among women with various types of APA

There is some evidence that high anti-β2GPI antibodies can present a risk factor for atherosclerosis, but more epidemiological data are required in order to confirm whether the pro-atherogenic properties of anti-phospholipid antibodies signifies an independent risk factor for atherosclerosis and its complications. We observed that women with anti-β2GPI antibodies had high cAI. Unfortunately, we could not perform statistical analysis because women with anti-β2GPI antibodies were small population.

It has been reported that a significantly high prevalence of anti-phosphatidylserine IgG was found in stroke patients (57.7%) (Kahles et al., 2005). Anti-phosphatidylserine antibodies have a strong predictive value and association for arterial thrombosis (Lopez et al., 2004). Antibodies against phosphatidylserine/prothrombin complex have been reported to be closely associated with clinical features of APS rather than antibodies against prothrombin alone (Atsumi et al., 2004). However, there are no reports on atherosclerosis in women with these antibodies. We observed no significant association between anti-phosphatidylserine antibodies or antibodies against phosphatidylserine-prothrombin complex and arterial stiffness.

Recent studies have shown that some patients with unexplained thrombophilic disorders may have anti-phosphatidylethanolamine antibodies as the sole basis for their hypercoagulable state (Sanmarco, et al., 2001). It is noteworthy that anti-phosphatidylethanolamine antibodies have been described as the sole antiphospholipid antibodies in patients with thrombotic diseases (Staub, et al., 1989; Karmochkine, et al., 1992; Berard, et al., 1996). However, there are little studies on association of anti-phosphatidylethanolamine antibodies and arterial stiffness or atherosclerosis.

We observed that cAI was significantly increased in RPL women with anti-phosphatidylethanolamine antibodies. Anti-phosphatidylethanolamine antibodies may be a risk factor for atherosclerosis in women with RPL. It has been reported that kininogen-dependent IgG anti-phosphatidylethanolamine antibodies markedly increases thrombin-induced platelet aggregation in vitro while kininogen independent IgG anti-phosphatidylethanolamine antibodies do not augment thrombin-induced platelet aggregation (Sugi et al, 1999). However, we observed that both two types of anti-phosphatidylethanolamine antibodies were associated with arterial stiffness.

Physical distribution of phosphatidylethanolamine is known to be at the blood-endothelium interface. The luminal phosphatidylethanolamine is a vulnerable to anti-phosphatidylethanolamine autoimmunity, which is consistent with the association between anti- phosphatidylethanolamine antibodies and elevated risk for idiopathic thrombosis (Zhixin et al., 2011).

Risk factors for atherosclerosis in SLE include traditional risk factors (mainly the Framingham risk factors). Moreover, specific antibodies to β2GPI; anticardiolipin antibodies; anti-oxidized low-density lipoprotein (oxLDL); and antibodies to heat shock proteins may be cardiovascular disease risk factors (Sherer et al., 2010). Immune complexes containing oxLDL, β2GPI, and/or CRP are known to be involved in atherosclerosis (Matsuura et al., 2006, Chekir et al, 2009). Autoantibodies to oxLDL/β2GPI complex were detected in SLE and APS patients, and were strongly associated with arterial thrombosis (Christodoulou et al., 2007). Further studies may help evaluating clinical usefullness of these autoimmune antibodies involving in progression of atherosclerosis in women RPL.

4.4 Women with PCOS

Previous study on arterial stiffness has shown that both baPWV and cAI are useful for risk stratification of hypertensive patients (Matsui et al., 2004). In this study, both of these indices are significantly correlated with age and systolic blood pressure and cAI is reported to be correlated with total cholesterol and LDL-C in hypertensive patients.

We have reported that women with PCOS in reproductive age have a significantly higher baPWV than that for the control women (Sasaki et al., 2011). Arterial stiffness evaluated using the baPWV and cAI in mildly-hypertensive women (systolic blood pressure ≥ 120 mmHg or diastolic blood pressure ≥ 90 mmHg) with PCOS was significantly higher than that in the control women or normotensive women with PCOS. Early changes in vascular function were detected in mildly-hypertensive women with PCOS.

4.5 Women with unexplained RPL

We observed that women with unexplained RPL showed increased baPWV and cAI in average as compared with control women (Figure 5, 6). Although ranges of these indices in women with unexplained RPL and those in control women were overlapped, at least a portion of women with unexplained RPL showed increased baPWV and cAI. These observations suggest that antiphospholipid antibodies or endocrinological disorders may not be the sole cause for arterial stiffness in women with RPL. Vascular dysfunction caused by various factors may be involved in at least a portion of women with unexplained RPL.

A portion of women with unexplained RPL should be considered as a high risk group for atherosclerosis and cardiovascular diseases. Measurement of baPWV or AI is a promising technique to assess vascular dysfunction in women with RPL.

5. Possible cardiovascular diseases in pregnant women with RPL

In pregnant women with RPL, who have early changes of systemic vasculatures, may suffer vascular complications during pregnancy because of physiological hypercoagulability and hemodynamic changes associated with pregnancy.

5.1 Venous thromboembolism (VTE)

Thrombophilia is a risk factor for venous thromboembolism (VTE) in pregnancy because of the hypercoagulability of pregnancy, which is further increased in the presence of thrombophilia. Vascular reactivity, which is believed to be increased during pregnancy, may also compound the risk.

Pregnant women are at increased risk of venous thromboembolism (VTE). Estimated incidence of VTE during pregnancy is about 1 event per 1000 pregnancies (Chauleur et al., 2007). Despite this low incidence, thromboembolic complications occurring during pregnancy and post-partum remain a major cause of maternal death. Although pregnant women have a higher risk of developing thromboembolic complications than non-pregnant women, treating all pregnant women to prevent these events is not recommended.

A scoring system for VTE risk in pregnant women (Chauleur et al., 2007) includes antiphospholipid antibodies and reproductive history of one stillbirth or at least three recurrent miscarriages, which are clinical features of women with APS (Bobba et al., 2007).

5.2 Coronary heart disease and stroke in pregnancy

The risk of acute myocardial infarction is known to be approximately 3 to 4 times higher in pregnancy. The incidence of pregnancy-related acute myocardial infarction is in the broad range of 3 to 10 per 100 000 deliveries that has been reported previously (James et al., 2006). Hypertension (odds ratio (OR) 21.7), thrombophilia including history of thrombosis and APS (OR 22.3), diabetes mellitus (OR 3.6), smoking (OR 8.4), transfusion (OR 5.1), postpartum infection (OR 3.2), and age 30 years and older remain as significant risk factors for pregnancy-related acute myocardial infarction in the multivariable analysis (James et al., 2006). The odds of acute myocardial infarction are 30-fold higher for women aged 40 years and older than for women 20 years of age.

Thrombophilia, gestational diabetes mellitus associated with PCOS, or age 30 years and older may increase the risk further in women with RPL.

There are few data on the risk of stroke in relation to the full range of outcomes of pregnancy (spontaneous or induced abortion, stillbirth, and live birth) (Kittner & Stern, 1996). One of the most important risks factors for stroke is advanced maternal age, which suggests arterial stiffness and atherosclerosis may affect on the incidence of stroke (Bushnell, 2008). The majority (48%) of pregnancy-related strokes occur in the postpartum period, versus 41% at delivery, and 11% antepartum (James et al., 2005). The Baltimore Washington Cooperative Young Stroke Study found that stroke rate was not increased in pregnant compared with nonpregnant women, but during the postpartum period, there was a fivefold increased risk of ischemic stroke (Kittner et al., 1996). Risk factors found to be associated with pregnancy-related stroke in the most recent analysis include thrombophilia (OR 16.0) and lupus (OR 15.2) (James et al., 2005). Preeclampsia and gestational hypertension, which are sometimes observed in women with RPL even during treatments, increase the risk of stroke during pregnancy as a result of severe hypertension and disturbed cerebral autoregulation.

6. Reproductive history and cardiovascular disease risk later in life

Adverse reproductive history and complications during pregnancy in women with RPL should to be considered as cardiovascular risk factors later in life. Physiological hypercoagulability, hemodynamic changes, and metabolic syndrome during pregnancy may provoke pregnancy complications including pregnancy loss, preeclampsia, placental abruption, preterm birth, or birth of an infant small for gestational age, or gestational diabetes mellitus in women with subclinical thrombophilia such as antiphospholipid antibodies or Factor V Leiden and/or subclinical endcrinological abnormalities such or PCOS. They could be considered a "failed stress test," possibly unmasking early or preexisting endothelial dysfunction and vascular or metabolic disease (Mosca, 2011).

6.1 Parity

Endothelial function is improved and asymmetrical dimethylarginine, an endogenous nitric oxide synthase inhibitor, decreased during pregnancy, both of which would be expected to slow the progression of atherosclerosis. In contrast, childbirth modified cardiovascular risk factors, most notably a redistribution of body fat to a phenotype characterized by increased abdominal adiposity and marked reductions in HDL-C and apoA-I.

There is an emerging body of literature examining the association between parity and cardiovascular disease. After adjustment for age, obesity, and family history of diabetes, increased parity was associated with a significantly increased risk of both non insulin dependent diabetes mellitus (NIDDM) (OR 1.16 per pregnancy) and impaired glucose tolerance (OR 1.10 per pregnancy) (Kritz-Silverstein et al., 1989).

Most of the studies on the association between parity and coronary heart disease have included only women. However, comparisons between men and women distinguish whether the mechanisms for the association between parity and atherosclerosis involve biological processes related to pregnancy or socioeconomic or lifestyle factors that are related to family size and child-rearing. It has been reported that increasing parity is associated with carotid atherosclerosis in women but not in men among a population with at least one risk factor for cardiovascular disease (Lawlor et al., 2003; Skilton et al., 2009; Skilton et al., 2010).

Lifestyle risk factors associated with child-rearing lead to obesity and result in increased coronary heart diseass in both sexes but biological responses of pregnancy may have additional adverse effects in women (Lawlor et al., 2003).

It is suggested that the association between childbirth and concurrent changes in IMT may be independent of traditional cardiovascular risk factors (Skilton et al., 2010). However, another study described no association between parity and either IMT or presence of plaques after adjustment for age in a population based cohort of 746 Finnish women (Kharazmi et al., 2007). The causality of the link between parity and early atherosclerosis is not concluded.

6.2 Pregnancy loss

Women who suffered one or more pregnancy losses have had pregnancies of shorter duration than usual and consequently they have received less/shorter estrogen exposure during pregnancy. The protective effect of estrogen, therefore, is potentially less than in the case of a full-term pregnancy (Kleijn & Schouw, 1999). However, it is more likely that cardiovascular disease risk in women with history of RPL may reflect common determinants, such as thrombophilic genetic defects, antiphospholipid antibodies, and endocrinological or metabolic disorders.

Women with subclinical cardiovascular disease could have a higher risk of pregnancy loss and cardiovascular events later in life. There have been various reports on association between pregnancy loss and coronary heart disease risk or pregnancy loss and stroke risk, which are inconclusive (de Kleijn & Schouw, 1999; La Vecchia et al., 1987; Smith et al, 2001).

It has been reported that a history of any spontaneous loss of early pregnancy before the first live birth was associated with an increased risk of ischemic heart diseases (Smith et al., 2003). The association was independent of maternal age at the time of first birth, height, socioeconomic deprivation, essential hypertension, and complications during the first pregnancy. By contrast, there was no association between therapeutic abortion and subsequent risk of ischemic heart diseases. Women who had experienced at least one spontaneous or induced abortion had either increased or similar risk of coronary heart disease than women who had never had an abortion (Bertuccioa et al., 2007).

There is a report describing that abortions, either spontaneous or induced, are not related to myocardial infarction risk, although underreporting cannot be excluded, because some women do not realize that early abortion may have occurred and because induced abortion may not be reported (Bertuccioa et al., 2007).

6.3 Recurrent pregnancy loss

In women 50–74 years of age who had experienced pregnancy, history of pregnancy loss tended to be associated with a higher risk of myocardial infarction (age-adjusted OR 2.1), and the risk increased significantly with the number of pregnancy loss (age-adjusted OR 1.4) (Kharazmi et al., 2010). This result suggests that women who experience RPL are likely to be at an increased risk of vascular disease later in life. Spontaneous RPL (>3) is associated with about five times higher risk of myocardial infarction after full adjustment (Kharazmi et al.,

2011). Women who experience spontaneous pregnancy loss are at a substantially higher risk of myocardial infarction later in life. Although women who had history of RPL (>3) tended to have a higher risk of stroke (adjusted OR 1.43), associations between RPL and cerebrovascular events including stroke are also inconclusive.

Several studies have shown associations between acquired and inherited thrombophilias and both spontaneous loss of early pregnancy and ischemic heart disease (Smith et al., 2003). High homocysteine levels in early pregnancy are another risk factor for pregnancy loss and preecclampsia (Dodds, et al., 2008). Elevated levels of homocysteine in the bloodstream can irritate the blood vessels, which may eventually lead to hardening of the arteries, stroke or heart attack.

Miscarriage can sometimes lead to infections which may also have some links with cardiovascular diseases (Kharazmi et al., 2011). For instance, chlamydia infection has been found to be associated with occurrence of miscarriage and also with atherogenesis. Inflammation and infection as known risk factors for cardiovascular diseases might be the underlying mechanisms that explain the association between miscarriage and cardiovascular disease.

It is possible that the cause of pregnancy loss is related to hemodynamic factors, such as preeclampsia, and therefore to cardiovascular risk or disease (de Kleijn & Schouw, 1999). This means that the causal relationship could be reversed: women with a cardiovascular disease risk could have a higher risk of pregnancy loss. Occult cardiovascular, microvascular, or haemostatic dysfunction result in pregnancy complications during reproductive years and in overt cardiovascular disease later in life (Smith et al., 2003).

6.4 Still birth

Stillbirth is known to be associated with an increased risk of death from coronary heart disease, all circulatory and renal causes (Calderon-Margalit et al., 2007). A history of stillbirth is reported to be associated with an increased age-adjusted risk of plaque (OR 3.43), but it lost its statistical significance in the fully adjusted model (Kharazmi et al., 2007). Recent study have reported that each stillbirth increased the risk of myocardial infarction 2.32 times after adjustment for age, smoking, alcohol consumption, body mass index, waist to hip ratio, physical activity, education, number of pregnancies, hypertension, hyperlipidaemia and diabetes mellitus (Kharazmi et al., 2011). Stillbirth is a strong sex-specific predictor for myocardial infarction and thus should be considered as important indicators for cardiovascular risk factors monitoring and preventive measures (Kharazmi et al., 2011).

7. Complications in women with RPL and cardiovascular diseases

Pregnancy complications such as preeclampsia, placental abruption, preterm birth, or birth of an infant small for gestational age, or gestational diabetes mellitus are characteristic in women with RPL. Women with RPL are also at increased risk for recurrent episode of major depressive disorder. These complications may be associated with vascular dysfunction in women with RPL.

7.1 Preeclampsia

Preeclampsia affects about 5–8% of all first pregnancies and is a major cause of maternal and fetal morbidity and mortality worldwide. Preeclampsia is associated with vascular dysfunction manifesting hypertension (Nakatsuka et al., 2002) and one of common complications observed in women with RPL even during treatment. We have reported that uterine, orbital, and brachial circulations are impaired in women with preeclampsia (Takata et al., 2002). Several studies focused on an attenuated vasodilatory response in large blood vessels by evaluating flow-mediated dilatation or venous occlusion plethysmography (Spaana et al., 2010). One study evaluated microvascular function several years after preeclampsia, observing a lower response to both endothelium-dependent and independent vasodilatation using laser Doppler imaging of the forearm 20 years after preeclampsia (Ramsay et al. 2003).

One of the most common risk factors for stroke in pregnancy, particularly postpartum, is preeclampsia/eclampsia (Bushnell & Chireau, 2011). A history of preeclampsia during pregnancy lead to an increased risk of stroke later in life (Bellamy et al, 2007). Biomarkers of endothelial dysfunction such as intercellular adhesion molecule-1 (ICAM-1) and vascular cell adhesion molecule-1 (VCAM-1) are known to be elevated in women preeclampsia. Women with a history of preeclampsia are more likely to have higher insulin levels compared to controls.

Although the symptoms of preeclampsia typically regress within a few days post partum, impaired vascular dilatation is still present several years after preeclampsia, suggesting persistent endothelial dysfunction, which may contribute to the development of cardiovascular disease in these women (Spaana et al., 2010). A recent large meta-analysis found that women with a history of preeclampsia have approximately double the risk for subsequent ischemic heart disease, stroke, and venous thromboembolic events over the 5 to 15 years after pregnancy (Moska, 2011). Preeclampsia, particularly in association with preterm delivery, has been identified as a risk factor for myocardial infarction and mortality from cardiovascular disease later in life (James et al., 2006).

As described in the meta-analysis and other longitudinal studies, hypertension is the risk factor for cerebrovascular disease that women with a history of preeclampsia and gestational hypertension are most likely to develop (Bellamy et al, 2007).

7.2 Anxiety and depression

Other factors, which are prevalent among women with RPL and may make special contributions to cardiovascular disease risk, include anxiety, depression, and other psychosocial risk factors (Blackmore et al., 2011).

Anxiety, which is often observed in women with RPL, is also suggested to be an independent predictor of adverse cardiovascular events (Olafiranye et al., 2011). Individuals with high levels of anxiety are at increased risk of coronary heart disease, congestive heart failure, stroke, fatal ventricular arrhythmias, and sudden cardiac death. Anxiety following a major cardiac event can impede recovery, and is associated with a higher morbidity and mortality.

Risk for an episode of major depressive disorder among miscarrying women in the 6 months following loss is compared with the 6-month risk among community women who have not been pregnant in the preceding year (Neugebauer et al., 1997). Among miscarrying women, 10.9% experience an episode of major depressive disorder, compared with 4.3% of community women. The overall relative risk (RR) for an episode of major depressive disorder for miscarrying women is 2.5 and is substantially higher for childless women (RR 5.0) than for women with children (RR 1.3).

Midlife women are particularly vulnerable to depressive mood; the changing hormonal milieu during the menopausal transition contributes to increased prevalence of depressive symptoms and to the worsening of the cardiovascular disease profile (Janssen et al., 2011). Among miscarrying women with a history of major depressive disorder, 54% experience a recurrence later in life.

Symptoms of depression and major depressive disorder have been identified as potential risk factors for coronary heart disease (Janssen et al., 2011). Longitudinal studies have consistently shown that persons with high levels of depressive symptoms, or with a history of major depressive disorders, are more likely to have clinical coronary events than persons without depression. Major depression and depressive symptoms are associated with cardiovascular disease, but the impact of depression on early atherogenesis is less well known (Janssen et al., 2011). Anxiety and/or depression may be a risk factor for cardiovascular diseases in women with RPL.

8. Vascular dysfunction in children of women with PRL

Previous studies suggested that the atherogenic process in humans has already started during fetal development (Napoli et al, 1997). Intrauterine exposure to maternal atherosclerotic risk factors may increases the susceptibility to atherosclerosis in adult life (Alkemade et al., 2007). In a morphometric postmortem analysis of atherosclerosis in fetuses and children (Fate of Early Lesions in Children Study), it is demonstrated that specifically maternal hypercholesterolemia is associated with a higher incidence of atherosclerotic lesions during the fetal period and a faster progression of these atherosclerotic lesions after birth even under conditions of normocholesterolemia in the offspring (Napoli et al, 1999).

8.1 Perinatal arterial ischemic stroke (PAS)

Perinatal arterial ischemic stroke (PAS), defined as a thromboembolic event occurring before age 28 days, is an increasingly recognized cause of neurological disabilities such as cerebral palsy, epilepsy, and cognitive abnormalities (Lee et al., 2005). PAS occurs at a frequency of 1/1600 to 1/5000 live births (Chabriera et al., 2010). Previous fetal loss, first pregnancy, primiparity, twin-gestation, cesarean and traumatic delivery, neonatal distress, male sex and premature rupture of membranes in PAS were statistically more common than in the general population (Chabriera et al., 2010).

PAS may result from thrombosis of intracranial vessels or from embolism from another site such as extracranial vessels, heart, umbilical vein, or placenta (Nelson, 2007). Although the site of origin is usually not clearly established, it is suspected that the fetal side of the placenta may often be the source. In addition to cerebral infarction, thrombosis in other sites, including kidney, heart, aorta, and limb arteries, is more common in neonates than at other times in childhood.

Antiphospholipid antibodies in women RPL may pass from mother to child via the placenta, can alter the placenta itself and may be a risk for PAS. The inherited thrombophilias both in mothers and fetuses may cause RPL and PAS in neonates (Nelson, 2007). It seems likely that maternal and perhaps infant thrombophilias can lead to complications of pregnancy, such as RPL, preeclampsia, placental abruption, placental vasculopathy, and fetal growth restriction, which are in turn risk factors for neonatal encephalopathy, stroke, or cerebral palsy (Nelson, 2007).

8.2 Genetic risk factors

Complications of pregnancy such as preeclampsia, which are observed in untreated and treated women with PRL, link to low birth weight. Previous studies have shown an association between an individual's birth weight and his or her subsequent risk of ischemic heart disease, hypertension, and diabetes mellitus (Hübinettea et al., 2001). Barker and colleagues have postulated that fetal adaptation to inadequate intrauterine nutrition, due to poor maternal diet or placental dysfunction, results in physiological programming of a "thrifty phenotype", which increases the risk of hypertension and ischemic heart disease in later life (Barker et al., 1989).

An alternative hypothesis is that common genetic factors predispose to fetal growth restriction, preterm birth, and ischemic heart diseases. Common genetic risk factors might explain the link between birthweight and risk of ischemic heart disease in both the mother and the child (Smith et al., 2001). A genetic link would be consistent with the much stronger association between birthweight and ischemic heart disease in the mother (11-fold) (Smith et al., 2001) than in the offspring (1.5–2.0-fold) (Barker et al., 1989). Maternal genes might modulate fetal growth both by affecting the intrauterine environment, for instance by effects on uterine blood flow, and by inheritance of genes from the mother that regulate fetal growth directly.

Epidemiological studies also provide evidence for common genetic links. Fathers of low-birthweight babies are at increased risk of coronary heart disease, hypertension, and diabetes (Smith et al., 2001). Children and their mothers, who experienced RPL, may have common genetic factors linked to cardiovascular diseases.

9. Treatment of pregnancy loss and prevention of cardiovascular diseases

Currently, low-dose aspirin treatment is used as an effective therapy for women with RPL associated with anti-phospholipid antibodies (Coulam et al., 1997). It has been reported that low-dose aspirin is effective in improving implantation and pregnancy rates in the IVF programme (Rubinstein et al., 1999). Two trials demonstrated that women without hereditary thrombophilia and at least three unexplained consecutive losses randomized to prophylactic low molecular weight heparin had higher live birth rates than those assigned to placebo or no treatment (Bates, 2010).

Antiphospholipid antibodies are more common in patients with thrombosis but a causal association is unproven and the clinical relevance of transient or low titer antiphospholipid antibodies remains uncertain (Lim et al., 2006). In patients with APS, moderate-intensity warfarin is effective for preventing recurrent venous thrombosis and perhaps also arterial thrombosis. Aspirin appears to be as effective as moderate-intensity warfarin for preventing recurrent stroke in patients with prior stroke and a single positive test result for antiphospholipid antibody. Many patients with myocardial infarction and antiphospholipid antibodies are treated by warfarin.

The relationship between preeclampsia and stroke involves shared risk factors for both disorders, including chronic endothelial dysfunction and increased risk for long-term hypertension following preeclampsia, one of the major risk factors for stroke (Bushnell & Chireau, 2010). Thrombophilic conditions and Vitamin D deficiency (Grant, 2009) has emerged as an important potentially modifiable risk factor for both preeclampsia and stroke. These overlaps provide insights into underlying pathophysiology and potential preventive strategies for both preeclampsia and stroke. For example, aspirin or Vitamin D may prevent both disorders.

Early changes in vascular function are detected in mildly-hypertensive women with PCOS (Sasaki et al., 2011). All women diagnosed with PCOS are not likely to share the same cardiovascular risk profiles and increased mortality and morbidity rates from cardiovascular disease in the PCOS population. However, lifestyle intervention such as diet and exercise should be the first-line of treatment in women with PCOS, particularly if they are hypertensive or overweight.

It is unlikely to treat all young women with aspirin following the occurrence of PRL without any other risk factors. Pharmacological therapies for hypertension, insulin resistance, or dyslipidemia are also available but should be tailored on an individual basis. It is important to evaluate arterial stiffness to identify women at early risk of cardiovascular disease and stroke and ultimately assess the risks and benefits of various prevention approaches.

10. Conclusion

Women who experienced RPL are at a substantially higher risk of vascular dysfunction, which leads to coronary heart disease, stroke, or VTE later in life. Reproductive history of obstetrical complications associated with RPL such as preeclampsia, premature delivery, fetal growth restriction, placental abruption, and gestational diabetes mellitus could be considered a "failed stress test," possibly unmasking early or preexisting vascular dysfunction and vascular or metabolic diseases. Therefore, these women should be carefully monitored and controlled. Healthcare professionals who meet women for the first time later in their lives should take a careful and detailed history of RPL and characteristic pregnancy complications.

Further studies will provide more information on association between PRL and vascular dysfunction, effective treatment for both women with PRL and their fetuses.

11. References

Abbott DH, Dumesic DA, Franks S: Developmental origin of polycystic ovary syndrome - a hypothesis. J Endocrinol 174:1-5, 2002.

Ajossa S, Guerriero S, Paoletti AM, Orru M, Melis GB: Hyperinsulinemia and uterine perfusion in patients with polycystic ovary syndrome. Ultrasound Obstet Gynecol 2:276-280, 2002.

Alcázar JL, Ruiz-Perez ML: Uteroplacental circulation in patients with first-trimester threatened abortion. Fertil Steril 73: 130-135, 2000.

Alkemade FE, Gittenberger-de Groot AC, Schiel AE, VanMunsteren JC, Hogers B, van Vliet LS, Poelmann RE, Havekes LM, Willems van Dijk K, DeRuiter MC: Intrauterine exposure to maternal atherosclerotic risk factors increases the susceptibility to atherosclerosis in adult life. Arterioscler Thromb Vasc Biol 27: 2228-2235, 2007.

Alves JD, Grima B: Oxidative stress in systemic lupus erythematosus and antiphospholipid syndrome: a gateway to atherosclerosis. Curr Rheumatol Rep 5: 383-390, 2003.

Ames PR, Antinolfi I, Scenna G, Gaeta G, Margaglione M, Margarita A. Atherosclerosis in thrombotic primary antiphospholipid syndrome. J Thromb Haemost 7: 537–542, 2009.

Ames PR, Margarita A, Delgado Alves J, Tommasino C, Iannaccone L, Brancaccio V: Anticardiolipin antibody titre and plasma homocysteine level independently predict intima media thickness of carotid arteries in subjects with idiopathic antiphospholipid antibodies. Lupus 11:208-214, 2002.

Anfossi G, Russo I, Doronzo G, Pomero A, Trovati M: Adipocytokines in atherothrombosis: focus on platelets and vascular smooth muscle cells. Mediators Inflamm 2010:174341. Epub 2010 Jun 28.

Atsumi T, Amengual O, Yasuda S, Koike T: Antiprothrombin antibodies--are they worth assaying? Thromb Res 114: 533-538, 2004.

Barker DJ, Winter PD, Osmond C, Margetts B, Simmonds SJ: Weight in infancy and death from ischaemic heart disease. Lancet 2: 577-580, 1989.

Baron MA, Khamashta MA, Hughes GR, D'Cruz DP: Prevalence of an abnormal ankle-brachial index in patients with primary antiphospholipid syndrome: preliminary data. Ann Rheum Dis 64 :144-146. 2005.

Bates SM: Consultative hematology: the pregnant patient pregnancy loss. Hematology Am Soc Hematol Educ Program 2010: 166-172, 2010.

Bellamy L, Casas JP, Hingorani AD, Williams DJ: Pre-eclampsia and risk of cardiovascular disease and cancer in later life: systematic review and meta-analysis. BMJ 335: 974. 2007.

Berard M, Chantome R, Marcelli A, Boffa MC: Antiphosphatidylethanolamine antibodies as the only antiphospholipid antibodies. I. Association with thrombosis and vascular cutaneous diseases. J Rheumatol 23: 1369-1374, 1996.

Bertuccio P, Tavani A, Gallus S, Negri E, La Vecchia C: Menstrual and reproductive factors and risk of non-fatal acute myocardial infarction in Italy. Eur J Obstet Gynecol Reprod Biol 134: 67-72, 2007.

Blacher J, Asmar R, Djane S, London GM, Safar ME. Aortic pulse wave velocity as a marker of cardiovascular risk in hypertensive patients. Hypertension 33: 1111-1117, 1999.

Blackmore ER, Côté-Arsenault D, Tang W, Glover V, Evans J, Golding J, O'Connor TG: Previous prenatal loss as a predictor of perinatal depression and anxiety. Br J Psychiatry 198: 373-378, 2011.

Bobba RS, Johnson SR, Davis AM: A review of the sapporo and revised Sapporo criteria for the classification of antiphospholipid syndrome. Where do the revised sapporo criteria add value? J Rheumatol 34: 1522-1527, 2007.

Brey RL Management of the neurological manifestations of APS--what do the trials tell us? Thromb Res 114: 489-499. 2004.

Burke GL, Evans GW, Riley WA, Sharrett AR, Howard G, Barnes RW, Rosamond W, Crow RS, Rautaharju PM, Heiss G: Arterial wall thickness is associated with prevalent cardiovascular disease in middle-aged adults. The Atherosclerosis Risk in Communities (ARIC) Study. Stroke 26: 386-391, 1995.

Bushnell C, Chireau M: Preeclampsia and Stroke: Risks during and after Pregnancy. Stroke Res Treat. 2011 Jan 20; 2011:858134.

Bushnell CD: Stroke in women: risk and prevention throughout the lifespan. Neurol Clin 26: 1161-1176, 2008.

Calderon-Margalit R, Friedlander Y, Yanetz R, Deutsch L, Manor O, Harlap S, Paltiel O: Late stillbirths and long-term mortality of mothers. Obstet Gynecol 109: 1301-1308, 2007.

Caruso A, De Carolis S, Ferrazzani S, Valesini G, Caforio L, Mancuso S. Pregnancy outcome in relation to uterine artery flow velocity waveforms and clinical characteristics in women with antiphospholipid syndrome. Obstet Gynecol 82:970-977, 1993.

Chabrier S, Saliba E, Nguyen The Tich S, Charollais A, Varlet MN, Tardy B, Presles E, Renaud C, Allard D, Husson B, Landrieu P: Obstetrical and neonatal characteristics vary with birthweight in a cohort of 100 term newborns with symptomatic arterial ischemic stroke. Eur J Paediatr Neurol 14: 206-213, 2010.

Chauleur C, Quenet S, Varlet MN, Seffert P, Laporte S, Decousus H, Mismetti P: Feasibility of an easy-to-use risk score in the prevention of venous thromboembolism and placental vascular complications in pregnant women: a prospective cohort of 2736 women. Thromb Res 122: 478-484, 2008.

Chekir C, Nakatsuka M, Kamada Y, Noguchi S, Sasaki A, Hiramatsu Y: Impaired uterine perfusion associated with metabolic disorders in women with polycystic ovary syndrome. Acta Obstet Gynecol Scand 84: 189-195, 2005.

Chekir C, Nakatsuka M, Sasaki A, Matsuda M, Kotani S, Sharula, Shimizu K, Kamada Y, Noguchi S, Hiramatsu Y, Matsuura E: Possible vascular dysfunction in endometriosis: An increase of oxidized LDL-β2GPI-CRP complex in serum. Reproductive Immunology and Biology 24: 34, 2009.

Christiansen OB, Nybo Andersen AM, Bosch E, Daya S, Delves PJ, Hviid TV, Kutteh WH, Laird SM, Li TC, van der Ven K: Evidence-based investigations and treatments of recurrent pregnancy loss. Fertil Steril 83:821-839, 2005.

Christodoulou C, Sangle S, D'Cruz DP: Vasculopathy and arterial stenotic lesions in the antiphospholipid syndrome. Rheumatology (Oxford) 46: 907-910, 2007.

de Kleijn MJ, van der Schouw YT, van der Graaf Y: Reproductive history and cardiovascular disease risk in postmenopausal women: a review of the literature. Maturitas 33: 7-36, 1999.

de Kleijn MJ, van der Schouw YT, van der Graaf Y: Reproductive history and cardiovascular disease risk in postmenopausal women: a review of the literature. Maturitas 33:7–36, 1999.

Dickey RP, Hower JF: Effect of ovulation induction on uterine blood flow and oestradiol and progesterone concentrations in early pregnancy. Hum Reprod 10: 2875-2879, 1995.

Diejomaoh M, Jirous J, Al-Azemi M, Baig S, Gupta M, Tallat A: The relationship of recurrent spontaneous miscarriage with reproductive failure. Med Princ Pract 12:107-111, 2003.

Dodds L, Fell DB, Dooley KC, Armson BA, Allen AC, Nassar BA, Perkins S, Joseph KS:. Effect of homocysteine concentration in early pregnancy on gestational hypertensive disorders and other pregnancy outcomes. Clin Chem 54: 326-334, 2008.

Doldi N, Gessi A, Destefani A, Calzi F, Ferrari A: Polycystic ovary syndrome: anomalies in progesterone production. Hum Reprod 13:290-293, 1998.

Dunaif A: Insulin resistance and the polycystic ovary syndrome: mechanism and implications for pathogenesis. Endocr Rev 18:774-800, 1997.

Dusse L, Godoi L, Kazmi RS, Alpoim P, Petterson J, Lwaleed BA, Carvalho M: Sources of thrombomodulin in pre-eclampsia: renal dysfunction or endothelial damage? Semin Thromb Hemost 37:153-157, 2011.

Ehrmann DA: Polycystic ovary syndrome. N Engl J Med 352: 1223–1236, 2005.

El-mashad AI, Mohamed MA, Farag MA, Ahmad MK, Ismail Y: Role of uterine artery Doppler velocimetry indices and plasma adrenomedullin level in women with unexplained recurrent pregnancy loss. J Obstet Gynaecol Res 37: 51-57, 2011.

Fenkci V, Fenkci S, Yilmazer M, Serteser M. Decreased total antioxidant status and increased oxidative stress in women with polycystic ovary syndrome may contribute to the risk of cardiovascular disease. Fertil Steril 80: 123-127, 2003.

Franks S: Polycystic ovary syndrome. N Engl J Med 333:853-861, 1995.

Galli M, Barbui T: Antiphospholipid syndrome: clinical and diagnostic utility of laboratory tests. Semin Thromb Hemost 31: 17-24, 2005.

Garruti G, Depalo R, Vita MG, Lorusso F, Giampetruzzi F, Damato AB, Giorgino F: Adipose tissue, metabolic syndrome and polycystic ovary syndrome: from pathophysiology to treatment. Reprod Biomed Online 19:552-563, 2009.

Glueck CJ, Awadalla SG, Phillips H, Cameron D, Wang P, Fontaine RN: Polycystic ovary syndrome, infertility, familial thrombophilia, familial hypofibrinolysis, recurrent loss of in vitro fertilized embryos, and miscarriage. Metabolism 48: 1589-1595, 1999.

Goswamy RK, Steptoe PC: Doppler ultrasound studies of the uterine artery in spontaneous ovarian cycles. Hum. Reprod 3: 721-726, 1988a.

Goswamy RK, Williams G. Steptoe PC: Decreased uterine perfusion-a cause of infertility. Hum. Reprod 3: 955-959, 1988b.

Grant WB: Role of vitamin D in up-regulating VEGF and reducing the risk of pre-eclampsia. Clin Sci (Lond) 116: 871, 2009.

Habara T, Nakatsuka M, Konishi H, Asagiri K, Noguchi S, Kudo T: Elevated blood flow resistance in uterine arteries of women with unexplained recurrent pregnancy loss. Hum Reprod 17: 190-194, 2002.

Hinson JP, Kapas S, Smith DM: Adrenomedullin, a multifunctional regulatory peptide. Endocrine Rev 21:138-167, 2000.

Huang J, Fu G, Yao Q, Cheng G: Relation of thrombomodulin, TFPI and plasma antioxidants in healthy individuals and patients with coronary heart disease. Acta Cardiol 63:341-346, 2008.

Hübinette A, Cnattingius S, Ekbom A, de Faire U, Kramer M, Lichtenstein P: Birthweight, early environment, and genetics: a study of twins discordant for acute myocardial infarction. Lancet 357: 1997-2001, 2001.

James AH, Bushnell CD, Jamison MG, Myers ER: Incidence and risk factors for stroke in pregnancy and the puerperium. Obstet Gynecol 106:509–516, 2005.

James AH, Jamison MG, Biswas MS, Brancazio LR, Swamy GK, Myers ER: Acute myocardial infarction in pregnancy: a United States population-based study. Circulation 113: 1564-1571, 2006.

Janssen I, Powell LH, Matthews KA, Cursio JF, Hollenberg SM, Sutton-Tyrrell K, Bromberger JT, Everson-Rose SA; SWAN study. Depressive symptoms are related to progression of coronary calcium in midlife women: the Study of Women's Health Across the Nation (SWAN) Heart Study. Am Heart J 161: 1186-1191, 2011.

Jauniaux E, Zaidi J, Jurkovic D, Campbell S, Hustin J: Comparison of colour Doppler features and pathological findings in complicated early pregnancy. Hum Reprod 9: 2432-2437, 1994.

Jougasaki M, Burnett JC Jr: Adrenomedullin: Potential in physiology and pathophysiology. Life Sci 66: 855–872, 2000.

Kahles T, Humpich M, Steinmetz H, Sitzer M, Lindhoff-Last E: Phosphatidylserine IgG and beta-2-glycoprotein I IgA antibodies may be a risk factor for ischaemic stroke. Rheumatology (Oxford) 44: 1161-1165, 2005.

Karakas M, Baumert J, Herder C, Rottbauer W, Meisinger C, Koenig W, Thorand B: Soluble thrombomodulin in coronary heart disease: lack of an association in the MONICA/KORA case-cohort study. J Thromb Haemost 9:1078-1080, 2011.

Karmochkine M, Cacoub P, Piette JC, Godear P, Boffa MC: Antiphosphatidylethanolamine antibody as the sole antiphospholipid antibody in systemic lupus erythematosus with thrombosis. Clin Exp Rheumatol 10: 603-605, 1992.

Kharazmi E, Moilanen L, Fallah M, Kaaja R, Kattainen A, Kahonen M, Jula A, Kesaniemi A, Luoto R: Reproductive history and carotid intima-media thickness. Acta Obstet Gynecol Scand 86: 995–1002, 2007.

Kharazmi E, Dossus L, Rohrmann S, Kaaks R: Pregnancy loss and risk of cardiovascular disease: A prospective population-based cohort study (EPIC-Heidelberg). Heart 97:49-54, 2011.

Kharazmi E, Fallah M, Luoto R: Miscarriage and risk of cardiovascular disease. Acta Obstet Gynecol Scand 89: 284-288, 2010.

Kittner SJ, Stern BJ, Feeser BR, Hebel R, Nagey DA, Buchholz DW, Earley CJ, Johnson CJ, Macko RF, Sloan MA, Wityk RJ, Wozniak MA: Pregnancy and the risk of stroke. N Engl J Med 335: 768-774, 1996.

Kritz-Silverstein D, Barrett-Connor E, Wingard DL: The effect of parity on the later development of non-insulin-dependent diabetes mellitus or impaired glucose tolerance. N Engl J Med 321: 1214-1219, 1989.

Kurjak A, Zalud I, Predanic M, Kupesic S: Transvaginal color and pulsed Doppler study of uterine blood flow in the first and early second trimesters of pregnancy: normal versus abnormal. J Ultrasound Med 1994; 13: 43-47.

Kutteh WH: Recurrent pregnancy loss (RPL): an update. Current Opinion Obstet Gynecol 11: 435-439, 1999.

Laurent S, Boutouyrie P, Asmar R, Gautier I, Laloux B, Guize L, Ducimetiere P, Benetos A: Aortic stiffness is an independent predictor of all-cause and cardiovascular mortality in hypertensive patients. Hypertension 37: 1236-1241, 2001 May.

La Vecchia C, Decarli A, Franceschi S, Gentile A, Negri E, Parazzini F: Menstrual and reproductive factors and the risk of myocardial infarction in women under fifty-five years of age. American Journal of Obstetrics & Gynecology 157: 1108–1112, 1987.

Lawlor DA, Emberson JR, Ebrahim S, Whincup PH, Wannamethee SG, Walker M, Smith GD; British Women's Heart and Health Study; British Regional Heart Study: Is the association between parity and coronary heart disease due to biological effects of pregnancy or adverse lifestyle risk factors associated with child-rearing? Findings from the British Women's Heart and Health Study and the British Regional Heart Study. Circulation 107: 1260-1264, 2003.

Lee J, Croen LA, Lindan C, Nash KB, Yoshida CK, Ferriero DM, Barkovich AJ, Wu YW: Predictors of outcome in perinatal arterial stroke: a population-based study. Ann Neurol 58: 303-308, 2005.

Legro RS. Polycystic ovary syndrome and cardiovascular disease: a premature association? Endocr Rev 24: 302-312, 2003.

Lim W, Crowther MA, Eikelboom JW: Management of antiphospholipid antibody syndrome: a systematic review. JAMA 295: 1050-1057, 2006.

Li TC: Recurrent miscarriage: principles of management. Hum. Reprod 13: 478-482, 1998.

London GM, Blacher J, Pannier B, Guerin AP, Marchais SJ, Safar ME: Arterial wave reflections and survival in end-stage renal failure. Hypertension 38: 434-438. 2001.

London GM, Cohn JN: Prognostic application of arterial stiffness: task forces. Am J Hypertens 15: 754-758. 2002.

Lopez LR, Dier KJ, Lopez D, Merrill JT, Fink CA: Anti- 2-glycoprotein I and antiphosphatidylserine antibodies are predictors of arterial thrombosis in patients with antiphospholipid syndrome. Am J Clin Pathol 121: 142-149, 2004.

Mackworth-Young CG: Antiphospholipid syndrome: multiple mechanisms. Clin Exp Immunol 136: 393-401, 2004.

Matsui Y, Kario K, Ishikawa J, Eguchi K, Hoshide S, Shimada K: Reproducibility of arterial stiffness indices (pulse wave velocity and augmentation index) simultaneously assessed by automated pulse wave analysis and their associated risk factors in essential hypertensive patients. Hypertens Res 27: 851-857, 2004.

Matsuura E, Kobayashi K, Tabuchi M, Lopez LR: Oxidative modification of low-density lipoprotein and immune regulation of atherosclerosis. Prog Lipid Res 45: 466-486, 2006.

Mok CC, Poon WL, Lai JP, Wong CK, Chiu SM, Wong CK, Lun SW, Ko GT, Lam CW, Lam CS: Metabolic syndrome, endothelial injury, and subclinical atherosclerosis in patients with systemic lupus erythematosus. Scand J Rheumatol 39:42-49, 2010.

Mosca L: Effectiveness-Based Guidelines for the Prevention of Cardiovascular Disease in Women—2011 Update A Guideline From the American Heart Association. Circulation 123: 1243-1262, 2011.

Nakatsuka M, Asagiri K, Kimura Y, Kamada Y, Tada K, Kudo T: Generation of peroxynitrite and apoptosis in placenta of patients with chorioamnionitis: possible implications in placental abruption. Hum. Reprod 14: 1101-1106, 1999a.

Nakatsuka M, Habara T, Noguchi S, Konishi H, Kudo T: Impaired uterine arterial blood flow in pregnant women with recurrent pregnancy loss. J Ultrasound Med 22:27-31, 2003a.

Nakatsuka M, Habara T, Noguchi S, Konishi H, Kudo T: Increased plasma adrenomedullin in women with recurrent pregnancy loss. Obstet Gynecol 102: 319-324, .2003b.

Nakatsuka M, Noguchi S, Kamada Y, Sasaki A, Chekir C, Lin H, Hiramatsu Y: Impaired vascular function in women with recurrent pregnancy loss: Involvement of antiphospholipid antibodies. Proceedings of the IX International Congress of Reproductive Immunology - ISIR: 97-100, 2004.

Nakatsuka M, Takata M, Tada K, Asagiri K, Habara T, Noguchi S, Kudo T: A long-term transdermal nitric oxide donor improves uteroplacental circulation in women with preeclampsia. J Ultrasound Med 21: 831-836, 2002.

Nakatsuka M, Tada K, Kimura Y, Asagiri K, Kamada Y, Takata M, Nakata T, Inoue N, Kudo T: Clinical experience of long-term transdermal treatment with NO donor for women with preeclampsia. Gynecol Obstet Invest 47:13-19, 1999b.

Napoli C, D'Armiento FP, Mancini FP, Postiglione A, Witztum JL, Palumbo G, Palinski W: Fatty streak formation occurs in human fetal aortas and is greatly enhanced by maternal hypercholesterolemia. Intimal accumulation of low density lipoprotein and its oxidation precede monocyte recruitment into early atherosclerotic lesions. J Clin Invest 100:2680 –2690, 1997.

Napoli C, Glass CK, Witztum JL, Deutsch R, D'Armiento FP, Palinski W. Influence of maternal hypercholesterolaemia during pregnancy on progression of early atherosclerotic lesions in childhood: Fate of Early Lesions in Children (FELIC) study. Lancet 354: 1234 –1241, 1999.

Nayak AK, Komatireddy G: Cardiac manifestations of the antiphospholipid antibody syndrome: a review. Mo Med 99:171-178, 2002.

Nelson KB: Perinatal ischemic stroke. Stroke 38: 742-745, 2007.

Neugebauer R, Kline J, Shrout P, Skodol A, O'Connor P, Geller PA, Stein Z, Susser M: Major depressive disorder in the 6 months after miscarriage. JAMA 277: 383-388, 1997.

Nichols WW: Clinical measurement of arterial stiffness obtained from noninvasive pressure waveforms. Am J Hypertens 18: 3S-10S. 2005.

Nicolo D, Monestier M: Antiphospholipid antibodies and atherosclerosis. Clin Immunol 112: 183-189, 2004.

Ogasawara M, Aoki K, Kajima S, Yagami Y: Are antinuclear antibodies predictive of recurrent miscarriage? Lancet 347: 1183-1184, 1996.

Olafiranye O, Jean-Louis G, Zizi F, Nunes J, Vincent M: Anxiety and cardiovascular risk: Review of Epidemiological and Clinical Evidence. Mind Brain 2: 32-37, 2011.

Petri M: The lupus anticoagulant is a risk factor for myocardial infarction (but not atherosclerosis): Hopkins Lupus Cohort. Thromb Res 114: 593-595, 2004.

Renaud SJ, Cotechini T, Quirt JS, Macdonald-Goodfellow SK, Othman M, Graham CH: Spontaneous pregnancy loss mediated by abnormal maternal inflammation in rats is linked to deficient uteroplacental perfusion. J Immunol 186:1799-1808, 2011.

Robson SC, Hunter S, Boys RJ, Dunlop W: Serial study of factors influencing changes in cardiac output during human pregnancy. Am J Physiol 256: H1060-H1065, 1989.

Rosendaal FR, Siscovick DS, Schwartz SM, Beverly RK, Psaty BM, Longstreth WT Jr, Raghunathan TE, Koepsell TD, Reitsma PH: Factor V Leiden (resistance to activated protein C) increases the risk of myocardial infarction in young women. Blood 89: 2817-2821, 1997.

Sabuncu T, Vural H, Harma M, Harma M. Oxidative stress in polycystic ovary syndrome and its contribution to the risk of cardiovascular disease. Clin Biochem 34: 407-413, 2001.

Sacks D, Bakal CW, Beatty PT, Becker GJ, Cardella JF, Raabe RD, Wiener HM, Lewis CA: Position statement on the use of the ankle-brachial index in the evaluation of patients with peripheral vascular disease: a consensus statement developed by the standards division of the society of cardiovascular & interventional radiology. J Vasc Interv Radiol 13: 353, 2002.

Salle B, Bied-Damon V, Benchaib M, Desperes S, Gaucherand P, Rudigoz RC: Preliminary report of an ultrasonography and colour Doppler uterine score to predict uterine receptivity in an in-vitro fertilization programme. Hum. Reprod 13: 1669-1673, 1998.

Sanmarco M, Alessi MC, Harle JR, Sapin C, Aillaud MF, Gentile S, Juhan-Vague I, Weiller PJ: Antibodies to phosphatidylethanolamine as the only antiphospholipid antibodies found in patients with unexplained thromboses. Thromb Haemost 85: 800–805, 2001.

Sasaki A, Emi Y, Matsuda M, Sharula, Kamada Y, Chekir C, Hiramatsu Y, Nakatsuka M: Increased arterial stiffness in mildly-hypertensive women with polycystic ovary syndrome. J Obstet Gynaecol Res ;37: 402-411, 2011.

Setji TL, Brown AJ: Polycystic ovary syndrome: diagnosis and treatment. Am J Med 120: 128-32, 2007.

Sherer Y, Shoenfeld Y: Antiphospholipid antibodies: are they pro-atherogenic or an epiphenomenon of atherosclerosis? Immunobiology 207:13-16, 2003.

Sherer Y, Zinger H, Shoenfeld Y: Atherosclerosis in systemic lupus erythematosus. Autoimmunity 43: 98-102, 2010.

Skilton MR, Sérusclat A, Begg LM, Moulin P, Bonnet F: Parity and carotid atherosclerosis in men and women: insights into the roles of childbearing and child-rearing. Stroke 40: 1152-1157, 2009.

Skilton MR, Bonnet F, Begg LM, Juonala M, Kähönen M, Lehtimäki T, Viikari JS, Raitakari OT: Childbearing, child-rearing, cardiovascular risk factors, and progression of carotid intima-media thickness: the Cardiovascular Risk in Young Finns study. Stroke 41: 1332-1337, 2010.

Slowińska-Srzednicka J, Zgliczyński S, Wierzbicki M, Srzednicki M, Stopińska-Gluszak U, Zgliczyński W, Soszyński P, Chotkowska E, Bednarska M, Sadowski Z: The role of hyperinsulinemia in the development of lipid disturbances in non-obese and obese women with the polycystic ovary syndrome. J Endocrinol Invest 14: 569-575, 1991.

Smith GC, Pell JP, Walsh D: Pregnancy complications and maternal risk of ischaemic heart disease: a retrospective cohort study of 129,290 births. Lancet 357: 2002-2006, 2001.

Smith GC, Pell JP, Walsh D: Spontaneous loss of early pregnancy and risk of ischaemic heart disease in later life: retrospective cohort study. BMJ 326: 423-424, 2003.

Soltesz P, Bereczki D, Szodoray P, Magyar MT, Der H, Csipo I, Hajas A, Paragh G, Szegedi G, Bodolay E: Endothelial cell markers reflecting endothelial cell dysfunction in patients with mixed connective tissue disease. Arthritis Res Ther 12:R78, 2010.

Spaan JJ, Houben AJ, Musella A, Ekhart T, Spaanderman ME, Peeters LL: Insulin resistance relates to microvascular reactivity 23 years after preeclampsia. Microvasc Res 80: 417-421, 2010.

Staub HL, Harris EN, Khamashta MH, Savidge G, Chahade WH, Hughes GR: Antibody to phosphatidylethanolamine in a patient with lupus anticoagulant and thrombosis. Ann Rheum Dis 48: 166-169, 1989.

Steel SA, Pearce JM, McParland P, Chamberlain GV: Early Doppler ultrasound screening in prediction of hypertensive disorders of pregnancy. Lancet 335: 1548-1551, 1990.

Steer CV, Tan AL, Mason BA, Campbell S: Midluteal-phase vaginal color Doppler assessment of uterine artery impedance in a subfertile population. Fertil. Steril 61: 53-58, 1994.

Sugi T, Katsunuma J, Izumi S, McIntyre JA, Makino T: Prevalence and heterogeneity of antiphosphatidylethanolamine antibodies in patients with recurrent early pregnancy losses. Fertil Steril 71:1060-1065, 1999.

Takata M, Nakatsuka M, Kudo T: Differential blood flow in uterine, ophthalmic, and brachial arteries of preeclamptic women. Obstet Gynecol 100: 931–939, 2002.

The Rotterdam ESHRE/ASRM-Sponsored PCOS consensus workshop group: Revised 2003 consensus on diagnostic criteria and long-term health risks related to polycystic ovary syndrome (PCOS). Hum Reprod 19:41-47, 2004.

van den Elzen HJ, Cohen-Overbeek TE, Grobbee DE, Quartero RW, Wladimiroff JW: Early uterine artery Doppler velocimetry and the outcome of pregnancy in women aged 35 years and older. Ultrasound Obstet Gynecol 5: 328-333, 1995.

van den Elzen HJ, Cohen-Overbeek TE, Grobbee DE, Wladimiroff JW. The predictive value of uterine artery flow velocity waveforms in miscarriage in older women. Br J Obstet Gynaecol 100: 762-764, 1993.

Venkat-Raman N, Backos M, Teoh TG, Lo WT, Regan L: Uterine artery Doppler in predicting pregnancy outcome in women with antiphospholipid syndrome. Obstet Gynecol 98: 235-242, 2001.

Vlachoyiannopoulos PG, Kanellopoulos PG, Ioannidis JP, Tektonidou MG, Mastorakou I, Moutsopoulos HM: Atherosclerosis in premenopausal women with antiphospholipid syndrome and systemic lupus erythematosus: a controlled study. Rheumatology (Oxford) 42: 645-651. 2003.

Weber T, Auer J, O'Rourke MF, Kvas E, Lassnig E, Berent R, Eber B: Arterial stiffness, wave reflections, and the risk of coronary artery disease. Circulation 109: 184-189, 2004.

Wang JX, Davies MJ, Norman RJ: Polycystic ovarian syndrome and the risk of spontaneous abortion following assisted reproductive technology treatment. Hum Reprod 16:2606-2609, 2001.

Wu KK: Soluble thrombomodulin and coronary heart disease. Curr Opin Lipidol 14:373-375, 2003.

Yokoyama H, Shoji T, Kimoto E, Shinohara K, Tanaka S, Koyama H, Emoto M, Nishizawa Y: Pulse wave velocity in lower-limb arteries among diabetic patients with peripheral arterial disease. J Atheroscler Thromb 10: 253-258. 2003.

Zaidi J, Jacobs H, Campbell S, Tan SL: Blood flow changes in the ovarian and uterine arteries in women with polycystic ovary syndrome who respond to clomiphene citrate: correlation with serum hormone concentrations. Ultrasound Obstet Gynecol. 12:188-196, 1998.

Zhixin Li, Wells CW, North PE, Kumar S, Duris CB, McIntyre JA, Ming Zhao: Phosphatidylethanolamine at the luminal endothelial surface--implications for hemostasis and thrombotic autoimmunity. Clin Appl Thromb Hemost 17: 158-163, 2011.

9

The Polycystic Ovary Syndrome Status – A Risk Factor for Future Cardiovascular Disease

Ioana Ilie, Razvan Ilie, Lucian Mocan, Carmen Georgescu, Ileana Duncea, Teodora Mocan, Steliana Ghibu and Cornel Iancu
"Iuliu Hatieganu" University of Medicine and Pharmacy Cluj-Napoca, Romania

1. Introduction

Polycystic ovary syndrome (PCOS) is a common endocrine disorder in women of reproductive age with a prevalence estimated at 4–8% (Azziz et al., 2004; Moran & Teede, 2009). It is associated with a range of reproductive, obstetric, metabolic and psychological features. Reproductive and obstetric manifestations include hyperandrogenism, menstrual dysfunction, infertility and pregnancy complications, such as early pregnancy loss, gestational diabetes, pregnancy-induced hypertensive disorders and neonatal complications (Boomsma et al., 2006). Additionally, women with PCOS cluster risk factors for cardiovascular disease (CVD) and type 2 diabetes mellitus (DM) as well as the metabolic syndrome (MS). As a consequence, metabolic complications and potential major long-term sequelaes include: an elevated risk of impaired glucose tolerance (IGT), type 2 DM (Legro, 1999, as cited in Moran & Teede, 2009), as well as an increased rate of hypertension and CVD (Shaw et al., 2008). Although there are still aspects to be cleared regarding the long-term consequences of these well-known cardiovascular (CV) risk factors, the research that has been conducted so far seems to indicate that patients with PCOS are at increased risk for adverse CV morbidity and mortality. Of utmost importance is the fact that these women are likely to develop CV disease early, and that even very young and nonobese patients may be affected (Moran & Teede, 2009; Lorenz & Wild, 2007).

However, there is a wide variety of diagnostic criteria generating several reproductive diagnostic phenotypes and the best diagnostic criteria for PCOS as well as the metabolic implications of newer non-National Institute of Health (NIH) PCOS phenotypes are still under intense debate. Although the prevalence of the MS is likely to vary according to PCOS and MS definition and ethnicity, its occurrence is estimated to be substantially higher in women with PCOS compared with the general population. Endothelial dysfunction and increased arterial stiffness are early markers of atherosclerosis, which has been recognized as a chronic inflammatory state. Increased carotid intima-media thickness (IMT) has been reported to occur relatively early in the atherosclerotic process and to represent a powerful predictor of coronary and cerebrovascular events. These alterations were first found in middle-aged women with PCOS and then demonstrated also in young ones. Moreover, coronary artery calcium, a radiographic marker for atherosclerosis, correlates with the extent of coronary atherosclerotic plaque. Up to the present, the results of the literature have been controversial as far as the presence of arterial structural and functional alterations or of chronic inflammation in PCOS are concerned. However, most lines of investigation point to increased CV risk and sustain the presence of sub-clinic CVD among women with PCOS. Therefore, medical intervention should target the reduction of the risk factors that cluster in women with this disorder. It has even been suggested that if pathologic values of IMT are found, these patients should be aggressively treated, starting with lifestyle programs and eventually with insulin-sensitizing or also statins (Carmina, 2009). Furthermore, the oral contraceptive pills (OCPs), the most common drugs used in PCOS, may exacerbate the metabolic profile of women with this disorder, as they were associated in some studies with a deterioration of carbohydrate metabolism and lipid profile. Women using OCPs have higher highly sensitive C-reactive protein (hsCRP) concentrations than non-users and the ethinyl-estradiol –cyproterne acetate pill has been shown to significantly increase serum CRP levels in PCOS subjects. Though controversies still exist, there are important reports providing suggestions that increased CV risk among women with PCOS indeed increases likelihood of them developing CVD and CV events (Shaw et al., 2008). PCOS thus constitutes a significant health and economic burden estimated at over $4 billion in the USA with ~40.5% of costs related to treatment of type 2 DM. (Azziz et al., 2005). If PCOS status were recognized as an independent risk factor for subsequent CV events, this would, then, justify earlier risk-factor intervention.

2. Phenotypes of the polycystic ovary syndrome and the risk for cardiovascular disease

Although it is widely recognised that PCOS is a diagnosis of exclusion, the optimal diagnostic criteria for PCOS remain controversial. Several definitions are in use today: one arising from an expert conference sponsored by the National Institute of Health (NIH1990 criteria) and the other from another expert conference sponsored by the European Society for Human Reproduction and Embryology (ESHRE) and the American Society for Reproductive Medicine (ASRM) in 2003 in Rotterdam (Rotterdam 2003 criteria). To date, there is limited understanding of the relative prevalence of risk factors for metabolic diseases (type 2 DM and CVD) across the reproductive diagnostic phenotypes of PCOS and clearly the prevalence and the long-term morbidity of PCOS will depend, to some degree, on the criteria used to define this disorder. Clarification of this will aid in determining whether to include non-NIH phenotypes as part of the complex condition of PCOS and in identifying if specific reproductive PCOS phenotypes have elevated metabolic risks (Moran & Teede, 2009).

NIH diagnostic criteria have been used for the past 15 years based on biochemical or clinical hyperandrogenism and anovulation (excluding other secondary causes including thyroid dysfunction, non-congenital adrenal hyperplasia or hyperprolactinaemia) (Zawdaki & Dunaif, 1992). According to these criteria, 4–8% of women in a general population have PCOS (Asuncion et al., 2000; Azziz et al., 2004; Diamanti-Kandarakis et al., 1999; Knochenhauer et al., 1998, as cited in Moran & Teede, 2009). The Rotterdam criteria (ESHRE/ASRM, 2004), which are more extensive, were formulated as two of the three criteria of hyperandrogenism, polycystic ovaries (PCO) on ultrasound and irregular anovulatory periods (Guastella et al., 2010). This introduced two new PCOS phenotypes (non-NIH PCOS) of hyperandrogenic ovulatory women with PCO or non-hyperandrogenic anovulatory women with PCO (2004) (Moran & Teede, 2009). The development of both the ESHRE/ASRM and the Androgen Excess Society (AES) criteria has introduced greater heterogeneity into PCOS from a reproductive and possibly from a metabolic perspective. In fact, according to these guidelines, the diagnosis of PCOS may present in patients with four different phenotypes: [1] hyperandrogenism, chronic anovulation, and PCO; [2] hyperandrogenism and chronic anovulation but normal ovaries; [3] hyperandrogenism and PCO but ovulatory cycles; and [4] chronic anovulation and PCO but no clinical or biochemical hyperandrogenism (Guastella et al., 2010). In 2006, the AES published a position statement which suggested that androgen excess is the key component of PCOS related to clinical presentation and long-term morbidity. The proposal of the AES was, therefore, to include in the diagnosis of PCOS only the first three phenotypes, excluding the phenotype of PCO and irregular cycles without hyperandrogenism (Azziz et al., 2006, 2009; Guastella et al., 2010; Moran & Teede, 2009).

For simplification, PCOS can be subdivided into four reproductive phenotypes: NIH-diagnosed PCOS either with (phenotype A) or without PCO (phenotype B); biochemical/clinical hyperandrogenism with PCO but no oligo/anovulation (phenotype C), or no biochemical/clinical hyperandrogenism with PCO and oligo/anovulation (phenotype D) (Moran & Teede, 2009).

There is an increasing body of literature devoted to examining the metabolic implications of the reproductive diagnostic phenotypes of PCOS. The majority of literature to date has focused on the NIH diagnosis of PCOS.

Hence, a very recent study performed in Brazil in order to assess the NIH PCOS phenotypes (A and B) for metabolic features indicated that PCOS diagnosis based on the presence of hyperandrogenism and ovulatory dysfunction, with or without PCO, is associated with a worse metabolic profile and more insulin resistance than that observed in ovulatory women with the hyperandrogenism +PCO phenotype or with isolated hirsutism, and in ovulatory control women without hirsutism, even after adjustment for BMI (because the prevalence of obesity was higher in the classic PCOS group) (Wiltgen & Spritzer, 2010). However, when weight-matched, the most of data suggest that the metabolic profile of the newer phenotypes is similar to the profile seen in NIH phenotypes (Moran & Teede, 2009). Interestingly, the adiponectin levels, which have been proposed as possible links between reproductive and metabolic anomalies in PCOS (Yilmaz et al., 2009), were significantly lower in groups 1 and 2 (classic PCOS) in comparison with the concentrations in women with the newer phenotype groups 3 and 4, added in accordance with the 2003 criteria. (phenotypes C and D), which were much higher, reaching those of control levels. It is worth mentioning that there was no significant difference in the waist circumference (WC), the waist-to-hip ratio (WHR) and, consequently, the amount of visceral fat between the five groups of women in the study. Thus, adiponectin levels could reflect the distinct PCOS phenotype (Karkanaki et al., 2009). Furthermore, the few studies specifically comparing NIH PCOS with or without PCO (phenotype A versus B) have generally shown similar risk of metabolic disease for the two phenotypes of NIH PCOS. (Dewailly et al., 2006; Diamanti-Kandarakis and Panidis, 2007; Hsu et al., 2007; Shroff et al., 2007, as cited in Moran & Teede, 2009; Moran & Teede, 2009).

Research on the metabolic implications of the newer phenotypes of PCOS introduced by the ESHRE/ASRM is only emerging.

Depending on the population recruited from, up to 18% of women with PCOS by ESHRE/ASRM criteria can have non-hyperandrogenic PCOS (D) and up to 25% of women can have ovulatory PCOS (C). This indicates an increasing number of women with PCOS who may experience different reproductive and metabolic risks, when compared with those who have NIH PCOS with potential implications for research, screening and clinical practice. There is emerging evidence that these two phenotypes have a less adverse metabolic profile than NIH PCOS (Moran & Teede, 2009).

Regarding the phenotype C and D, particularly, compared with NIH PCOS, the literature, although scarce, suggests less adverse metabolic profiles for both hyperandrogenic ovulatory PCOS and non-hyperandrogenic anovulatory PCOS. Reduced adiposity and abdominal adiposity contribute to a more favourable metabolic profile in these two non-NIH phenotypes. These patients presented with most of the PCOS characteristics but in a milder form. In fact, patients with ovulatory PCOS had intermediate values (between classic PCOS and controls) of BMI, WC, testosterone, insulin, and quantitative insulin sensitivity index (QUICKI) (Guastella et al., 2010; Moran & Teede, 2009). As far as the specific PCOS phenotype- hirsute ovulatory patients with PCO are concerned, there are data indicating a lower prevalence of CV risk factors in hirsute ovulatory patients with PCO and normal androgen levels than with the classic PCOS phenotype, being similar in that regard to women with isolated hirsutism. However, obesity might be implicated in increased susceptibility to insulin resistance in hirsute women, and the monitoring of this group for metabolic comorbidities and CV risk factors is warranted even in the presence of androgen levels within the normal range (Wiltgen & Spritzer, 2010). All in all, both non-NIH (hyperandrogenic ovulatory) PCOS (phenotype C) and non-hyperandrogenic PCOS (phenotype D) generally have lower body weight and body mass index (BMI) and better metabolic profiles compared with NIH PCOS (phenotypes A/B). However, non-NIH (phenotype C and D) PCOS and weight-matched NIH PCOS appear to present with similar metabolic risk profiles, particularly where abdominal fat and total fat are similar between subjects (Moran & Teede, 2009).

In comparison to controls, although not universally observed, women with non-NIH (hyperandrogenic ovulatory) PCOS (phenotype C) seem to be more adversely metabolically affected and this appears to be strongly related to the presence of adiposity and specifically abdominal adiposity. Additionally, some evidence exists to suggest that non-hyperandrogenic anovulatory PCOS matched for abdominal obesity have an adverse metabolic profile compared with controls.

There are even fewer studies comparing the non-NIH phenotypes of hyperandrogenic ovulatory PCOS (phenotype C) and non-hyperandrogenic anovulatory PCOS (phenotype D) and from this limited and conflicting literature, non-hyperandrogenic anovulatory PCOS seems not to display improved metabolic risk factors compared with hyperandrogenic ovulatory PCOS. There is, thus, currently limited evidence to support the exclusion of non-hyperandrogenic PCOS as a phenotype of PCOS based on metabolic presentation (Moran & Teede, 2009).

The current evidence shows that patients with NIH PCOS, who are hyperandrogenic and generally insulin resistant, have the most severe metabolic features. The adverse metabolic profile is strongly connected to obesity and abdominal obesity, the latter being more severe in NIH PCOS than in other non-NIH phenotypes. Both hyperandrogenism and insulin resistance play a role in the adverse metabolic profiles and both may establish the metabolic phenotypes of women with PCOS, either directly or through a high inclination towards abdominal obesity. The metabolic profile of newer reproductive phenotypes appears to be milder than that of NIH PCOS, but more adverse than that of controls and, again, strongly related to abdominal adiposity. While the ovulatory subgroup is more hyperandrogenic, evidence suggests non-hyperandrogenic women as having a similar metabolic profile to ovulatory PCOS with limited evidence even suggesting they present with more severe IR and dyslipidaemia (Norman et al., 1995a, as cited in Moran & Teede, 2009). In the setting of either hyperandrogenism or insulin resistance, metabolic abnormalities are observed. Consequently, the literature has been, so far, sustaining the inclusion of both newer phenotypes of PCOS based on the ESHRE/ASRM Rotterdam diagnostic criteria, suggesting that these phenotypes are milder forms of PCOS.

There are, however, serious limitations of the literature on the metabolic features of PCOS, such as: ethnic diversity, recruitment sources of participants, consistency in the use of end-points and inconsistently defined controls or the use of CV risk factors instead of clinical disease outcomes (e.g. type 2 DM, coronary artery disease, subclinical or clinical atherosclerosis), to name but a few. Taking all these into account, it has become obvious that we need rigorous, well designed studies with well-defined controls and longitudinal follow-up to efficiently grasp clinical outcomes in order to clarify many of the ambiguous aspects of the metabolic phenotype of PCOS (Moran & Teede, 2009).

3. Cardiovascular risk factors in PCOS

3.1 Traditional cardiovascular risk factors

Several studies have examined the presence of CV risk factors in premenopausal women with PCOS. It has long been established that women with PCOS have an unfavorable cardiometabolic risk profile. Based on National Cholesterol Education Program guidelines, traditional CV risk factors include age > 55 years, current cigarette smoking, diabetes, history of premature coronary artery disease in first-degree relatives (men < 55 years, women < 65 years), hypertension, and dyslipidemia. (Birdsall et al., 1997; Dahlgren et al., 1992; Solomon et al., 2002, as cited in Dokras, 2008).

3.1.1 High blood pressure

The patient's risk is determined by the levels of both systolic (SBP) and diastolic blood pressure (DBP). In fact, of the two readings, the SBP may best predict all the complications related to hypertension.

In spite of the fact that blood pressures (BP) are generally within the normal range in young women with PCOS and not very different from that of age and weight matched controls (Dokras, 2008) abnormalities in the regulation of BP are common in these patients. Prehypertension, defined as SBP 120 to 139 mm Hg or DBP 80 to 89 mm Hg, is associated with a twofold increased risk of CV mortality (Chobanian et al., 2003, as cited in Dokras, 2008). 24-hour ambulatory BP readings showed that women with PCOS have an increased risk of prehypertension (Holte et al., 1996, as cited in Dokras, 2008; Lo et al.,2006). Moreover, although both SBP and DBP are normal in PCOS women in many studies, there are reports in which mean arterial pressures and ambulatory SBP (e.g. Holte et al., 1996, as cited in Cho et al., 2007) or the prevalence of hypertension (Cho et al., 2007) are increased in women with PCOS compared with controls (Hoffman & Ehrmann, 2008). Confirming these results, both mean arterial BP and the risk of preeclampsia have been found to be higher in women with PCOS (Akram et al., 2010; Boomsma et al., 2006).

According to a study carried out in 2005, there is no difference in ambulatory or office-based BP measurements between women with PCOS and control individuals; however, women with PCOS had a less significant overnight drop in mean arterial BP, a phenomenon also noted in obese adolescents with PCOS (Wild et al., 2005, as cited in Hoffman & Ehrmann, 2008). A Taiwanese study showed that the characteristic hyperandrogenemia in PCOS is associated with an elevated SBP and DBP independent of age, insulin resistance, obesity, or dyslipidemia (Chen et al., 2003). Overall, it appears that elevated SBP is detected after the third decade of life and may be independent of obesity (Dokras, 2008). Moreover, in a very recent study that targeted 113 PCOS women, the frequency of women with BP values above the normal limit was significantly higher in the PCOS group than in the control group. In the PCOS group, the values of SBP and DBP were positively correlated with age, BMI, WC, and triglycerides (TG) ($p<0.05$) to a significant degree. These results underline the importance of preventive strategies in PCOS women in anticipating pathological events related to the cardiovascular system (Azevedo et al., 2011).

Women with PCOS are under an increased risk of developing hypertension later in life, as proved by retrospective data. Follow-up data from the Pittsburgh case-control study proved physician-diagnosed hypertension in 23% of women with PCOS whereas the percentage of cycling control women in this situation was of only 6.9% (Talbott et al., 2001). In an earlier retrospective cohort study of 33 older women with histopathology consistent with PCOS on wedge resection 22 to 31 years earlier, Dahlgren et al. (1992) found the diagnosis of hypertension to be three times more common in women with PCOS than in normal age-matched controls (Dahlgren et al., 1992, as cited in Sukalich & Guzick, 2003). Preliminary data from the Nurses' Health Study demonstrate that the risk of developing hypertension was twice higher in women with increased or highly irregular menstrual cycle length (a possible surrogate for a clinical diagnosis of PCOS) than in women with regular cycles (Rich-Edwards et al., 1998, as cited in Sukalich & Guzick, 2003). A significant difference in the prevalence of hypertension was still noted after correction for BMI.

In spite of noted characteristics that typically accompany PCOS (e.g. insulin resistance, obesity etc.) the exact mechanisms responsible for hypertension in women with PCOS are yet to be clarified. Insulin resistance causes secondary hyperinsulinemia. Hyperinsulinemia may produce enhanced sodium retention (Zavaroni et al., 1995, as cited in Cho et al., 2007), increasing intracellular sodium and calcium and augmenting sympathetic activity (Reaven et al., 1996, as cited in Sukalich & Guzick, 2003) which may have a role in the development of hypertension (Sukalich & Guzick, 2003). Insulin also stimulates the release of insulin-like growth factor (IGF-1) that may contribute to the development of hypertension by determining vascular smooth muscle hypertrophy (Cho et al., 2007). Furthermore, the obesity that is common in PCOS adds to the risk of hypertension. The higher level of androgens seems to be strongly related to BP in women with PCOS who are not obese. Although the mechanisms by which hyperandrogenemia mediates the higher BP in women with PCOS remain to be determined, it is possible that androgens may directly stimulate endothelin-1 (ET-1) or may stimulate the rennin-angiotensin system (RAS) to increase ET-1, thus leading to the expression of two powerful vasoconstrictors that could impact BP in these women (Reckelhoff, 2007).

In conclusion, PCOS women seem to be at increased risk for hypertension development, if not during their reproductive years, then at least later in life (Hoffman & Ehrmann, 2008). Accordingly, very recently (2010), the AE-PCOS Board committee *has been recommending* a BP routine check at each visit. Ideal BP is 120 mm Hg systolic and 80 mm Hg diastolic or lower, and prehypertension should be detected and treated (Cushman, 2007). BP control has the largest benefit for reducing CVD (Wild et al., 2010).

3.1.2 High blood cholesterol and related lipid problems

Dyslipidemia is a major determinant of progression of atherosclerosis. Atherosclerosis starts at a very young age, and PCOS may represent an important model of lipid alterations starting during adolescence or fertile age (Wild et al., 1985; Wild et al., 2011). Actually, lipid abnormalities have been reported in up to 70% of PCOS patients and displayed different patterns, depending on several factors such as: the PCOS phenotype, the presence of obesity and the associated effects of IR and hyperandrogenism that combine with environmental (diet, physical exercise) and genetic factors (Essah et al., 2008; Valkenburg et al., 2008; Wild et al., 2011). The dyslipidaemia occurs independent of BMI (Wild et al., 1985; Wild & Bartholomew, 1988, as cited in Teede et al., 2010a; Talbott et al., 1995, as cited in Sukalich & Guzick, 2003; Teede et al., 2010a) and several studies have confirmed adverse lipid alterations in both obese and nonobese women with PCOS compared with weight-matched control women (Sukalich & Guzick, 2003). Consequently, PCOS might be considered the most common cause of dyslipidemia in women under 40.

Wild and colleagues (Wild et al., 1985) were the first to present data suggesting that women with PCOS had a more adverse lipid profile than control subjects and there are many studies that have analyzed this aspect ever since. Lipid abnormalities include low high-density lipoproteins cholesterol (HDL-C), high low-density lipoprotein cholesterol (LDL-C), high TG levels and small dense LDL particles (Lambrinoudaki, 2011; Wild et al., 2011), a combination closely linked to insulin resistance and an independent predictor of myocardial infarction (MI) and CVD. Increased TG/HDL-C ratio is also a marker for atherogenic, small, dense LDL-C particles and it may be also used as a simple metabolic marker to identify overweight individuals who are insulin-resistant (McLaughlin et al., 2003, Brehm et al., 2004, as cited in Dokras, 2008). This relationship has been demonstrated in women with PCOS by identifying a negative correlation between TG/HDL-C and QUICKI (Dokras et al., 2005). Recently, it has been proved that TG/HDL C > 3.2 and respectively > 3.5 identify both the MS as well as insulin-resistant and dyslipidemic patients whose chances to be at an increased risk for CVD are extremely high (Dokras, 2008). As mentioned earlier, prevalent MS in women with PCOS (Apridonidze et al., 2005; Dokras et al., 2005; Moran et al., 2010) has concentrated attention of most authors on changes in TG and HDL-C (that are components of the metabolic syndrome) with relatively little attention to other lipid changes, although LDL-C and nonHDL-C are considered to be the primary and secondary targets to reduce CVD and atherosclerosis as described by the National Cholesterol Education Program Adult Treatment Panel III (NCEP-ATP III) guidelines (NCEP-ATP III, 2002, as cited in Wild et al., 2011). However, qualitative disorders of LDL-C have also been identified in women who have PCOS and there have been a large number of studies during the past decade who found increased LDL-C levels in women with this disorder (Carmina et al., 2005; Legro et al., 2001; Rizzo et al., 2009; Wild et al., 2011) and LDL particles smaller than in matched controls (Dejager et al., 2001). Small, dense LDL particles are associated with increase in cardiovascular risk independent of total LDL (Austin et al., 1988, as cited in Sukalich & Guzick, 2003). However, the wide variability of LDL-C values between individual studies indicate that LDL-C values are influenced by many variables, including ethnic groups, severity of the syndrome (anovulatory versus ovulatory forms), quality of food, and body weight (Essah et al., 2008; Wild et al., 2011). When subset analyses including only BMI-matched patients were performed, LDL-C was still higher in women with PCOS. It clearly indicates that PCOS per se is responsible for increased lipid values, although the absolute value and the related cardiovascular risk may be different among individual patients (Wild et al., 2011).

Only one study reported mean values of LDL-C <100 mg/dL. Four studies reported mean concentrations in PCOS women ≥130 mg/dL, whereas no study showed mean LDL-C values >130 mg/dL in control subjects. Considering the reported variances, it is not uncommon for individual PCOS patients to have LDL concentrations >160 mg/dL. Elevated nonHDL-C was reported as a common abnormality in PCOS women included in the studies. 21 of the 31 comparisons, registered nonHDL-C >130 mg/dL and the mean difference was still considerably higher with BMI matching (16 mg/dL vs. control subjects). Similarly to what was found for LDL-C, higher nonHDL-C levels were generally reported in PCOS subjects whose mean BMI was higher. There were clear differences with PCOS even when the BMI was in the nonobese or nonoverweight categories. This suggests that obesity or overweight (and higher insulin resistance) is not the only factor that accounts for elevated LDL-C and nonHDL-C in PCOS (Carmina, 2009; Wild et al., 1985).

However, though decreased HDL-C (particularly HDL2, the most antiatherogenic HDL subtype) (Legro et al., 2001; Diamanti-Kandarakis et al., 2007, as cited in Hoffman & Ehrmann, 2008) may represent the most common lipid alteration in PCOS (Essah et al., 2008), and many studies have reported elevated levels of TG as compared to controls, a very recent meta-analysis performed by Wild et al. (2011) shows that altered levels of TG are not commonly identified in many populations (Carmina et al., 2003, as cited in Wild et al., 2011; Essah et al., 2008). Only three studies reported TG concentrations that exceeded 150 mg/dL, and these were found in women who were overweight or obese (Wild et al., 2011).

However, two main patterns of lipid alteration were described separately or combined (Wild et al., 2011). The most common pattern is probably classic atherogenic dyslipidemia (increased TG, low HDL-C, and increased small dense LDL subclasses + increased nonHDL-C). This lipid pattern is similar to that found in type 2 DM, and it is mainly the consequence of insulin resistance that impairs the ability of insulin to suppress lipolysis, thereby increasing mobilization of free fatty acids (FFA) from adipose stores. Consequently, increased hepatic delivery of FFAs impairs insulin inhibition of hepatic very low-density lipoprotein 1 synthesis, causing altered catabolism of very low-density lipoprotein (Brunzell et al., 2003 as cited in Wild et al., 2010). Additionally, the ability of insulin resistance to alter the expression of lipoprotein lipase and hepatic lipase may also contribute to this lipid pattern (Wild et al., 1985). Sustaining this hypothesis, insulin resistance was linked with hyperlipidemia in most of the studies including women with PCOS (Slowinska-Srzednicka et al., 1991, as cited in Sukalich & Guzick, 2003). Due to the fact that excessive adipose tissue increases insulin resistance, this pattern is likely to be found in obese patients with PCOS. These lipid abnormalities are further augmented among those women who develop glucose intolerance in association with PCOS. The magnitude of androgen elevation, race and ethnicity are considered additional modifiers of dyslipidemia in women with PCOS (Ehrmann et al., 2006, as cited in Hoffman & Ehrmann, 2008). The lipid profile of both lean and obese women with PCOS is improved by treatment with the androgen-receptor blocker flutamide. Moreover, both in vitro and in vivo studies have included hyperandrogenemia in the pathogenesis of low HDL-C levels, possibly by upregulating the genes involved in the catabolism of HDL-C (Hoffman & Ehrmann, 2008). However, Wild et al. found that hyperinsulinemia has a more significant effect on lipids than hyperandrogenemia in hirsute women (Wild et al., 1992, as cited in Sukalich & Guzick, 2003). This lipid pattern was reported in about 70% of American women with classic PCOS but is less commonly met in other countries where mean body weight is lower (Essah et al., 2008). However, also in Mediterranean countries, about one half of women with PCOS have low HDL-C and a small dense LDL phenotype. However, because of the common increase of LDL-C, a second mechanism related to altered LDL quality has been demonstrated (Wild et al., 2010). Many studies have also demonstrated an increase in LDL-C in women with PCOS (Essah et al., 2008; Legro et al., 2001; Valkenburg et al., 2008). However, its prevalence in PCOS is generally lower than that found for the atherogenic dyslipidemia and ranges from 24 to 40% (Essah et al., 2008; Valkenburg et al., 2008). It depends on body weight to a lesser extent and may be at least partially related to the hyperandrogenism (Wild et al., 2010). In fact, several studies have shown that in female postmenopausal populations, increased circulating values of LDL are related to higher testosterone and free androgen index (Mudali et al., 2005, Liu et al., 2001, as cited in Wild et al., 2011).

In conclusion, dyslipidemia is likely to be found in women with PCOS. Consequently both the American College of Obstetricians and Gynecologists (ACOG) (ACOG, 2009 as cited in Wild et al., 2011) and the Androgen Excess and PCOS Society (Wild et al., 2010) guidelines have recently pointed to the fact that an individual CV risk assessment in women with PCOS is highly necessary and that the CV risk assessment of patients with this disorder should include a complete fasting lipid and lipoprotein evaluation including LDL-C and nonHDL-C, as well as for TG and HDL-C. In addition, the Androgen Excess and PCOS Society guidelines have indicated different LDL-C cutoff values depending on the degree of CV risk of PCOS patients (Wild et al., 2010). In the prevention of CV risk, the first goal is to bring LDL-C to normal levels by using lifestyle intervention and medication if necessary. The second goal is keeping nonHDL-C reduced (Wild et al., 2011).

3.1.3 Obesity

Obesity and excess weight are among the most widely met chronic diseases in the Western world countries. The prevalence of increased BMI ranges between 30% and 80% among women with PCOS (Vribkova & Hainer, 2009). Moreover, it has been widely proved that 50–60% of women with PCOS have a body fat distribution of the android type irrespective of their BMI (Barber et al., 2006) and that patients with PCOS had a central fat excess independent of total fat mass (Lambrinoudaki, 2011; Puder et al., 2005; Ilie et al., 2008).

Obesity also increases hyperandrogenism, hirsutism, insulin resistance and metabolic disorders, infertility and pregnancy complications both independently and by exacerbating PCOS phenotypic expression (Balen et al., 1995, Kiddy et al., 1990, as cited in Teede et al., 2010a). Therefore, in spite of the lack of epidemiological data, the increasing epidemic of obesity worldwide is thought to facilitate the high prevalence of PCOS in the general population. It is of utmost importance to underline the fact that the defining characteristic of PCOS is visceral fat, rather than subcutaneous one, as visceral fat plays an important role in the proinflammatory response. Accumulation of visceral fat leads to insulin resistance, endothelial dysfunction and a proinflammatory status through fat-derived metabolic products, hormones (adiponectin, resistin, FFA) and cytokines (interleukin-1 (IL-1), interleukin-6 (IL-6), interleukin-18 (IL-18), tumor necrosis factor-α (TNF-α). Although many researches (Puder et al., 2005; Cascella et al., 2008; Svendsen et al., 2008, as cited in Penaforte et al., 2011) have advanced the idea that women with PCOS accumulate fat mainly in the upper body compared to controls matched for weight and age (Gambineri et al., 2002, as cited in Penaforte et al., 2011), other studies, including ours, did not detect any differences in total body fat, abdominal fat, visceral fat or trunk fat (Faloia et al., 2004; Glintborg et al., 2006; Barber et al., 2008, as cited in Penaforte et al., 2011; Carmina et al., 2007; Ilie et al., 2011), or trunk to peripheral fat (arm fat + leg fat + head fat) ratio in obese women with and without the syndrome (Svendsen et al., 2008, as cited in Penaforte et al., 2011), either.

We have already underlined the fact that the presence of obesity has a big impact on the development and expression of PCOS (for instance, in a woman who has PCO but does not meet diagnostic criteria for PCOS, obesity can cause disorders such as: menstrual irregularity and hirsutism, thus completing the PCOS diagnosis) (Kiddy et al., 1990 as cited in Farrel &.Antoni, 2010). There is evidence that molecules secreted by adipose tissue such as leptin, TNF-α, IL-6 might also influence adrenal and ovarian function (Escobar-Morreale et al., 2007). In fact, PCO is present in approximately 20% of all women and many of these women do not display other syndrome features (i.e., hirsutism, irregular menstrual cycles, and elevated testosterone), which would likely appear if a PCO woman were to become overweight or obese (Polson et al., 1998 as cited in Farrel &.Antoni, 2010). The prevention of obesity, then, can be a crucial factor against the increased incidence of PCOS and its associated physiological abnormalities, especially during childhood and preadolescent years (Farrel & Antoni, 2010). Whether obesity represents a factor amplifying intrinsic hormonal and metabolic components of PCOS or, alternatively, whether it has a direct pathophysiological role is still a matter of debate. However, overall, all the reports suggest that obesity (especially abdominal obesity) and PCOS interact to promote premature atherosclerosis and increase CV mortality (Guzick et al., 1996; Birdsall et al., 1997; Christian et al., 2003, as cited in Amato et al., 2011; Pierpoint et al., 1998; Wild et al., 2000; Shaw et al., 2008).

3.1.4 Insulin resistance, glucose intolerance, diabetes mellitus

The American Heart Association and American Diabetes Association (ADA) consider the diagnosis of DM a CV disease equivalent to a prior MI. Insulin resistance is considered one of the main pathogenic factors behind the development of PCOS (Svendsen et al., 2010). Hyperandrogenism and insulin resistance were first linked in 1921 when Achard and Thiers (1921) published their classic description of a bearded woman with diabetes. This link has been confirmed ever since by many investigators (Legro, 2006; Svenden et al., 2010) and insulin resistance is now considered the main pathogenic factor in the development of PCOS. Many of the late complications of PCOS, primarily diabetes, dyslipidemia, and CVD also seem to be connected to insulin resistance (Dunaif, 1997, as cited in Svendson et al., 2010). Moreover, IGT and MS, as predictors of type 2 DM and premature CVD mortality, are more widely met in women with PCOS (odds ratio, approximately 4:1) (Ehrmann et al., 1999, Legro et al., 1999, as cited in Wild et al., 2010).

3.1.4.1 Insulin resistance and abnormal glucose metabolism

Insulin resistance occurs in around 50% to 80% of women with PCOS (Wild et al., 2000, as cited in Wild et al., 2010), and in 95% of obese women with PCOS (Carmina & Lobo, 2004, DeUgarte et al., 2005, as cited in Wild et al., 2010), primarily in the more severe NIH diagnosed PCOS. Lean women and milder Rotterdam diagnosed PCOS seem to be less affected by severe insulin resistance. Ethnicity may also be an independent factor that contributes to the risk for insulin resistance and glucose intolerance. For example, though there are few data related to the relatively higher prevalence of PCOS among women of South Asian origin, there is some evidence that the latter group of women are more likely to be affected by insulin resistance than Caucasian women (Rodin et al., 1998, Wijeyaratne et al., 2002, Balen et al., 2005, Bhathena, 2007, as cited in Bathena, 2011). Women with PCOS manifest IR independently and additively with obesity, with PCOS and obesity acting synergistically to impair insulin sensitivity (Dunaif et al., 1989, as cited in Wild et al., 2010).

A family history of type 2 diabetes is also more widely met among PCOS women with IGT or type 2 DM compared with those with normal glucose tolerance (Ehrmann et al., 2005, as cited in Dokras, 2008). Furthermore, in spite of the variability in reports concerning the prevalence of prediabetes and DM among women with PCOS, most studies confirm that women with PCOS, especially obese PCOS women, have a higher prevalence of impaired fasting glucose (IFG), IGT and DM (Chang & Wild, 2009), and a risk to develop the disease at an earlier age than the general population (Sukalich & Guzick, 2003). PCOS is now recognized by the ADA as a leading risk factor for DM screening in adolescent girls (Palmert et al., 2002, as cited in Dokras, 2008) and premenopausal women irrespective of race and ethnicity (Dokras, 2009).

Mechanisms involved in insulin resistance are likely to be complex with genetic and environmental contributors. Specific abnormalities of insulin metabolism identified in PCOS include reductions in secretion, reduced hepatic extraction, impaired suppression of hepatic gluconeogenesis and abnormalities in insulin receptor signaling. Interestingly, there is a paradoxical expression of insulin resistance in PCOS whereby insulin-stimulated androgen production persists while its role in glucose metabolism is impaired (Dunaif, 1997). Therefore, insulin resistance in PCOS results in hyperinsulinaemia with its associated diverse and complex effects on regulating lipid metabolism, protein synthesis and modulation of androgen production.

Lean women with PCOS often have abnormalities of insulin secretion and action compared to weight-matched control subjects. An overweight woman with PCOS may also demonstrate extrinsic insulin resistance associated with adiposity, which can be mechanistically distinct from the insulin resistance present in lean women with PCOS. Only a subgroup of women with insulin resistance and PCOS develops coexistent pancreatic insufficiency with β cell failure followed by type 2 (non-insulin-dependent) DM. In this setting, insulin output cannot overcome resistance and hyperglycaemia develops (Dunaif et al., 1989, Dunaif and Finegood, 1996, Ehrmann et al., 1999, Legro et al., 1999, Kelly et al., 2000, Goodarzi and Korenman, 2003, Balen et al., 2005, Ehrmann, 2005, as cited in Bahthena, 2011).

3.1.4.2 Impaired glucose tolerance (IGT) and type 2 diabetes mellitus

Overall, the risk of IGT in premenopausal PCOS women in the United States may be 25 to 40% and that of type 2 DM 4 to 10%, irrespective of race (Dokras, 2008). Solomon et al.

examined the risk for type 2 DM development in the 106,052 women enrolled in the Nurses' Health Study. Women with menstrual cycles greater than 40 days or irregular cycles had an age-adjusted relative risk of type 2 DM of 2.42 (95% confidence interval, 1.81-3.24) compared with normally cycling controls (Solomon et al., 1998, as cited in Sukalich & Guzick, 2003). But do women with PCOS switch to DM at higher rates?

Women with PCOS in the United States who have IGT have been reported to convert to DM anywhere from 6% over 3 years to 13.4% over 8 years in older women (Ehrmann et al., 1999, Legro et al., 2005, as cited in Chang & Wild, 2009). Smaller samples have reported rates of 29% (4 of 14) over 2 years and 54% (7 of 13) after 6 years (Norman et al., 2001, as cited in Chang & Wild, 2009).

Additionally, the rate of conversion from IGT to type 2 DM in a general Australian population was estimated in the large cohort Australian Diabetes, Obesity and Lifestyle (AusDiab) study at 2.9% per year for young females (Barr et al., 2005, as cited in Teede et al., 2010a). Another Australian study has reported a substantially higher conversion rate (8.7% per year over 6.2 years) in women with PCOS (Norman et al., 2001, as cited in Teede et al., 2010a). However, this has not been uniformly reported (Legro et al., 2005, as cited in Teede et al., 2010a). In the United States, women with normal glucose tolerance at baseline had a 16% conversion to IGT per year, and those with baseline IGT had a 6% conversion rate over ~3 years, or 2% per year (Legro et al., 2005, as cited in Dokras, 2009). In another study, classic PCOS patients had a 5-fold risk of developing type 2 DM over 8 yr *vs.* age- and weight-matched controls, although only 12% of PCOS patients without obesity developed glucose abnormalities (Wild et al., 2010).

Comparatively, other studies reported conversion rates to DM of 25% and 66% over 5 and 10 years in the high-risk Pima Indian population (Saad et al., 1988, as cited in Chang & Wild, 2009) and 50% over 5 years in Latina women with a previous history of gestational diabetes (Kim et al., 2002, as cited in Chang & Wild, 2009). Conversion rates for normoglycemic women to IGT vary from 9 to 16%, to as high as 40% (Chang & Wild, 2009). Collectively, these data may support high rates of conversion from IGT to DM and normal glucose tolerance to IGT, but the rates are not higher than those of other at-risk populations. These data are also incomplete due to the fact that the presence or absence of PCOS status according to race has not been defined in the populations referred to. Finally, with the RR of developing DM 6.90 (95% CI, 4.35 to 10.94) over 8 years in women with the MS (established in much larger cohorts though also among older women), the assessment of the MS and the prevention of conversion to DM are of high clinical relevance for women with or without PCOS (Chang & Wild, 2009).

Alarmingly, IGT and type 2 DM are highly prevalent among PCOS adolescents (Palmert et al., 2002, as cited in Wild et al., 2010). Although incident data are not rigorous, up to 40% of women with classic PCOS develop IGT or type 2 DM by the fourth decade of life and their glycemic control is seriously affected by age and weight gain. (Boudreaux et al., 2006, Legro et al., 2005, Norman et al., 2001, as cited in Wild et al., 2010).

Women with PCOS also have higher gestational diabetes (GDM) risk, with a recent meta-analysis reporting an odds ratio (OR) of 2.94 (Boomsma et al., 2006). The risk of GDM occurs both independent of and is exacerbated by obesity (Boudreaux et al., 2006, Legro et al., 1999, as cited in Teede et al., 2010a). Though there are few studies to adequately assess the natural history of IGT, DM2 and CVD in PCOS and further research is needed, the International Diabetes Federation (IDF) has identified PCOS as a major non-modifiable risk factor associated with type 2 DM (Alberti et al., 2007, as cited in Teede et al., 2010a).

It has become more and more obvious that IGT has significant clinical relevance and its early identification and intervention improve long-term outcomes and can prevent IGT progression to DM, including in high-risk PCOS women.

There are currently no generic guidelines for IGT screening, only for type 2 DM based on fasting glucose or more recently on HbA1c as a first line. However, impaired fasting glucose cannot accurately predict IGT in women, in general, and in PCOS (Teede et al., 2010a). As a consequence, and taking into account the high prevalence of insulin resistance, IGT and type 2 DM in PCOS, as well as their implications in the pathogenesis of this disease and especially in the onset of type 2 DM and of CVD, recently, the AE-PCOS Board recommend that a 2-h post 75-g oral glucose challenge be performed in PCOS women with a BMI greater than 30 kg/m^2, or alternatively in lean PCOS women with advanced age (>40 yr), personal history of GDM, or family history of type 2 DM (Salley et al., 2007). Those with IGT should be screened annually for developing type 2 DM, acknowledging efficacy of treating IGT, but not necessarily impaired fasting glucose, to prevent type 2 DM (Salley et al., 2007). Hemoglobin A1c above 6.5% has been proposed as the defining criterion for diabetes (Lorenzo & Haffner, 2010). This criterion was proposed for risk assessment, but further studies will be needed to determine whether this criterion is useful in implementing lifestyle interventions and medical management for CVD prevention (Wild et al., 2010).

3.2 Other risk factors-nontraditional cardiovascular risk factors

Besides the traditional CVD risk factors, a large number of markers that have been proposed as "nontraditional" CVD risk factors (adiponectin, leptin, CRP, IL-6, plasminogen activator inhibitor 1 (PAI-1) or serum amyloid A) and were shown to contribute to accelerated atherosclerosis in diabetes might also be involved in the pathogenesis of vascular disease in PCOS. Platelet function abnormalities, alterations in the coagulation cascade or a prothrombotic state (reduced fibrinolysis and raised level of PAI-1 or elevated clotting factors such as fibrinogen) can be seen with diabetes and hyperinsulinemia. Elevated levels of CRP, or of inflammatory cytokines such as TNF-α and IL-6, IL-18, of matrix metalloproteinases, fibrinogen, ET-1, of white blood cell and platelet counts have been reported in women with PCOS (Wild et al., 2010; Jovanovic et al., as cited in Lambrinoudaki, 2011; Lorenz & Wild et al., 2007; Essah et al., 2007). Talbott et al. also identified significantly increased mean PAI-1 levels in women with PCOS (28 ng/mL) compared with controls (19 ng/mL), a relationship that remained after adjustments for BMI and insulin levels (Talbott et al., 2000b). Moreover, the increased level of PAI activity in PCOS was directly correlated with insulin resistance and it decreased with improvement in insulin sensitivity, either through weight loss or through the use of sensitizing agents, thus implicating it as a contributing cardiovascular risk factor (Cho et al., 2007). No differences, however, in PAI-1 between women with PCOS and controls have been identified by other studies (Atiomo et al., 2000, Yarali et al., 2001, as cited in Sukalich & Guzick, 2003). Further research regarding PAI-1 in women with PCOS is needed to resolve this discrepancy.

Elevated concentrations of circulating homocysteine have been identified as another cardiovascular risk factor, causing endothelial oxidative stress and platelet aggregation and consequently leading to atherosclerosis. Significantly elevated concentrations of homocysteine have been documented in both lean and obese women with PCOS versus normal controls (Yarali et al., 2001, as cited in Sukalich & Guzick, 2003; Lorenz & Wild, 2007). Several but not all studies have found insulin resistance to be the most important predictor of increased homocysteine (Lorenz & Wild, 2007).

Adiponectin, a crucial adipocytokine, may also have a protective role in vascular damage in PCOS. Adiponectin has been shown to inhibit endothelial inflammation, to stimulate the production of NO in the endothelium, protecting blood vessels from the damage associated with insulin resistance. The majority of studies performed on women with PCOS demonstrate decreased level of adiponectin, compared to controls (Escobar-Morreale et al., 2006; Ardawi et al., 2005; Carmina et al., 2006b). Moreover, it was shown that hypoadiponectinemia is present in PCOS independent of BMI, with WHR, WC and free testosterone levels as the major determinants of decreased concentrations of adiponectin (Escobar-Morreale et al., 2006; Gulcelik et al., 2008; Ilie et al., 2008). These studies suggest that abdominal adiposity is characteristically associated with hypoadiponectinemia; hyperandrogenemia may also have a role, probably by facilitating an abdominal deposition of fat. A negative correlation was found between levels of adiponectin and IMT in a PCOS group compared with matched controls, apparently independent of the well known association of carotid change with insulin resistance and BMI, suggesting that the decrease in adiponectin may be an independent risk factor for the development of endothelial damage in PCOS (Carmina et al., 2006b).

Obstructive sleep apnea (OSA) is an independent CV risk factor and women with PCOS are 5-30 times more likely to have this disorder than are controls (Hoffman & Ehrmann, 2008). Moreover, it was suggested that the prevalence of OSA among women with PCOS is equal to, or may even exceed that in men. As previously noted, OSA is characterized by the combination of episodic sleep disruption and hypoxemia, each of which can trigger at least three major hormonal responses: activation of the hypothalamic-pituitary-adrenal (HPA) axis with increased cortisol production/secretion, increased catecholamine output from sympathetic nervous system stimulation, and increased release of adipokines from adipose tissue. These responses appear to contribute to the metabolic abnormalities associated with OSA, particularly to the decline in insulin sensitivity and glucose tolerance (Nitsche & Ehrmann, 2010).

The risk of OSA is increased as a function of both total body fat mass as well as body fat distribution. Visceral fat appears to be more metabolically active and the quantity of visceral fat has been shown to highly correlate with OSA risk (Nitsche & Ehrmann, 2010). Furthermore, disordered breathing during sleep has been found to be more common in PCOS than controls, even when controlled for BMI (Gopal et al., 2002; Fogel et al., 2001, as cited in Cho et al., 2007). In two studies (Vgontzas et al., 2001, Gopal et al., 2002, as cited in Nitsche & Ehrmann, 2010), the severity of sleep apnea did not correlate with BMI and in a third one (Fogel et al., 2001, as cited in Nitsche & Ehrmann, 2010), even after controlling for BMI, PCOS women were as much as 30 times more likely to have sleep disordered breathing and 9 times more likely than controls to have daytime sleepiness (Nitsche & Ehrmann, 2010). Overall, all these data indicate that the high prevalence of OSA in women with this disorder cannot be fully attributed to excess adiposity and that additional factors (e.g. hyperandrogenemia that is characteristic of PCOS or insulin resistance) might explain the high prevalence. These factors are particularly relevant to the pathogenesis of OSA in women with PCOS (Nitsche & Ehrmann, 2010). Both WHR, a measure of central obesity, and circulating total testosterone were correlated with AHI. The androgenization of the PCOS women promotes development of central obesity, which has been established in other studies as a predictor for OSA. However, others have suggested that insulin resistance was the strongest predictor of OSA, stronger than were age, BMI or circulating testosterone (Vgontzas et al., 2001, as cited in Cho et al., 2007).

Nitsche (2010) has even proposed that there may be two "subtypes" of PCOS, i.e. PCOS with or without OSA, and these two subtypes may be associated with distinct metabolic and endocrine abnormalities. PCOS women with OSA may be at much higher risk for diabetes and CVD than PCOS women without OSA and may benefit from therapeutic interventions targeted to decrease the severity of OSA (Nitsche & Ehrmann, 2010).

4. Metabolic syndrome in PCOS

Metabolic syndrome is a conglomeration of multiple interrelated risk factors for CVD and type 2 DM, occurring 'more often than by chance alone'. These include atherogenic dyslipidemia, elevated blood pressure and blood glucose levels, along with central obesity (Bhattacharya, 2011). Although there is a general agreement regarding the main components of the MS, at least six diagnostic definitions have been proposed, including those formulated by the Adult Treatment Panel-III (ATP-III), the IDF and the World Health Organization (WHO). This variation requires different cut-off points and inclusion criteria (Day, 2007, as cited in Kandaraki et al., 2009). The definition proposed by the National Cholesterol Education Program Adult Treatment Panel III (NCEP ATPIII) (Grundi et al., 2004, as cited in Kandaraki et al., 2009) is the most commonly used for clinical and research purposes. The IDF has proposed the most recent criteria, which resemble the NCEP ones, with the exception that central obesity, assessed according to ethnicity-specific cut-offs, is an integral part of the IDF definition (Kandaraki et al., 2009).

Along with the epidemic of obesity, the prevalence of MS is increasing worldwide, both in the developing and developed countries. As noted previously, MS is associated with a risk of CVD and is a common early abnormality in the development of type 2 DM. In addition, MS plays a well-recognised role in the development of OSA, erectile dysfunction, PCOS and malignant tumours (Baranova et al., 2011).

MS and PCOS are undoubtedly common afflictions in women of reproductive age in the general population. The significant interconnection between MS and PCOS when studied in combination is noteworthy. Namely, MS is significantly more prevalent in women with PCOS than in their age-matched counterparts from the general population. This PCOS-MS overlap is not singularly met in Caucasian women with PCOS. A highly prevalent MS has also been identified in Brazilian, Chinese, Korean, Indian and in multiracial PCOS populations, at least in overweight/obese patients, in spite of the fact that there are variations in the MS prevalence rates dependent on ethnic/racial regions, age, the diagnostic criteria and the comparison group studied (Fig.1) (Soares et al., 2008; Cheung et al., 2008; Park et al., 2007; Bhattacharya, 2008; Glueck et al., 2003; Apridonidze et al., 2005; Ehrmann et al., 2006; Dokras et al., 2005).

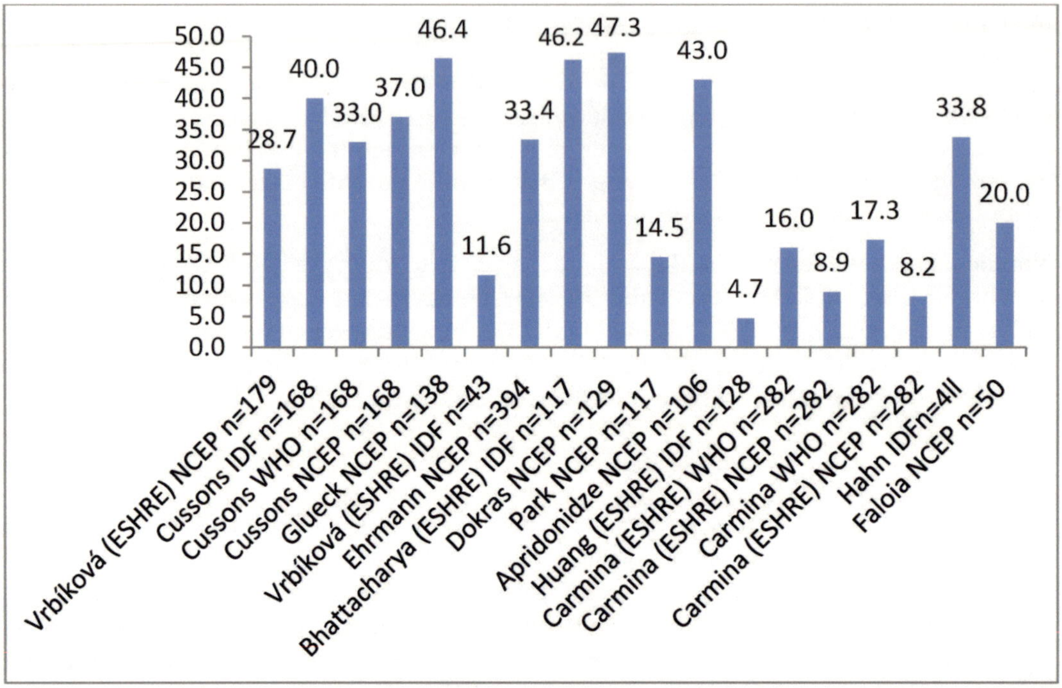

Fig. 1. The prevalence of metabolic syndrome in studies of PCOS

Data are presented as %. Studies are listed on the pattern: first author - the definition of the MS - the number of participants included in the study. Wherever unspecified (in the brackets), the criteria used for the diagnosis of PCOS were the NIH criteria. Except for the studies of Carmina, who examined both NIH and ESHRE/ASRM criteria, the rest of the mentioned researches used either NIH or ESHRE criteria (as mentioned). NIH, National Institute of Health; ESHRE/ASRM, European Society for Human Reproduction and Embryology/American Society for Reproductive Medicine

Four US studies in predominantly obese women with PCOS have reported that 33.4% to 47.3% of these women fulfill the NCEP ATPIII criteria for MS (Glueck et al., 2003; Apridonidze et al., 2005; Ehrmann et al., 2006; Dokras et al., 2005). Apridonidze et al. (2005) performed a study on 106 women with PCOS and recorded a 43% prevalence rate, which is twice higher than the age-adjusted rate of 24% in women of all ages in the general population based on data from the Third National Health and Human Examination Survey III (NHANES III). The prevalence of MS in PCOS women, divided by decade of life registered the following values: women between ages 20 and 29 - 45% and women between ages 30 and 39 - 53%, compared with 6% and 15%, respectively, in women in the general US population of the same age ranges. Notably, the prevalence rate of the MS in women with PCOS between ages 30 and 39 (53%) was even higher than the reported 44% rate observed in women aged 60 to 69 years from the NHANES III study. Similar results were reported by Dokras et al. (2005) who discovered, in a retrospective study carried on 129 women with PCOS and 177 normal controls, that the age-adjusted prevalence rate of the MS was 47.3% compared with a 4.3% rate in controls. They also observed that when compared by age group, MS was significantly more prevalent in PCOS subjects than in controls (Essah et al.,

2007). Despite being obviously higher than the US population-based estimates, these prevalence rates may, to some extent, reflect the impact of the high prevalence of obesity in the above populations - independently of PCOS per se (Glueck et al., 2003; Apridonidze et al., 2005; Ehrmann et al., 2006; Dokras et al., 2005). Furthermore, in three of the above US studies, the included control groups were not specifically selected (Glueck et al., 2003; Apridonidze et al., 2005; Ehrmann et al., 2006). In another US study (Dokras et al., 2005), the apparent preponderance of MS in the PCOS group was eliminated when non-obese PCOS patients were compared with age and BMI- matched controls, while the difference between the obese subgroups of patients and controls was reduced to non-significant levels. Thus, the actual impact of MS in women with PCOS as compared to controls, evenly matched for age and BMI, awaits further investigation.

Moreover, European studies among PCOS populations with lower BMI and also other non-US studies have reported significantly lower prevalence rates of MS than the ones reported by the US studies (Carmina et al., 2006a; Vural et al., 2005; Vrbikova et al., 2005). In spite of these different results, in some studies (Carmina et al., 2006a, c; Vural et al., 2005), but not all (Vrbikova et al., 2005), the MS has been shown to be more prevalent in European PCOS patients than in controls of similar ethnicity and age.

For instance, in Italy, where women with PCOS have a lower mean body weight and less frequently increased serum TG than US PCOS, MS is less common but still 4 times more frequent in PCOS patients than in the general female population of similar age. Patients with mild PCOS phenotype (ovulatory PCOS) have a lower prevalence of MS but, in these patients too, MS is twice more frequent than in the normal population (Carmina, 2006c). Carmina et al. (2006a) sought to determine the prevalence of MS in Italian women using both the ATP-III and the WHO criteria. Using ATP-III criteria, the prevalence of MS was 8.2% and, using WHO criteria, it was 16% in Italian women with PCOS, higher than in controls, where the prevalence was 2.4% using both methods. Regarding the influence of the way in which PCOS is diagnosed, the MS prevalence was higher (8.9% by ATP-III, 17.3% by WHO) in classic PCOS patients than in ovulatory PCOS (5% and 10.6% respectively). Body weight significantly modified prevalence rates (Carmina et al., 2006a). Furthermore, in a very recent study, the same researchers found a relatively low prevalence of MS (7.1%) in Mediterranean PCOS, but higher than in normoweight and BMI-matched controls (2.4% and 3.5%, respectively) (Rizzo et al., 2011). Additionally, in a Czech study, MS (defined by IDF adolescent criteria) was present in five adolescents (11,62%) with PCOS (defined according to the ESHRE criteria) in comparison with one healthy girl. When comparing the prevalence of adolescents with at least one feature of MS, there was no difference between PCOS (17 out of 43) and healthy controls (27 out of 48) (Vrbĺková et al., 2010a). Moreover, using ATP III criteria this time, MS was detected in 28.7% of those 179 women with PCOS. The most frequent features were an increased WC, decreased concentration of HDL - C (both in 96%), and increased BP (88%). Increased TG (49%) and impaired fasting blood glucose or type 2 DM (37.3%) were less common (Vrbĺková et al., 2010b).

Another study performed on Caucasian women also found an approximate 4-fold increase in the prevalence of MS in women with PCOS compared with the age-matched female population (33% by WHO, 37% by NCEP-ATP-III and 40% by IDF criteria in PCOS subjects, compared with 10% by NCEP-ATP-III and 13% by IDF in controls) (Cussons et al., 2008). A similar prevalence was found also in a German study using IDF criteria (Hahn et al., 2007, as cited in Cussons et al., 2008). The most common individual component of the MS present in the PCOS group was an elevated WC, followed by reduced HDL, then insulin resistance indicated by the homeostasis model assessment of insulin resistance (HOMA-IR). The least prevalent individual component was an elevated fasting glucose (Cussons et al., 2008). The adverse metabolic milieu of the syndrome can affect not only adults but also adolescents with PCOS (Diamanti-Kandarakis et al., 2008, as cited in Kandaraki et al., 2009). This is extremely likely to generate an increased prevalence of MS in this age group of patients, too. To explore this intuitively plausible concept, a few studies have addressed the prevalence of MS in adolescents with PCOS and the results are contradictory (Coviello et al., 2006, Rossi et al., 2008, as cited in Kandaraki et al., 2009). In an Indian study, MS (defined by IDF criteria) was found in 46.2% of females with PCOS, with both adolescent and adults being similarly affected. Regarding the individual component of the MS, dyslipidaemia and elevated BP were more common than fasting glucose abnormalities in both the adolescents and adults groups (Bhattacharya, 2008). Furthermore, the first study from India utilizing the 2009 "joint interim criteria" reported recently that the adolescents with PCOS were reported to have 4.26 times more chances of developing MS compared to those without (Bhattacharya, 2011). The prevalence of MS, diagnosed by IDF criteria, was 4.7% in the studied Chinese adolescents with PCOS. Metabolic disorders were common in these adolescents as more than one third of them exhibited at least one component of MS. Central obesity and dyslipidemia were the two most common metabolic features, which was also the case in adult PCOS patients according to a previous study (Huang et al., 2010). And finally, compared with Caucasians and Chinese women in Westernized societies, mainland Chinese women with PCOS were found to have a low risk of MS, as, overall, the prevalence of MS was 6.4% and its presence does not vary across the specific four PCOS phenotypes, according to the 2003 Rotterdam consensus criteria (range of 2.3-12.2%) (Guo et al., 2010).

However, there are some important limitations that should be mentioned. Most of these studies have not included patients and controls properly matched for age and BMI. Thus, not only the presence of PCOS but also BMI differences may have contributed to the above findings. The ethnic variations in the rates of MS reported by different studies may be attributable not only to anthropometric differences between diverse ethnicity, but also to differences in the criteria used for PCOS diagnosis. The selection of PCOS patients was based on NIH criteria in studies from the United States, but mostly on Rotterdam criteria in European or other non-US countries. The patients fulfilling the NIH definition of PCOS are expected to be more severely metabolically affected than the patients selected by Rotterdam criteria. Consequently, the MS rates were lower in women with hyperandrogenism and polycystic ovarian morphology, but normal ovulation, as well as in those with anovulation and PCO, but normal androgen levels when compared with women with classic PCOS (Kandaraki et al., 2009). The NCEP-ATP III criteria have been implemented for the diagnosis of MS by the majority of worldwide PCOS studies. However, there was one study that has employed both the WHO (gives more importance to the presence of insulin resistance or glucose intolerance) and the NCEP ATP III criteria, and has proposed the former set as more discriminating and more appropriate for the evaluation of MS in PCOS women with lower degrees of obesity (Carmina et al., 2006a). Accordingly, another study reported a significantly higher MS prevalence in PCOS women than in controls when using the WHO criteria, while the NCEP criteria identified a considerably lower MS in PCOS women, and thus could not show any difference between PCOS women and controls (Vural et al., 2005).

However, in a more recent study carried on a mixed population of obese and non-obese Caucasian PCOS women, comparable rates of MS have been reported, irrespective of the criteria used for MS diagnosis (NCEP, the WHO or the IDF criteria) (Cussons et al., 2008). Last but not least, the use of the 2009 "joint interim criteria" has just begun. The retrospective design is another weakness of the majority of the available studies. Differences in the exclusion criteria of each study should be also considered in the interpretation of their varying results (Kandaraki et al., 2009).

5. Markers of sub-clinical cardiovascular disease

It has been shown that women with PCOS have high CV risk factors. Whether this risk means an increased clinical disease is still debatable (Sukalich & Guzick, 2003).

- Functional studies
    - Ventricular function
    - Arterial stiffness
    - Endothelial function
        - Vascular tone
            - Vascular reactivity
            - Vasoconstrictors: ET-1
            - Vadsodilators: products of nitric oxide
        - Markers of endothelial activation
            - Adhesion molecules (sVCAM, sICAM, E- and P-selectin), ADMA
        - Markers of coagulation/fibrinolysis
            - PAI-1, tPA, fibrinogen, trombomodulin, vWF
        - Markers of inflammation
            - hs-CRP, TNF-α , IL-1, IL-6, ferritine, homocysteine
        - Hormones and substrates with known vascular effects
            - Adiponectin, resistin, visfatin, FFA, leptin, ghrelin
- Morphological studies
    - Carotid wall thickness
    - Arterial calcification

Note: ET-1 = endothelin-1, sVCAM = soluble vascular cell adhesion molecules; sICAM = soluble intercellular adhesion molecule; ADMA = asymmetric dimethylarginine; PAI = plasminogen activator inhibitor-1; tPA = tissue plasminogen activator, vWF = vonWillebrand factor; hs-CRP = highly sensitive C reactive protein; TNF-α = tumor necrosis factor alpha; IL-1 = interleukin 1; IL-6 = interleukin 6; FFA = free fatty acid

Table 1. Studies of markers of subclinical cardiovascular disease

Atherosclerosis is a systemic process the main characteristics of which is chronic inflammation, a disorder that affects all vascular territories and modifies their structure and function, ultimately leading to arterial thrombosis. Due to the fact that there is a long latency phase before clinical symptoms manifest during the progression of this disorder, the possibility of assessing arterial function before angiographically detectable atherosclerotic plaques appear could have a significant role in the early detection and evaluation of the risk for CVD (Soares et al., 2009).

This early detection of CVD risk can be performed with the help of noninvasive methods that permit the assessment of arterial structure and function. Currently, several such approaches exist; echographic measurements of arterial elasticity, IMT and endothelial function are clinically useful techniques for assessing arterial structure and function (Table 1). As a first approximation to studying the translation of risk factors into disease, data are accumulating on "preclinical" CVD of the carotid and coronary arteries as well as changes in vascular function (Sukalich & Guzick, 2003).

5.1 Functional studies

Vascular damage plays a key role in the development and progression of atherosclerosis and has been evaluated as an early risk marker of atherosclerosis and an independent predictor of future cardiac events (Sasaki et al., 2011).

5.1.1 Ventricular function

Left ventricular (LV) diastolic dysfunction is an early manifestation of diabetic cardiomyopathy and atherosclerotic CVD and has been shown to identify hypertensive patients at increased risk of CV events (Cussons et al., 2006). Its aetiology is multifactorial and relates to coronary artery disease, hypertension, autonomic neuropathy, microangiopathy, dyslipidaemia, insulin resistance, endothelial dysfunction and oxidative stress (Aurigemma et al., 2004, as cited in Cussons et al., 2006). Specific myocardial mechanisms include altered cardiomyocyte substrate metabolism and bioenergetics, altered collagen metabolism, inflammation and fibrosis (Watts et al., 2003, as cited in Cussons et al., 2006). Ventricular systolic and diastolic dysfunction may be an early finding for coronary heart disease in patients with PCOS (Kosmala et al., 2008).

In a case-control, echocardiographic study, women with PCOS were found to have an increased isovolumetric relaxation time (IVRT), an index of early LV diastolic dysfunction, and lower ejection fraction (EF) compared with weight matched controls (Tiras et al., 1999, as cited in Cussons et al., 2006). These changes were linked to the presence of a non-restrictive type of diastolic dysfunction and LV stiffness in patients with PCOS. However, E/A ratio, and DT were not significantly different between patients with PCOS and control. A significant direct relationship between plasma insulin levels and IVRT was demonstrated in the PCOS group. These findings were consistent with another report showing an independent correlation between hyperinsulinaemia and LV mass (Orio et al., 2004, as cited in Cussons et al., 2006). The existing studies sustain the hypothesis that insulin resistance may contribute to myocardial dysfunction in PCOS. Moreover, one study also predicted impaired coronary flow reserve and decreased myocardial glucose utilisation in PCOS related to insulin resistance and type 2 DM (Iozzo et al., as cited in Cussons et al., 2006).

Orio et al. studied the prevalence of LV hypertrophy and diastolic filling and systolic performance by echocardiography in a selected cohort of young women with PCOS. These authors found that patients with PCOS had significantly higher interventricular septum, left ventricle posterior wall thickness, end-systolic volume and lower LV EF, E/A ratio than controls. Nevertheless, all patients had normal LV EF and only two out of 30 patients with PCOS had abnormal E/A ratio (Orio et al., 2004, as cited in Tekin et al., 2009). Yarali et al. assessed systolic and diastolic function in 30 women with PCOS and 30 controls with echocardiography (Yarali et al., 2001, as cited in Sukalich & Guzick, 2003). They reported that patients with PCOS had slower mitral E velocity, a lower mitral E/A ratio and shorter IVRT than a group of healthy controls, suggesting that LV diastolic function was impaired in PCOS. However, in this study, patients with PCOS were older and had higher LDL cholesterol and BMI than those found in other patients (Tekin et al., 2009). Of note, they did not report BPs measures of the study population. Thus, it is unclear whether the impaired diastolic function could be attributed to presence of PCOS, per se, or to the inclusion of sicker subjects in PCOS group. On the contrary, Tekin et al. (2009) reported that there were no significant differences between patients with PCOS and control subject with respect to EF, mitral E/A, DT, IVRT and pulmonary velocity. They showed that the tissue doppler profiles of patients with PCOS and controls were also not significantly different. Topcu et al. assessed coronary flow reserve in patients with PCOS, similar in terms of age, BMI, total cholesterol, smoking status and BP with the women in the study of Tekin et al. (2009), by using echocardiographically determined colour Doppler flow mapping of left anterior descending artery. They ended up with normal coronary flow reserve in patients with PCOS who had no associated CV risk factors. They also noticed that mitral E velocity, mitral A velocity and E/A were not significantly different between patients with PCOS and controls (Topcu et al., 2006, as cited in Tekin et al., 2009). Selcoki et al.(2010) also suggest that there are no significant differences in certain conventional and tissue Doppler echocardiographic measures of cardiac function between patients with PCOS and control groups. However, their PCOS populations have low BMI, normal BP, low TG, LDL and total cholesterol. Furthermore, no significant differences were found in insulin, HOMA-IR, HDL, LDL and total cholesterol, and TG levels between the two groups. Hence, these echocardiographic findings support previous reports (Topcu et al., 2006, as cited in Tekin et al., 2009) Tekin et al., (2009) indicating that diastolic function is preserved in young patients with PCOS who have no associated CV risk factors. Risk reduction regimens may be particularly important to those with other recognized risk factors for CVD to herald the progression of the disease. Further studies with obese, older and dyslipidemic subjects are needed.

5.1.2 Arterial stiffness

One of the major contributing factors to CV morbidity and mortality in patients with hypertension is arterial stiffness. The reduced elasticity of central arteries may play an important role in the early changes that predispose to the development of major vascular disease (Sasaki et al., 2011). Reduced arterial compliance and increased arterial stiffness represent independent risk factors for CVD and may favour the development and progression of hypertension, LV hypertrophy, MI and heart failure (Safar &London, 2000, as cited in Soares et al., 2008).

The ankle-brachial index (ABI) - the ratio of ankle-to-brachial systolic blood pressure (SBP) - is a simple, non-invasive, reliable method to estimate the presence of peripheral arterial occlusive disease. The brachial-ankle pulse wave velocity (baPWV) is known to be a marker for both the severity of vascular damage and the prognosis of atherosclerotic vascular diseases in patients with hypertension, end-stage renal failure and DM. The carotid augmentation index (cAI), which is augmentation expressed as a percentage of the pulse pressure and influenced by the vascular tone of the small muscular arteries, is associated with the presence and severity of coronary artery disease, particularly in younger and middle-aged male patients. Recently, these indices can be measured easily by simultaneous oscillometric measurement of pulse waves and they are widely used as arterial stiffness indices (Sasaki et al., 2011).

In a small case-control study, Kelly et al. reported increased pulse wave velocity of the brachial artery, but not of the aorta, in a young obese PCOS group (Kelly et al., 2002, as cited in Cussons et al., 2006). Similarly, Lakhani et al. demonstrated increased stiffness of both internal and external carotid arteries in woman with both PCOS and PCO (ultrasonographic polycystic ovaries alone) compared with controls (Lakhani et al., 2000, as cited in Cussons et al., 2006).), even if BP and BMI were taken into account. However, this study did not show an independent relationship between insulin resistance or other CV risk factors and arterial stiffness and, as the patients with PCOS studied by these investigators had higher BMIs and arterial pressures and basal insulinaemia than the remaining participants, it was unclear whether the presence of PCOS *per se*, as opposed to the comorbidities of this syndrome, was responsible for this difference. Pulse wave velocity over the carotid-femoral tract, another method for the assessment of arterial distensibility, also demonstrated unfavourable results for young obese women with PCOS in a previous study. A significant relationship between PWV and BP and between PWV and both insulin and glucose has been detected during a glucose tolerance test (Meyer et al., 2005a). However, some possible confounding factors, such as smoking, insulin resistance and hypertriglyceridaemia, were not excluded in this research and no adjustments were made for BP or BMI.

Moreover, in the study by Sasaki et al. (2011), women with PCOS had a significantly higher brachial–ankle pulse wave velocity (baPWV) than that of the controls whereas there was no significant difference in the carotid augmentation index (cAI) as well as ABI between the two groups. There was no significant difference in age or BMI between the controls and the women with PCOS. These women with PCOS had a significantly higher serum testosterone and CRP levels and showed insulin resistance and dyslipidemia. The mean BP in women with PCOS was within the normal range, but still significantly higher than those in the controls. Stepwise multiple regression analysis revealed that BP influences the baPWV in women with PCOS. Arterial stiffness evaluated using the baPWV in mildly-hypertensive women (SBP ≥120 mmHg or DBP ≥90 mmHg) with PCOS was significantly higher than that in the controls or normotensive women with PCOS, suggesting early changes in vascular function in mildly-hypertensive women with PCOS. Furthermore, among the women with PCOS, obese women had significantly higher baPWV as compared to normal-weight women although no significant difference was observed in the ABI and cAI. Hence, it appears that obesity and elevation of BP within subclinical levels in women with PCOS may have adverse effects on vascular functions (Sasaki et al., 2011).

In view of these results, PCOS has been suggested to be associated with arterial stiffening. The question remains whether the risks conferred by obesity and other CV risk factors, commonly found in PCOS subjects and PCOS, are additive. The drawback of other studies that have evaluated nonobese women with PCOS (Arikan et al., 2009, Orio et al., 2004) is the fact that they did not analyse these markers simultaneously so they did not identify those linked specifically with the presence of PCOS and not simply triggered by the metabolic dysfunctions so common in these patients. Thus, Soares et al. (2008) evaluated the subclinical markers of CVD (echographic and serum markers of chronic inflammation) in nonobese women with PCOS but without comorbidities. Common carotid artery stiffness index (β) (CCA β) was higher in PCOS than in control women and CCA distensibility was lower, indicating that young women with PCOS exhibit changes in vascular elasticity even in the absence of classical risk factors for CVD, such as hypertension, obesity and type 2 DM. These data suggest that patients with PCOS may be at higher risk for CVD, because their arterial distensibility is already reduced during atheroma formation and thus represents a subclinical sign of atherosclerosis (Mattsson et al., 2008, as cited in Soares et al., 2008). However, as the women from this study did not present with hyperglycaemia or hyperinsulinaemia, the increased stiffness index and the reduced distensibility of the carotid artery detected in PCOS women might be attributed to the hyperandrogenism inherent to PCOS and not to comorbid conditions associated with the syndrome (Soares et al., 2008).

On the contrary, and sustaining the results of Muneyyirci-Delate et al., Ketel et al. (2010) demonstrated in a small study that (central) obesity, but not PCOS, is associated with greater arterial stiffness (Muneyyirci-Delate et al., 2007, as cited in Ketel et al., 2010). Beside the fact that most of the studies have not distinguished the effects of obesity from those of PCOS, they also have not taken into consideration the fact that stiffness of elastic (e.g. the carotid) and muscular (e.g. the femoral) arteries may differ in their association with obesity and potentially PCOS. The study of Ketel et al. (2010) is the first comprehensive study taking into account stiffness in both elastic and muscular arteries in both lean and obese women with and without PCOS. Previous investigations, which investigated one type of artery, pulse wave velocity over elastic and (or) muscular vascular regions, or small and large arterial compliance, showed somehow discordant results. Nevertheless, in their research, Ketel et al. (2010) demonstrated that PCOS was not associated with stiffening of either muscular or elastic arteries.

In conclusion, current studies suggest that differences in vascular function between normal women and women with PCOS may be very small if both are young, of normal weight and have normal BP. However, they showed that slightly increased BP, which weakly correlated with BMI, can be rightfully considered a risk factor for arterial stiffness in young women with PCOS. It has not been yet established whether these adverse effects of mild hypertension on arterial stiffness are characteristic to women with PCOS. We thus need further research on arterial stiffness in young women with mild hypertension caused by the other diseases (Sasaki et al., 2011). The mechanism for increased arterial stiffness reported in some studies of PCOS have not been cleared but, as in the metabolic syndrome and insulin resistance, may involve endothelial dysfunction and altered artery wall collagen metabolism (Cussons et al., 2006).

5.1.3 Endothelial dysfunction

Endothelial dysfunction can be defined as the partial or complete loss of balance between vasoconstrictors and vasodilators, growth promoting and inhibiting factors, pro-atherogenic and anti-atherogenic factors, and pro-coagulant and anti-coagulant factors. Endothelial dysfunction is the initiating event in the development of atherogenesis and has been shown to precede the development of clinically detectable atherosclerotic plaques in the coronary arteries, being also implicated in the development of microvascular complications in diabetes (Caballero, 2005). Therefore, the assessment of endothelial function by different methods has emerged as a tool for detection of preclinical CVD. A common approach to the evaluation of endothelial function is the assessment of blood flow and vascular reactivity which allows the investigator to evaluate the status of the endothelial cells as well as that of the underlying vascular smooth muscle cells. A lot of invasive and noninvasive techniques are available for evaluating these functions such as catheterization, ultrasound, positron emission tomography, laser Doppler flowmetry, and plethysmography (Caballero, 2005).

Measurement of post-ischemic flow mediated dilatation (FMD) of the brachial artery with high resolution ultrasonography is an established method to assess endothelial function of conduit arteries and correlates with measures of coronary endothelial dysfunction (Meyer et al., 2005b). Most of the studies performed in women with PCOS showed altered endothelial function in women with this disorder either using non-invasive methods (endothelium-dependent FMD or endothelium-independent, glyceroltrinitrate (GTN)-mediated dilatation vascular responses of the brachial artery) or invasive methods (Orio et al., 2004; Kravariti et al., 2005; Diamanti-Kandarakis et al., 2005, 2006a; Tarkun et al., 2004; Sorensen et al., 2006; Dagre et al., 2006) as compared to the control group. Impaired FMD is associated with insulin resistance, total cholesterol and CRP levels, while relationship to testosterone levels is controversial (Cussons et al., 2006; Kravariti et al.; Tarkun et al., 2004). However, it is not clear yet if the endothelial dysfunction found in women with PCOS is independent of obesity and insulin resistance that characterize so often this disorder. Therefore, Cussons et al. (2009) performed a study in nonobese, noninsulin resistant women with PCOS, assessing endothelial function (with FMD of the brachial artery) and arterial stiffness (with PWV and augmentation index (AI)). Although there were no significant differences between PCOS and control subjects in terms of BMI, BP, HOMA-IR, lipids, oestradiol and markers of arterial stiffness, the PCOS subjects had significantly lower FMD of the brachial artery compared with the controls. On the contrary, others suggested that middle-aged patients with PCOS display signs of endothelial dysfunction in comparison to age-matched controls, but that this is largely due to the increased prevalence of independent risk factors for CVD found in this group (Hudecova et al., 2010). On the other hand, there are also reports which do not sustain an association between PCOS and impaired endothelial function (assessed by FMD of the brachial artery) (Arikan et al., 2009; Brinckworth et al., 2006; Mather et al., 2000). Hence, Arikan et al. (2009) could not find a deteriorated endothelial function in young nonobese women with PCOS in spite of a significant insulin resistance in PCOS patients. They suggest that the existence of insulin resistance alone may not be an adequate factor for deterioration of endothelial function and carotid IMT in young, nonobese patients with PCOS. Other factors such as duration of insulin resistance, older age, presence of obesity, and inflammatory markers may play an important role in this process.

Endothelial dysfunction of the microcirculation and resistance vessels in PCOS has also been proved by invasive studies employing intra-arterial infusion of vasoactive agents with thermodilutional or plethysmographic assessment of limb blood flow. In a study by Paradisi et al., leg blood flow (LBF) was measured by means of an intravenous thermodilution catheter in a group of obese women with PCOS showing impaired LBF responses to methacoline and to hyperinsulinemia during an euglycaemic clamp compared with the control group. However, it should be mentioned that LBF response to sodium nitroprusside, an endothelium independent vasodilator, was not assessed, meaning that the demonstrated defect could not necessarily be localized to the endothelial cell as opposed to smooth muscle. Impaired endothelium-dependent vasodilatation was related to both androgen levels and insulin resistance (Paradisi et al., 2001). Using the same techniques, an improvement in the endothelial dysfunction was noted after 3 months of treatment with rosiglitazone in PCOS subjects compared with controls and this improvement was associated with a decrease in insulin resistance, testosterone and PAI-1 level (Paradisi et al., 2003). In an ex vivo study, the contractile response of gluteal resistance arteries to norepinephrine before and after incubation with insulin was measured, thus confirming the above results, namely that there is a resistance to the vasodilator effects of insulin in PCOS (Kelly et al., 2002), which proved to be present even in the absence of other risk factors. The defect in the resistance arterioles revealed in this study appears to be specific to the action of insulin, as constriction to norepinephrine and relaxation to Ach were not different between the PCOS group and the control group. In contrast, Bickerton et al.(2005), using venous occlusion plethysmography to assess differences in reactive hyperemia of the forearm microcirculation, found no evidence of endothelial dysfunction in women with PCOS compared with age- and weight-matched controls without PCOS. Carmassi et al. (2005), who studied PCOS women with and without insulin resistance, demonstrated a blunted vasodilatory response to insulin and an abolished expression of tissue plasminogen activator (t-PA) exclusively in insulin-resistant patients, suggesting that insulin resistance, rather than PCOS status, confers endothelial dysfunction in this vascular bed.

The measurement of plasma levels of several markers of endothelial activation (e.g. soluble vascular cell adhesion molecules (sVCAM), soluble intercellular adhesion molecule (sICAM), E- and P-selectin), coagulation and/or fibrinolysis (e.g. PAI-1, tPA, fibrinogen, von Willebrand factor), vascular tone (e.g. ET-1, products of nitric oxide), inflammation and other products, cytokines and hormones associated with vascular function also represent common approaches to evaluate endothelial function in humans (Caballero, 2005) (Table 1).

Endothelin-1 has endothelial mitogenic effects (Dubin et al., 1989, as cited in Ilie et al., 2008) and seems to play a role in the early events of endothelial dysfunction. Therefore, it can be used as a marker of abnormal vascular reactivity. Diamanti-Kandarakis et al. were the first ones to demonstrate elevated ET-1 levels in PCOS compared with controls. A positive correlation of ET-1 with free testosterone levels was shown, as well as a negative correlation of ET-1 with glucose utilization, which might indicate an involvement of hyperinsulinemia and insulin resistance as well as of hyperandrogenemia in the abnormal endothelial status (Diamanti-Kandarakis et al., 2001). It appears that early impairment of endothelial structure and function is present even in young women with PCOS as suggested by significantly higher ET-1 levels in normal-weight, non-dyslipidemic and non-hypertensive women with PCOS than in BMI-matched healthy controls (Orio et al., 2004). The metformin therapy appeared to have beneficial effects, decreasing ET-1 levels (Diamanti-Kandarakis et al., 2001; Orio et al., 2005, as cited in Ilie et al., 2008). Consistent with others results, we also clearly demonstrated in a previous report that young, euglycaemic, eulipidemic and normotensive women with PCOS have evidence of endothelial dysfunction as assessed by both hemodynamic (FMD) and biochemical methods (ET-1). Impaired vascular reactivity and increased level of ET-1 were linked to markers of hyperandrogenemia in our study (Ilie et al., 2011). Interestingly, visfatin, an adipokine predominantly expressed in, and secreted from visceral adipose tissue, has also been shown to play a role in the pathogenesis of endothelial dysfunction in PCOS, independent of additional risk factors, since circulating visfatin was significantly related to brachial artery FMD and free testosterone (Pepene, 2011).

In healthy vessels, an infusion of an endothelium-dependent vasodilatator, such as acetylcholine, induces a nitric oxide (NO)-mediated vasodilatory response; however, in patients with endothelial dysfunction, this effect is blunted or paradoxical vasoconstriction may occur (Verma et al., 2003, as cited in Ilie et al., 2008). Nacul et al. are the first who evaluated the concentration of nitrite/nitrate (as index of endothelium-derived NO) in a PCOS group compared to an age-matched control group and found similar levels of nitrite/nitrate and fibrinogen in the two groups. A negative, BMI-independent correlation between NO and insulin resistance was seen in PCOS patients only, but no association was observed between NO and BMI, WC, WHR or androgens suggesting that in PCOS endothelial dysfunction is related to the presence of insulin resistance (Nacul et al., 2007). Moreover, in a very recent study, Battaglia et al. (2010) demonstrated that young women with PCOS displayed levels of nitrite/nitrate within normal range and similar with those found in controls, which preserved the endothelium-dependent vasodilatation, which was also similar in both groups. There are also reports which, on the contrary, found lower levels of nitrites/nitrates in PCOS and subjects with polycystic ovaries (Battaglia et al., 2008) as well as in normal weight, eumenorrheic, nonhirsute daughters of patients with PCOS (Battaglia et al., 2009) compared with controls, which suggests that PCOS is a condition associated with an increased vascular risk.

Overall, data from the literature support the presence of endothelial dysfunction in women with PCOS, including those who are young and apparently not displaying CV risk factors. So far, insulin resistance appears to be the major responsible factor related to endothelial dysfunction in PCOS subjects. Additionally, there are also reports indicating an association of endothelial dysfunction with obesity, hsCRP and, less consistently, with hyperandrogenemia. The slight differences among the obtained results might be explained either through the different methodology used for the investigation of vascular reactivity and endothelial dysfunction, or through the different metabolic status of the recruited patients. Additionally, small sample sizes, bias in case-control designs, and the use of different criteria to define PCOS might also contribute to discrepancies amongst some studies.

5.2 Morphological studies

The two major anatomic markers for sub-clinical cardiovascular disease are carotid IMT, assessed by ultrasonography or angiography and coronary artery calcifications (CAC) evaluated by electron beam tomography (Essah et al., 2007). Increased carotid IMT has been reported to occur relatively early in the atherosclerotic process and has been linked with traditional CV risk factors, such as increasing age, obesity and adverse lipid profile, as commonly observed in PCOS (Talbott et al., 2004a). Several studies demonstrated the role of carotid IMT in predicting coronary and cerebrovascular events, with increasing carotid IMT associated with an elevated age-adjusted cardiovascular risk (Cussons et al., 2006). In particular, Talbott et al. demonstrated a difference in carotid IMT between middle-aged women with PCOS (≥45 years) and age-matched controls, but not in younger women (group aged 30 to 45 years) (Talbott et al., 2000a). However, there are also reports showing significantly higher carotid IMT values also in young, normal weight PCOS women compared with controls (Carmina et al., 2006b; Orio et al., 2004, Luque-Ramirez et al., 2007). Increased carotid IMT was found to be related to insulin resistance and lower adiponectin levels (Carmina et al., 2006b) or correlate with free androgen index or TT (Costa et al., 2008; Orio et al., 2004; Luque-Ramirez et al., 2007) and DHEAS (Pamuk et al., 2008), thus suggesting a contribution of hyperandrogenemia to the progression of atherosclerosis in PCOS (Ilie et al., 2008). By contrast, other studies showed that increased carotid IMT was inversely correlated with plasma DHEAS and androstendion levels suggesting an intriguing vasculoprotective effect of hyperandrogenemia in PCOS. However, further researches are needed to confirm whether elevated DHEAS actually protects against atherogenesis in PCOS (Cussons et al., 2006). As inflammation has been implicated as a novel risk factor in the development and progression of atherosclerosis, the same Talbott et al. investigated the elevated CRP, as a marker of inflammation, as a possible determinant of increased IMT in middle-aged women with PCOS. They noted, however, that although CRP was significantly higher in PCOS patients than in controls, it did not appear to appreciably mediate the influence of PCOS on IMT (Talbott et al., 2004b). On the contrary, in another study, elevated serum IL-18 levels were associated with greater carotid IMT in patients with PCOS, suggesting a link between IL-18 and carotid atherosclerosis in patients with this disorder (Kaya et al., 2009). In line with other studies (Arikan et al., 2009; Costa et al., 2008; Meyer et al., 2005a), we could not find evidence of altered arterial structure in our group of young subjects with PCOS, as compared to controls (Ilie et al., 2011).

Coronary artery calcifications, both radiographic markers for coronary atherosclerotic plaque and predictors of clinical events were found more prevalent in premenopausal obese women with PCOS aged 30-45 years in comparison to controls (Christian et al., 2003, as cited in Ilie et al., 2008). In a nine year follow-up study, an increased incidence of CAC was described in middle-aged women with PCOS; the degree of calcification was dependent on central obesity, elevated BP, dyslipidemia and thus insulin resistance (Talbott et al., 2004a). Furthermore, the prevalence of coronary artery calcium (CAC) was significantly higher also in young, obese women with PCOS, as compared with age and weight matched controls, even though the majority of subjects with detectable coronary artery calcification did not have traditional CV risk factors. The finding supports the idea that the presence of PCOS status per se appeared to contribute to this increased risk of CAC (Shroff et al., 2007). These reports suggest that women with PCOS have morphological evidence of coronary atherosclerosis and that insulin resistance, in particular, is the major causal factor. While the morphological changes in the vascular wall seem to be more evident in middle-aged and older women with PCOS, endothelial dysfunction is more likely a feature of the vasculopathy of young women with PCOS. This is not surprising, as endothelial dysfunction has been shown to occur earlier in the atherosclerosis development and progression, preceding the onset of increased carotid IMT (Meyer et al., 2005a, b).

5.3 Low-grade chronic inflammation

Recent evidence has been focused on a state of low-grade chronic inflammation, which has been described in PCOS as a potential link between hyperandrogenism, insulin resistance or abdominal adiposity and the metabolic and CV long-term complications of the syndrome.

Low-grade inflammation can be defined as a condition characterized by increased circulation levels of several mediators of inflammation triggered by a noxious stimulus, such as classic molecules (TNF-α, IL-1, IL-6, CRP), or white blood cell (WBC) count (Repaci et al., 2011). Obesity, particularly the visceral phenotype, has been defined as a state of low-grade inflammation because visceral adipose tissue is able to produce cytokines (TNF-α, IL-6, and IL-1), chemokines (interferon-inducible protein-10 (IP-10), IL-8, IL-18, monocyte chemotactic protein-1 (MCP-1)) and other adipokines (FFA, PAI-1, leptin, resistin, visfatin, and adiponectin) that act, directly or indirectly, as mediators of systemic inflammation. Interestingly, the adipo-cytokines and, overall, the chronic inflammatory state associated with obesity are also related to the insulin resistance state (Sell & Eckel, 2009, as cited in Repaci et al., 2011), type 2 DM or CVD due to the development of hypertension, dyslipidemia, and endothelial dysfunction (Yudkin et al., 1999, as cited in Repaci et al., 2011) (Fig. 2). Furthermore, accumulating evidence suggests that atherosclerosis represents a chronic inflammatory process and that the inflammation at the level of the vessel wall plays a pivotal role in atherosclerotic lesion formation, progression, and eventual rupture.

There is much evidence sustaining that high levels of IL-6, TNF-α, and leptin, and reduced levels of adiponectin inhibit the expression and activity of nitric oxide synthase (eNOS), leading to decreased NO synthesis and reduced vasodilation and consequently promoting endothelial dysfunction (Rizvi, 2007, 2009, as cited in Repaci et al., 2011) (Fig. 2). The release of cytokines and chemokines, such as TNF-α, MCP-1, and IL-18 has been demonstrated to promote the recruitment of macrophages from the bloodstream which, through the production of adhesion molecules, in turn accelerate adhesion, arrest, and diapedesis of inflammatory cells through the endothelium with the consequent infiltration of the lipid core. These inflammation mediators also promote the proliferation of smooth muscle cells and their migration from the tunica media to the tunica intima (Sengenès et al., 2007, as cited in Reapaci et al., 2011), leading to the formation of atherosclerotic plaque. Hence, chronic inflammation is responsible of early and late atherosclerotic processes.

5.3.1 Classic and non-classic markers of low-grade inflammation in PCOS

A classic and widely studied marker of low-grade inflammation is CRP, which has been shown to significantly predict the incidence of peripheral vascular diseases, endothelial dysfunction, MI, stroke, and sudden death (Ridker, 2003, as cited in Repaci et al., 2011). Recent data suggests that CRP is not only an inflammatory marker of atherosclerosis, but it may have some direct deleterious effects in the vascular wall, contributing to the pathogenesis of lesion formation, plaque rupture, and coronary thrombosis by interacting with and altering the endothelial cell phenotype (Verma et al., 2003, as cited in Ilie et al., 2008). CRP may directly promote endothelial dysfunction by increasing the expression of endothelial cell adhesion molecules (CAMs), the MCP-1 secretion and macrophage LDL-uptake. Also it appears that CRP directly influences the production of endothelium-derived vasoactive factors: it decreases the NO production while augmenting production of the potent endothelium-derived vasoconstrictor ET-1 as well as of PAI-1 (Devaraj et al., 2003, as cited in Ilie et al., 2008). Additionally, CRP facilitates endothelial cell apoptosis and attenuates angiogenesis. The most published data, but not all (Capoglu et al., 2009; Mohlig et al., 2005; Shroff et al., 2007), demonstrate increased levels of hsCRP in women with PCOS (Diamanti-Kandarakis et al., 2006a, b; Talbott et al., 2004b; Tarkun et al., 2004). However, many studies, including our previous report, have demonstrated that in women with PCOS the CRP values are primarily dependent to upon co-existent obesity and fatty mass or insulin resistance (Kelly et al., 2001, as cited in Ilie et al., 2008; Benson et al., 2008, as cited in Repaci et al., 2011; Ilie et al., 2011), rather than to PCOS status per se. Hence, increased serum CRP levels were found in obese and non-obese PCOS compared to controls (Tarkun et al., 2004; Talbott et al., 2004b; Kelly et al., 2001, Orio et al., 2005, as cited in Ilie et al., 2008) with significantly higher values in obese than in non-obese PCOS subjects (Morin-Papunen et al., 2003), decreasing after metformin (Morin-Papunen et al., 2003). Regarding hyperandrogenemia, in PCOS subjects, either no correlation (Tarkun et al., 2004; Puder et al., 2005) or a positive association between increased androgen levels and indices of chronic inflammation (Diamanti-Kandarakis et al., 2006a, b) were described. Diamanti-Kandarakis et al. (2006a) demonstrated that serum CRP concentrations were positively related to BMI and negatively related to FMD values and insulin sensitivity indices. Furthermore, FMD was statistically higher in PCOS population with CRP≤1mg $^{-1}$ when compared with PCOS population with CRP≥1mg $^{-1}$. The finding that the increased levels of CRP are consistent with the severity of endothelial dysfunction supports the hypothesis that chronic inflammation contributes to endothelial dysfunction (Diamanti-Kandarakis et al., 2006a).

Other classic markers of low-grade inflammation, which are significantly increased in PCOS, although not constantly (Shroff et al., 2007) are IL-18 (Escobar-Morreale et al., 2004, as cited in Repaci et al., 2011; Kaya et al., 2008), TNF-α and IL-6 (Gonzalez et al., 1999, as cited in Repaci et al., 2011; Tarkun et al., 2006). Like CRP, these cytokines have been related to the risk of developing type 2 DM and CVD and are strongly associated with insulin resistance and body fat amount (Repaci et al., 2011; Tarkun et al., 2006).

Accordingly, an increase of WBCs, particularly lymphocytes and monocytes (Orio et al., 2005a, as cited in) or neutrophils (Ibanez et al., 2005, as cited in Ilie et al., 2008) which have been demonstrated to be strongly associated with insulin resistance (Orio et al., 2007; Ibanez et al., 2005) has also been noted in PCOS. Metformin and the combination flutamide-metformin had a beneficial effect on low-grade inflammation, attenuating WBC (Orio et al., 2007, as cited in Ilie et al., 2008) and hyperneutrophilia (Ibanez et al., 2005, as cited in Ilie et al., 2008), that further supports a link between hyperleukocytosis and insulin resistance (Ilie et al., 2008). A high expression of other classic markers, such as IL-6, MCP-1 and matrix metallopeptidase-2 (MMP2), have also been described in PCOS. Whether this relationship may be attributable to increased adiposity, particularly to the visceral phenotype, or, conversely, may depend on other factors is, however, still debatable (Vgontzas et al., 2006; Hu et al., 2006; Lewandowki et al., 2006; Orio et al., 2004b; Gonzalez et al., 2006a,b, 2009; Glintborg et al., 2009, as cited in Repaci et al., 2011).

Endothelial dysfunction triggers the expression of cell adhesion molecules on the surface of endothelial cells and leukocytes to handle the intricate process of leukocyte rolling, adhesion, and transmigration into the sub-intimal space. Last but not least, in several studies, PCOS has been shown to associate with high levels of adhesion molecules, such as sICAM-1, sVCAM-1, ET-1, and sE-selectin, (Ley and Huo, 2001; Pai et al., 2004; Meigs et al., 2004; Roldan et al., 2003; Corti et al., 2004; Kowalska et al., 2002; Kadoand Nagata, 1999; Diamanti-Kandarakis et al., 2006b, as cited in Repaci et al., 2011). An interesting fact reported was that all these adhesion molecules were positively associated not only with insulin resistance (Diamanti-Kandarakis et al., 2006b), but also with the degree of hyperandrogenemia in PCOS (Diamanti-Kandarakis et al., 2001, 2006a). This association makes androgen excess a potential factor in the development of endothelial dysfunction. This hypothesis is confirmed by a recent in vitro study which proved that high levels of dihydrotestosterone favored the development of atherosclerotic lesions by inducing the expression of sVCAM on endothelial cell surface through a NF-κB dependent mechanism, which finally induces the adhesion of monocytes to endothelial cells (Death et al., 2004).

Among the non-classic markers of low-grade inflammation, increased levels of ferritin have been described in obesity, type 2 DM and the MS (Fernandez-Real et al., 2002, as cited in Repaci et al., 2011) as well as in PCOS, where it was associated with obesity and insulin excess (Escobar-Morreale et al., 2005, Botella-Carretero et al., 2006; Luque-Ramirez et al.,

2007b, as cited in Repaci et al., 2011). Osteoprotegerin (OPG) has both anti-inflammatory and antiapoptotic effects, particularly at the level of endothelial cells, where it exerts a protective role in the development of atherosclerotic plaque and plaque rupture (Scatena and Giachelli, 2002; Schoppert et al., 2002; Kiechl et al., 2007; Kim et al., 2005, as cited in Repaci et al., 2011). Reduced levels of OPG have been observed in obesity and in the presence of insulin resistance (Ugur-Altun et al., 2005; Holecki et al., 2007, as cited in Repaci et al., 2011), as well as in PCOS (Escobar-Morreale et al., 2008), where they were related to the androgen excess (Escobar-Morreale et al., 2008). Interestingly, we have demonstrated very recently that circulating OPG was negatively and significantly correlated with FMD and, moreover, that PCOS women in the upper OPG quartile group (> 2.65 pmol/l) presented significantly altered endothelial function compared to all the rest. Nevertheless, it is unclear whether the relationship between OPG and FMD found here reflects a compensatory response of the endothelium to injury or if it should rather be regarded as a direct involvement of OPG in the pathogenesis of endothelial dysfunction. In previous studies, elevated plasma OPG concentrations, reported in several states associated with vascular damage, were negatively related to endothelium-dependent arterial dilation in newly diagnosed diabetes and hypothyroidism (Shin et al., 2006, Rasmussen et al., 2006, Guang-da et al., 2008, as cited in Pepene et al., 2011). Coming back to our results, since patients with important insulin resistance and severely impaired FMD presented with the highest OPG levels, we might speculate that in PCOS, OPG may link disturbances in insulin sensitivity to impaired endothelial dysfunction and progression of atherosclerosis, independently from hyperandrogenemia. Moreover, confirming previous results (Escobar-Morreale et al., 2008) that suggest a deleterious effect of androgen excess on OPG, the latter was negatively related to FT in our study (Pepene et al., 2011). Finally, PCOS has been associated with high levels of advanced glycation endproducts (AGEs), which is described to act as oxidants and inflammatory mediators as well as increased levels of platelet mean volume (MPV), an indicator of platelet activation and aggregation (Repaci et al., 2011).

5.3.2 Androgen excess and low-grade chronic inflammation

As far as the relationship between androgen excess and low-grade chronic inflammation is concerned, there are still debates whether molecules involved in the low-grade inflammatory state are involved in the pathogenesis of hyperandrogenemia or, conversely, whether androgen excess might promote the inflammatory state. Either no correlation (Tarkun et al., 2004; Puder et al., 2005; Cascella et al., 2008; Tosi et al., 2009) or a positive association between increased androgen levels and indices of chronic inflammation (Diamanti-Kandarakis et al., 2006a, b) were described in PCOS subjects. The in vitro studies support the hypothesis that the state of low-grade inflammation influences androgens, showing that TNF-α stimulates the proliferation and steroidogenesis of theca cells (Spaczynski et al., 1999, as cited in Repaci et al., 2011), whereas IL-6 is capable of stimulating human adrenal cells, thereby increasing adrenal steroidogenesis (Path et al., 1997, as cited in Repaci et al., 2011).

In spite of the fact that the role of androgens in low-grade inflammation is yet to be demonstrated, vast evidence has accumulated to suggest that androgens could, however, play an indirect role in the development of low-grade inflammation through the impact on the adipose tissue. In fact, androgens seem to have a stimulatory effect on the hypertrophy of adipocytes by influencing the expression of enzymes and proteins involved in lipid and carbohydrate metabolism, in oxidative stress and in the differentiation of pre-adipocytes into mature adipocytes. Additionally, androgens enhance lipolysis, determining an increased release of FFA (Cortón et al., 2007, Xu et al., 1991, as cited in Repaci et al., 2011). Briefly, there still are aspects that need to be cleared regarding the bidirectional relationship between low-grade inflammation and androgen excess in PCOS, and much more research should, thus, be performed in this exciting area.

Several polymorphisms of cytokines have been studied for the possible association with PCOS. In particular, Escobar-Morreale et al. showed the association between one polymorphism at the level of the promoter of TNF-α [−308 A] and increased androgen circulating levels in both hyperandrogenic and healthy women, independent of the presence of obesity and insulin resistance (Escobar-Morreale et al., 2001).

Additionally, some studies have demonstrated the association between adipokines and androgens. One of these adipokines is visfatin, whose mRNA levels are increased in the adipose tissue of women with PCOS (Panidis et al., 2008, as cited in Repci et al., 2011; Carmina et al., 2009) and who has recently been shown to be positively associated with LH, androstenedione, and free testosterone levels, and negatively with SHBG (Panidis et al., 2008; Kowalska et al., 2007; Gen et al., 2009, as cited in Repaci et al., 2011; Pepene CE, 2011). Adiponectin and leptin are another two adipokines involved in the mediation of systemic inflammation, whose relationship with androgens is the subject of conflicting results (Page et al., 2005; Seftel, 2005; Yilmaz et al., 2009, as cited in Repaci et al., 2011). Regarding leptin in particular, some studies failed to demonstrate any relationship with androgens (Vicennati et al., 1998; Pehlivanov and Mitkov, 2009; El Orabi et al., 1999, as cited in Repaci et al., 2011), whereas others showed a positive relationship between leptin circulating levels and androgens (Hislop et al., 1999; Castrogiovanni et al., 2003; Pardo et al., 2004, as cited in Repaci et al., 2011). More convincing results have been obtained by the analysis of the ratio adiponectin/leptin, considered a good marker of a state of inflammation in PCOS (Xita et al., 2007), that was found to be positively related with SHBG. Reduced adiponectin (Carmina et al., 2006b), and increased leptin (Gomez-Ambrosi et al., 2002, as cited in Repaci et al., 2011) may also contribute to the development of endothelial dysfunction in PCOS, as shown by some reports. Finally, circulating levels of ghrelin and androgens, particularly androstenedione, have been found to be negatively connected in women with PCOS. These results have been further confirmed by the observation that a short-term treatment with flutamide, a drug with anti-androgenic properties, triggered a significant increase in ghrelin circulating levels (Glintborg et al., 2006; Pagotto et al., 2002; Panidis et al., 2005; Gambineri et al., 2003, as cited in Repaci et al., 2011).

In conclusion, PCOS is associated with a low-grade of chronic inflammation mainly attributable to the accumulation of visceral fat, although an effect of insulin resistance cannot be excluded. The impact of hyperandrogenemia can be restricted so far to the influence of androgens on the development and distribution of the adipose tissue, which is, in fact, a true endocrine gland. A vicious circle is established with a continuous release of inflammatory mediators that are responsible for the development of insulin resistance, dyslipidemia, endothelial dysfunction, and metabolic and CV long-term complications. In addition, through the impact on the regulation of the synthesis and secretion of androgens in the ovary and in the adrenal, the state of low-grade inflammation also seems able to contribute to the maintenance of the syndrome (Repaci et al., 2011).

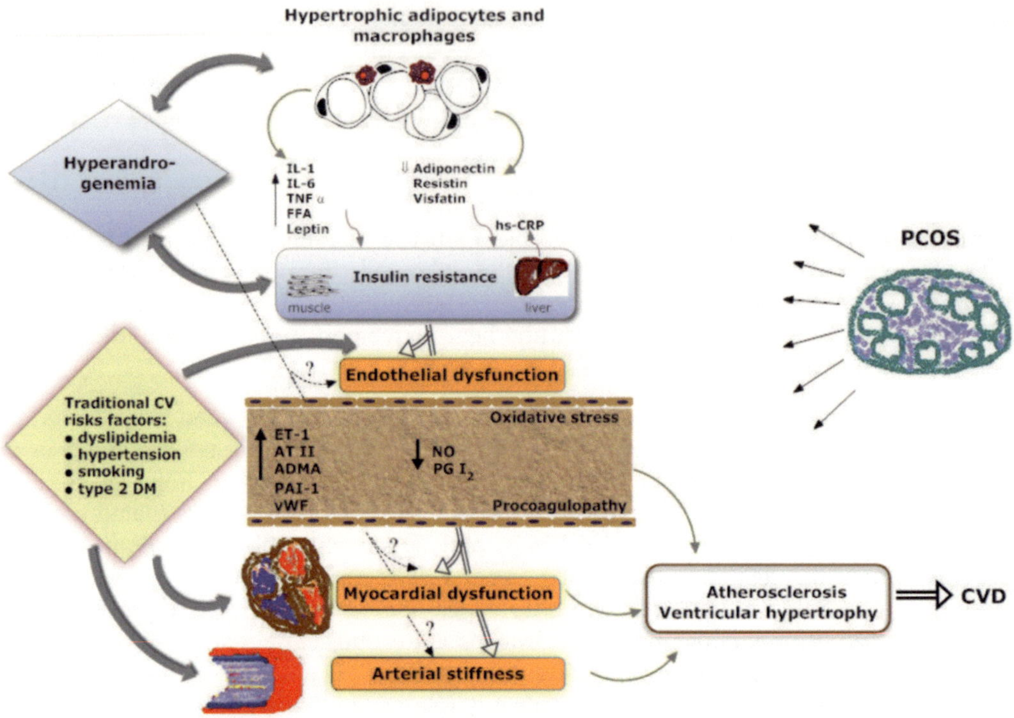

Fig. 2. Some hypothetical pathways for the development of cardiovascular disease in women with PCOS

Several traditional and non-traditional cardiovascular risk factors commonly met in PCOS play a role either directly or indirectly by developing insulin resistance (in the liver and the muscles). The latter definitely has a major influence, beside other mechanisms, in the development of subclinic cardiovascular disease, eventually leading to cardiovascular disease. The hypertrophic adipocytes secrete various molecules, including inflammatory markers and adipokines, which may, in turn, determine the development of insulin resistance, an increase of the hepatic production of hsCRP, an increase of ovarian and adrenal androgens production which may further aggravate central adiposity distribution and may even directly act to determine vascular injury. It is not, yet clear if androgen excess (the marker of PCOS) has a direct influence in the development of atherosclerosis and preclinic cardiovascular disease. TNF-α = tumor necrosis factor alpha; IL-1 = interleukin 1; IL-6 = interleukin 6; PAI-1 = plasminogen activator inhibitor-1; IL-18 = interleukin 18; FFA = free fatty acids; hsCRP = highly sensitive C reactive protein; ET-1=endothelin-1; AT II= angiotensin II; ADMA= asymmetric dimethylarginine; vWF= vonWillebrand factor; NO=nitric oxide; PG I2 = prostacyclin; CVD=cardiovascular disease.

6. Oral contraceptives may further exacerbate the metabolic profile of women with PCOS

Since its introduction in 1960, the combined oral contraceptive (COC) pill has become one of the most widely and frequently used methods of contraception worldwide. COC also have a long history of use in patients with PCOS, where they are prescribed for obtaining a regular menstrual cycle and for improving the clinical signs of hyperandrogenism. Although highly effective, COC, in particular early formulations, were associated with significant adverse effects and unacceptable CV risk. In addition, a decade after the advent of oral hormonal contraception, epidemiologic research confirmed an increased risk for cardiovascular events, particularly venous thromboembolism (VTE), in women using the high-dose COCs or COCs containing the newer gonane progestins desogestrel and gestodene (commonly referred to as "third-generation" progestins) (Burkmana et al., 2011). Research indicates also that COC use is associated with an increased risk of MI, particularly in women who smoke and are older than 35 years and in those who have underlying risk factors for coronary artery disease, such as hypertension (Burkman et al., 2011). Different estrogens and progestins exert different metabolic and CV effects. Estrogen component is almost always ethinyl estradiol (EE) in doses ranging from 15 to 50 μg. The progestin component is of variable potency and androgenicity. Hence, while in combined COCs the EE component seems to be responsible for the slight changes in the procoagulation and fibrinolytic balance, most progestins appear not to affect the coagulation factors and liver proteins when given alone (Sitruk-Ware & Nath, 2011). However, the metabolic effects of pills are extremely variable; for example estrogens impair insulin action dose-dependently and the associated progestins may modify these effects (Nader & Diamanti-Kandarakis, 2007). It was suggested that when a dose of EE < 50 μg/day is used, the effects of the COCs on the lipid and glycoinsulinemic metabolism is related to the progestin used in the combination (Mancini et al., 2010). Hence, the estrogen component of hormonal contraceptives when administered orally tends to increase the production of lipoproteins such as, the very low density lipoprotein (VLDL) and HDL levels while decreasing LDL levels (Sitruk-Ware & Nath, 2011). Non-androgenic or anti-androgenic progestins exert minimal influence on the lipid profile and carbohydrate metabolism, which lessens the risk of developing coronary heart disease while androgenic progestins have shown an adverse effect over total and HDL cholesterol (Nath & Sitruk-Ware, 2009, as cited in Sitruk-Ware & Nath, 2011). Over the past half century, COCs have undergone a number of evolutionary steps, involving modifications of hormone doses and types, dosage regimens and administration schedules (Burkmana et al., 2011) in order to improve the safety profile, particularly the metabolic and cardiovascular safety. In young women, the risk of CVD is very low but can be strongly influenced by smoking and the presence of other risks factors, such as hypertension, obesity, and DM or PCOS, specially for women over 35 (Farley et al., 1998, 1999, as cited in Sitruk-Ware & Nath, 2011).

As a special subgroup of COCs users, women with PCOS have an increased risk for IGT and as COCs are often prescribed as first-line treatment, a worsening of the metabolic outcomes in this population (e.g. insulin resistance, glucose tolerance, lipid profile or chronic inflammation) would be of concern. In the literature, there are conflicting reports about the CV effects of OCPs on PCOS patients (Battaglia et al., 2010; Meyer et al., 2007). Some of these reports support the beneficial effects of OCPs on the CV system in PCOS patients (Luque-Ramirez et al., 2009; Mancini et al., 2010). However, a recent meta-analysis suggested that OCPs may have negative effects on CV events in healthy individuals and these effects may be aggravated in patients displaying increased CV risk, such as PCOS (Baillargeon et al., 2005, as cited in Gode et al., 2010; Nader & Diamanti-Kandarakis, 2007). The outcome of the studies evaluating the effects of OCPs on carbohydrate metabolism in PCOS has been extremely variable, their results covering all possibilities: improvement, no change, deterioration (Nader & Diamanti-Kandarakis, 2007). Different OCPs used with different dosage of estrogen, type of progestin and formulation of the pill, different laboratory methods used to assess these effects represent, however, few but important limitations of these studies which should be mentioned.

Hence, Nader & Diamanti-Kandarkis (2007) concluded that the effects of OCPs on carbohydrate metabolism in PCOS will be determined by the degree of androgenicity of the woman and the androgen-lowering effect of the pill, genetically determined endogenous insulin sensitivity of the individual, anthropometric differences that can affect insulin action and by the natural history of PCOS or environmental influences and by other factors, such as puberty, which is associated with decreased insulin sensitivity (Moran et al., 1999, as cited in Nader & Diamanti-Kandarakis, 2007).

These concepts are represented in a few studies. Thus, Cagnacci et al. compared a monophasic 35-µg EE/cyproterone acetate (CPA) pill, widely used in PCOS with a biphasic 40/30 EE/desogestrel pill. The results were contradictory: insulin sensitivity improved with the CPA pill (lowering of androgens with a pill containing the most potent antiandrogenic progesterone) and deteriorated with the desogestrel pill (a more androgenic pill and/or a different formulation with a higher initial dose of estrogen) (Cagnacci et al., 2003, as cited in Nader & Diamanti-Kandarakis, 2007). Ibanez & de Zegher (2004a) also demonstrated the effect of different progestins of potentially different androgenicity. They included post-adolescent PCOS subjects who were already taking flutamide and metformin along with a 20-µg EE-/gestodene-containing OCP in their study and, after some months of this treatment, they randomized subjects to replacement of the gestodene OCP with a drospirenone (DRP) OCP containing 30 µg of EE. The patients who were switched DRP presented a reduced total and abdominal fat and an increased lean body mass (a less androgenic OCP reduced the abdominal fat and potentially improved the metabolic profile in spite of the higher dose of estrogen in the drospirenone pill) as compared with those who remained on gestodene.

As far as lipid metabolism is concerned, HDL -C and TG generally increase after OCP treatment in PCOS and this effect varies with the progestin. Higher TG concentrations are seen with less androgenic progestins (Mastorakos et al., 2002, as cited in Nader & Diamanti-Kandarakis, 2007). Ibanez & de Zegher (2004b) demonstrated that abnormal adipocytokines (increased IL-6 levels and decreased adiponectin levels), hypertriglyceridaemia and body adiposity deteriorated in a group of adolescents and young women with PCOS who were administered EE/DRP, and improved towards the norm after flutamide and metformin were added. They also showed that flutamide and metformin have beneficial effects on these adverse factors either taken individually or together (Ibanez et al., 2004; Ibanez & de Zegher, 2005, as cited in Nader & Diamanti-Kandarakis, 2007).

Furthermore, Halperin et al. (2011) undertook a meta-analysis of published observational studies to investigate the association between COC use and dysglycemia, dyslipidemia and insulin resistance in women with PCOS. COC use was significantly associated with an increase in HDL-C and TG, but was not associated with changes in fasting glucose or fasting insulin. The authors concluded that the use of COCs in women with PCOS was not associated with clinically significant adverse metabolic consequences (Halperin et al., 2011). Additionally, according to the findings in the literature, OCPs seem to have neutral or negative effects on endothelial function among healthy individuals (Gode et al., 2010).

Regarding different OCPs components, FMD appears to increase when circulating levels of estrogens augment naturally or synthetically and this beneficial vasodilator effect of estrogens on the arterial function might be antagonized by some certain types of progestins e.g. levonorgestrel, desogestrel (Torgrimson et al., 2007), but not by DRP, a progestin with antiandrogenic and antimineralocorticoid activity (Meendering et al., 2010). Consistent with these findings, it has been demonstrated that endothelial function was less in women using either a levonorgestrel combined OCP or medroxyprogesterone acetate (MPA) (a highly androgenic progestin) compared to nonusers (Meendering et al., 2010). However, controversial results have been reported in PCOS, suggesting that OCPs may have deteriorating, neutral or improving effects on endothelial function (Battaglia et al., 2010; Mancini et al., 2010; Meyer et al., 2007). In the study of Mancini et al. (2010), hypocaloric diet was prescribed to the obese patients in addition to OCPs and a significant weight reduction was observed after the treatment. In lean patients with PCOS, the DRP/EE30µg did not seem to affect endothelial function, whereas in overweight PCOS women it did not seem to counteract the loss of weight due to healthier lifestyle changes, which was associated with an improvement of insulin sensitivity and FMD. Therefore, it may be hypothesized that life style implementation may hinder the negative effects of treatment or natural progression of PCOS. In another recent study, there was a tendency of reduction in FMD in PCOS women during the 6-month treatment with EE and CPA combination. In addition, the significant alteration, which was observed particularly in the overweight group, supports the previous reports, which emphasize the independent role of obesity in CV risk (Vural et al., 2005, Mancini et al., 2009, as cited in Gode et al., 2010). Raised plasma concentrations of the endogenous nitric oxide synthase inhibitor asymmetric dimethylarginine (ADMA) have been associated with a higher prevalence of CV risk factors and CVD in different populations, including PCOS women (Dahlgren et al., 1992). Interestingly, ADMA levels were significantly decreased in PCOS subjects, after the administration for a longer period of time-12 months -of natural or synthetic estrogens, combined with anti-androgens (CPA or desogestrel), to levels comparable with those in the control group, in accordance with previous reports on ADMA concentrations in young and healthy women. A borderline but interesting decrease in ET-1 was also observed, possibly further indicating the beneficiary effect estrogens, combined with antiandrogens, have on endothelial function in women with this syndrome. The results of the present study are in agreement with previously published evidence regarding an inhibitory effect of estrogenic compounds on ADMA production (Charitidou et al., 2008).

Regarding carotid IMT, a non-significant tendency toward a decrease in carotid IMT was reported with EE/CPA treatment in PCOS subjects (Luque-Ramirez et al., 2009). The remarkable aspect of the study was that a diet and physical activity were prescribed to all patients in addition to the ongoing treatment. The results of Gode et al. (2010) were contrary to the above mentioned study, and reported a significant increase in both right and left carotid IMTs in both the normal weight and the overweight groups after the 6-month follow-up of PCOS patients given OCP containing CPA. It is possible that the significant change in carotid IMT was triggered by increased lipid taking into account the fact that, with the exception of HDL, all lipid profile components were significantly augmented in the normal-weight patients while only TG levels were significantly increased in the overweight patients and endothelial dysfunction and increased IMT coexist with abnormal lipid profile (Karasek et al., 2006, as cited in Gode et al., 2010). Moreover, a recent study reported a CIMT progression rate of 0.015 ± 0.024 mm per year among healthy young women (Johnson et al., 2007, as cited in Gode et al., 2010). However, the increase in carotid IMT in PCOS patients was 0.03 ± 0.01 mm at the end of the 6 month-period, a value which is four times higher than that reported in the healthy young women of that study. The quick advance of these CV risk parameters draws the attention to the importance of close follow-up in PCOS patients. However, due to the fact that the study included only one type of pill, to explain the deterioration of arterial structure through CPA would be a rushed conclusion. Another possibility is that EE plays a role in this fast progression of atherosclerosis. Therefore, we need additional studies to include different types of OCPs to provide clear and accurate results.

In previous studies, a CRP greater than 3 mg/L was accepted to be correlated with CVD (Boulman et al., 2004, as cited in Gode et al., 2010). In the same study performed by Gode et al. (2010), there was also a tendency toward increment in hCRP after 6 months treatment with EE/CPA. Sustaining these observations, the use of OCPs (EE−Desogestrel combination) in obese and nonobese patients with PCOS with impaired glucose tolerance resulted in significantly higher ADMA and hs-CRP levels compared to pretreatment values, thus creating an increase in the metabolic risk (Kilic et al., 2010). The hsPCR levels increased after a 6 month-treatment with COC in young, obese PCOS patients even though CO included progestatives with antiandrogenic activity (Morin-Papunen et al., 2003; Teede et al., 2010b). Both estrogens and progestin content and dosage appear to be implicated in CRP regulation, even though the role of oestrogen might be more important than that of progestin (Haarala et al., 2009). It was noted that COCs stimulate hepatocytes directly to synthesize CRP, and not via IL-6-mediated inflammation. Furthermore, there are studies that demonstrate that DRP/EE30µg monotherapy additionally deteriorated the already increased levels of IL-6 and the decreased levels of adiponectin as well as the adiposity of young PCOS female patients, whereas the treatment with flutamide-metformin reduced all studied indices towards normal levels (Ibanez L & de Zegher, 2006).

To date combined oral contraceptive pills (OCPs) have been the first-line treatment for PCOS. They induce predictable cyclic menses, reduce luteinizing hormone secretion, lower ovarian androgen production and ameliorate androgenic symptoms, increase sex hormone binding globulin thus reducing free androgens and protecting the endometrium. Taken together, until further definitive results are available, these findings revealed that OCPs may not be protective against the progression of CV risk parameters in PCOS. Thus, in some PCOS patients, such as the obese or pubertal, this additional metabolic risk should be considered when OCPs are prescribed, and appropriate surveillance is advisable, as is concomitant use of agents that modify these effects, such as metformin. Some additional treatment modalities such as life style implementation may be added to the treatment, especially in overweight PCOS patients too. Additionally, it is preferable to evaluate CV risk factors of PCOS patients under treatment with OCP, especially the obese ones. Long-term studies with larger populations are needed to confirm how specific OCP formulations affect vascular function of the arterial system in young women.

7. Do cardiovascular risk factors in PCOS result in more cardiovascular events?

The high prevalence of CV risk factors and signs of early atherosclerosis (e.g. increased IMT or altered endothelial reactivity) in young women with PCOS may determine an increased rate of CVDs in postmenopausal women affected by PCOS. However, in spite of the fact that risk factors have accumulated, we still need evidence to indicate that the high risk increases events and available studies have not ascertained, yet, a uniform association between PCOS and CVD. This is because of the lack of adequate PCOS characterization, appropriate CV disease measurement, and sufficient duration of follow-up or a true lack of association.

Initial studies on the prevalence of CVDs in postmenopausal women who were probably affected by PCOS indicated an increased risk for developing MI (Dahlgren et al., 1992). It was calculated that postmenopausal women with previous PCOS have a 7.1 higher risk than non-PCOS women of developing MI (Carmina, 2009). In a Pittsburgh cohort of 162 Caucasian women with PCOS who were followed up for CV events for up to 12 years, 5 women reported MI, angina pectoris, and/or coronary bypass or angioplasty, whereas no events were observed among 142 control women who were similarly followed (Talbott et al., 2004c). Additionally, a 4-fold risk in cardiac events among women with PCOS was reported in a cohort from the Czech Republic (Cibula et al., 2000). On the other hand, reviewing death certificates of 786 women in the United Kingdom who were diagnosed with PCOS at an average age of 26.4 years and followed for an average duration of 30 years, Pierpoint et al. (1998) failed to show a statistically significant increase in CV mortality. This study has been criticized because the diagnosis of PCOS was based on historical records over a very long period and was not supported by hormonal studies or ovarian morphology. Additionally, interpretation of their data is constrained by the fact that PCOS cases were diagnosed mainly on the basis of hospital records related to wedge resection and by the absence of a matched control cohort. Wedge resection can correct the anovulation and metabolic changes that are observed in PCOS for long periods of time, and this method of case identification may under-ascertain PCOS cases as defined by clinical characteristics. Probably, a more important criticism is that the study evaluated the causes of death of relatively young women. However, in a later report, the same authors (Wild et al., 2000) noted a higher prevalence of cerebrovascular accidents in women who had PCOS during their fertile age. The history of coronary heart disease was, on the contrary, not significantly more common in women with PCOS. On the other hand, in the Nurses' Health Study, which followed 82 439 women for 14 years, it was noted that the women with very irregular menses, which can be considered a surrogate marker for PCOS, had a significantly increased relative risk of 1.5 (95% confidence interval (CI) 1.3–1.9) for coronary heart disease and 1.9 (95% CI 1.3–2.7) for fatal MI compared with eumenorrheic women (Dawber et al., 1951, as cited in Carmina, 2009). More recently, a sub-study of the Women's Ischemia Evaluation Study (WISE) confirmed that women with PCOS have a larger number of CV events. In this study, 104 postmenopausal women with PCOS and a control group of 286 matched normal postmenopausal women were followed prospectively for close to 10 years; multi-vessel angiographic coronary artery disease was observed in 32% of PCOS women compared to 25% of non-PCOS women (odds ratio 1.7) and correlated with several factors, including increased free testosterone. In addition, the event-free survival (including fatal and non-fatal events) was significantly lower in PCOS compared to non- PCOS women. The difference between the two groups was higher when cerebrovascular accidents were also considered, confirming the association of PCOS with stroke. Moreover, women with clinical features of PCOS with increased hsCRP concentrations had a 12.2-fold higher risk of CV death or nonfatal MI than women without clinical features of PCOS and lower levels of hsCRP, suggesting that the independent adverse association between PCOS status and postmenopause CV events may act vis-à-vis inflammatory pathway (Shaw et al., 2008).

While other studies are needed to confirm and expand the available information, PCOS seems, however, to be associated with an increased risk for cerebrovascular events (stroke) and probably also for fatal and non-fatal coronary heart disease, that is independent of their underlying clinical risk, indicating that PCOS-related protracted hyperandrogenism may be one possible mechanism for their CV risk. Consequently, identification of clinical features of PCOS in postmenopausal women may provide an opportunity for risk factor intervention for the prevention of CV disease and CV events.

Nevertheless, there is a clear need for longitudinal, prospective study of a large cohort of well-characterized premenopausal PCOS, along with an appropriate cohort of matched control women that can be followed into menopause. Studies like these will provide a more categorical analysis of the increased CV risk in PCOS and a more accurate assessment of the risk for CV events and mortality in a way that could apply to the overall population of women with PCOS.

8. PCOS status - A major cardiovascular risk factor in women

Taken all together, there is no doubt that the diagnosis of PCOS implies increased cardiac risk. Moreover, in a previous research, we noted that the regression analysis performed on our subjects (women with PCOS and healthy age-matched controls) revealed a predictive value of PCOS status on both FMD and ET-1 values (Ilie et al., 2011). Therefore, in line with others who have suggested PCOS as a major unrecognized CV risk factor in women (Alexander et al., 2009), we proposed that PCOS status should be regarded as a predictor marker of CV risk, beside other well-known CV risk factors, e.g. insulin resistance, dyslipidemia.

The common clustering of CV risk factors with PCOS in reproductive young women might become a public health concern if proved to trigger an increased risk for the development of CVD. Hence, there is a need for longitudinal, prospective, case-control, more rigorous, large sample size studies in young women with PCOS, all of which should be not only long term so as to go beyond menopause, but also homogeneous in terms of both prevalence and degree of obesity as well as the methodology used for evaluating vascular injury or insulin resistance in order to document the early presence of vascular abnormalities and chronic inflammation and to establish whether these CV risk factors subsequently lead to CV events. These are also especially important because it was hypothesized that differences in risk factors between women with PCOS and controls may diminish with increasing age as a consequence of both spontaneous decrease in androgen secretion after the age of 35 years in normal women and in those with PCOS as well as decrease in the polycystic ovary prevalence with age (Labrie et al., 1997, Koivunen et al., 1999, as cited in Carmina, 2009). This might account for the possible overestimation of CV risk in young women with PCOS or for failure to detect excess risk of CV mortality among women with this disorder. However, these is very unlikely since at least one-third of PCOS patients present with increased levels of non-HDL C (Berneis et al., 2009, as cited in Carmina, 2009) and/or display several other traditional and nontraditional CV risk factors. Moreover, short-term trials of pertinent interventions, for example OCPs, insulin sensitizers, on surrogate CV outcomes are warranted, since their effect on CV risk factors and events are not clearly settled. We need accurate studies to establish CV screening guidelines for women with

PCOS. Early CV screening and treatment of all modifiable CV risk factors may be clinically considered a secondary preventing intervention. Recognition of PCOS as an independent risk factor for subsequent CV events would then justify earlier risk-factor intervention.

9. References

Achard C & Thiers J. (1921). Le virilisme pilaire et son association á l`insuffisance glycotique (diabete des femmes á barbe). BullAcad Natl Méd (Paris) Vol. 86, pp. 51-56.

Akram T, Hasan S, Imran M, Karim A & Arslan M. (2010). Association of polycystic ovary syndrome with cardiovascular risk factors. Gynecol Endocrinol, Vol. 26, pp. 47–53.

Alexander CJ, Tangchitnob EP & Lepor NE. (2009). Polycystic ovary syndrome: a major unrecognized cardiovascular risk factor in women. Rev Obstet Gynecol Vol. 2, No. issue 4, pp. 232-9.

Amato MC, Verghi M, Galluzzo A & Giordano C. (2011). The oligomenorrhoic phenotypes of polycystic ovary syndrome are characterized by a high visceral adiposity index: a likely condition of cardiometabolic risk. Hum Reprod. Vol. 26, No. issue 6, pp.1486-94

Apridonidze T, Essah P, Iuorno M & Nestler JE. (2005). Prevalence and characteristics of metabolic syndrome in women with polycystic ovary syndrome. J Clin Endocrinol Metab, Vol. 90, No. issue 4, pp. 1929-1935.

Ardawi MS & Rouzi AA. (2005). Plasma adiponectin and insulin resistance in women with polycystic ovary syndrome, Fertil. Steril., Vol. 83, pp. 1708-1716

Arikan S, Akay H, Bahceci M, Tuzcu A & Gokalp D. (2009). The evaluation of endothelial function with flow-mediated dilatation and carotid intima media thickness in young nonobese polycystic ovary syndrome patients; existence of insulin resistance alone may not represent an adequate condition for deterioration of endothelial function. Fertil Steril, Vol. 91, pp. 450-455

Azevedo MF, Costa EC, Oliveira AI, Silva IB, Marinho JC, Rodrigues JA & Azevedo GD. (2011). Elevated blood pressure in women with polycystic ovary syndrome: prevalence and associated risk factors. Rev Bras Ginecol Obstet. Vol.33, No. issue 1, pp. 31-36

Azziz R, Carmina E, Dewailly D, Diamanti-Kandarakis E, Escobar-Morreale HF, Futterweit W, Janssen OE, Legro RS, Norman RJ, Taylor AE & Witchel SF. (2006). Positions statement: criteria for defining polycystic ovary syndrome as a predominantly hyperandrogenic syndrome: an Androgen Excess Society guideline. J Clin Endocrinol Metab, Vol. 91, pp. 4237-4245

Azziz R, Carmina E, Dewailly D, Diamanti-Kandarakis E, Escobar-Morreale HF, Futterweit W, Janssen OE, Legro RS, Norman RJ, Taylor AE & Witchel SF. (2009). The Androgen Excess and PCOS Society criteria for the polycystic ovary syndrome: the complete task force report. Fertil Steril, Vol.91, pp. 456-488.

Azziz R, Marin C, Hoq L, Badamgarav E & Song P. (2005). Health care-related economic burden of the polycystic ovary syndrome during the reproductive life span. J Clin Endocrinol Metab, Vol. 90, pp. 4650-4658

Azziz R, Woods KS, Reyna R, Key TJ, Knochenhauer ES & Yildiz BO. (2004). The prevalence and features of the polycystic ovary syndrome in an unselected population. J Clin Endocrinol Metab, Vol.89, pp. 2745–2749

Baranova A, Tran TP, Birerdinc A & Younossi ZM. (2011). Systematic review: association of polycystic ovary syndrome with metabolic syndrome and non-alcoholic fatty liver disease. Aliment Pharmacol Ther, Vol. 33, No. issue 7, pp. 801-14

Barber TM, McCarthy MI, Wass JAH & Franks S. (2006). Obesity and polycystic ovary syndrome. Clin. Endocrinol, Vol. 65, pp. 137–145

Battaglia C, Mancini F, Cianciosi A, Busacchi P, Facchinetti F, Marchesini GR, Marzocchi R & de Aloysio D. (2008) Vascular risk in young women with polycystic ovary and polycystic ovary syndrome. Obstet Gynecol, Vol.111, pp. 385-395

Battaglia C, Mancini F, Cianciosi A, Busacchi P, Persico N, Paradisi R, Facchinetti F, de Aloysio D. (2009). Cardiovascular risk in normal weight, eumenorrheic, nonhirsute daughters of patients with polycystic ovary syndrome: a pilot study. Fertil Steril, Vol 92, pp.240-249

Battaglia C, Mancini F, Fabbri R, Persico N, Busacchi P, Facchinetti F, Venturoli S. (2010). Polycystic ovary syndrome and cardiovascular risk in young patients treated with drospirenone-ethinylestradiol or contraceptive vaginal ring. A prospective, randomized, pilot study. Fertil Steril, Vol 94, pp.1417-1425

Bhathena RK. (2011). Insulin resistance and the long-term consequences of polycystic ovary syndrome. J Obstet Gynaecol, Vol. 31, No. issue 2, pp. 105-110

Bhattacharya S M & Jha A. (2011), Prevalence and risk of metabolic syndrome in adolescent Indian girls with polycystic ovary syndrome using the 2009 'joint interim criteria'. J Obstet Gynaecol Res. 2011 May 3, n.d.

Bhattacharya SM. (2008). Metabolic syndrome in females with polycystic ovary syndrome and International Diabetes Federation criteria. J Obstet Gynaecol Res, Vol. 34, No. issue 1, pp. 62-66.

Bickerton AS, Clark N, Meeking D, Shaw KM, Crook M, Lumb P, Turner C & Cummings MH. (2005). Cardiovascular risk in women with polycystic ovarian syndrome (PCOS), J. Clin. Pathol, Vol. 58, pp. 151–154.

Boomsma CM, Eijkemans MJ, Hughes EG, Visser GH, Fauser BC & Macklon NS. (2006). A meta-analysis of pregnancy outcomes in women with polycystic ovary syndrome. Hum Reprod Update, Vol. 12, pp. 673-683

Boomsma CM, Fauser BC & Macklon S. (2008). Pregnancy complications in women with polycystic ovary syndrome. Semin Reprod Med Vol. 26 , pp. 72–84.

Brinkworth GD, Noakes M, Moran LJ, Norman R & Clifton PM. (2006) Flow-mediated dilatation in overweight and obese women with polycystic ovary syndrome. BJOG Vol. 113, pp. 1308-1314

Burkman R, Bell C & Serfaty D. (2011). The evolution of combined oral contraception: improving the risk-to-benefit ratio. Contraception, Vol. 84, No.issue1, pp. 19-34

Caballero AE. (2005). Metabolic and vascular abnormalities in subjects at risk for type 2 diabetes: the early start of a dangerous situation. Arch Med Res, Vol.36, pp. 241-249

Capoglu I, Erdem F, Uyanik A & Turhan H. (2009). Serum levels of resistin and hsCRP in women with PCOS, Cent Eur J Med, Vol. 4, No. issue 4, pp. 428-432

Carmassi F, Negri FD, Fioriti R, De Giorgi A, Giannarelli C, Fruzzetti F, Pedrinelli R, Dell'Omo G & Bersi C.(2005). Insulin resistance causes impaired vasodilation and hypofibrinolysis in young women with polycystic ovary syndrome, Thromb Res, Vol. 116, pp. 207–214.

Carmina E , Bucchieri S , Esposito A , Del Puente A , Mansueto, P, Orio, F, Di Fede G & Rini GB. (2007). Abdominal fat quantity and distribution in women with polycystic ovary syndrome and extent of its relation to insulin resistance. J Clin Endocrinol Metab, Vol. 92, pp. 2500–2505.

Carmina E, Bucchieri S, Mansueto P, Rini G, Ferin M & Lobo RA. (2009). Circulating levels of adipose products and differences in fat distribution in the ovulatory and anovulatory phenotypes of polycystic ovary syndrome. Fertil. Steril, Vol.91 , No.issue 4 (Suppl.), pp. 1332–1335.

Carmina E, Chu MC, Longo RA, Rini GB & Lobo RA. (2005). Phenotypic variation in hyperandrogenic women influences the findings of abnormal metabolic and cardiovascular risk parameters. J Clin Endocrinol Metab, Vol.90, pp. 2545–2549

Carmina E, Napoli N, Longo RA, Rini GB, Lobo RA. (2006a). Metabolic syndrome in polycystic ovary syndrome (PCOS): lower prevalence in southern Italy than in the USA and the influence of criteria for the diagnosis of PCOS. Eur J Endocrinol, Vol 154 No. issue 1, pp. 141-5.

Carmina E, Orio F, Palomba S, Longo RA., Cascella T, Colao A, Lombardi G, Rini GB & Lobo RA. (2006b). Endothelial dysfunction in PCOS: role of obesity and adipose hormones. Am. J. Medicine, Vol. 119, No. issue 4, pp. 356.e1-356.e6

Carmina E. (2006c). Metabolic syndrome in polycystic ovary syndrome. Minerva Ginecol, Vol 58, No. issue 2, pp. 109-14.

Carmina E. (2009). Cardiovascular risk and events in polycystic ovary syndrome. Climacteric, I2 (Suppl I), pp.22-25

Cascella T, Palomba S, De Sio I, Manguso F, Giallauria F, De Simone B, Tafuri D, Lombardi G, Colao A & Orio F. (2008). Visceral fat is associated with cardiovascular risk in women with polycystic ovary syndrome. Hum Reprod, Vol. 23, pp. 153-159

Chang AY & Wild RA. (2009). Characterizing cardiovascular risk in women with polycystic ovary syndrome: more than the sum of its parts? Semin Reprod Med, Vol. 27, No. issue 4, pp. 299-305

Charitidou C, Farmakiotis D, Zournatzi V, Pidonia I, Pegiou T, Karamanis N, Hatzistilianou M, Katsikis I & Panidis D. (2008). The administration of estrogens, combined with anti-androgens, has beneficial effects on the hormonal features and asymmetric dimethyl-arginine levels, in women with the polycystic ovary syndrome. Atherosclerosis, Vol. 196, pp. 958-965

Chen MJ, Yang WS, Yang JH, Chen CL, Ho HN & Yang YS. (2007). Relationship between androgen levels and blood pressure in young women with polycystic ovary syndrome. Hypertension. Vol. 49, pp. 1442-1447

Cheung LP, Ma RC, Lam PM, Lok IH, Haines CJ, So WY, Tong PC, Cockram CS, Chow CC & Goggins WB. Cardiovascular risks and metabolic syndrome in Hong Kong Chinese women with polycystic ovary syndrome. Hum Reprod, Vol. 23, No. issue 6, pp. 1431-1438.

Cho LW, Randeva HS & Atkin SL. (2007). Cardiometabolic aspects of polycystic ovarian syndrome. Vasc Health Risk Manag, Vol. 3, No. issue 1, pp. 55-63

Cibula D, Cífková R, Fanta M, Poledne R, Zivny J, Skibová J. (2000). Increased risk of non-insulin dependent diabetes mellitus, arterial hypertension and coronary artery disease in perimenopausal women with a history of the polycystic ovary syndrome. Hum Reprod, Vol.15, No. issue 4, pp. 785-9.

Costa LO, dos Santos MP, Oliveira M & Viana A. (2008). Low-grade chronic inflammation is not accompanied by structural arterial injury in polycystic ovary syndrome. Diabetes. Res. Clin. Pract, Vol. 81,pp. 179-183.

Cushman WC. (2007). JNC-7 guidelines: are they still relevant? Curr Hypertens Rep, Vol. 9, pp. 380–386

Cussons AJ, Watts GF & Stuckey BG. (2009). Dissociation of endothelial function and arterial stiffness in nonobese women with polycystic ovary syndrome (PCOS). Clin Endocrinol (Oxf), Vol. 71, No. issue 6, pp. 808-14.

Cussons AJ, Watts GF, Burke V, Shaw JE, Zimmet PZ & Stuckey BG (2008). Cardiometabolic risk in polycystic ovary syndrome: a comparison of different approaches to defining the metabolic syndrome. Hum Reprod, Vol. 23, No. issue 10, pp. 2352-2358

Dagre A, Lekakis J, Mihas C, Protogerou A, Thalassinou L, Tryfonopoulos D, Douridas G, Papamichael C & Alevizaki M. (2006). Association of dehydroepiandrosterone-sulfate with endothelial function in young women with polycystic ovary syndrome. Eur J Endocrinol, Vol. 154, pp. 883-890

Dahlgren E, Janson PO, Johansson S, Lapidus L & Odén A. (1992). Polycystic ovary syndrome and risk for myocardial infarction. Evaluated from a risk factor model based on a prospective population study of women. Acta Obstet Gynecol Scand, Vol. 71, No. issue 8, pp. 599-604

Death AK, McGrath KC, Sader MĂ, Nakhla S, Jessup W, Handelsman DJ & Celermajer DS. (2004). Dihydrotestosterone promotes vascular cell adhesion molecule-1 expression in male human endothelial cells via a nuclear factor-kappaB-dependent pathway. Endocrinology, Vol.145, pp. 1889-1897

Dejager S, Pichard C, Giral P, Bruckert E, Federspield MC, Beucler I & Turpin G. (2001). Smaller LDL particle size in women with polycystic ovary syndrome compared to controls. Clin Endocrinol (Oxf), Vol.54, pp. 455-462

Diamanti-Kandarakis E, Alexandraki K, Protogerou A, Piperi C, Papamichael C, Aessopos A, Lekakis J & Mavrikakis M. (2005). Metformin administration improves endothelial function in women with polycystic ovary syndrome. Eur J Endocrinol, Vol. 152, pp. 749-756

Diamanti-Kandarakis E, Spina G, Kouli C & Migdalis I (2001). Increased endothelin-1 levels in women with polycystic ovary syndrome and the beneficial effect of metformin therapy, J Clin Endocrinol Metab, Vol. 86, pp. 4666–4673.

Diamanti-Kandarakis E., Alexandraki K., Piperi C., Protogerou A., Katsikis I., Paterakis T., et al. (2006a). Inflammatory and endothelial markers in women with polycystic ovary syndrome, Eur J Clin Invest, Vol 36, pp.691-697

Diamanti-Kandarakis E., Paterakis T., Alexandraki K., Piperi C., Aessopos A., Katsikis I., et al. (2006b). Indices of low-grade chronic inflammation in polycystic ovary syndrome and the beneficial effect of metformin, Hum Reprod, Vol 21, pp.1426-1431

Dokras A, Bochner M, Hollinrake E, Markham S, Vanvoorhis B & Jagasia DH (2005). Screening women with polycystic ovary syndrome for metabolic syndrome. Obstet Gynecol, Vol. 106, No. issue 1, pp. 131-137.

Dokras A. (2008). Cardiovascular Disease Risk Factors in Polycystic Ovary Syndrome. Semin Reprod Med, Vol. 26, No. issue 1, pp. 39-44

Dunaif A. (1997). Insulin resistance and the polycystic ovary syndrome: mechanism and implications for pathogenesis. Endocr Rev, Vol. 18, No. issue 6, pp. 774-800

Ehrmann D, Liljenquist D, Kasza K, Azziz R, Legro R, Ghazzi M & PCOS/Troglitazone Study Group. (2006). Prevalence and predictors of the metabolic syndrome in women with polycystic ovary syndrome. J Clin Endocrinol Metab, Vol. 91, No. issue 1, pp. 48-53.

Escobar-Moreale HF & San Millan JL. (2007). Abdominal adiposity and the polycystic ovary syndrome. Trends in Endocrinology and Metabolism, Vol.18, pp. 266-272

Escobar-Morreale H F , Villuendas G , Botella-Carretero J I , Álvarez-Blasco F , Sanchón R & Luque-Ramírez M. (2006). Adiponectin and resistin in PCOS: a clinical, biochemical and molecular genetic study. Human Reproduction, Vol 21, pp. 2257-2265

Escobar-Morreale HF, Botella-Carretero JI, Martínez-García MA, Luque-Ramírez M, Alvarez-Blasco F & San Millán JL. (2008). Serum osteoprotegerin concentrations are decreased in women with the polycystic ovary syndrome. Eur J Endocrinol, Vol.159, No.issue 3, pp. 225-32.

Escobar-Morreale HF, Calvo RM, SanchoJ & San Millàn, JL. (2001). TNF-a and hyperandrogenism: a clinical, biochemical and molecular genetic study. J Clin Endocrinol Metab, Vol. 86, No.issue 8, pp. 3761–3767.

Essah P, Nestler JE & Carmina E. (2008). Differences in dyslipidemia between American and Italian women with polycystic ovary syndrome. J Endocrinol Invest, Vol. 31, pp. 35–41

Essah PA, Wickham EP & Nestler JE. (2007). The metabolic syndrome in polycystic ovary syndrome. Clin Obstet Gynecol Vol. 50, pp. 205-225

Farell K & Antoni M. (2010). Insulin resistance, obesity, inflammation, and depression in polycystic ovary syndrome: biobehavioral mechanisms and interventions. Fertil Steril, Vol. 94, No. issue 5, pp. 1565-1574

Glueck CJ, Morrison JA, Goldenberg N & Wang P. (2009). Coronary heart disease risk factors in adult premenopausal white women with polycystic ovary syndrome compared with a healthy female population. Metabolism, Vol.58, pp. 714-721

Glueck CJ, Papanna R, Wang P, Goldenberg N & Sieve-Smith L. (2003). Incidence and treatment of metabolic syndrome in newly referred women with confirmed polycystic ovarian syndrome. Metabolism, Vol. 52, No. issue 7, pp. 908-15.

Gode F, Karagoz C, Posaci C, Saatli B, Uysal D, Secil M & Akdeniz B. (2010). Alteration of cardiovascular risk parameters in women with polycystic ovary syndrome who were prescribed to ethinyl estradiol-cyproterone acetate. Arch Gynecol Obstet. 2010 Dec 8 n.d.

Guastella E, Longo R & Carmina E. (2010). Clinical and endocrine characteristics of the main polycystic ovary syndrome phenotypes. Fertil Steril, Vol. 94, No. issue 6, pp. 2197-2201

Gulcelik NE, Aral Y, Serter R & Koc G. (2008). Association of hypoadiponectinemia with metabolic syndrome in patients with polycystic ovary syndrome. J Natl Med Assoc, Vol. 100, pp. 64-68

Guo M, Chen ZJ, Macklon NS, Shi YH, Westerveld HE, Eijkemans MJ, Fauser BC, & Goverde AJ. (2010). Cardiovascular and metabolic characteristics of infertile Chinese women with PCOS diagnosed according to the Rotterdam consensus criteria. Reprod Biomed Online, Vol. 21, No. issue 4, pp. 572-580.

Haarala A, Eklund C, Pessi T, Lehtimaki T, Huupponen R, Jula A, et al. (2009). Use of combined oral contraceptives alters metabolic determinants and genetic regulation of C-reactive protein. The Cardiovascular Risk in Young Finns Study. Scand J Clin Lab Invest, Vol. 69, pp. 168-174.

Halperin IJ, Kumar SS, Stroup DF & Laredo SE. The association between the combined oral contraceptive pill and insulin resistance, dysglycemia and dyslipidemia in women with polycystic ovary syndrome: a systematic review and meta-analysis of observational studies. Hum Reprod. 2011, Vol.26, pp. 191–201.

Hoffman LK & Ehrmann DA. (2008). Cardiometabolic features of polycystic ovary syndrome. Nat Clin Pract Endocrinol Metab, Vol. 4, pp. 215-222

Huang J,1 Ni R, Chen X, Huang L, Mo Y & Yang D. (2010). Metabolic abnormalities in adolescents with polycystic ovary syndrome in south china. Reprod Biol Endocrinol, Vol. 8: 142.

Hudecova M, Holte J, Olovsson M, Lind L & Poromaa IS. (2010). Endothelial function in patients with polycystic ovary syndrome: a long-term follow-up study. Fertil Steril, Vol. 94, No. issue 7, pp. 2654-2658

Ibanez L & De Zegher F. (2004 b). Ethinylestradiol-drospirenone, flutamide-metformin, or both for adolescents and women with hyperinsulinemic hyperandrogenism: opposite effects on adipocytokines and body adiposity. J Clin Endocrinol Metab, Vol. 89, pp. 1592-1597

Ibanez L & De Zegher F. (2004 a). Flutamide-metformin plus an oral contraceptive (OC) for young women with polycystic ovary syndrome: switch from third- to fourth-generation OC reduces body adiposity. Hum Reprod , Vol. 19, pp. 1725-1727

Ibanez L & De Zegher F. (2006). Low-dose flutamide-metformin therapy for hyperinsulinemic hyperandrogenism in non-obese adolescents and women. Hum Reprod Update, Vol.12, pp. 243-252

Ilie IR, Georgescu C, Duncea I, Ilie IR. (2008). Vascular abnormalities and low-grade chronic inflammation in women with polycystic ovary syndrome: relationships with insulin resistance, obesity and hyperandrogenemia, Central European Journal of Medicine, Vol 3, pp. 257-270

Ilie IR, Pepene CE, Marian I, Mocan T, Hazi G, Drăgotoiu G, Ilie R, Mocan L and Duncea I. (2011). The polycystic ovary syndrome (PCOS) status and cardiovascular risk in young women, Central European Journal of Medicine, Vol 6, No. issue 1, pp. 64-75

Kandaraki E, Christakou C & Diamanti-Kandarakis E. (2009). Metabolic syndrome and polycystic ovary syndrome... and vice versa. Arq Bras Endocrinol Metabol, Vol.53, No. issue 2, pp. 227-237

Karkanaki A, Piouka A, Katsikis I, Farmakiotis D, Macut D & Panidis D. (2009). Adiponectin levels reflect the different phenotypes of polycystic ovary syndrome: study in normal weight, normoinsulinemic patients. Fertil Steril, Vol 92, No. issue 6, pp. 2078-2081

Kaya C, Pabuccu R, Berker B & Satiroglu H. (2010). Plasma interleukin-18 levels are increased in the polycystic ovary syndrome: relationship of carotid intima-media wall thickness and cardiovascular risk factors, Fertil. Steril, Vol.93, No. issue 4, pp. 1200-1207.

Kelly CJ, Speirs A, Gould GW, Petrie JR, Lyall H & Connell JMC (2002). Altered vascular function in young women with polycystic ovary syndrome. J Clin Endocrinol Metab, Vol.87, pp. 742–746.

Ketel I J ,Stehouwer C D, Henry RM, Serne EH, Hompes P, Homburg R, Smulders YM & Lambalk CB. (2010). Greater Arterial Stiffness in Polycystic Ovary Syndrome (PCOS) Is an Obesity- But Not a PCOS-Associated Phenomenon. J Clin Endocrinol Metab Vol.95, pp. 4566-4575

Kilic S, Yilmaz N, Zulfikaroglu E, Erdogan G, Aydin M & Batioglu S. (2011). Inflammatory-metabolic parameters in obese and nonobese normoandrogenemic polycystic ovary syndrome during metformin and oral contraceptive treatment. Gynecol Endocrinol, Vol. 27, No.issue 9, pp. 622-9

Kosmala W, O'Moore-Sullivan TM, Plaksej R, Kuliczkowska-Plaksej J, Przewlocka-Kosmala M & Marwick TH. (2008). Subclinical impairment of left ventricular function in young obese women: contributions of polycystic ovary disease and insulin resistance. J Clin Endocrinol Metab, Vol. 93, No. issue 10, pp. 3748-3754

Kravariti M, Naka KK, Kalantaridou SN, Kazakos N, Katsouras CS, Makrigiannakis A, Paraskevaidis EA, Chrousos GP, Tsatsoulis A & Michalis LK (2005). Predictors of endothelial dysfunction in young women with polycystic ovary syndrome. J Clin Endocrinol Metab, Vol.90, pp. 5088-5095

Lambrinoudaki I. (2011). Cardiovascular risk in postmenopausal women with the polycystic ovary syndrome. Maturitas, Vol.68, No. issue 1, pp. 13-6.

Legro RS, Kunselman AR & Dunaif A. (2001). Prevalence and predictors of dyslipidemia in women with polycystic ovary syndrome. Am J Med, Vol.111, pp. 607–613

Legro RS. (2006). Type 2 diabetes and polycystic ovary syndrome. Fertil Steril, Vol. 86 (Suppl 1), pp. S16–S17

Lo JC, Feigenbaum SL, Yang J, Pressman AR, Selby JV & Go AS. (2006). Epidemiology and adverse cardiovascular risk profile of diagnosed polycystic ovary syndrome. J Clin Endocrinol Metab, Vol.91, pp. 1357-1363

Lorenz LB & Wild RA. (2007). Polycystic ovarian syndrome: an evidence-based approach to evaluation and management of diabetes and cardiovascular risks for today's clinician. Clin Obstet Gynecol, Vol. 50, pp. 226-243

Lorenzo C & Haffner SM. (2010). Performance characteristics of the new definition of diabetes: the insulin resistance atherosclerosis study. Diabetes Care Vol. 33, pp. 335–337

Luque-Ramirez M, Mendieta-Azcona C, Alvarez-Blasco F & Escobar-Morreale HF. (2007). Androgen excess is associated with the increased carotid intima-media thickness observed in young women with polycystic ovary syndrome. Hum Reprod Vol.22, pp. 3197-3203

Luque-Ramirez ML, Mendieta-Azcona C, Alverez-Blasco F & Escobar-Morreale HF. (2009). Effects of metformin versus ethinyl-estradiol plus cyproterone acetate on ambulatory blood pressure monitoring and carotid intima media thickness in women with the polycystic ovary syndrome. Fertil Steril, Vol. 91, pp. 2527–2536

Mancini F, Cianciosi A, Persico N, Facchinetti F, Busacchi P & Battaglia C. (2010). Drospirenone and cardiovascular risk in lean and obese polycystic ovary syndrome patients: a pilot study. Am J Obstet Gynecol, Vol. 202, No. issue 2, 169 e1-8.

Mather KJ, Verma S, Corenblum B & Anderson TJ. (2000). Normal endothelial function despite insulin resistance in healthy women with the polycystic ovary syndrome. J Clin Endocrinol Metab, Vol. 85, pp. 1851-1856

Meendering JR, Torgrimson BN, Miller NP, Kaplan PF& Minson CT. (2010). A combined oral contraceptive containing 30 mcg ethinyl estradiol and 3.0 mg drospirenone does not impair endothelium-dependent vasodilation. Contraception, Vol. 82, pp. 366-372.

Meyer C, McGrath BP & Teede HJ. (2005a). Overweight women with polycystic ovary syndrome have evidence of subclinical cardiovascular disease. J Clin Endocrinol Metab, Vol. 90, pp. 5711-5716

Meyer C, McGrath BP & Teede HJ. (2007). Effects of medical therapy on insulin resistance and the cardiovascular system in polycystic ovary syndrome. Diabetes Care Vol.30, pp. 471–478

Meyer C, McGrath BP, Cameron J, Kotsopoulos D & Teede HJ. (2005b). Vascular dysfunction and metabolic parameters in polycystic ovary syndrome. J Clin Endocrinol Metab, vol. 90, pp. 4630-4635

Mohlig M, Spranger J, Osterhoff M, Ristow M, Pfeiffer AF, Schill T, Schlösser HW, Brabant G & Schöfl C. (2004). The polycystic ovary syndrome per se is not associated with increased chronic inflammation. Eur J Endocrinol, Vol. 150, pp. 525-532.

Moran LJ, Misso ML, Wild RA & Norman RJ. (2010). Impaired glucose tolerance, type 2 diabetes and metabolic syndrome in polycystic ovary syndrome: a systematic review and meta-analysis. Hum Reprod Update, Vol. 6, pp. 347–363

Moran L & Teede H. (2009). Metabolic features of the reproductive phenotypes of polycystic ovary syndrome. Hum. Reprod, Vol.15, No.4, pp. 477–488

Moran LJ, Pasquali R, Teede HJ, Hoeger KM & Norman RJ. (2009). Treatment of obesity in polycystic ovary syndrome: a position statement of the Androgen Excess and Polycystic Ovary Syndrome Society. Fertil Steril, Vol.92, pp. 1966-1982

Morin-Papunen L, Rautio K, Ruokonen A, Hedberg P, Puukka M & Tapanainen JS. (2003). Metformin reduces serum C-reactive protein levels in women with polycystic ovary syndrome. J Clin Endocrinol Metab, Vol. 88, pp. 4649-4654

Nacul AP, Andrade CD, Schwarz P, Homem de Bittencourt Jr PI & Spritzer PM. (2007) Nitric oxide and fibrinogen in polycystic ovary syndrome: associations with insulin resistance and obesity. Europ. J. Obstet. Gynecol, Vol. 133, pp. 191-196

Nader S & Diamanti-Kandarakis E. (2007). Polycystic ovary syndrome, oral contraceptives and metabolic issues: new perspectives and a unifying hypothesis. Hum Reprod, Vol. 22, pp. 317-322.

Nitsche K & Ehrmann DA. (2010). Obstructive sleep apnea and metabolic dysfunction in polycystic ovary syndrome. Best Pract Res Clin Endocrinol Metab, Vol. 24, No. issue 5, 717-730

Orio F, Jr., Palomba S, Cascella T, De Simone B, Di Biase S, Russo T, Labella D, Zullo F, Lombardi G & Colao A. (2004). Early impairment of endothelial structure and function in young normal-weight women with polycystic ovary syndrome. J Clin Endocrinol Metab Vol.89, pp. 4588-4593

Pamuk BO, Torun AN, Kulaksizoglu M, Ertugrul D, Ciftci O, Kulaksizoglu S, Yildirim E & Demirag NG. (2008). Asymmetric dimethylarginine levels and carotid intima-media thickness in obese patients with polycystic ovary syndrome and their relationship with metabolic parameters. Fertil Steril, Vol. 93, No.issue 4, pp. 1227-1233.

Paradisi G, Steinberg HO, Hempfling A, Cronin J, Hook G, Shepard MK & Baron AD. (2001). Polycystic ovary syndrome is associated with endothelial dysfunction. Circulation Vol.103, pp. 1410-1415

Paradisi G, Steinberg HO, Shepard MK, Hook G & Baron AD (2003). Troglitazone therapy improves endothelial function to near normal levels in women with polycystic ovary syndrome, J. Clin. Endocrinol. Metab, Vol. 88, pp. 576-580

Park HR, Choi Y, Lee HJ, Oh JY, Hong YS & Sung YA. (2007). The metabolic syndrome in young Korean women with polycystic ovary syndrome. Diabetes Res Clin Pract, Vol. 77, Suppl 1, pp. S243-246.

Penaforte FR, Japur CC, Diez-Garcia RW & Chiarello PG. (2011). Upper trunk fat assessment and its relationship with metabolic and biochemical variables and body fat in polycystic ovary syndrome. J Hum Nutr Diet, Vol. 24, No. issue 1, pp. 39-46.

Pepene CE, Ilie IR, Marian I &Duncea I. (2011). Circulating osteoprotegerin and soluble receptor activator of nuclear factor κB ligand in polycystic ovary syndrome: relationships to insulin resistance and endothelial dysfunction. Eur J Endocrinol. Vol. 164, No. issue 1, pp. 61-68

Pepene CE. (2011). Evidence for serum visfatin but not adiponectin or resistin as an independent predictor of endothelial dysfunction in polycystic ovary syndrome. Clin Endocrinol (Oxf). 2011 Jul 9. n.d.

Pierpoint R, McKeigue PM, Isaacs AJ, Wild SH & Jacobs HS. (1998). Mortality of women with polycystic ovary syndrome at long- term follow-up. J Clin Epidemiol, Vol. 51, pp. 581-586

Puder JJ, Varga S, Kraenzlin M, De Geyter C, Keller U & Muller B. (2005). Central fat excess in polycystic ovary syndrome: relation to low-grade inflammation and insulin resistance. J Clin Endocrinol Metab, Vol. 90, pp. 6014-6021

Reckelhoff JF. (2007). Polycystic ovary syndrome: androgens and hypertension. Hypertension, Vol. 49, pp. 1220-1221

Repaci A, Gambineri A & Pasquali R. (2011). The role of low-grade inflammation in the polycystic ovary syndrome. Mol Cell Endocrinol, Vol. 335, pp. 30–41

Rizzo M, Berneis K, Hersberger M, Pepe I, Di Fede G, Rini GB, Spinas GA, Carmina E. (2009). Milder forms of atherogenic dyslipidemia in ovulatory versus anovulatory polycystic ovary syndrome phenotype, Hum Reprod, Vol. 24, pp. 2286–2292

Rizzo M, Longo RA, Guastella E, Rini GB & Carmina E. (2011). Assessing cardiovascular risk in Mediterranean women with polycystic ovary syndrome. J Endocrinol Invest, Vol.34, No. issue 6, pp. 422-426

Rotterdam ESHRE/ASRM Sponsored PCOS Consensus Workshop Group. (2004). Revised 2003 consensus on diagnostic criteria and long-term health risks related to polycystic ovary syndrome, Fertil Steril, Vol. 81 , pp. 19–25.

Salley KE, Wickham EP, Cheang KI, Essah PA, Karjane NW & Nestler JE. (2007) Glucose intolerance in polycystic ovary syndrome—a position statement of the Androgen Excess Society. J Clin Endocrinol Metab Vol. 92, pp. 4546–4556

Sasaki A, Emi Y, Matsuda M, Sharula, Kamada Y, Chekir C, Hiramatsu Y & Nakatsuka M. (2011). Increased arterial stiffness in mildly-hypertensive women with polycystic ovary syndrome. J Obstet Gynaecol Res, Vol. 37, No. issue 5, pp. 402-411.

Selcoki Y, Yilmaz OC, Carlioglu A, Onaran Y, Kankilic MN, Karakurt F & Eryonucu B. (2010). Cardiac flow parameters with conventional and pulsed tissue Doppler echocardiography imaging in patients with polycystic ovary syndrome. Gynecol Endocrinol. Vol. 26, No. issue 11, pp. 815-818

Shaw LJ, Bairey Merz CN, Azziz R, Stanczyk FZ, Sopko G, Braunstein GD, Kelsey SF, Kip KE, Cooper-Dehoff RM, Johnson BD, Vaccarino V, Reis SE, Bittner V, Hodgson TK, Rogers W & Pepine CJ. (2008). Postmenopausal women with a history of irregular menses and elevated androgen measurements at high risk for worsening cardiovascular event-free survival: results from the National Institutes of Health--National Heart, Lung, and Blood Institute sponsored Women's Ischemia Syndrome Evaluation. J Clin Endocrinol Metab, Vol. 93, pp. 1276-1284

Shroff R, Kerchner A, Maifeld M, Van Beek EJ, Jagasia D & Dokras A. (2007). Young obese women with polycystic ovary syndrome have evidence of early coronary atherosclerosis. J Clin Endocrinol Metab, Vol. 92, pp. 4609-4614

Sitruk-Ware R & Nath A. (2011). Metabolic effects of contraceptive steroids. Rev Endocr Metab Disord, Vol.12, No.issue 2, pp. 63-75.

Soares EM, Azevedo GD, Gadelha RG, Lemos TM & Maranhão TM. (2008). Prevalence of the metabolic syndrome and its components in Brazilian women with polycystic ovary syndrome. Fertil Steril, Vol. 89, No. issue 3, pp. 649-55

Soares GM, Vieira CS, Martins WP, Franceschini SA, dos Reis RM, Silva de Sá MF, Ferriani RA. (2009). Increased arterial stiffness in nonobese women with polycystic ovary syndrome (PCOS) without comorbidities: one more characteristic inherent to the syndrome? Clin Endocrinol (Oxf), Vol. 71, No. issue 3, pp. 406-11.

Sorensen MB, Franks S, Robertson C, Pennell DJ & Collins P. (2006). Severe endothelial dysfunction in young women with polycystic ovary syndrome is only partially explained by known cardiovascular risk factors. Clin Endocrinol (Oxf, Vol. 65, pp. 655-659

Sukalich S & Guzick D. (2003). Cardiovascular health in women with polycystic ovary syndrome. Semin Reprod Med, Vol. 21, No. issue 3, pp. 309-316

Svendsen PF, Madsbad S & Nilas L. (2010). The insulin-resistant phenotype of polycystic ovary syndrome. Fertil Steril. Vol. 94, No. issue 3, pp. 1052-1058

Talbott EO, Guzick DS, Sutton-Tyrrell K, McHugh-Pemu KP, Zborowski JV, Remsberg KE & Kuller LH. (2000a). Evidence for association between polycystic ovary syndrome and premature carotid atherosclerosis in middle-aged women. Arterioscler Thromb Vasc Biol,Vol. 20, pp. 2414-2421.

Talbott EO, Zborowski JV, Boudreaux MY, McHugh-Pemu KP, Sutton-Tyrrell K, Guzick DS. (2004b). The relationship between C-reactive protein and carotid intima-media wall thickness in middle-aged women with polycystic ovary syndrome. J Clin Endocrinol Metab, Vol 89, pp.6061-6067

Talbott EO, Zborowski JV, Rager JR, Boudreaux MY, Edmundowicz DA, Guzick DS. (2004a). Evidence for an association between metabolic cardiovascular syndrome and coronary and aortic calcification among women with polycystic ovary syndrome. J Clin Endocrinol Metab, Vol 89, pp.5454-5461

Talbott EO, Zborowskii JV& Boudraux MY. (2004c) Do women with polycystic ovary syndrome have an increased risk of cardiovascular disease? Review of the evidence. Minerva Ginecol, Vol. 56, No. issue 1, pp. 27-39.

Talbott E, Zborowski J, Guzick D. et al.(2000b). Increased PAI-1 levels in women with polycystic ovary syndrome: evidence for a specific "PCOS effect" independent of age and BMI. In: Programs and Abstracts of the 40th Annual Conference on Cardiovascular Disease Epidemiology and Prevention, American Heart Association, San Diego, p 13

Talbott E, Zborowski J, Sutton-Tyrrell K, McHugh-Pemu KP & Guzick DS. (2001). Cardiovascular risk in women with polycystic ovary syndrome. Obstet Gynecol Clin North Am, Vol. 28, pp. 111-133

Tarkun I, Arslan BC, Canturk Z, Turemen E, Sahin T & Duman C. (2004). Endothelial dysfunction in young women with polycystic ovary syndrome: relationship with insulin resistance and low-grade chronic inflammation. J Clin Endocrinol Metab, Vol. 89, pp. 5592-5596

Tarkun I, Cetinarslan B, Turemen E, Canturk Z & Biyikli M. (2006). Association between Circulating Tumor Necrosis Factor-Alpha, Interleukin-6, and Insulin Resistance in Normal-Weight Women with Polycystic Ovary Syndrome. Metab Syndr Relat Disord Vol. 4, pp. 122-128

Teede H, Deeks A & Moran L. (2010a). Polycystic ovary syndrome: a complex condition with psychological, reproductive and metabolic manifestations that impacts on health across the lifespan. BMC Med, Vol. 8:41.

Teede HJ, Meyer C, Hutchison SK, Zoungas S, McGrath BP, Moran LJ. (2010b) Endothelial function and insulin resistance in polycystic ovary syndrome: the effects of medical therapy. Fertil Steril, Vol.93, pp. 184-191

Tekin A, Tekin G ,Çölkesen Y , B. Kılıçdağ E , Başhan İ , Sezgin AT & Müderrisoğlu H. (2009). Left Ventricular Function in Patients with Polycystic Ovary Syndrome: A Doppler Echocardiographic Study. Exp Clin Endocrinol Diabetes, Vol.117, No. issue 4, pp. 165-169

Torgrimson BN, Meendering JR, Kaplan PF & Minson CT. (2007). Endothelial function across an oral contraceptive cycle in women using levonorgestrel and ethinyl estradiol. Am J Physiol Heart Circ Physiol, Vol. 292, No.issue 6, H2874-2880 n.d.

Tosi FDR, Castello R, Maffeis C, Spiazzi G, Zoppini G, Muggeo M & Moghetti P. (2009). Body fat and insulin resistance independently predict increased serum C-reactive protein in hyperandrogenic women with polycystic ovary syndrome. Eur J Endocrinol, Vol. 161, pp. 737-745.

Valkenburg O, Steegers-Theunissen RP, Smedts HP, Dallinga-Thie GM, Fauser BC, Westerveld EH & Laven JS. (2008). A more atherogenic serum lipoprotein profile is present in women with polycystic ovary syndrome: a case-control study. J Clin Endocrinol Metab, Vol. 93, pp. 470–476

Vrbikova J & Hainer V. (2009). Obesity and polycystic ovary syndrome, Obes Facts, Vol.2, pp. 26–35

Vrbíková J, Hill M, Dvoráková K, Stanická S, Stárka L. (2010b) [The prevalence of metabolic syndrome in women with polycystic ovary syndrome], Cas Lek Cesk, Vol 149, No.issue 7, pp.337-9

Vrbikova J, Vondra K, Cibula D, Dvorakova K, Stanicka S, Sramkova D, , Sindelka G, Hill M, Bendlová B & Skrha J. (2005). Metabolic syndrome in young Czech women with polycystic ovary syndrome. Hum Reprod, Vol. 20, No. issue 12, pp. 3328-3332.

Vrbíková J, Zamrazilová H, Sedláčková B, Snajderová M. (2010a). Metabolic syndrome in adolescents with polycystic ovary syndrome, Gynecol Endocrinol, nd

Vural B, Caliskan E, Turkoz E, Kilic T & Demirci A. (2005). Evaluation of metabolic syndrome frequency and premature carotid atherosclerosis in young women with polycystic ovary syndrome. Hum Reprod, Vol. 20, No. issue 9, pp. 2409-2413

Wild RA, Carmina E, Diamanti-Kandarakis E, Dokras A, Escobar-Morreale HF, Futterweit W, Lobo R, Norman RJ, Talbott E & Dumesic DA. (2010). Assessment of cardiovascular risk and prevention of cardiovascular disease in women with the polycystic ovary syndrome: a consensus statement by the Androgen Excess and Polycystic Ovary Syndrome (AE-PCOS) Society. J Clin Endocrinol Metab, Vol. 95, No. issue 5, pp. 2038-2049

Wild RA, Rizzo M, Clifton S & Carmina E. (2011). .Lipid levels in polycystic ovary syndrome: systematic review and meta-analysis. Fertil Steril, Vol. 95, No. issue 3, pp. 1073-9.e1-11

Wild RA, Painter PC, Coulson PB, Carruth KB & Ranney GB. (1985). Lipoprotein lipid concentrations and cardiovascular risk in women with polycystic ovary syndrome. J Clin Endocrinol Metab, Vol. 61, pp. 946-951

Wild S, Pierpoint T, McKeigue P & Jacobs H. (2000). Cardiovascular disease in women with polycystic ovary syndrome at long-term follow-up: a retrospective cohort study. Clin Endocrinol (Oxf), Vol.52, No. issue 5, pp. 595-600.

Wiltgen D & Spritzer PM. (2010). Variation in metabolic and cardiovascular risk in women with different polycystic ovary syndrome phenotypes. Fertil Steril, Vol 94, No. issue 6, pp. 2493-2496

Xita, N, Papassotiriou I, Georgiou I, Vounatsou M, Margeli A & Tsatsoulis A. (2007). The adiponectin-to-leptin ratio inwomenwith polycystic ovary syndrome: relation to insulin resistance and proinflammatory markers. Metab Clin Exp, Vol. 56, No.issue 6, pp. 766–771

Yilmaz M, Bukan N, Demirci H, Oztürk C, Kan E, Ayvaz G & Arslan M. (2009). Serum resistin and adiponectin levels in women with polycystic ovary syndrome. Gynecol Endocrinol, Vol. 25, pp. 246–252

Zawdaki J, Dunaif A. Diagnostic criteria for polycystic ovary syndrome: towards a rational approach. In: Dunaif A, Givens J, Haseltine F, Marrian G, editors. Polycystic Ovary Syndrome. Current Issues in Endocrinology and Metabolism. Vol. 4. Boston: Blackwell Scientific; 1992. pp. 377-384.

10

Premature Atherosclerosis Long After Kawasaki Disease

Nobutaka Noto and Tomoo Okada
Department of Pediatrics and Child Health, Nihon University School of Medicine, Tokyo, Japan

1. Introduction

Kawasaki disease (KD) is a systemic vasculitis of unknown etiology in infants and children. First described in Japan in 1967, KD has been described worldwide among children of all races and ethnicities (Kawasaki, 1967). More than 4000 hospitalizations associated with KD were reported in 2000 and KD is the leading cause of acquired heart disease in childhood in the United State (Taubert et al., 1991). In Japan, the national survey of KD has performed every 2 years since 1970. From the most recent 20th survey dealt with the years 2007 and 2008, the number of new cases of KD in those years was 11,581 and 11,756, respectively. As of 2008, the total number of patients since 1970 was 249,019 (Nakamura et al., 2010). Therefore, patients diagnosed with KD in the sixties and seventies have already reached adulthood. The increased incidence of young adults who experience KD during childhood has been accompanied by a new problem of an association between post-KD lesions and atherosclerosis.

In this chapter, we would like to review and verify with regarding to the propensity of "Premature atherosclerosis long after Kawasaki disease" from several cutting edges such as epidemiologic features, dyslipidemia, non-invasive diagnostic methods for evaluating atherosclerosis such as flow-mediated dilatation (FMD) of brachial artery, carotid intima-media thickness (IMT), pulse wave velocity (PWV), invasive diagnostic method such as intravascular ultrasound imaging (IVUS) and pathological features along with the findings of our recent studies.

2. Epidemiology of Kawasaki disease

The incidence rate and number of patients with KD in Japan continue to increase. The 20th nationwide survey of KD in Japan was conducted in 2009, and included patients treated for the disease in 2007 and 2008 (Nakamura et al., 2010). Hospitals specializing in pediatrics, and hospitals with pediatric departments and 100 or more beds, were asked to report all patients with KD during the 2 survey years. From a total of 1540 departments and hospitals, 23,337 patients (11 581 in 2007 and 11 756 in 2008) were reported: 13,523 boys and 9814 girls. The annual incidence rates were 215.3 and 218.6 per 100,000 children aged 0-4 years in 2007 and 2008, respectively. This incidence was approximately 10 to 25 times higher than that of the United States and the United Kingdom. These were the highest annual KD incidence rates ever recorded in Japan. The age-specific incidence rate showed a monomodal distribution with a peak at age 9-11 months. The prevalence of both cardiac lesions during the acute phase of the disease and cardiac sequelae were higher among infants and older age groups. During the acute phase, 2577 (11.0%) patients had a cardiac lesion(s): 58 (0.25%) had giant coronary aneurysms, 282 (1.21%) had coronary aneurysms less than 8 mm in diameter, 1992 (8.54%) had coronary dilatations, 8 (0.03%) had coronary stenoses, 3 (0.01%) had myocardial infarction, and 383 (1.64%) had valvular lesions. A total of 746 patients (3.2%) had cardiac sequelae 1 month after the onset of KD: 59 (0.25%) had giant coronary aneurysms, 188 (0.81%) had coronary aneurysms less than 8mm in diameter, 435 (1.86%) had coronary dilatations, 5 (0.02%) had coronary stenoses, 2 (0.01%) had myocardial infarction, and 114 (0.49%) had valvular lesions. The proportion of patients with cardiac sequelae has decreased year by year. The proportion was 7.0% in the 15th nationwide survey in 1997–1998, 5.9% in the 16th (1999–2000), 5.0% in the 17th (2001–2002), 4.4% in the 18th (2003–2004), and 3.8% in the 19th survey. 87% of patients received intravenous immunoglobulin therapy (IVIG). Of those, 16.5% of patients received additional IVIG therapy, 5.0% of patients were treated with steroids, 0.35%of patients received infliximab, and 0.23% of patients were treated with immunosuppressive agents. Although the incidence of coronary sequelae has gradually been decreasing, the rate of severe sequelae, such as giant aneurysms, has not been decreasing as expected (Figure 1). Patients with persistent coronary aneurysms, stenoses, and regressed aneurysms have suffered the most severe arterial insult. In such patients, the possibility of early progression to atherosclerosis occurs. It is therefore important to determine the factors concerning with how to reduce the patients with severe sequelae.

3. Fate of coronary sequelae in Kawasaki disease

Kato et al. demonstrated the angiographic outcome of coronary aneurysms in KD (Kato et al., 1996). This fundamental work has led to the current understanding that coronary artery lesions (CALs) change markedly with time into a variety of forms. These lesions may regress, stay unchanged, progress to stenosis or obstructive lesions with or without recanalization, and on very rare occasions, rupture, develop new lesions, or expand. These structural changes may modified the early progression of atherosclerosis long after KD.

3.1 Regression

Many aneurysms formed in the acute phase demonstrate a shrinking tendency in the convalescent phase and thereafter. The phenomenon in which the aneurysm resolves normally and disappears on coronary angiography is described as regression, and commonly occurs 1 to 2 years after disease onset. Regression frequently occurs for small-to-medium-sized aneurysms, and 32-50% of patients with CALs (Sasaguri& Kato, 1982) (Suzuki et al., 1994). Regression is mainly the results of smooth muscle cell infiltration and proliferation in the intima.

3.2 Occlusion

Thrombotic occlusion is often seen in medium-sized or large coronary aneurysms. Suzuki et al. have reported that 16% of coronary aneurysms are occluded at follow-up, 78% of those became occluded within 2 years from onset (Suzuki et al., 1997). Whereas, acute myocardial infarction and sudden death have been caused by coronary artery occlusion, two-thirds of cases with occlusion have no symptomatic episodes due to the consequence of post-occlusion recanalization and development of collateral vessels. Tsuda et al. reported the clinical features of 50 adult patients (mean age 28 years old) who had an acute coronary syndrome caused by coronary artery lesions due to KD from 1980 to 2008. Of the 50 patients, 43 had thrombotic occlusion of an aneurysm and 40 had giant coronary aneurysms. Based on these evidences, it is likely that patients with known aneurysms during the acute phase of KD will have some cardiovascular morbidity and mortality as young adults (Tsuda et al., 2011).

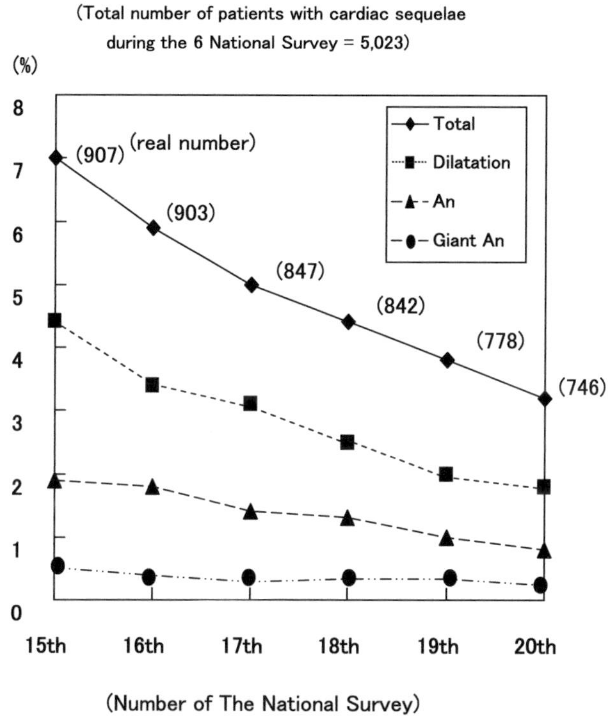

Fig. 1. Transition of the number of patients with cardiac sequelae in KD
An, coronary aneurysm; Dilatation, coronary dilatation.

3.3 Recanalization (segmental stenosis)

New vessels after occlusion are called as segmental stenosis. Segmental stenosis has been observed in 14.8% of patients with KD sequelae, 90% of which occurred in the right coronary artery. The right coronary artery is occluded or recanalized more easily than the left coronary artery (Suzuki et al., 1997).

3.4 Localized stenosis

At coronary angiography, localized stenosis is reported to occur at a frequency from 12% to 4.7% (Kato et al.,1996). Localized stenosis is often seen especially in the territory of the left anterior descending coronary artery, and usually occurs in both the inflow and outflow shoulder of the aneurysm. It is caused mainly by inward luminal intimal thickening.

3.5 Coronary artery with no aneurysm formation

Coronary arteries that appear normal from the onset of KD have been regarded as normal as yet. Even in coronary arteries in which there is no aneurysm formation in the acute phase, mild intimal thickening may be seen in some patients (Takahashi et al.,2001). Therefore, there is some debate about the possibility that a history of KD might be a risk factor in the progression of atherosclerosis.

4. Dyslipidemia in Kawasaki disease

It is well known that the process of atherosclerosis is enhanced in the presence of cardiovascular risk factors (CRFs). Undoubtedly, one of the strongest CRFs for atherosclerosis is dyslipidemia. Among patients characteristics that influence vascular health, dyslipidemia is prevalent in patients with KD with or without overt coronary artery sequelae well beyond the time that the clinical disease has resolved. Earlier studies have shown that high-density lipoprotein cholesterol (HDL-C) levels may be depressed in the acute phase of KD (Okada T et al, 1990) (Newberger JW et al., 1991). However, there is controversy whether this decrease persists over the long time. In the convalescent phase, McCrindle et al. showed that KD patients 10 to 20 years of age had lower apolipoprotein A1 levels than the healthy control subjects (McCrindle et al., 2007). Mitani et al. showed that there were no differences between patients with KD 10 years after the onset and the control subjects with regard to total cholesterol (T-C) and HDL-C levels (Mitani et al., 2005). Cheung et al. reported that KD patients around 10 years old with or without coronary artery lesion (CAL) had significantly higher levels of apolipoprotein B and lower levels of HDL-C compared with control subjects (Cheung et al., 2004). Therefore, no consensus has been reached whether dyslipidemia in KD patients over the term after clinical resolution causes a higher risk of atherosclerosis than that in the general population. In epidemiological studies of children, the best correlation with adult cholesterol levels was obtained from cholesterol levels measured during the late teen years, suggesting that subtle adverse lipoprotein profiles obtained at this age could be predictive of future dyslipidemia in young adulthood (Strong WB et al., 1992). Since young adults often become much less active once they leave school and physical activities are generally restricted in KD patients at AHA risk levels IV to V with giant coronary aneurysms and stenoses, it is likely that subtle risk factors cluster in individual patients. Hence, we suggest that even in subtle abnormalities of lipid profile in post-KD patients with CALs may contribute to further endothelial dysfunction and the propensity for subclinical atherosclerosis in the future.

5. Inflammatory examinations in Kawasaki disease

Atherosclerosis is an inflammatory disease as demonstrated in animal models and human. Clinical or subclinical inflammation of the coronary and systemic arteries may form the substrate for long-term functional and structural abnormalities and increase the risk of premature atherosclerosis. Serum high-sensitivity C-reactive protein (hs-CRP) and serum amyloid-A (SAA), have recently been regarded as reliable clinical markers for the prediction of coronary events, independent of other known CRFs (Mitani et al., 2005). In fact, serum high-sensitivity C-reactive protein (hs-CRP) level in patients with CALs is significantly higher than those seen in normal age-matched control or among patients with KD without aneurysms or regressed aneurysms. C-reactive protein inhibits NO production by endothelial cell and increases the endothelial expression of adhesion molecules. Inflammatory mediators, such as hs-CRP, may themselves promote atherosclerosis. Therefore, we suspect that in patients with CALs chronic low grade inflammation may continue after the acute phase of KD. Whereas, several studies suggest that oxidative stress may promote endothelial dysfunction through increased production of reactive oxygen species (ROS) (Griendling et al., 2003). Urinary 8-iso-prostaglandin F2α is increased long after the onset of KD, as well as after acute phase KD. Oxidative stress, evidenced by significant higher levels of malonyldialdehyde (MDA) and hydroperoxides, is increased in KD patients with CALs compared with those in control subjects and is associated with carotid intima-media thickness and stiffness (Cheung et al., 2008).

6. Endothelial function in Kawasaki disease

6.1 Non-invasive method for evaluating endothelial function

A number of noninvasive methods have been developed to study endothelial function and structural changes suggestive of atherosclerosis. Brachial artery flow-mediated dilatation (FMD) has been studied widely and applied to varied group of patients including children. The %FMD reflects endothelial NO-dependent vasodilatation. Decreased %FMD reflects endothelial cell dysfunction, and a significant decrease in %FMD is a common feature of early marker in adult atherosclerosis. Decreased %FMD in patients with KD has been reported by many facilities (Niboshi et al., 2008). Ikemoto et al. demonstrated endothelial dysfunction, as indicated by decreased %FMD, only among patients with persistent CALs (Ikemoto et al., 2005). Endothelial dysfunction is worst among patients with coronary artery aneurysms (Dhillon et al.,1996) (Noto et al., 2009) (Figure 2). Abnormalities of systemic endothelial function are present many years after resolution of acute KD, even in patients without detectable early coronary involvement. In contrast, McCrindle et al. reported that patients with KD, compared with healthy control subjects, had similar systemic endothelial function, assessed by %FMD. Furthermore, FMD was not significantly related to either patient or KD characteristics (McCrindle et al., 2007). With respect to the noninvasive method investigating endothelial dysfunction after KD, data are not consistent.

6.2 Invasive method for evaluating endothelial function

The coronary artery response to acetylcholine or isosorbide has been well documented as a marker for endothelial dysfunction. Isosorbide induces dilatation of arteries in an endothelium-independent manner. On the other hand, acetylcholine dilates arteries in an endothelium-dependent manner. The reaction to acetylcholine of normal-appearing coronary arteries in patients with KD is equivalent to that of the control. However, the response to acetylcholine of coronary arteries with aneurysms or stenoses or both is poor dilatation or even constriction (Yamakawa et al., 1998)(Iemura et al., 2000) .

7. Diagnostic methods for assessment of atherosclerosis in Kawasaki disease

7.1 Carotid intima-media thickness

Structural arterial abnormalities are indicated by cartid intima-media thickness (IMT) measured by B-mode ultrasonography. Increased IMT has been shown to reliably indicate the presence of atherosclerosis. In KD patients with persistent CALs, compared with control patients, the carotid arterial wall has been reported to have a higher IMT and lower distensibility (Noto et al., 2001&2007) (Figure 3). Carotid IMT, expressed as both unadjusted dimension and z-score, was greater among patients with KD than control subjects; within the KD group, patients with CALs had greater carotid IMT than those without CALs (Della Pozza et al., 2007). Cheung et al. found increased carotid IMT even among patients with KD with normal coronary arteries, compared with control subjects (Cheung et al., 2007). However, some investigators have found no difference in carotid IMT between patients with KD and control subjects, consistent with the hypothesis that functional abnormalities might precede those of structure (McCrindle et al., 2007).

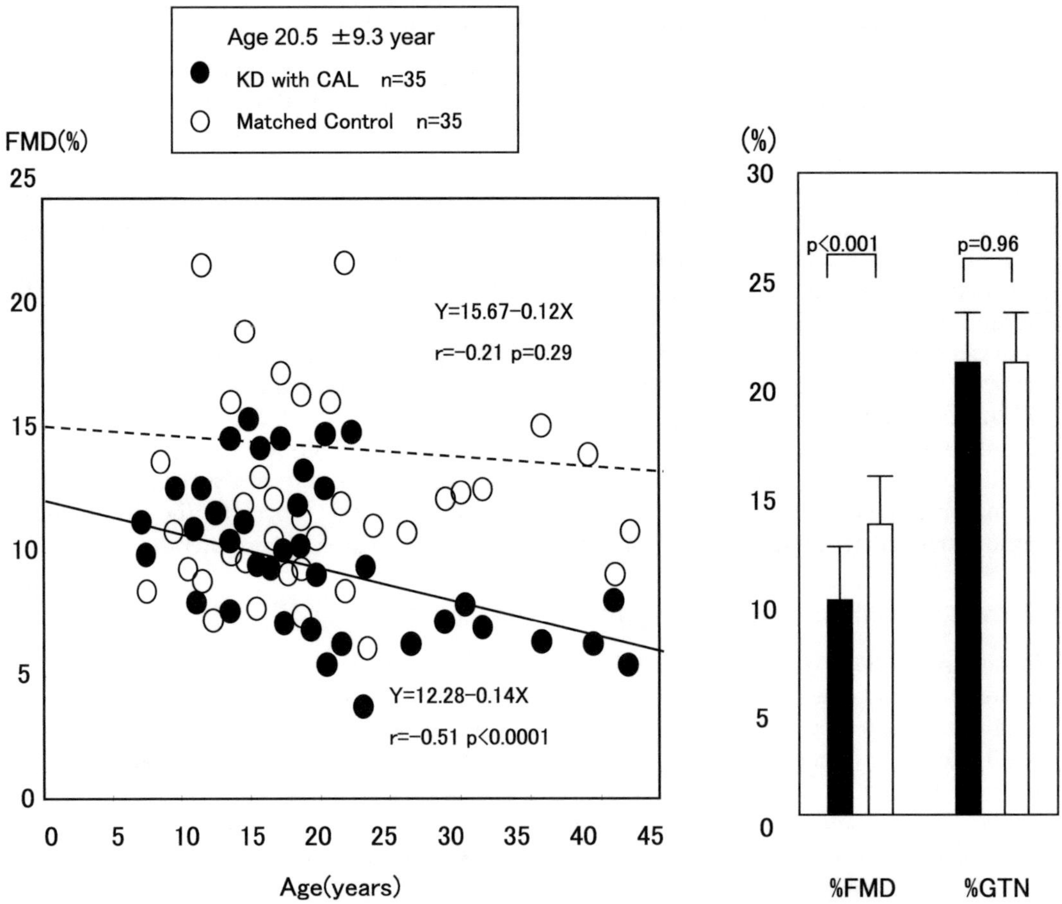

Fig. 2. Endothelial dysfunction in KD patients with CALs . (Left) Scatter plot of FMD% versus age in the subjects with KD(•) and the control subjects(○). Regression lines for subjects with KD and controls are represented by a solid and dashed line, respectively. (Right) %FMD and %GTN in KD (black bar) and control subjects (white bar). FMD, flow mediated dilatation;
GTN, sublingual glyceryl trinitrate.

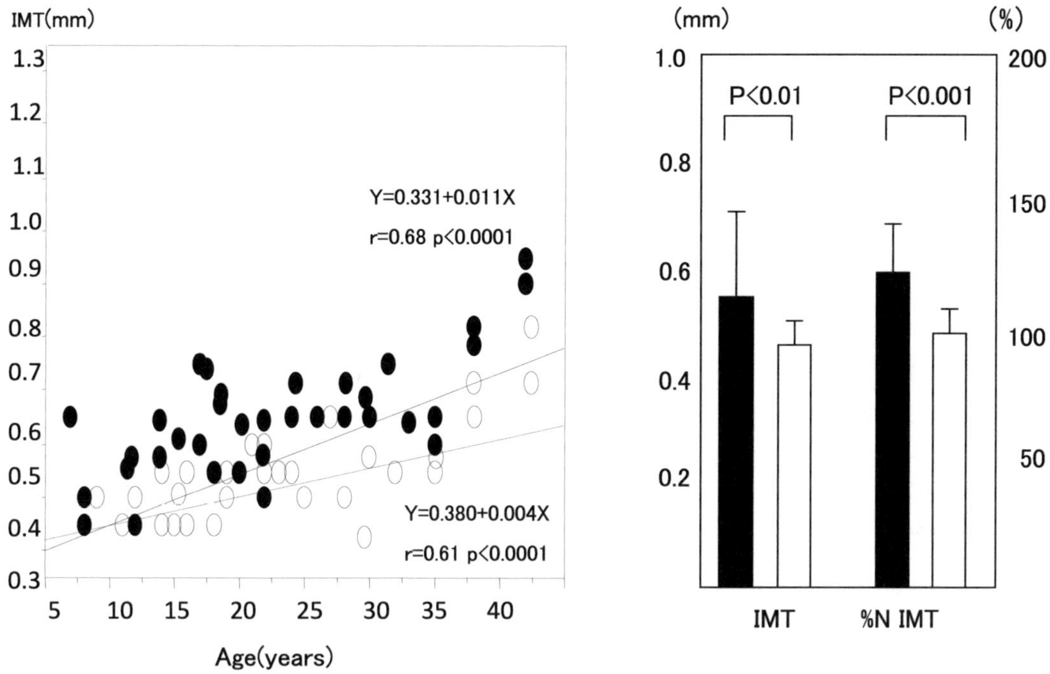

Fig. 3. Intima-media thickness (IMT) and % normal predicted IMT (%N IMT) in KD patients and control subjects. (Left) Scatter plot of IMT versus age for subjects with KD(•) and control subjects (○). Regression lines for subjects with KD and controls are represented by a solid and dashed line, respectively. A significant correlation ($r=0.61$, $p<0.001$) between age and IMT was observed. (Right) Bar graphs of IMT and % N IMT in KD patients (black bar) and control subjects (white bar). The normal predicted IMT value (np-IMT) and percent normal predicted IMT value (%N IMT) were calculated from the following formula: np-IMT=0.381+0.004×age, %N IMT=100×measured IMT/np-IMT.

7.2 Pulse wave velocity

An alternative noninvasive method is measurement of arterial stiffness by pulse wave velocity (PWV). The PWV is simple to measure and is a powerful marker for the risk of atherosclerosis in adults. It has been reported that PWV is especially high in patients with KD who have CALs. Patients with a history of KD have a higher PWV than control subjects, moreover there is no significant difference in the PWV between the KD patients with or without CALs (Cheung et al., 2004). However, in other study PWV does not differ significantly between KD patients with normal-appearing coronary arteries and healthy controls (Ooyanagi et al., 2004). Data are conflicting.

7.3 Intravascular ultrasound imaging

Iemura et al have shown the evidence of persisting abnormal vascular wall morphology and vascular dysfunction at the site of regressed coronary aneurysms in patients with KD by intravascular ultrasound imaging using intracoronary infusion of acetylcholine and isosorbide dinitrate (Iemura et al., 2000). More recently, Mitani et al have demonstrated the plaque composition and morphology in CALs after KD using a virtual histology-intravascular ultrasound imaging (VH-IVUS). Qualitatively, the normal coronary segment had no or trivial intravascular ultrasound-visible plaque area. While, the CALs exhibited a heterogeneous plaque area with the components (fibrous, fibrofatty, necrotic core, and dense calcium) in different amounts and proportions. VH-IVUS findings in KD suggest that arteriosclerotic lesions found in CALs but not in the normal segment in patients with KD are characterized by a heterogeneous intimal area, distinct from a purely fibrotic area (Mitani et al., 2009). These findings may give new insight into the potential role of atherosclerosis in CALs long after KD.

8. Histological examinations in Kawasaki disease

8.1 Pathological features

In the acute phase of KD, histopathological investigations has shown that inflammatory cells invade the intima and destroy the internal elastic lamina and continue to infiltrated the tunica media. With inflammatory cell invasion from the adventitia, panvasculitis develops (Naoe et al., 1991).In the convalescent phase, even in clinically normal coronary artery of a child, who died of unrelated causes, pathological studies in autopsy cases showed a slightly thickened intima and the disrupted lamina interna in some parts and many α-actin-positive smooth muscle cells were observed in the intima (Suzuki et al., 2004). In fact, the lamina interna serves as a barrier for cells and macromolecules migration between the intima and the media in the vascular wall. Therefore, one can easily expect that KD patients with CALs might have a vulnerability to more easily develop atherosclerotic changes in early adulthood according to these structural alterations. Whereas, current histological studies showed that there was no significant macrophage infiltration or foamy cell formation in the intima in KD coronary arteries with localized stenosis several years after the onset of KD (Suzuki et al., 2000). Likewise, no atheromatous plaques were found in seemingly normal coronary arteries distal to aneurysmsin 10 autopsied adults KD patients (Burns et al., 1996). On the contrary, Takahashi et al. reported that 3 patients who were 15, 20, and 39 years of age had new intimal thickening, including atheroma-like bright areas and foamy macrophages in CALs (Takahashi et al., 2001). Also, Negoro et al. showed that a substantial lipid core with cholesterol crystals and macrophages was found in an atherectomy specimen from a stenotic lesion in a 32-year-old man who presented with acute coronary syndrome (Negoro et al., 2003). Due to conflicting results, we speculate that there is some heterogeneity on the propensity of atherosclerosis in individual including such as age, the latent CRFs and the given degree of structural changes after vascular remodeling in KD with CALs. At least, aneurysms are present, a history of KD in children become a risk factor for atherosclerosis later in life. Thus, a study of coronary arteries more than a decade after being afflicted with KD is greatly needed.

8.2 Immunohistological features

Current immunohistological studies using antibodies against vascular growth factors (GFs), such as transforming growth factor β1, platelet-derived growth factor-A, basic fibroblast growth factor, and vascular endothelial growth factor, demonstrated that GFs were strongly expressed in the newly formed microvessels within the intima and some GFs were also expressed in adventitial vasa vasorum in the localized and recanalized vessels of KD children with CALs (Suzuki et al., 2000). Furthermore, vascular senescence, demonstrated as increased β-galactosidase activity, adhesion molecules and pro-inflammatory cytokines, as well as a reduction of normal physiological vascular proteins, such as eNOS, was increased in KD with CALs. These findings were more remarkable in intima as well as in vasculature of vasa vasorum (Fukazawa et al., 2007). Inevitably, adult atherosclerosis originates from the intimal side of the arteries. In contrast, arteriosclerotic changes characterized by active vascular remodeling including with luxuriant intimal proliferation and neoangiogenesis in KD with CALs may develop earlier from the both sides of the intima and adventitia of the arteries.

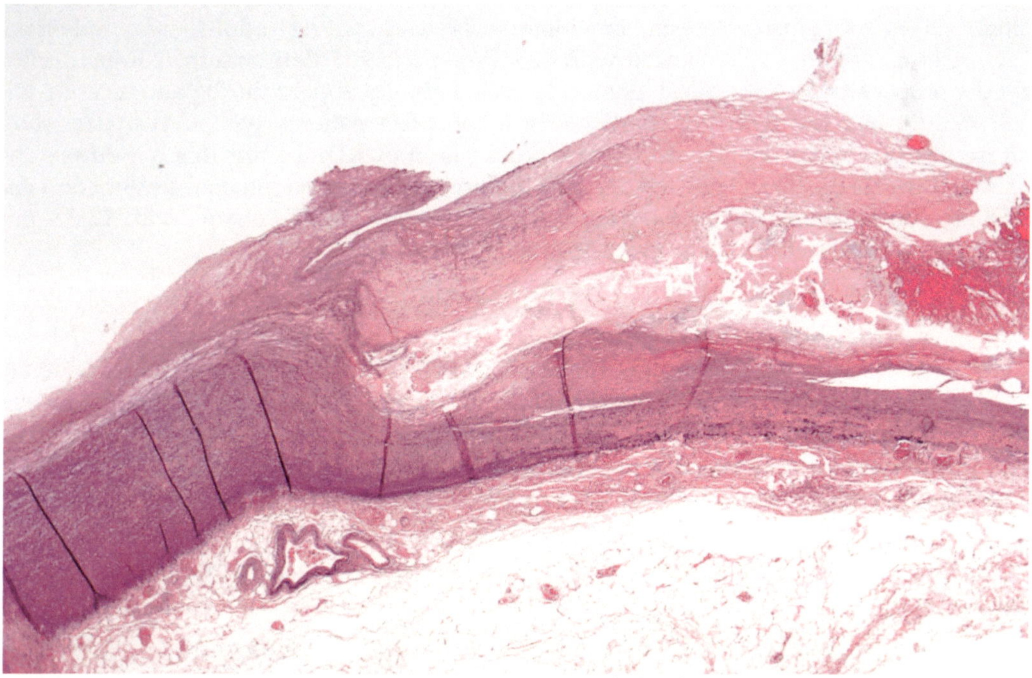

Takahashi K, et al. Pediatr Cardiol, 2001.

Fig. 4. Complicated atherosclerotic lesion in the orifice of the left coronary artery. (Elastica-HE, ×10). Right side is the orifice of the left coronary artery. Left side is aorta.

9. Experimental model of coronary arteritis

Recently, Ozawa et al. developed an animal model of KD, which is similar to the model of vasculitis in juvenile rabbits. Allergic coronary arteritis in rabbits induced by serial horse serum injections showed typical panarteritis characterized by inflammatory cell invasion of both sides from intima and adventitia, medial edema, and destruction of internal elastic lamina. When a high fat diet was being fed to this allergic arteritis rabbits models, typical atherosclerotic plaque appeared significantly (Ozawa et al., 2006). This experimental result suggests that post arteritis tissue may more easily develop atherosclerosis. Intriguingly, they also demonstrated the anti-inflammatory activities of HMG-CoA reductase inhibitors against the progress of acute arteritis (Hamaoka et al., 2010).

10. The propensity for atherosclerosis in KD

Due to conflicting previous reports dealing with the endothelial function and non-invasive diagnostic methods in KD, concerns have been raised as to whether KD patients are really at risk for premature atherosclerosis later in adulthood. Although the exact reasons for these conflicting results remain undetermined, differences in study populations, methodology, and latent CRFs including age, pubertal status, systemic inflammation may play a role. Age is of particular interest because the atherosclerotic process begins in childhood. Additionally, a strong association exists between the adverse lipoprotein levels and the initial stages of atherosclerosis in adolescents and young adults, and advanced atherosclerotic lesions are enhanced with age. We speculated that endothelial dysfunction and the propensity for subclinical atherosclerosis gradually appear during adolescence, and then rapidly increase with age, particularly in post-KD patients with CALs, who show diffuse vascular inflammation during the acute phase of KD. To test this hypothesis, we examined the relationship between age and the progression of endothelial dysfunction and subclinical atherosclerosis in case-control study using post-KD patients with CALs and healthy control subjects across a wide age range (Noto et al 2009).

10.1 Study design

A case-control study was performed that included 35 post-KD subjects across a wide age range (range 8-42 years) without traditional cardiovascular risk factors (CRFs) and 35 age- and sex-matched healthy control subjects (Cont). Flow-mediated dilatation (FMD) of the brachial artery induced by reactive hyperemia, intima-media thickness (IMT), and the elastic modulus (Ep) of the common carotid artery were compared between KD and Cont subjects assessed against age.

10.2 Results

KD subjects had slightly higher levels of BMI, lipid profile, and HbA1c than Cont subjects, but the differences were not significant. The mean IMT ($p<0.001$), age-adjusted % normal IMT (%N IMT) ($p<0.0001$), and Ep ($p<0.001$), were significantly higher in KD than Cont subjects, and the peak FMD% ($p<0.01$) was significantly lower in KD than Cont subjects. There were significant correlations between FMD% and age ($r= -0.51$ $p<0.0001$), IMT and age ($R=0.68$ $p<0.001$), and Ep and age ($r=0.58$ $p<0.01$) in KD but not Cont subjects. When the difference in FMD% between KD and matched Cont subjects (ΔFMD%) was plotted against age, no significant relationship was found, although significant correlations between ΔIMT and age ($r=0.52$, $p<0.01$) as well as ΔEp and age ($r=0.46$, $p<0.05$) were observed. When we defined values that were +2.0 SD over the mean control values (i.e. %N IMT $\geq$ 120% and or Ep $\geq$ 50KPa) as markers of subclinical atherosclerosis, 15 subjects met the criteria. Subjects over the age of 22 years were more likely to be (OR=16.54, $p=0.0001$) subclinical atherosclerosis in this cohort (Figure 5)(Figure 6)(Figure 7). Our results suggest that endothelial dysfunction and the development of premature atherosclerosis were accelerated in adult post-KD than Cont subjects.

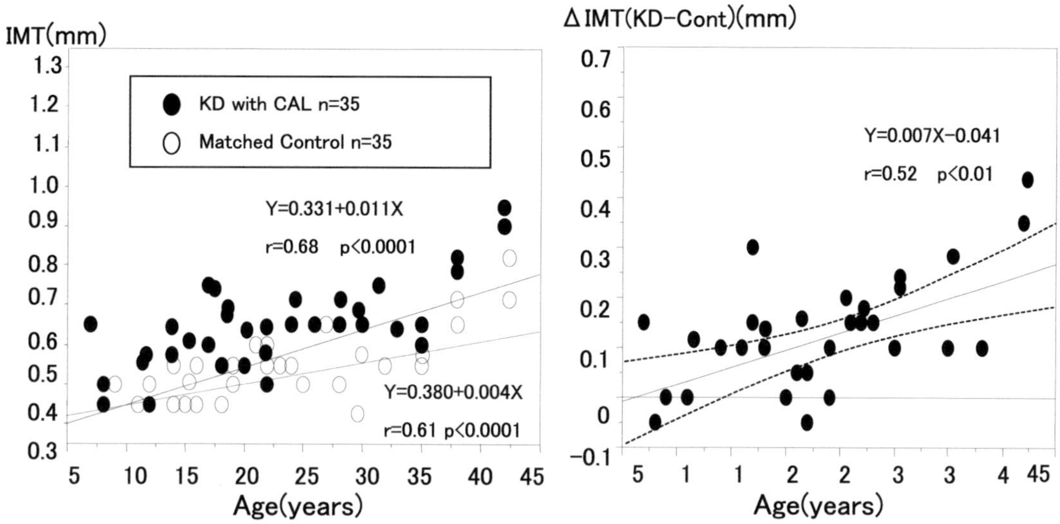

Fig. 5. Relationship between IMT and the age in KD patients and control subjects. (Left) Scatter plot of IMT versus age for subjects with KD(•) and control subjects(○). Regression lines for subjects with KD and controls are represented by a solid and dashed line, respectively. (Right) Difference in IMT(ΔIMT) and 95% CI between subjects with KD and controls plotted against age. Mean=solid line, 95% CI=dashed lines.

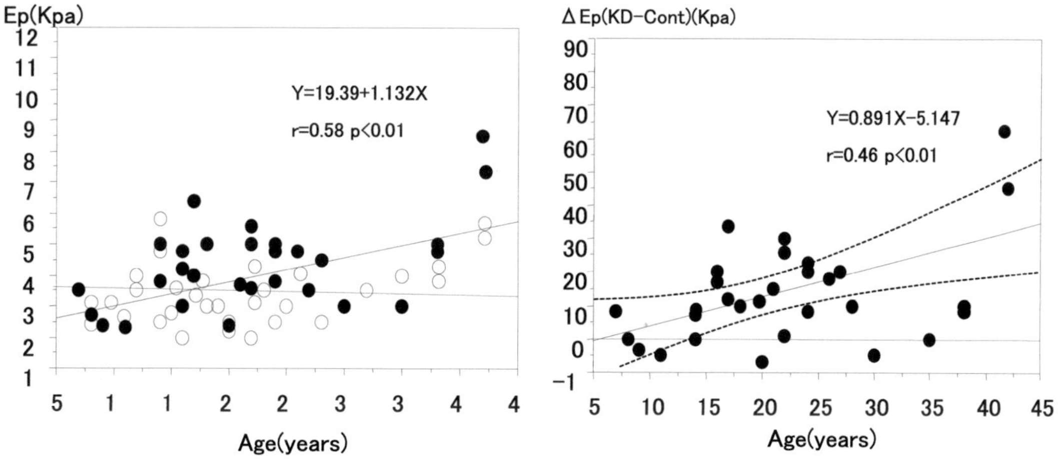

Fig. 6. Relationship between Ep and the age in KD patients and control subjects. (Left) Scatter plot of Ep versus age for subjects with KD(•) and control subjects(○). Regression lines for subjects with KD and controls are represented by a solid and dashed line, respectively. (Right) Difference in Ep(ΔEp) and 95% CI between subjects with KD and controls plotted against age. Mean=solid line, 95%CI=dashed lines.

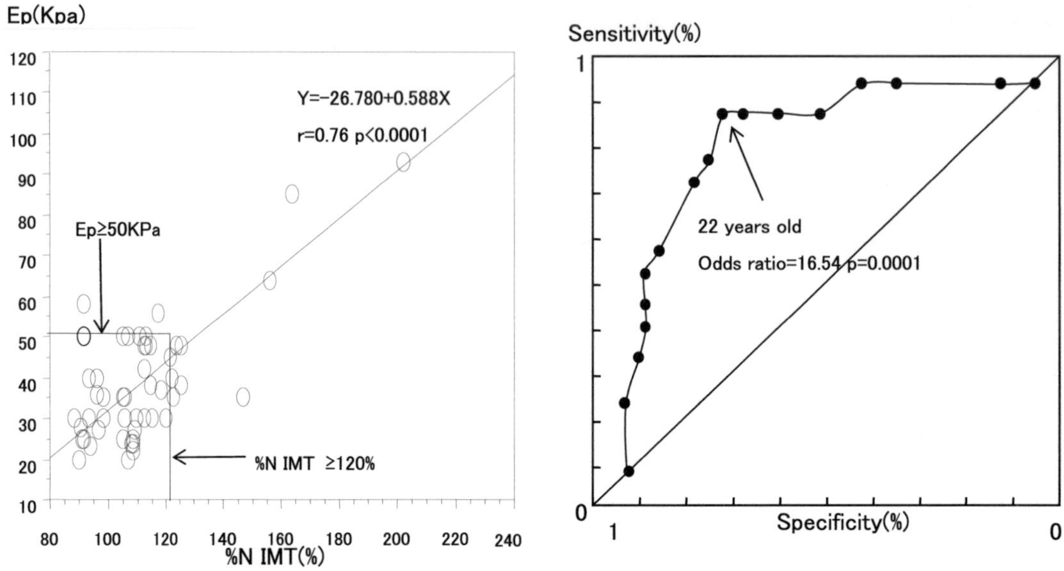

Fig. 7. Relationship between %N IMT and Ep and ROC Curve in KD patients and Control Subjects. (Left) Regression line for all subjects is represented by a solid line. Arrows represent the cut-off points of %N IMT ≥ 120% and or Ep ≥ 50KPa as markers of subclinical atherosclerosis. (Right) Receiver-operating characteristic curve for the prediction of subclinical atherosclerosis against age in all subjects. Arrow indicates 22 years of age with a high odds ratio (OR=16.54, p=0.0001).

11. Future perspective: Detection of earlier atherosclerotic involvement in KD patients with CALs

It remains unclear whether the vascular remodeling process of atherosclerosis in KD differs from that in adults. In particular, major concern has been raised as to whether the vessels with predisposed arteriosclerotic changes in KD patients with CALs may more easily develop atherosclerotic changes. Several studies showed that carotid IMT, a surrogate of atherosclerotic vessel wall change, is sensitive to risk intervention and constitutes a reliable indicator of clinical outcome in adult subjects, even in children with familial hypercholesterolemia (FH) (Jarvisalo et al., 2001). Furthermore, these changes in the arterial wall occur earlier in the carotid arteries than in the coronary circulation, making the carotid arteries an ideal site for detection of premature atherosclerotic disease (Bland et al., 1986). In addition, current study has demonstrated that textural changes in the carotid intima-media complex (IMC) by B-mode ultrasound were associated with early atherosclerotic involvement in patients with FH (Noto et al., 2011) (Figure 8). We speculated that changes in the textural characteristics of carotid IMC by B-mode ultrasound could be indicative of the earlier involvement of carotid atherosclerosis in KD patients with CALs. To test this hypothesis, we assessed the ultrasonic textural parameters of the IMC by first-order statistics, second-order statistics in KD patients with CALs without CRFs, age-matched healthy control subjects and age-matched FH subjects and findings were compared among the 3 groups.

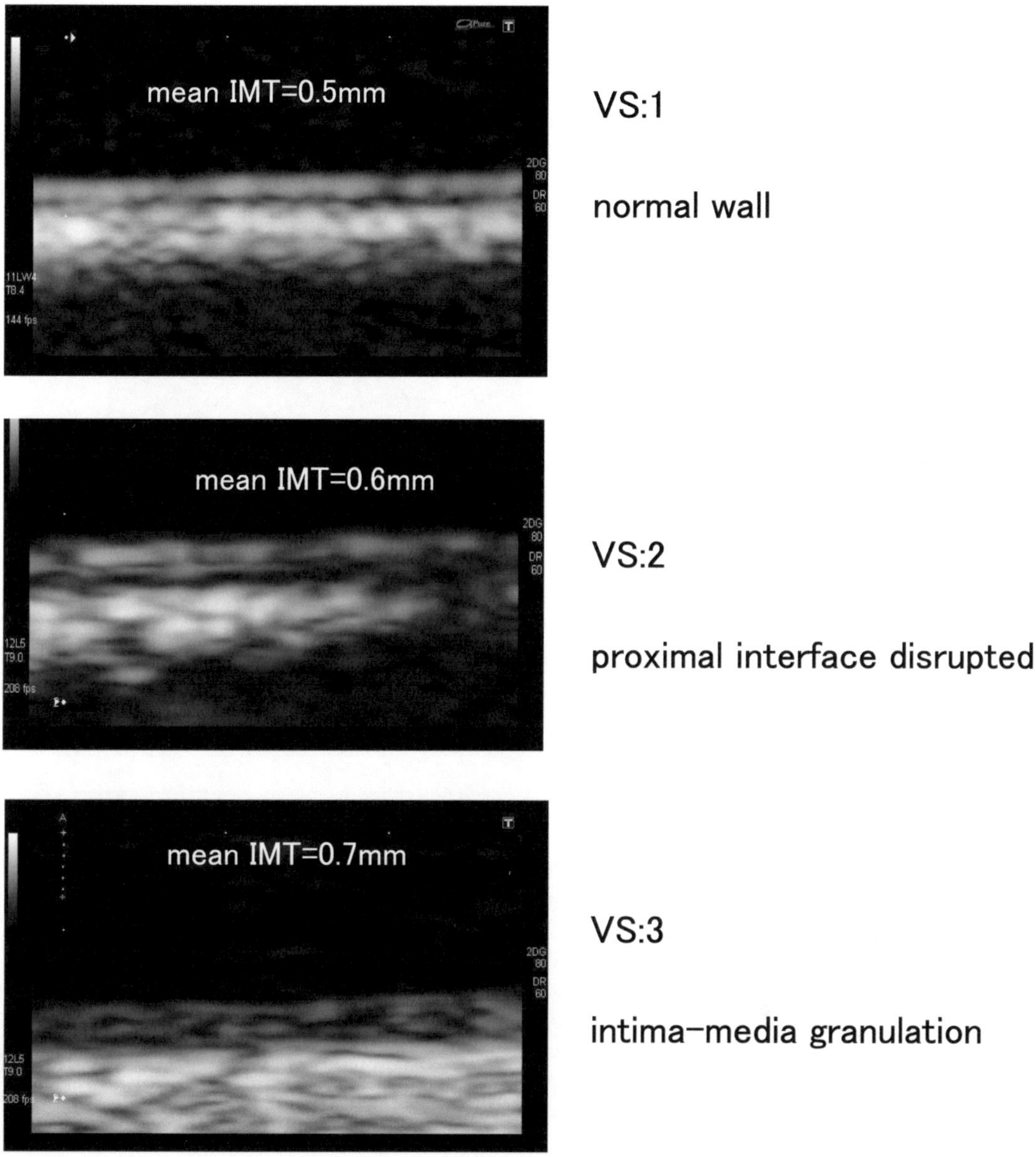

Fig. 8. Representative typical Visual Scoring (VS) by magnified B-mode ultrasound images of the intima-media complex (IMC) in heterozygous familial hypercholesterolemia (FH). Visual Scoring 1: normal wall (intima media and adventitia clearly separated); Visual Scoring 2: proximal interface disrupted by hypoechoic components in the proximal echogenic layer; Visual Scoring 3: intima-media granulation with mixed hypoechoic and echogenic components. According to the increased IMT with medial infiltration of lipids, VS progresses from proximal interface disruption to intima-media granulation (Noto et al., J Am Soc Echocardiog 2011).

11.1 Study design

To test the hypothesis that textural changes in the carotid intima-media complex (IMC) by B-mode ultrasound are associated with the earlier atherosclerotic involvement, 12 patients with KD and CALs without cardiovascular risk factors (mean age 20.5 years), 12 patients with heterozygous familial hypercholesterolemia (FH) (mean age 18.6 years) and age-matched 9 healthy control subjects (Cont) were assessed for intima-media thickness (IMT), first- and second-order statistics, and plot profile curve (PC) for regional analysis of the alteration of gray value in IMC, and were compared among 3 groups.

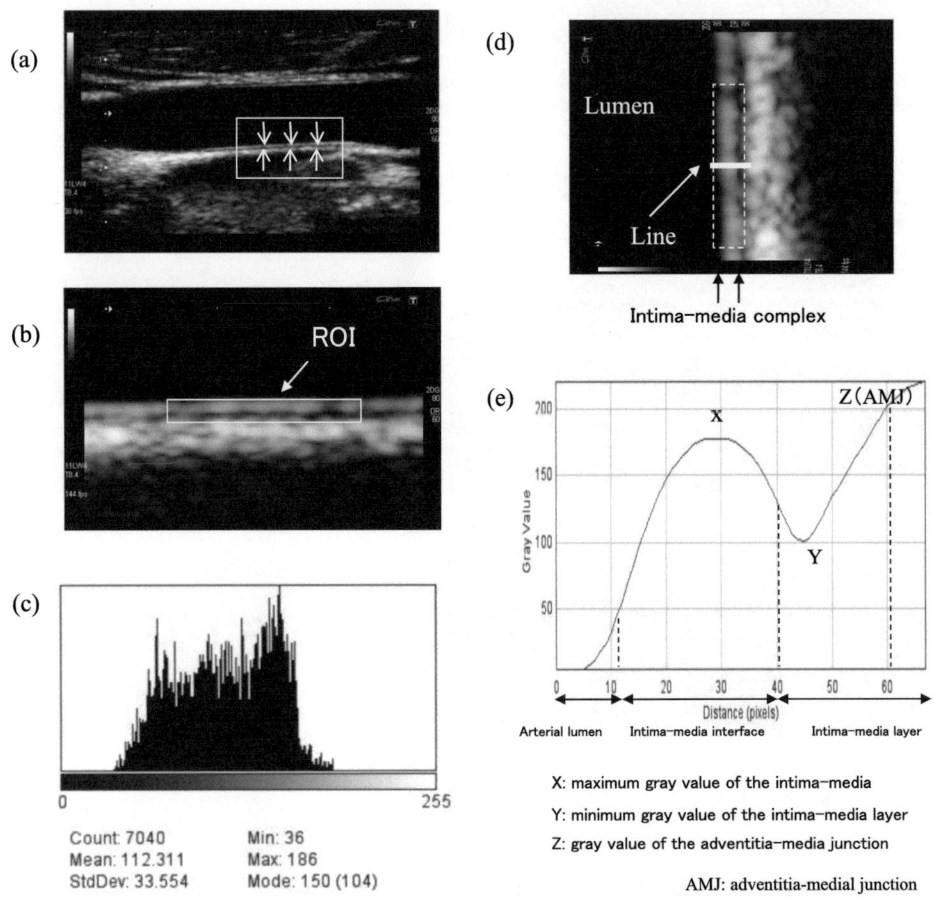

Fig. 9. Measurement of the textural parameters and gray value by plot profile curve
(a) Conventional B-mode image of common carotid artery (CCA). Rectangle indicates the magnified portion around the far wall of CCA. (b) Maximal magnified B-mode image (×8.6). Rectangle indicates the region of interest (ROI) in the far wall of the intima-media complex (IMC). (c) Histogram of ROI. This feature was automatically extracted by Image J 1.38x software. (d) Maximal magnified B-mode image (×8.6). *Line* indicates the portion of measurement of plot profile curve located center of ROI in the far wall of the intima-media complex (IMC). (e) Plot profile curve of gray values of the pixels along a 0.7mm line over the IMC.

11.2 Results

The mean IMT was significantly higher in FH ($p<0.0001$) and KD ($p=0.005$) than Cont. KD showed significantly higher gray-scale median (GSM) than FH ($p=0.027$) and Cont ($p=0.048$), however, there were no significant differences in Skewness, Kurtosis and Contrast among 3 groups. While, KD ($p<0.0001$) and FH ($p=0.004$) showed significantly higher Entropy than Cont. Furthermore, KD ($p=0.0041$) and FH ($p=0.001$) showed significantly lower Angular second moment (ASM) than Cont, but no significant difference was found between KD and FH. As for PC, KD showed significantly higher gray value both at the minimum point in IMC ($p<0.01$) and at the adventitia-media junction ($p<0.01$) than FH and Cont. These findings demonstrate that higher GSM in KD may indicate alteration of tissue component and heterogeneity IMC, suggesting sclerotic vascular remodeling after vasculitis. In contrast, decreased GSM may indicate atherotic vascular remodeling often observed in FH patients.

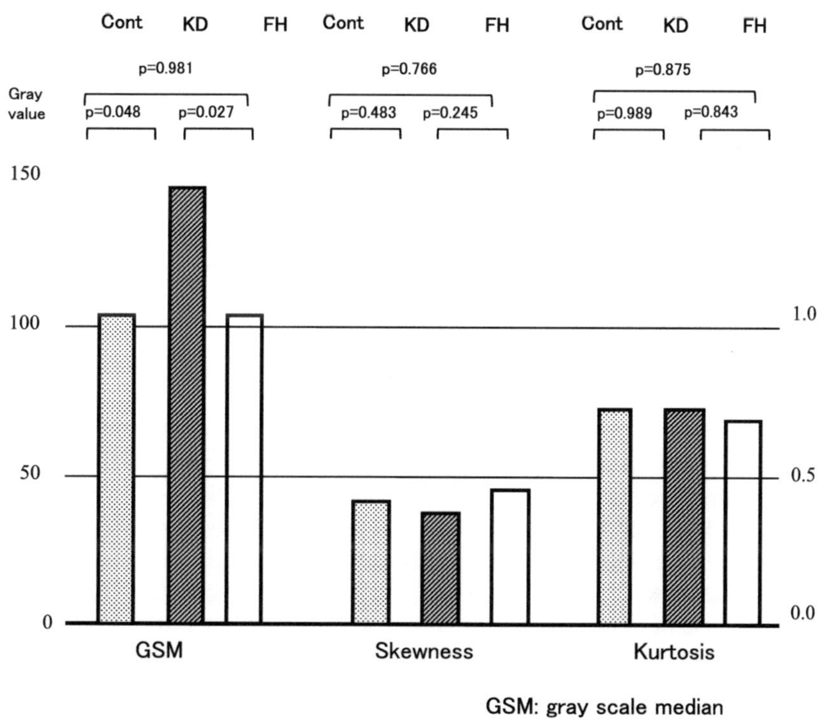

Fig. 10. Histogram variables among KD patients, Familial hypercholesterolemia, and control subjects.

12. Conclusion

We reviewed the recent several problems concerning with the propensity of atherosclerosis in patients long after KD. Among KD patients with CALs, impairments of coronary artery structure and function have been well documented. However, it is still too early to determine the conclusion whether post-KD patients in whom coronary abnormalities were never detected are at risk for premature atherosclerosis later in adulthood until the early

Japanese cohort reaches middle and older age. To date, all patients with a history of KD should be carefully assessed for factors promoting atherosclerosis, including hypercholesterolemia, obesity, systemic hypertension, and smoking.

13. References

Burns JC, Shike H, Gordon JB, Malhotra A, Schoenwetter M, & Kawasaki T. (1996). Sequelae of Kawasaki disease in adolescents and young adults. J Am Coll Cardiol, Vol. 28, pp. 253-257.

Cheung YF, Young TC, Ho MH, & Chau AK. (2004). Novel and traditional cardiovascular risk factors in children after Kawasaki disease. J Am Coll Cardiol, Vol. 43, pp. 120-124.

Cheung YF, Ho MH, Tam SCF, & Young TC. (2004). Increased high sensitivity C reactive protein concentrations and increased arterial stiffness in children with a history of Kawasaki disease. Heart, Vol. 90, pp. 1281-1285.

Cheung YF, Wong SJ, & Ho MH. (2007). Relationship between carotid intima-media thickness and arterial stiffness in children after Kawasaki disease. Arch Dis Child, Vol. 92, pp. 43-47.

Cheung YF, O K, Woo CW, Armstrong S, Siow YL, Chow P, & Cheung EW. (2008). Oxidative stress in children late after Kawasaki disease: relationship with carotid atherosclerosis and stiffness. BMJ Pediatrcs, Vol.8, pp. 20.

Della Pozza R, Bechtold S, Urshel S, Kozlik-Feldmann R, & Netz H. (2007). Subclinical atherosclerosis, but normal autonomic function after Kawasaki disease. J Pediatr, Vol. 151, pp. 239-43.

Dhillon R, Clarkson P, Donald AE, Powe AJ, Nash M, Novelli V, Dillon MJ, & Deanfield JE. (1996). Endothelial dysfunction late after Kawasaki disease. Circulation, Vol. 94, pp. 2103-2106.

Fukazawa R, Ikeman E, Watanabe M, Hajikano M, Kamisago M, Katsube Y, Yamauchi H, Ochi M, & Ogawa S. (2007). Coronary artery aneurysm induced by Kawasaki disease in children show features typical senescence. Circ J, Vol. 71, pp. 709-715.

Griending KK, & FitzGerald GA. (2003). Oxidative stress and cardiovascular injury: Part 2: Animal and human studies. Circulation, Vol. 108, pp.2034-2040.

Hamaoka A, Hamaoka K, Yahata T, Fujii M, Ozawa S, Toiyama K, Nishida M, & Itoi T. (2010). Effects of HMG-CoA reductase inhibitors on continuous post-inflammatory vascular remodeling late after Kawasaki disease J Cardiol, Vol. 56, pp. 245-253.

Iemura M, Ishii M, Sugimura T, Akagi T, & Kato H. (2000). Long-term consequences of regressed coronary aneurysms after Kawasaki disease: vascular wall morphology and function. Heart, Vol. 83, pp. 307-311.

Ikemoto Y, Ogini H, Teraguchi M, & Kobayashi Y. (2005). Evaluation of preclinical atherosclerosis by flow-mediated dilatation of the brachial artery and carotid artery analysis in patients with a history Kawasaki disease. Pediatr Cardiol, Vol. 26, pp. 782-786.

Jarvisalo MJ, Jartti L, Nanto-Saloren K, Irjala K, Ronnemaa T, & Hartiala JJ. (2001). Increased aortic intima-media thickness: a marker of preclinical atherosclerosis in high-risk children. Circulation, Vol. 104, pp.:2943-2947.

Kato H, Sugimura T, Akagi T, Sano N, Hashino K, Kazunc T, Eto G, & Yamakawa R. (1996). Long-term consequences of Kawasaki disease: A 10- to 21-year follow-up study of 594 patients. Circulation, Vol. 94, pp. 1379-1385.

Kawasaki T. (1967). Acute febrile muco-cutaneous lymph node syndrome in youngchildren with unique digital desquamation. Jpn J Allergol, Vol.16, pp. 178-222.

McCrindle BW, McIntyre S, Kim C, Lin T, & Adeli K. (2007). Are patients after Kawasaki disease at increased risk for accelerated atherosclerosis? J Pediatr, Vol. 151, pp. 244-248.

Mitani Y, Sawada H, Hayakawa H, Aoki K, Ohashi H, & Matsumura M. (2005). Elevated levels of hight-sensitivity C-reactive protein and serum amyloid-A late after Kawasaki disease: association between inflammation and coronary sequelae in Kawasaki disease. Circulation, Vol. 111, pp. 38-43.

Mitani Y, Ohashi H, Sawada H, Ikeyama Y, Hayakawa H, Takabayashi S, Maruyama K, Shimpo H, & Komada Y. (2009). In vivo plaque composition and morphology in coronary artery lesions in adolescents and young adults long after Kawasaki disease: a virtual histology intra vascular ultrasound study. Circulation, Vol. 119, pp. 2829-36.

Nakamura Y, Yashiro M, Uehara R, Sadakane A, Chihara I, Aoyama Y, Kotani K, & Yanagawa H. (2010). Epidemiologic features of Kawasaki disease in Japan: results of the 2007-2008 nationwide survey. J Epidemiol, Vol.20, pp. 302-307.

Naoe S, Takahashi K, Masuda H, & Tanaka N. (1991). Kawasaki disease. With particular emphasis on arterial lesions. Acta Pathol Jpn, Vol. 41, pp. 785-97.

Negoro N, Nariyama J, Nakagawa A, Katayama H, Okabe T, Hazui H, Yokota N, Kojima S, Hoshiga M, Morita H, Isihara T, & Kanafusa T. (2003). Successful catheter interventional therapy for acute coronary syndrome secondary to Kawasaki disease in young adults. Circ J, Vol. 67, pp. 362-365.

Newberger JW, Burns JC, Beiser AS, & Loscalzo J. (1991). Alterd lipid profile after Kawasaki syndrome. Circulation, Vol. 84, pp. 625-631.

Niboshi A, Hamaoka K, Sakata K, & Yamaguchi N. (2008). Endothelial dysfunction in adult patients with a history of Kawasaki disease. Eur J Pediatr, Vol. 167, pp. 189-196.

Noto N, Okada T, Yamasuge M, Taniguchi K, Karasawa K, Ayusawa M, Sumitomo N, & Harada K. (2001). Noninvasive assessment of the early progression of atherosclerosis in adolescents with Kawasaki disease and coronary artery lesions. Pediatrics, Vol. 107, pp. 1095-99.

Noto N, Okada T, Karasawa K, Ayusawa M, Sumitomo N, Harada K, & Mugishima H. (2009). Age-related acceleration of endothelial dysfunction and subclinical atherosclerosis in subjects with coronary artery lesions after Kawasaki disease. Pediatr Cadiol, Vol. 30, pp. 262-268.

Noto N, Okada T, Abe Y, Miyashita M, Kanamaru H, Karasawa K, Ayusawa M, Sumitomo N, & Mugishima H. (2011). Changes in the textural characteristics of intima-media complex in young patients with familial hypercholesterolemia: Implication for visual inspection on B-mode ultrasound. J Am Soc Echocardiogr, Vol. 24, pp. 438-443.

Okada T, Karada K, & Okuni M. (1982). Serum HDL-cholesterol and lipoprotein function in Kawasaki disease (acute mococutaneous lymph node syndrome). Jpn Circ J, Vol. 46, pp. 1039-1044.

Ooyanagi R, Fuse S, Tomita H, Takamuro M, Horita N, Mori M, & Tsutsumi H. (2004). Pulse wave velocity and ankle brachial index in patients with Kawasaki disease. Peditr Int, Vol. 46, pp. 398-402.

Ozawa S, & Hamaoka K. (2006). HMG-CoA refuctase inhibitors are effective for prevention of acute coronary injury in a rabbit model of Kawasaki disease. J Am Coll Cadiol, Vol. 46(Suppl A), pp.244A.

Sasaguri Y, & Kato H. (1982). Regression of aneurysms in Kawasaki disease: a pathological study. J Pediatr, Vol. 100, pp. 225-231.

Suzuki A, Kamiya T, Arakaki Y, Kinoshita Y, & Kimura K. (1994). Fate of coronary arterrial aneurysms in Kawasaki disease. Am J Cardiol, Vol. 74, pp. 822-824.

Suzuki A, Kamiya T, Tsuda E, & Shinya T. (1997). Natural history of coronary arterial lesions in Kawasaki disease. Prog Pediatr Cardiol, Vol. 6, pp. 211-218.

Suzuki A, Miyagawa-Tomita S, Komatsu K, Nishikawa T, Sakomura Y, Horie T, & Nakazawa M. (2000). Active remodeling of the coronary arterial lesions in the late phase of Kawasaki disease: Immunohistochemical study. Circulation, Vol. 101, pp. 2935-41.

Suzuki A, Miyagawa-Tomita S, Komatsu K, Nakazawa M, Fukaya T, Baba K, & Yutani C. (2004). Immunohistochemical study of apparently intact coronary artery in a child after Kawasaki disease. Pediatrics International, Vol. 46, pp. 590-596.

Strong WB, Deckelbaum RJ, Gidding SS, Kavey RE, Washinton R, Wilmore JH & Perry CL. (1992). Integreted cardiovascular health promotion in childhood. A statement for health profrssionals from the subcommittee on atherosclerosis and hypertension in childhood of the council on cardiovascular disease in the young, American Heart Association. Circulation., Vol. 85, pp. 1638-50.

Takahashi K, Oharaseki T, & Naoe S. (2001). Pathological study of postcoronary arteritis in adolescents and young adults: with reference to the relationship between sequelae of Kawasaki disease and atherosclerosis. Pediatr Cardiol, Vol. 22, pp. 138-142.

Taubert KA, Rowley AH, & Shulman ST. (1991). Nationwide survey of Kawasaki disease and acute rheumatic fever. J Pediatr, Vol. 119, pp. 279-282.

Tsuda E, Abe T, Tamaki W. (2011). Acute coronary syndrome in adult patients with coronary artery lesions caused by Kawasaki disease: review of case reports. Cardiol Young, Vol 21, pp.74-82.

Yamakawa R, Ishii M, Sugimura T, Akagi T, Eto G, Iemura M, Tsutsumi T, & Kato H. (1998). Coronary endothelial dysfunction after Kawasaki disease: evaluation by intracoronary injection of acetylcholine. J Am Coll Cardiol, Vol.31, pp.1074-1080.

11

Dysmetabolic Syndrome

Craiu Elvira, Cojocaru Lucia, Rusali Andrei,
Maxim Razvan and Parepa Irinel
*Ovidius University of Constantza, Faculty of Medicine,
Romania*

1. Introduction

The dysmetabolic syndrome (DMS) reunites a cluster of interrelated and important risk factors and/or medical conditions or disorders which act and worsen each other, aggravate and provoke each other, promoting the development of atherosclerotic vascular disease and type 2 diabetes (DM).

Although it has been termed „a syndrome or a disease-state", the prevalence of metabolic syndrome has risen dramatically in all societies over the past two decades; therefore, DMS should be analyzed as „an educational concept that focuses attention on complex multifactorial health problems", but in relation „to four key areas: pathophysiology, epidemiology, clinical work and public health" (Ford et all., 2002; Simmons et all., 2010). This aspect must be well deepened by doctors and understood by patients, because the patients with DMS are at a much higher risk for many and serious medical conditions (atherogenic dyslipidemia, elevated blood pressure, elevated plasma glucose, proinflammatory and prothrombotic states, and so on).

This review evaluates the multiple similarities and differences between several concepts and definitions of DMS, in an attempt to clarify its practical and clinical usefulness, amid many exciting controversies. The clinical significance of DMS, as a distinct entity, has been debated in the past years. Initially, DMS was scarcely used as a practical tool for clinical management, educational concept or pre-morbid condition, until 1988, when GM Reaven brought it to the attention of clinicians and theorists in "Banting Lecture"; thus, GM Reaven remains the main author who has developed and strengthened this „clinical and pathological concept", identifying insulin resistance as the central pathophysiologic feature (Reaven, 1988).

DMS is known under many names: „Metabolic syndrome" (World Health Organisation [WHO], 1998; National Cholesterol Education Program [NCEP], 2002; International Diabetes Federation [IDF], 2005), „Insulin resistance syndrome", „Dysmetabolic syndrome", „Cardiometabolic syndrome", „Syndrome X" (Reaven, 1988), „Plurametabolic syndrome", „Deadly Quartet: upper-body obesity, glucose intolerance, hypertriglyceridemia, and hypertension" (Kaplan, 1989), "Atherometabolic Syndrome", „Sindrom dismetabopres" (Buşoi G, 2005), „CHAOS" (in Australia), and so on.

2. History

The history of DMS was not an easy one; we will present, in chronological order, the most important events (Isomaa et al., 2001).

Between 1920-1923, Kylin (as cited in Lau, 2009), a Swedish physician, described for the first time a constellation of metabolic disturbance and the clustering of hypertension, hyperglycemia, and gout. After Kylin, J Vague, from the University of Marseille, reported that body fat topography, respectively upper-body obesity, causes the predisposition to diabetes mellitus, atherosclerosis, gout, and renal calculi, and that its anatomical distribution differs according to gender. Vague used the term "android obesity" to define the pattern of fat distribution with an accumulation of adipose tissue over the trunk and the term "gynoid obesity" for adipose tissue that accumulates mostly around the hips and thighs, commonly found in women (Vague et al., 1947). As the research continued, after 1960, a link between obesity, insulin-resistance and related complications was suggested. Albrink and Meigs reported an association between trunk fat and hypertriglyceridemia (Meigs et al., 2003). In 1975-1977, Haller used the term "metabolic syndrome" for an association of obesity, diabetes mellitus, hyperlipoproteinemia, hyperuricemia, and hepatic steatosis, and describes the additional role of these risk factors on the cardiovascular disease (CVD) (Haller, 1977). In 1977-1978, Singer and Phillips developed the concept that risk factors for myocardial infarction, respectively a "constellation of associated abnormalities" (i.e. glucose intolerance, hyperinsulinemia, hypercholesterolemia, hypertriglyceridemia, and hypertension) are associated with CVD, aging, obesity, sex hormones, and other clinical states (Singer, 1977; Phillips, 1978). In 1988, Reaven, describes "Syndrome X" in his famous Banting Lecture; this is a critical moment, subject to many controversies in the literature; more and more risk factors (RF) (hypertension, hyperglycemia, glucose intolerance, elevated triglycerides, and low HDL-cholesterol), as well as many metabolic disturbances, especially insulin resistance, are incriminated in the pathogeny of CVD (Reaven, 1988). In 2005, Kahn draws attention to several unresolved questions about the metabolic syndrome, many of them still unresolved even now:

- Metabolic syndrome name?
- Existence of metabolic syndrome?
- More than some of its parts?
- Metabolic sindrome vs. prediabetes & type 2 diabetes
- Diagnostic utility? Pathogenesis? Clinical utility?

3. Definitions of dysmetabolic syndrome

In 1998-1999, WHO defines metabolic syndrome (MS) as a clustering of arterial hypertension, dyslipidemia, obesity with high waist to hip ratio, microalbuminuria, glucose intolerance or insulin resistance, or type 2 diabetes; at the same time, it recognizes „CVD as the primary outcome of the metabolic syndrome" (table 1).

The criteria for the diagnosis of MS are: the presence of one of diabetes mellitus, impaired glucose tolerance, impaired fasting glucose or insulin resistance, AND two of the following:

1. blood pressure ≥ 140/90 mmH
2. dyslipidemia: triglycerides (TG) ≥ 1.695 mmol/L and high-density lipoprotein cholesterol (HDL-C) ≤ 0.9 mmol/L (in males) or ≤ 1.0 mmol/L (in females);

Parameters	NCEP ATP3 2005	IDF 2005	EGIR 1999	WHO 1999	AACE 2003
Required		Waist ≥94 cm (men) or ≥80 cm (women)*	Insulin resistance or fasting hyperinsulinemia in top 25 percent	Insulin resistance in top 25 %•; glucose ≥6.1 mmol/L (110 mg/dL); 2-hour glucose ≥7.8 mmol/L (140 mg/dL)	High risk of insulin resistanceΔ or BMI ≥25 kg/m^2 or waist ≥102 cm (men) or ≥88 cm (women)
Nr. of abnormalities	≥3 of:	And ≥2 of:	And ≥2 of:	And ≥2 of:	And ≥2 of:
Glucose	≥5.6 mmol/L (100 mg/dL) or drug treatment for elevated blood glucose	≥5.6 mmol/L (100 mg/dL) or diagnosediabetes	6.1-6.9 mmol/ (110-125 mg/dL)		≥6.1 mmol/L (110 mg/dL); ≥2-hour glucose 7.8 mmol/L (140 mg/dL)
HDL cholesterol	<1.0 mmol/L (40 mg/dL) (men); <1.3 mmol/L (50 mg/dL) (women) or drug treatment for low HDL-C◊	<1.0 mmol/L (40 mg/dL) (men); <1.3 mmol/L (50 mg/dL) (women) or drug treatment for low HDL-C	<1.0 mmol/L (40 mg/dL)	<0.9 mmol/L (35 mg/dL) (men); <1.0 mmol/L (40 mg/dL) (women)	<1.0 mmol/L (40 mg/dL) (men); <1.3 mmol/L (50 mg/dL) (women)
TGs	≥1.7 mmol/L (150 mg/dL) or drug treatment for elevated triglycerides◊	≥1.7 mmol/L (150 mg/dL) or drug treatment for high TGs	or ≥2.0 mmol/L (180 mg/dL) or drug treatment for dyslipidemia	or ≥1.7 mmol/L (150 mg/dL)	≥1.7 mmol/L (150 mg/dL)
Obesity	Waist ≥102 cm (men) or ≥88 cm (women)§		Waist ≥94 cm (men) or ≥80 cm (women)	Waist/hip ratio >0.9 (men) or >0.85 (women) or BMI ≥30 kg/m^2	
HTA	≥130/85 mmHg or drug treatment for HTA	≥130/85 mmHg or drug treatment for HTA	≥140/90 mmHg or drug treatment for hypertension	≥140/90 mmHg	≥130/85 mmHg

* For South Asia and Chinese patients, waist ≥90 cm (men) or ≥80 cm (women); for Japanese patients, waist ≥90 cm (men) or ≥80 cm (women).
• Insulin resistance measured using insulin clamp.
Δ High risk of being insulin resistant is indicated by the presence of at least one of the following: diagnosis of CVD, hypertension, polycystic ovary syndrome, non-alcoholic fatty liver disease or acanthosis nigricans; family history of Type 2 diabetes, hypertension of CVD; history of gestational diabetes or glucose intolerance; nonwhite ethnicity; sedentary lifestyle; BMI 25 kb/m2 or waist circumference 94 cm for men and 80 cm for women; and age 40 years.
◊ Treatment with one or more of fibrates or niacin. § In Asian patients, waist ≥90 cm (men) or ≥80 cm (women).

Table 1. Five current definitions of the metabolic syndrome (Meigs, 2006).

3. central obesity: waist:hip ratio > 0.90 (in males) and > 0.85 (in females), or body mass index > 30 kg/m2 ;
4. microalbuminuria: urinary albumin excretion ratio ≥ 20 μg/min. or albumin:creatinine ratio ≥ 30 mg/g.

We can see a potential disadvantage of the WHO criteria, namely the need for the routine assessment of the glycemic metabolism. (Simmons et al., 2010; Alberti & Zimmet, 1998).

The European Group for the Study of Insulin Resistance (EGIR, 1999), designed to be used in non diabetics only, requires two or more of the following:

1. central obesity: waist circumference ≥ 94 cm (male), ≥ 80 cm (female);
2. dyslipidemia: TG ≥ 2.0 mmol/L and/or HDL-C < 1.0 mmol/L or treated for dyslipidemia;
3. hypertension: blood pressure ≥ 140/90 mmHg or antihypertensive medication;
4. fasting plasma glucose (FPG) ≥ 6.1 mmol/L (table 1).

In 2001-2002, the National Cholesterol Education Program and Adult Treatment Panel (ATPIII) provides a clinical definition of metabolic syndrome, "a multiplex risk factor for cardiovascular disease (CVD) and identifies" six components of the metabolic syndrome that relate to CVD: abdominal obesity, atherogenic dyslipidemia, raised blood pressure, insulin resistance ± glucose intolerance, proinflammatory state, prothrombotic state". It also states that "the presence of type 2 DM does not exclude a diagnosis of metabolic syndrome" and the definition does not require evidence of insulin or glucose abnormalities, although „abnormal glycemia is one of the criteria". The US NCEP and ATP III require at least three of the following:

1. central (abdominal) obesity: waist circumference ≥ 102 cm (40 inches) (male), ≥ 88 cm (35 inches) (female);
2. dyslipidemia:
   - TG ≥ 150 mg/dL (1.7 mmol/L), or drug treatment for elevated triglycerides;
   - HDL-C < 40 mg/dL (1 mmol/L) (male), < 50 mg/dL (1,3 mmol/L) (female), or drug treatment for low HDL-C;
3. blood pressure ≥ 130/85 mmHg, or drug treatment for elevated blood pressure;
4. FPG ≥100 mg/dL (5.6 mmol/L) or drug treatment for elevated blood glucose (table 1).

We can see that:

- the WHO criteria consider both central obesity ("waist-to-hip ratio") and overall obesity (defined by the "BMI");
- the NCEP ATP III criteria consider only central obesity ("waist circumference"),
- the presence of type 2 DM does not exclude the diagnosis of metabolic syndrome;
- elevated microalbuminuria is a component in the WHO definition, while it is not considered for NCEP ATP III (NCEPT ATPIII, 2001, 2002).

In 2005, ADA (American Diabetes Association) and EASD (European Association for the Study of Diabetes) discourage the use of the term "metabolic syndrome" in the field literature, questioning "whether this constellation of clinical findings constitutes a syndrome" and "whether that constellation, in and of itself, is an entity of medical concern above and beyond the individual components", and so on (Beaser & Levy, 2007).

The IDF (International Diabetes Federation) releases in 2005 the "Consensus worldwide definition" of the metabolic syndrome, which mentions the following criteria needed for the diagnosis:

1. central obesity is an essential element (defined as waist circumference with race/ethnicity specific values) and any two of the following:
2. raised triglycerides: > 150 mg/dL (1.7 mmol/L) or specific treatment for this lipid abnormality;
3. reduced HDL cholesterol: < 40 mg/dL (1.03 mmol/L) in males, < 50 mg/dL (1.29 mmol/L) in females, or specific treatment for this lipid abnormality;
4. raised blood pressure: systolic BP > 130 mmHg or diastolic BP >85 mmHg, or treatment of previously diagnosed hypertension;
5. raised fasting plasma glucose : > 100 mg/dL (5.6 mmol/L), or previously diagnosed type 2 diabetes. (table 1 and 2).

It can be noted that:

- if FPG > 5.6 mmol/L or 100 mg/dL, oral glucose tolerance test (OGTT) is strongly recommended, but is not necessary to define presence of the MS;
- if BMI is > 30 kg/m^2, central obesity can be assumed and waist circumference does not need to be measured (Alberti et al., 2005, 2006).

ADDITIONAL METABOLIC IDF CRITERIA (for research)
Abnormal body fat distribution: - general body fat distribution, - central fat distribution (CT/MRI), - adipose tissue biomarkers: leptin, adiponectin, - liver fat content.
Atherogenic dyslipidaemia (beyond elevated triglyceride and low HDL): - ApoB (or non-HDL-C), - small LDL particles.
Dysglycaemia: Oral glucose tolerance test (OGTT).
Insulin resistance (other than elevated fasting glucose): - fasting insulin/proinsulin levels, - insulin resistance, - elevated free fatty acids (fasting and during OGTT).
Vascular dysregulation (beyond elevated blood pressure): - measurement of endothelial dysfunction, - microalbuminuria.
Proinflammatory state: - elevated high sensitivity C-reactive protein, - elevated inflammatory cytokines (eg TNF-alpha, IL-6), - decrease in adiponectin plasma levels.
Prothrombotic state: - fibrinolytic factors (PAI-1 etc), - clotting factors (fibrinogen etc).
Hormonal factors: pituitary-adrenal axis.

Table 2. IDF: Additional metabolic criteria (for research) -„platinum standard" definition (www.idf,org)

After a brief period of time, AHA (American Heart Association) and NHLB (National Heart, Lung, and Blood Institute) state the opposite and consider MS:

- a "multidimensional risk condition" for both atherosclerotic cardiovascular disease (ASCVD) and type 2 diabetes;
- as "multiple risk factors that are metabolically interrelated";
- as "multifactorial in origin, with underlying causes and exacerbating factors".

The confusion generated by AHA/NHLBI is clarified by AHA/Updated NCEP ATP III, which gives the following criteria of diagnosis:

1. elevated waist circumference:
   - men — greater than 40 inches (102 cm);
   - women — greater than 35 inches (88 cm);
2. elevated triglycerides - equal to or greater than 150 mg/dL (1.7 mmol/L);
3. reduced HDL ("good") cholesterol:
   - men — less than 40 mg/dL (1.03 mmol/L);
   - women — less than 50 mg/dL (1.29 mmol/L);
4. elevated blood pressure:
   - equal to or greater than 130/85 mm Hg or
   - use of medication for hypertension;
5. elevated fasting glucose:
   - equal to or greater than 100 mg/dL (5.6 mmol/L) or use of medication for hyperglycemia.

The following notes are made:

- lowering the threshold for abnormal fasting glucose to 100 mg/dL, corresponding to the ADA criteria for impaired fasting plasma glucose;
- the inclusion of diabetes in the hyperglycemia trait definition;
- the therapeutic control of dyslipidemia and arterial hypertension (table 1) (Grundy et al., 2004, 2005; Beilby, 2004).

Following this statement, AACE (American Association of Clinical Endocrinologists) propose a "third set of clinical criteria for the insulin resistance syndrome", in fact ''a hybrid of those of ATP III and WHO metabolic syndrome'', but with „clinical value as a diagnosis".

As a disease entity, MS is recognized by the American Society of Endocrinology, NCEP, and WHO, among others. The above mentioned set has some complicated aspects:

- it does not state the number of RF;
- the diagnosis is left to clinical judgment;
- the term „insulin resistance syndrome" is not applied when the patient has MD, but „high risk of being insulin resistant" is indicated by the presence of at least one of the following:
  - diagnosis of CVD, hypertension, polycystic ovary syndrome, non-alcoholic fatty liver disease or acanthosis nigricans;
  - family history of type 2 diabetes, hypertension or CVD;
  - history of gestational diabetes or glucose intolerance;
  - non-white ethnicity; sedentary lifestyle; BMI 25 kb/m2 or waist circumference 94 cm for men and 80 cm for women; and

- age 40 years (table 1) (Kahn, 2005).

Now the DMS has been recognized as a proinflammatory, prothrombotic state, with elevated levels of C-reactive protein, interleukin (IL)-6, and plasminogen activator inhibitor (PAI)-1, and so on. Therefore, in the near future, many other diagnostic criteria will arise; for example, if high-sensitivity c-reactive protein (hs-CRP) can be used as a marker to predict coronary vascular diseases in DMS and as a predictor for non-alcoholic fatty liver disease, in correlation with serum markers that indicate the disturbance of the lipid and glucose metabolism (Kogiso et al., 2009).

These sets of defining criteria for DMS are similar but they also have many important differences (clinical, etiopathogenic, ethnical, geographical, and so on) (tables 1,2,3). In fact, these five definitions of DMS illustrate "its complexity and heterogeneity", although they are not unanimously accepted.

ATP III / IDF
Atherogenic dyslipidemia Elevated blood pressure Elevated plasma glucose Prothrombotic state Proinflammatory state
ADA / EASD
Atherogenic dyslipidemia Prediabetes Elevated plasma glucose Prothrombotic state Proinflammatory state

Table 3. Clustering or constellation of the metabolic risk factors (3+) in definition of the metabolic syndrome

The DMS is an insulin-resistant state with a cluster of cardiovascular risk factors, including various combinations and substantial additional CV risk, which occur in the same individual, but the question is "how to integrate the DMS into concepts of insulin resistance, pre-diabetes, and type-2 diabetes". Insulin resistance is a component of obesity, it favors the onset of type 2 DM and is found in many cases of hypertension and hypertriglyceridaemia with low levels of HDL-cholesterol (Reaven, 1988), in association with correlated metabolic abnormalities recognized as CV risk factors that are present prior to the onset of diabetes. If insulin resistance evolves with many other characteristics (abdominal obesity, dyslipidemia, hypertension, non-dipper pattern of blood pressure, salt sensitivity, glucose intolerance, history of gestational DM, increased PAI-1/ platelets and so on), can all of these be seen as cardiovascular RF in various combinations? Which and how many of these RF carry the greatest impact? (Johnson & Weinsstock, 2006).

In all definitions of DMS, the abdominal adiposity is underlined and not the body weight. It is indeed the visceral adipocytes that are metabolically active, leading „to elevated plasma free fatty acids that result in elevated triglycerides and lower HDL cholesterol, and contribute to elevated plasma glucose"; is this explication enough to consider that this type of obesity is the RF with the greatest impact? (Beaser & Levy, 2005).

In addition to age, race, and weight are there other RF associated with an increased risk of DMS? Indeed, in NHANES III trial, other RF have emerged (postmenopausal status, smoking, low household income, high carbohydrate diet, no alcohol consumption, and physical inactivity); should these RF be included in the DMS? And when other RF for CVD will arise, which RF will not be components of the DMS? We should not forget that the notion of DMS ignores „other several strong risk factors" for cardiovascular disease (like cigarette smoking and elevated levels of low-density lipoprotein cholesterol, for example). (Palaniappan et al., 2004).

Is the treatment of the DMS different, next to the treatment for each of its components? It is obvious that the presence of a DMS component will lead to its evaluation and optimal treatment, but it is also important to look for and evaluate all the individual components of DMS from all the definitions. If a patient has certain characteristics included in one of the definitions for DMS (large waist circumference, high triglycerides and high fasting glucose) and another patient has other characteristics (high blood pressure, low HDL, and high triglycerides), both of them will be diagnosed with DMS, but will they benefit from different therapeutic strategies? Because there is no unique mechanism for DMS, thereby there won't be a unique treatment (Bayturan et al., 2010).

If we accept that "the Framingham score for the risk" is a better "short-term" (10 year) risk tool, does it mean that the metabolic syndrome was meant to identify individuals at "higher long-term risk"? Are there other risk factors for CVD, which are not components of the metabolic syndrome, such as inflammatory markers, which may have equal or greater bearing on risk? (Grundy, 2006). Is the CVD risk associated with the metabolic syndrome higher than the sum of its individual components? (Sundstorm et al., 2006).

The setting of diagnostic criteria for DMS is very difficult with numerous controversies and uncertainties. Therefore, is the DMS:

1. a true syndrome?
2. a simple collection of things with "an identifiable pattern" ?
3. a clustering of certain signs and symptoms that tend to occur under certain circumstances?
4. three or more related diagnostic entities associated with any morbid process? And so on (Kahn et al., 2005; Balta, 2010).

This research showed that the SM is a most complex problem, a focus of much research and clinical interest, involving:

- symptoms that are associated,
- diseases that occur as a result of this condition,
- multiple risk factors representing the factors of metabolic origin (table 4).

Metabolic syndrome affects 44% of the U.S. population older than age 50; the percentage of women having the syndrome is higher than that of men; the age dependency of the syndrome's prevalence is seen in most populations around the world. The „clustering" of CV and metabolic abnormalities in the same person will lead to an additional CV risk „over and above the sum of the risks associated with each abnormality" (Golden et al, 2002).

Thus, it is necessary:

- to define and validate a „single, universally accepted diagnostic tool";
- to adopt a „global and practical consensus" for using a single "adequate terminology that will guarantee the correct understanding of the etiopathogeny, morphological and metabolic substrate of the multiple complex phenomena of cardiometabolic syndrome";
- to realize a comprehensive "platinum standard" list of criteria, which could be easily used in clinical practice and be sufficiently comprehensive in the following clinical trials.

CLINICAL SYNDROMES ASSOCIATED WITH INSULIN RESISTANCE
Type 2 diabetes
CVD
Essential hypertension
Polycystic ovary syndrome
Nonalcoholic fatty liver disease
Certain forms of cancer
Sleep apnea

Table 4. Clinical syndromes associated with insulin resistance

4. Etiopathogeny of dysmetabolic syndrome

Endothelial dysfunction (ED) is a key event in the pathogenesis of atherosclerosis. The possibility of early identification of individuals at risk and achieving an objective control of the effectiveness of treatment in clinical practice become an attractive goal of therapeutic strategies useful to reduce cardiovascular morbid-mortality, and the endothelium is the logical "window" for the next evolution of atherosclerosis.

Given that DMS includes „an atherogenic dyslipidaemia, an insulin resistance state leading to a disturbed plasma glucose/insulin homeostasis, a abdominal obesity, especially visceral obesity, a thrombotic and inflammatory profile, as well as an endothelial dysfunction could substantially increase the risk of coronary heart disease (CHD) and type 2 diabetes" (Alexander et al., 2003; Kahn R, et al., 2005; Grundy, 2006).

K. Watson draws attention to the practicality of cardiometabolic risk management, particularly attractive to lower morbidity and mortality but also the economic costs for health, particularly if the disease or diseases and/or it's complications are identified early, especially in the subclinical phase (Watson, 2007).

The key to identification of cardiometabolic risk is the recognition that a patient with one or 2 clinically evident risk factors likely has additional factors, as these risk factors have been shown to „cluster"; this cluster effect is not specific for DMS; it remains a concept on the basis of which the results of future research will show new perspectives.

Meigs et al. refined the concept of the metabolic syndrome "by outlining the function of distinct clusters of risk factors", actually "three factors underlie the clustering of risk variables", risk factors that are still topical:

1. a "metabolic" factor, including BMI, waist circumference, 2-hour glucose tolerance, triglycerides, insulin sensitivity, and plasminogen activator inhibitor;

2. an "inflammation" factor, including BMI, waist circumference, fibrinogen, C-reactive protein, and insulin sensitivity ; and
3. a "blood pressure" factor, including systolic and diastolic blood pressure)" (Meigs et al., 1997).

Wilcox, presenting the much-disputed „Z syndrome" still in the concept of „cluster", cautions that „in populations at risk of vascular disease, many patients who experience a cardiovascular event either do not have identifiable risk factors or have disease severity which appears to be out of proportion to their known risk factors. Since these risk factors have been shown to be independent predictors of adverse events, they will show at least additive effects in combination and possibly potentiate each other" (Wilcox et al., 1998).

The metabolic syndrome „is a cluster of the most dangerous heart-attack risk factors:

- diabetes and pre-diabetes,
- abdominal obesity,
- high cholesterol and
- high blood pressure".

The clustering of CVD risk factors that marks the metabolic syndrome is now considered to be „the driving force for a CVD epidemic" (Stern et al., 2004).

The exact mechanisms of the complex syndrome are not yet completely known and elucidated. Presently, the main etiologic factors for DMS obesity and the dysfunctional adipose tissue are present in clinical situations determined by insulin resistance; this process also „prevents the efficient conversion of food into energy because of a vastly reduced number of insulin receptors on the cell wall", thus inducing „an increase in blood levels of insulin". In addition, there is a multiple „set of risk factors" that commonly appear together in MS, but confer „a substantial additional CV risk, over and above the sum of the risks associated with each abnormality" (Golden et al., 2002).

The etiopathogenesis of the DMS is not entirely known and understood.

There are three potential etiological categories: obesity and disorders of adipose tissue, insulin resistance and a number of independent factors that mediate specific components of the DMS;

It is an established fact that "all components of metabolic syndrome are strongly interconnected and so they cannot be treated separately".

Questioning if and when "the whole is greater than the sum of its parts?" and „what factors comprise the syndrome?", Kahn argue with several answers:

- „diagnosing the metabolic syndrome adds nothing beyond each individual risk factor for predicting cardiovascular disease or diabetes";
- „the definition should include all the factors clearly associated with that underlying pathophysiology, such that there is little ambiguity regarding the etiology of the clustering";
- "if the etiology is unclear, it becomes much more difficult to decide what factors to include in the definition, since the word "cluster" itself can be ambiguous" (Kahn et al., 2005).

There is debate "whether obesity or insulin resistance are the causes of the DMS or if they are consequences of a more far-reaching metabolic derangement".

The multiple risk factors represent factors of metabolic origin, and can be grouped in several syndromes, each of which are metabolic risk factors;

Both insulin resistance and central obesity are considered significant factors. It is necessary to specify that insulin resistance is not synonymous with type 2 diabetes mellitus. Insulin resistance is not a disease, but remains the "primary mediator of metabolic syndrome". Insulin resistance does not necessarily lead to the clinical syndromes or to obesity; obesity is a „physiologic variable that increases the likelihood that an individual will be insulin resistant". It appears long before the diagnosis of diabetes and suggests an increased risk for the latter. Unlike type 2 diabetes, in the case of insulin resistance, the pancreas produces too much insulin as a compensatory mechanism and does not require drug treatment, but only diet and exercise. The combination of insulin resistance with compensatory hyperinsulinemia will determine an increased risk for CVD (table 4, 5) (Nakamura et al., 1994; Nesto, 2003, Matsuzawa et al., 2002). Present studies maintain „the central obesity and insulin resistance" as „main etiological factors" in DMS (Matsuzawa et al., 2002).

Fasting insulin (Insulin Assay):	10 IU/mL and below is optimal; over 10 IU/mL is high.
High sensitive CRP (C-Reactive Protein):	Less than 1.0 µU/ml is optimal.
Triglycerides:	50-100 mg/dL is optimal, 100-150 mg/dL is moderate and over 150 mg/dL is high.
Homocysteine:	Less than 6 µmol.L is optimal; greater than 9 µmol/L is high.
Cholesterol:	HDL 40 mg/dL is good, although higher is even better. In studies, women with HDL of 70 mg/dL had low cardiac risk. LDL of less than 100 mg/dL is good. Total cholesterol should be less than 200 mg/dL or under.
Fasting glucose:	Normal is 74-106 mg/dL. Values of 100-125 mg/dL are indicative of Pre-Diabetes. Values greater than or equal to 126 mg/dL are indicative of Type 2 Diabetes.
Oral glucose tolerance (with 75 gr. Glucose load):	Results greater than or equal to 200 at 2 hours following the oral glucose tolerance test indicate Type 2 Diabetes.
(PAI -1):	Greater than 31
Fibrinogen:	This test is a general measure of inflammatory processes; the results vary greatly with the patient's age, gender and test method. Results that are both too high and too low are problematic.

Table 5. Lab exams in DMS (Grundy et al., 2005)

4.1 Central obesity

It has been demonstrated that the central obesity is by far the most prevalent form of the MS and a major component of the MS. Reaven points out that insulin resistance does not cause obesity; rather, obesity causes insulin resistance and has a key role in the pathophysiology of metabolic disorders; but insulin resistance also occurs in 10% to 15% of people who are not overweight. Basically, abdominal (visceral) obesity:

- represents the accumulation of central fat,
- plays a key role in the pathophysiology of metabolic disorders,
- has potential negative effects on metabolic and CV risk,
- is associated with insulin resistance, but is independently associated with each of the other MS components, including insulin resistance,
- predicts the development of type 2 DM,
- is easily measured, either by waist circumference or by waist-to-hip ratio;
- this measurement estimates the CV risk (table 3)
- has "remarkable heterogeneity"(Weisberg et al., 2003; Nesto, 2003; Grundy et al., 2005).

These affirmations are sustained by the following arguments:

- there is a linear correlation between waist circumference and visceral fat; but, subcutaneous fat is metabolically and cardiovascularly inert, exerting a possible protective function;
- insulin resistance of visceral fat is linked to dislipidemia, hypertension, hyperglycemia and inflammation, complex phenomenon representing DMS ;
- adipocyte (fat cells of the visceral fat) dysfunction may be either „intrinsic or secondary to immune dysregulation, inflammation, hypothalamic-pituitary adrenal dysfunction, local glucocorticoid dysregulation within visceral fat, or, possibly, stress or energy imbalance"; adipocytes hypertrophy is followed by macrophage infiltration, inflammation, and so on, with the alteration of different functions (TNFα, resistin, PAI-1, etc.), which contributes to a prothrombotic state;
- hypoadiponectinemia has been shown to increase insulin resistance, and is considered to be a risk factor for developing and worsening MS;
- the visceral, abdominal fat tissue releases inflammatory cytokines that increase insulin resistance in the body's skeletal muscles, and is also associated with a decreased production of adiponectin, which is the adipose-specific, collagen-like molecule with anti diabetic, anti-atherosclerotic and anti-inflammatory functions;
- TNFα presence can increase production of inflammatory cytokines and may lead to insulin resistance during a very complex process. (Grundy et al., 2004; Matsuzawa et al., 2004a, 2004b).

The distribution of adipose tissue appears to affect its role in metabolic syndrome. While visceral, intra-abdominal fat correlates with inflammation, subcutaneous fat does not. Only abdominal fat produces potentially harmful levels of cytokines (tumor necrosis factor, adiponectin, leptin, resistin, and plasminogen activator inhibitor). Only visceral fat accumulation and insulin-resistance have been associated with a cluster of dyslipidaemic features (i.e., elevated plasma triglyceride, increased very low density lipoprotein /VLDL, presence of small dense LDL particles, with decreased of HDL-cholesterol, and so on).

In conclusion, central obesity:

1. is independently associated with each of the other metabolic syndrome components, including insulin resistance
2. contributes to hypertension, dyslipidemia (high serum cholesterol, low HDL-c) and hyperglycemia, and is independently associated with higher CVD risk. (Anderson et al., 2001; Zimmet et al., 2001).

The increased flow of free fatty acids through the liver leads to accelerated synthesis of VLDL-C, hypertriglyceridemia, endothelial dysfunction, and vasoconstriction, leading to an increase in blood pressure; also, through this mechanism, insulin resistance may exert an atherogenic effect (Fonseca, 2005).

4.2 Inflammation

A number of markers of systemic inflammation, including C-reactive protein, are often increased, as are fibrinogen, interleukin 6 (IL–6), tumor necrosis factor-alpha (TNFα), and others.

CVD and diabetes are associated with elevated levels of inflammatory biomarkers, including C-reactive protein (CRP).

At the same time, CRP is the best-studied inflammatory marker of atherothrombotic risk, placed among the parameters used in "Framingham Risk Score".

C-reactive protein is present in the MS; its plasma levels increase with the number of metabolic risk factors, and also with other inflammatory markers; these associations are „purely correlative, not causative, and do not imply a mechanistic action" (table 2)

The mechanisms that lead to the increase of CRP are complex and only partially understood; we take this opportunity to remind that only excessive fatty tissue releases inflammatory cytokines and determines higher CRP levels; adipose cell enlargement and infiltration of macrophages into adipose tissue will lead to the release of proinflammatory cytokines and promote insulin resistance. It increases the thrombogenicity of circulating blood, in part by raising plasminogen activator type 1 and adipokine levels, and it causes endothelial dysfunction (Grundy et al., 2004; Ridker et al., 2004).

4.3 The prothrombotic and proinflammatory states

The prothrombotic and proinflammatory states may be metabolically interconnected by "plasma plasminogen activator inhibitor (PAI)-1 and fibrinogen", "in response to a high-cytokine state" (Grundy et al., 2004)

4.4 Atherogenic dyslipidemia

Atherogenic dyslipidemia represents the combination of raised triglycerides (TG), low HDL-C, elevated apolipoprotein B (ApoB), small dense LDL and small HDL particles, and so on; all are independently atherogenic and are observed in type 2 DM and DMS. Low HDL-c is considered to be „a particularly key risk factor for CVD in both non-diabetic and diabetic individuals", „an independent contributor to CVD, in both men and women". Low HDL-c and high TG levels are frequently found in insulin resistance, with or without type 2 diabetes, and both are risk factors for CVD (table 3) (Robins et al., 2003; Brunzell & Ayyobi, 2003).

5. Diagnosis of DMS

Although the present review does not have as purpose the detailed presentation of the way in which the diagnosis of DMS is made, we consider that few remarks are necessary in order to manage it correctly.

The literature of the past years regarding the management of this concept agrees upon the necessity of a team research, especially in the population of high risk, on national criteria, with subsequent establishment of a realistic management programme.

S Julius (and not only him) supports this point of view because "the clinical spectrum of the Metabolic Syndrome is variable and influenced by gender, ethnicity, and genetic susceptibility", especially in arterial hypertension, and even in borderline hypertension (Julius & Nesbitt, 1996). Paul Zimmet, from Australia, draws attention to the need of a "careful definition and management of the "tick test" in the DMS", which must rely on „evidence-based criteria"; he adds: "Tackling diabetes and obesity is likely to be the single most important challenge for Australia's public health in the 21st century. It is a battle that we can and must win!" (Eckel et al., 2005; Barr et al., 2006). More recently, a Joint Scientific Statement was necessary "in an attempt to unify criteria", to underline the fact that DMS is a "multifaceted, but distinct entity", and that "further progress depends in part on interdisciplinary dissemination of knowledge" (Table 6); moreover, "various diagnostic criteria have been proposed by different organizations over the past decade", which often led to confusion.

Simmons RK and collaborators evaluated the utility of metabolic syndrome from several points of view: pathophysiology, epidemiology, clinical work and public health, but also educational; the authors conclude that they agree with this „concept that focuses attention on complex multifactorial health problems", but they accept it only as „a diagnostic or management tool" with a limited practical utility (Simmons et al., 2010).

To gave up the widespread term of DMS that Sindrom metabolic, which is used for many years for this „cluster of risk factors", " is an unrealistic act, even impossible to fulfill, because the term is rooted in the medical literature"; DMS is: „a heterogeneous entity, composed of abnormal situations involved in the production of a metabolic imbalance with common metabolic links, but also with important differences in the etiopathogenesis of its components" (Balta, 2010).

Despite numerous criticisms of the concept by many authors, Kahn and collegues express „our recommendations to clinicians":

„All CVD risk factors should be individually and aggressively treated"

„Pharmacological therapy to reduce insulin resistance will be beneficial to patients with the metabolic syndrome"

„An aggressive research agenda to identify the underlying cause(s) of the CVD risk factor clustering"

..."it remains to be demonstrated that the impact of the syndrome exceeds that of the sum of its individual components" and so on (Kahn et al., 2005).

David Nathan (Massachusetts General Hospital, Boston) described the situation as "a firestorm about nothing" and adds about DMS:

- "it was raised from a research view",
- "it captured a confluence of clinical conditions that can occur together"
- "an important concept from an epidemiology view and to investigate whether these conditions had a single underling cause".

Hypertriglyceridaemic waist phenotype estimated prevalence: 20-25%
- Atherogenic metabolic triad (fasting hyperinsulinaemia, elevated apolipoprotein B levels and increased proportion of small LDL particles
- Elevated total cholesterol/HDL cholesterol ratio
- Postprandial hyperlipidaemia
– Fasting hyperinsulinaemia
– Glucose intolerance
– Increased risk of type 2 diabetes
– Increased cardiovascular risk

Table 6. Hypertriglyceridaemic waist phenotupe association with features of metabolic syndrome

We note some compelling conclusions regarding the current global state of DMS:

- "DMS is common and it has a rising prevalence worldwide.
- Now, DMS is both a public health and a clinical problem.
- The DMS is a complex of interrelated risk factors for CVD, DM.
- Three abnormal findings out of 5 would qualify a person for the metabolic syndrome.
- The term "metabolic syndrome" is acceptable for the condition of the presence of multiple metabolic risk factors for CVD and DM.
- The metabolic syndrome is not an absolute risk indicator.
- The metabolic risk factors are atherogenic dyslipidemia, elevated blood pressure, and elevated plasma glucose.
- The risk associated with a particular waist measurement will differ in different populations. We recommend the use of waist measurement as a useful screening tool in many primary populations"(Alberti et al., 2009).

Even if now we assign to DMS multiple metabolic risk factors and/or a complex of interrelated risk factors for CVD and DM, although we know that DMS substantially increases the risk of CHD, we do not know which of its defining characteristics (insulin resistance/ hyperinsulinaemia, small LDL particles, reduced adiponectin levels, increased CRP, etc.) are "critical therapeutic targets for the optimal management of CHD and type 2 diabetic risk" (Hu et al., 2001). We need to globally asses the individual risk of these patients in order to optimally manage the dyslipidaemic state in this high-risk population. In the context of the current knowledge regarding the DMS, the patients diagnosed with arterial hypertension, DLP, or hyperglycemia will be actively investigated for DMS. We must insist upon the realisation of a complete diagnosis, specifying the risk score for CV and/or metabolic disorders that we found (table 5, 6).

Given the susceptibility to many other pathological conditions, we must use all clinical and paraclinical methods needed in order to establish a positive and differential diagnosis (ex. polycystic ovary syndrome, fatty liver, cholesterol gallstones, asthma, sleep disturbances, some forms of cancer), especially if they are sugested by the familial genetic aspect, by the signs and simptoms and so on. The mesurement that are needed (weight, height, waist circumference or waist/hip ratio) for initial diagnosis of DMS and for follow-up will be taken in a proper manner, following the current guidelines (by gender, etnicity, etc.). It is estimated that the introduction of "waist circumference rather than the body mass index has been "a major conceptual leap", because it recognizes the much greater causal role of abdominal obesity than general obesity. (www.metabolicsyndromeinstitut/information /screeningdiagnosis/procedures-for-the-measurement-of-the-waist-circumference.php).

The canadian researchers Lemieux I, Pascot A, Couillard C et al., introduce a new notion, namely: „HYPERTRIGLYCERIDEMIC WAIST": a marker of the atherogenic metabolic triad: hyperinsulinemia, hyperapolipoprotein B, and small, dense LDL, in men. We note the depth of this interesting concept, its validation in a trial (Québec Health Survey) and its practical usefulness, at least from two points of view:

- first, the possibility of identifying men at high risk, with normal glucose levels or impaired fasting glucose state;
- secondly, because it avoids the exact procedure for measuring visceral fat by sophisticated and costly methods, such as magnetic resonance or computed tomography.

„The hypertriglyceridaemic waist phenotype significantly increased the odds of finding CAD in men, whereas impaired fasting glucose was not predictive of CAD in the absence of hypertriglyceridaemic waist":

- "the simultaneous measurement and interpretation of waist circumference and triglyceride level", "the hypertriglyceridaemic waist", may be a simple tool to identify individuals at high risk";
- "men characterised by the hypertriglyceridaemic waist phenotype had a substantially elevated total cholesterol/HDL-cholesterol ratio compared with those without this phenotype";
- results suggest that the hypertriglyceridaemic waist phenotype may be useful in the screening of patients with many features of DMS (Table 7), such as an elevated total cholesterol/HDL-cholesterol ratio, postprandial hyperlipidaemia, fasting hyperinsulinaemia and additional risk factors.

Identified by the simultaneous measurement of waist circumference and fasting triglyceride levels, this approach can be "a simple and inexpensive marker to better identify individuals at high risk of CVD and/or type-2 diabetes and to evaluate CHD risk in individuals with abdominal obesity"(Lemieux et al., 2002; Blackburn et al. 2003).

There are multiple laboratory tests and many of them are vital (glycaemic profile, lipids, inflammatory tests); we must not forget about exploring the thyroid function or investigating other systems (cerebrovascular, hepatic or renal). The new guidelines recognize the importance of elevated triglycerides and of reduced HDL cholesterol concentrations as useful lipid markers of the presence of an atherogenic "dysmetabolic" milieu. In DMS, the lipidic profile can vary, and so can the therapeutic options; they can be prescribed together with dietary changes or sustained physical effort.

Here are a few patterns:

- when there is a high LDL-cholesterol level, the use of statins as the drug of choice is preferred to reduce the risk of a first or recurrent CHD event;
- if we have a "normal" LDL-cholesterol level and typical dyslipidaemia, a fibrate is preferred as the first therapeutic option;
- if LDL-cholesterol and triglycerides are elevated, together with a relatively low HDL-cholesterol, patients are considered under "high risk" and combination therapy with both a statin and a fibrate is indicated, because of the high risk atherogenic profile - "atherogenic dyslipidemia" (Sacks, 2002).

Interventions which can improve insulin sensitivity, especially lifestyle modifications, weight loss, Mediterranean diet, and increased physical activity, remain the elements of choice in DMS, because of their favorable impact on DMS components. (Hu et al., 2001)

As an example for the complexity of what we call DMS, Zeller, Steg et al. insist that "fasting hyperglycaemia is the most important risk factor for development of severe heart failure in patients with metabolic syndrome"; these situations are associated with „a higher in-hospital case fatality rate"; strict control of glycemic levels in patients with DMS with or without a critical state is recommended by many authors and by the algorithm of the American Diabetes Association and the European Association for the Study of Diabetes (2006) (Zeller et al. 2005; Nathan et al., 2006).

Similarly, for a correct and complete diagnosis, Enzo Bonora et al. proposed a short list of novel (non-traditional) risk factors in order to emphasise the fact that, in the "metabolic syndrome approach", it is necessary to prove the "existence of underlying pathogenic disorders of the cluster, i.e. central obesity and insulin resistance"; to this end, the authors present a "systematization of biomarkers" that are useful in DMS and in clinical trials:

- chronic mild inflammation (e.g. C-reactive protein, CRP, white blood cells, WBC, erythrocyte sedimentation rate, ESR),
- increased oxidant stress (e.g. oxidized LDL, reactive exigent species, ROS),
- thrombophilia (e.g. fibrinogen, plasminogen activator inhibitor-1, PAI-1), - endothelial dysfunction (e.g. E-selectin, intercellular adhesion molecule-1, ICAM-1,
- vascular cell adhesion molecule-1, VCAM-1),
- adipose tissue derangement (e.g. adiponectin, leptin, resistin).

The authors consider that a better diagnosis and treatment of "several classic and ancillary components of the metabolic syndrome" will accomplish "a substantial reduction of the cardiovascular risk" (Bonora et al., 2003).

Matsuzawa Y, Funahashi T, and many others emphasize the importance of adiponectin; "one of these adipocytokines which we identified in human adipose tissue"; it circulates abundantly in human plasma, and has both anti-atherogenic and anti-diabetic effects. In addition, a series of clinical and experimental studies suggest that adiponectin may become a novel 'hot' marker of the Metabolic Syndrome (Matsuzawa et al., 2004).

Based on complicated lab research, Kumada M, Kihara S, Ouchi N et al. suggest the results above and conclude that „plasma adiponectin may become a novel biomarker for atherosclerotic vascular diseases, as well as plasma cholesterol and glucose levels" (Kumada et al., 2004).

The significance of adiponectin as „a negative risk for diabetes and its dual protective capacity", both against diabetes and atherosclerosis, makes the subject of much prestigious research; we are talking about „adipocytokines", considering the remark that "reduction of adiponectin may facilitate coronary plaque rupture" but, at the same time, adiponectin „suppresses both the atherosclerotic process and the production of an inflammatory cytokine," and so on.

Based on all these observations, it is obvious why „body weight reduction, physical exercise, and lifestyle changes" can raise plasma adiponectin levels. In addition, agents such as "thiazolidinediones, renin-angiotensin system blockers and glimepiride" have been reported to increase adiponectin concentrations (Weyer et al., 2001).

Wiecek et al. reported that plasma adiponectin levels are negatively correlated with mean blood pressure (BP) in patients with essential hypertension (Adamczak et al., 2003).

Some well known Japanese authors point out the association of obesity with increased risk for breast and endometrial cancers; also, high serum adiponectin levels are associated with an increased risk for breast cancer (Miyoshi et al., 2003).

Imaging tests are not routinely indicated, but they can be performed when previous examinations suggest cardiovascular complications.

Adverse clinical consequences and/or target organ damage appear during long term evolution of DMS; all these elements will be periodically investigated and quantified by specific methods. The most frequent example is represented by arterial hypertension, which evolves with very important target organ damage (left ventricular hypertrophy, progressive peripheral arterial disease, and renal dysfunction).

Using the NCEP/ATP III definition, Mulè et al. investigated the efect of SXM on markers of target organ damage, and they have demonstrated that these lesions can explain „the enhanced cardiovascular risk associated with the Metabolic Syndrome". The authors also conclude that there must be a global evaluation of the „influence of the SXM on some cardiac, renal, and retinal markers of target organ impairment" (Mulè et al., 2005).

We must not overlook the complications associated with DMS, representing short and long-term prognosis factors; there can be cardiovascular (coronary heart disease, atrial fibrillation, heart failure, aortic stenosis , ischemic stroke, and so on) or extra cardiac complications (nonalcoholic fatty liver disease, obstructive sleep apnea, breast cancer, cancer of the colon, gallbladder, kidney, prostate gland, and so on).

6. Management of DMS

Because DMS is associated with dramatically higher risk of DCV, diabetes, and so on, its recognition and follow-up have become a major issue in preventive cardiology.

According to the DMS concept and the recognition of its defining combinations (hypertriglyceridemia, hyperglycemia, hypertension, low HDL-C level, and greater waist circumference / adiposity) there are:

- a clinical method for identifying CVD risk and symptoms of an underlying disease or condition;
- the variation of cardiovascular and metabolic risk according to which syndrome components are present, their duration, and existing complications.

These elements represent the foundation of DMS complex management. (Ding et al., 2010).

6.1 Primary prevention

Primary prevention consists in a healthy life style, smoking cessation, caloric restriction, and a modified daily diet. A moderate increase of physical activity and a 7-10% weight loss over 6-12 months are also indicated.

Low caloric diet and moderate but sustained exertion are considered "the most important initial steps in treating metabolic syndrome" (Ford et al., 2002).

If we analyze each individual component of DMS reporting it to the DMS diagnosis, a greater chance of progression was observed, especially if we consider that hyperglycemia, hypertension, and low HDL-C level are the main risk factors; consequently, these risk factors represent a potential target for active and individual cardiovascular prevention in these patients (Després et al., 2008).

6.2 Secondary prevention

Secondary prevention is addressed to patients for whom lifestyle change is not enough and who are considered to be at high risk for CVD; these patients will receive medical treatment together with lifestyle changes.

All these will act "as a whole" on the basic mechanisms of DMS in order to reduce the evolutionary impact of all risk factors and all "metabolic and cardiovascular consequences", on short and long-term evolution.

Separate, incomplete or inconsistent approach of individual components of DMS is to be avoided; the emphasis will be laid on sustained reduction of individual risk, especially in patients with several DMS components and complications; only, in this way, we can really reduce „the overall impact on CVD and DM risk". (Lindström et al., 2003; Tuomilehto et al. 2001).

After the complete diagnosis is established, the management of DMS must be more comprehensive and more aggressive compared to other clinical situations, in order to reduce the risk for CVD and DM; thereby, a complete evaluation of cardiovascular risk according to present guidelines of medical practice is of outmost importance.

Framingham risk scoring (or other risk scores, although they include different components) will be used to estimate „10-year atherosclerotic disease risk" and may guide the use of medication therapy (Spellman & Chemitiganti, 2010; Nicholls et al., 2007).

6.3 Medical care

The initial management of metabolic syndrome involves lifestyle modifications (changes in diet and exercise habits).

The choice of drug and dose should be individualized to the patient and titrated to achieve guideline-recommended goals.

Diets that promote the consumption of fruits, vegetables, and low-fat dairy products ("DASH-style diet") help lower blood pressure and may lower risk of stroke. The consumption of products with high-glycemic-index will be avoided.

Increasing physical activity is associated with a reduction in the risk of stroke, at least 30 minutes of moderate intensity activity on a daily basis, maintaining long-term adherence.

Weight reduction among overweight and obese persons is recommended to reduce blood pressure and risk of stroke.

Bianchi C et al. stipulates the basics of food diet for prevention and treatment of DMS:

- protein for 10-20% of total daily energy;
- saturated fatty acids and trans-unsaturated fatty acids ≤ 10% of total energy, and further lowered to < 8%, if serum LDL-cholesterol level is increased;
- cholesterol intake: 300 mg or less per day;
- carbohydrates: 45-60% of total energy, vegetables, legumes, fruits, and whole-grain cereals: the most appropriate sources of carbohydrates;
- foods rich in dietary fiber: ≥ 40 g/d (or 20 g/1000 kcal/d), about half in soluble form;
- sodium restriction can reduce systolic blood pressure in hypertensive patients;
- 30 minutes of walking a day: all overweight subjects;
- pharmacotherapy may be necessary for cardiovascular risk factors: LDL-cholesterol, hypertension, T2DM, and obesity (Bianchi et al., 2006).

The medical care is represented by "a multi-drug treatment", in order to reduce morbidity and prevent DMS complications; the treatment must be with metabolic and glucidic neutrality, with respect to the accompanying disturbances of the DMS":

- angiotensin converting enzyme inhibitors (ACEI) or/and angiotensin-II-receptor blockers;
- anti-diabetic treatments to improve glycemic control, with metformin and thiazolidinediones, representing "a rational first-line treatment of patients with type 2 diabetes mellitus ";
- obesity and visceral obesity can respond to certain drugs with "the potential possibility of ameliorating the metabolic aspects in obese patients": Sibutramine, Orlistat and Rimonabant (the first inhibitor of CB1 receptors);
- although a therapeutic class of drugs capable of reducing the "inflammatory state" from DMS has not been established, there are many classes of drugs indicated in these patients (statins, fibrates, ACEIs, and thiazolidinediones), with an anti-inflammatory action;

- the procoagulative state in these patients, associated with elevation of the circulating levels of fibrinogen, factor VII, PAI-1, together with an increased platelet aggregation, determine the introduction of low-dose aspirin, with or without other anti-inflammatory agents (Antithrombotic Trialists' Collaboration, 2002).

In dyslipidemia, primary aims for therapy are:

1. lower TG (as well as lowering ApoB and non-HDL cholesterol),
2. raise HDL-c levels,
3. reduce LDL-c levels (elevated levels represent a high risk in the metabolic syndrome).

Fibrates (PPAR alpha agonists) improve all components of atherogenic dyslipidaemia (elevated triglyceride and low HDL-C levels), especially in overweight patients, and reduce the risk for cardiovascular disease in DMS,

For patients with elevated triglyceride levels, the addition of omega-3 fatty acids is likely to produce added benefit (according to clinical trials).

Statins are administered in order to reduce all apoB-containing lipoproteins and to achieve ATP III goals for LDL-cholesterol, as well as for non-HDL-Cholesterol; the multiple benefits are confirmed through many clinical trials „at all indicated ranges", the pleiotropic and metabolic effects being an "undisputed reality".

Management of reduced high-density lipoprotein cholesterol (HDL-C) remains controversial, not yet having a specific treatment; some measures have proved a positive influence: dietary changes, sustained physical efort, some statins (ex. Rosuvatatin), etc.

The latest guidelines insist on LDL-cholesterol being „the primary target of treatment by adequate use of statins"; although high levels of LDL-cholesterol are not necessarily associated with DMS, they will be properly quantified and treated, for reducing the cardiovascular risk.

Fibric-acid derivatives, bile acid sequestrants, and ezetimibe may be useful in patients who have not achieved target LDL with statin therapy or cannot tolerate statins (Eckel et al., 2005; Alberti et al., 2009; Robins et al., 2003; Heart Protection Study Collaborative Group, 2003; The Task Force for the management of dyslipidaemias of the European Society of Cardiology (ESC) and the European Atherosclerosis Society 2011).

Hypertension remains a clinical target according to present guidelines; regular blood pressure screening, lifestyle modification, and drug therapy are recommended. The focus must be on clinical situations associated with target organ damage, diabetes, or renal complications. Hypertension and diabetes, both components of metabolic syndrome, are known to be associated with renal dysfunction; oxidative stress and inflammation mediated by renin-angiotensin system activation are the most frequently involved mechanisms. Other mechanisms acting singly or in combination, linking obesity to chronic kidney disease, have been proposed: renal adaptation to increased body mass, with an increased excretory load, sodium retention, insulin resistance, renal lipotoxicity, etc. (Praga, 2002).

Microalbuminuria, however, was more common in subjects who had a constellation of all 3 components of metabolic syndrome than in those without. Presently, microalbuminuria is an early marker of renal dysfunction due to hypertension, predicts the onset of kidney disease in diabetic and nondiabetic subjects, and reflects widespread endothelial dysfunction, microvascular damage, and possibly inflammation. (Gerstein et al., 2001; Festa et al., 2000). The precise pathogenetic basis of microalbuminuria in metabolic syndrome is not known; it is, however, possible that microalbuminuria in metabolic syndrome reflects renin-angiotensin system activation and resultant oxidant stress, inflammation, and endothelial injury.

Dzau VJ, Safar ME, amongst many other elite scientists, have shown that hypertension, dyslipidemia, and insulin resistance are associated with renin-angiotensin system activation and generation of large amounts of angiotensin II (Dzau & Safar, 1988; Shinozaki et al., 2004).

Angiotensin converting enzyme inhibitors and angiotensin receptor blockers are useful antihypertensive drugs; some clinical trials suggest that they have advantages over other drugs, in patients with diabetes, and that the risk reduction associated with antihypertensive drugs is „the result of blood pressure lowering per se, and not due to a particular type of drug" (Chobanian et al., 2003).

Diabetes mellitus, recognized as „a true cardiovascular disease", raises particular problems of follow-up and treatment; the periodic screening with the assessment of end-organ complications is required even from the beginning of its evolution;

- the sustained control of blood pressure and dyslipidemia, along with diet, regular physical exercise, and the maintaining of normal body weight is recommended;
- as in hypertension, for DM, medical practice guidelines come with many details for each of „these pursue matters" (ex. JNC 7, update 2009).

Medical treatment of hyperglycemia in DMS begins with an insulin-sensitizing agent (ex. metformin), which proved that it can reverse the complications DMS, especially together with fibrates and thiazolidinediones.

Multiple research have shown the possibility that drugs that reduce insulin resistance will delay the onset of type 2 diabetes and will reduce CVD risk, when DMS is present (ex. „Diabetes Prevention Program" (DPP) with metformin, thiazolidinedione in delaying or preventing type 2 diabetes in impaired glucose tolerance (IGT) and insulin resistance) (www.idf.org).

Of course, we should not avoid prescribing aspirin for its well-deserved preventive actions, especially in patients with a high CV risk given by DMS, unless contraindicated.

Many other recommendations are necessary:

- patients with diabetes should be referred to a diabetic nutritionist, if not an endocrinologist;
- patients with high CV risk should be referred to a cardiologist for primary or secondary prevention of CVD;
- patients who are at high risk for obesity-associated morbidity and mortality with BMI greater than 40 kg/m2 or with BMI >35 kg/m2 plus one or more significant co-morbid conditions may be referred for consideration of bariatric surgery, when less invasive methods of weight loss have failed, etc., for more than 5 years;
- liposuction is used for cosmetic weight loss, but evidence shows that liposuction of abdominal subcutaneous fat (with no removal of visceral fat) has little effect on cardiometabolic risk parameters.

Moreover, it is required to follow up the effect/effects of the prescribed treatment, especially in cases of hypertension, DLP and DM, with a periodic assessment of patient adherence to treatment; attention will be directed to prescribe optimal combination regimens, respectively those recognized in reducing the CV risk.

Of course that the management of DMS is impossible to be wholly presented; it is a subject of great practical interest, but its defining elements are found in specialized literature and guides.

7. Conclusions

With all these questions, different opinions and debates, "the metabolic syndrome serves as a call to action for practitioners to focus more carefully on risk prevention above and beyond traditional ...". (Smith, 2006).

Jean Pierre Després (Institut Universitaire de Cardiologie et de Pneumologie de Québec) presents the DMS as "a work in progress" and adds :« I think it should be redefined as a constellation of metabolic abnormalities associated with visceral fat and insulin resistance; this would simply things and clarify a lot of confusion over this." (Després, 2008)

DMS was and remains an attractive subject in many ways, theoretical and practical, as demonstrated by all of the research so far; it remains a concept with great practical use, a heterogeneous entity based on a metabolic imbalance that has not yet found the best definition, the optimal nosological framing, widely accepted, even if it will reach soon 100 years of existence.

We propose the terminology of CARDIOVASCULAR DISMETABOLIC SYNDROME (CV DMS) which express a metabolic disorder, multifactorial entity that require the participation of several medical specialties (even over 10 specialities) in order to quantify and consolidate the defining elements of cardiometabolic risk and defining appropriate management in real time.

In order to reduce the confusion in the medical community, universal agreement on the definition and clinical tools to assess the DMS would be very helpful and eforts for additional international consensus activities have been made; all this research will determine all the "preventive and screening strategies for the dismetabolic syndrome".

Theoreticians and practitioners, laboratory doctors, lipidologists, diabetologists, nutritionists, or hypertensiologists, cardiologists, nephrologists, neurologists, endocrinologists, but also pediatricians, geneticists, family doctors and so on all participate in this complex process, because only teamwork can, indeed, to define actively, to monitor and improve multiple abnormal components of this entity called CARDIOVASCULAR DISMETABOLIC SYNDROME (CV DMS).

8. References

[1] Adamczak, M,; Wiecek, A. & Funahashi, T. (2003). *Decreased plasma adiponectin concentration in patients with essential hypertension.* Am J Hypertens;16:72-5

[2] Alberti, KG.; Zimmet, P. & Shaw, J. (2006). *Metabolic syndrome-a new world-wide definition. A Consensus Statement from the International Diabetes Federation.* Diabet Med, 23(5):469-80.

[3] Alberti, KG.; Zimmet, P. & Shaw, J. (2005). IDF Epidemiology Task Force Consensus Group. *The metabolic syndrome: a new worldwide definition.* Lancet; 366: 1059-62.

[4] Alberti KG, Zimmet PZ. (1998) *Definition, diagnosis and classification of diabetes mellitus and its complications." Part 1: "Diagnosis and classification of diabetes mellitus provisional report of a WHO consultation."* Diabet Med; 15: 539-53.

[5] Alberti KG., Eckel RH.,Grundy SM. (2009) *Joint Scientific Statement, Harmonizing the Metabolic Syndrome Circulation.*; 120: 1640-1645

[6] Alberti, KG, Eckel, RH, Scott M, Grundy SM et al. (2009*) Joint Scientific Statement: Harmonizing the Metabolic Syndrome Circulation.*; 120: 1640-1645

[7] Alexander CM, Landsman PB, Teutsch SM, et al. (2003) *NCEP-defined metabolic syndrome, diabetes, and prevalence of coronary heart disease among NHANES III participants age 50 years and older.* Diabetes 52:1210–1214;

[8] Anderson PJ, Critchley JAJH, Chan JCN et al. *"Factor analysis of the metabolic syndrome: obesity vs insulin resistance as the central abnormality."* International Journal of Obesity 2001;25:1782.

[9] Antithrombotic Trialists' Collaboration. (2002) *Collaborative meta-analysis of randomised trials of antiplatelet therapy for prevention of death, myocardial infarction, and stroke in high risk patients.* Br Med J;324:71-86

[10] Baltå N. (2010) *Some considerations on the denomination and concept of metabolic syndrome. Revista Medicalå Românå,* vol. LVII, nr. 3, 134-157

[11] Barr ELM, Magliano DJ, Zimmet PZ, et al. (2006*) AusDiab 2005, the Australian Diabetes, Obesity and Lifestyle Study. Tracking the accelerating epidemic: its causes and outcomes.* Melbourne, Australia: International Diabetes Institute, 2006

[12] Bayturan O, Tuzcu EM, Lavoie A, et al. (2010) *The metabolic syndrome, its component risk factors, and progression of coronary atherosclerosis.* Arch Intern Med; 170:478.

[13] Beaser RS., Levy Ph. (2007) *A Work in Progress, but a Useful Construct* Circulation; 115: 1812-1818.

[14] Beilby J. (2004*). Definition of Metabolic Syndrome: Report of the National Heart, Lung, and Blood Institute/American Heart Association Conference on Scientific Issues Related to Definition (reviewed).* Circulation;109:433–8

[15] Bianchi C, Penno G, Malloggi L, et al. (2006). *Non-traditional markers of atherosclerosis potentiate the risk of coronary heart disease in patients with type 2 diabetes and metabolic syndrome.* Nutr Metab Cardiovasc Dis

[16] Blackburn P, Lamarche B, Couillard C, et al. (2003*). Postprandial hyperlipidemia: another correlate of the "hypertriglyceridemic waist" phenotype in men.* Atherosclerosis; 171:327-36

[17] Bonora E, Kiechl S, Willeit J, et al. (2003). *The metabolic syndrome: epidemiology and more extensive phenotypic description. Cross-sectional data from the Bruneck Study.* Int J Obes;27:1283-89

[18] Brunzell JD, Ayyobi AF. (2003) *Dyslipidemia in the metabolic syndrome and type 2 diabetes mellitus.* Am J Med 2003;115 Suppl 8A:24S-28S.

[19] Chobanian AV, Bakris GL, Black HR et al. (2003). *Seventh report of the Joint National Committee on prevention, detection, evaluation, and treatment of high blood pressure.* Hypertension; 42(6):1206-52

[20] David C. W. Lau. (2009). *Metabolic syndrome: Perception or reality?* Current Atherosclerosis Reports, Volume 11, Number 4, 264-271.

[21] Després JP, Lemieux I, Bergeron J; et al. (2008) *Abdominal obesity and the metabolic syndrome: contribution to global cardiometabolic risk.* Arterioscler Thromb Vasc Biol.; 28(6):1039-1049

[22] Ding EL.; Smit LA.; Frank B. Hu FB. et al. (2010) *The Metabolic Syndrome as a Cluster of Risk Factors: Is the Whole Greater Than the Sum of Its Parts? Comment on "The Metabolic Syndrome, Its Component Risk Factors, and Progression of Coronary Atherosclerosi.* Arch Intern Med.;170(5):484-485

[23] Dzau VJ, Safar ME. (1988). *Large conduit arteries in hypertension: role of the vascular renin-angiotensin Circulation;77:947–54.*

[24] Eckel RH, Grundy SM, Zimmet PZ. (2005). *The metabolic syndrome.* Lancet; 365:1415-28;

[25] Expert Panel On Detection, Evaluation, And Treatment Of High Blood Cholesterol In Adults. (2001) *Executive Summary of the Third Report of the National Cholesterol Education Program (NCEP) Expert Panel on Detection, Evaluation, and Treatment of High Blood Cholesterol in Adults (Adult Treatment Panel III).* JAMA: the Journal of the American Medical Association, 285 (19): 2486–97.

[26] Festa A, D'Agostino R, Howard G, et al (2000). *Inflammation and microalbuminuria in nondiabetic and type 2 diabetic subjects: the Insulin Resistance Atherosclerosis* Study Kidney Int; 58:1703–10

[27] Fonseca VA. (2005) *The metabolic syndrome, hyperlipidemia, and insulin resistance.* Clin Cornerstone; 792:61–72.

[28] Ford ES, Giles WH, Dietz WH. (2002). *Prevalence of the metabolic syndrome among US adults: findings from the third National Health and Nutrition Examination Survey.* JAMA; 287:356–9.

[29] Gerstein HC, Mann JF, Yi Q, et al. (2001) *HOPE Study Investigators Albuminuria and risk of cardiovascular events, death, and heart failure in diabetic and nondiabetic individuals* JAMA;286:421–6.

[30] Golden SH, Folsom AR, Coresh J et al. (2002). *Risk factor grouping related to insulin resistance and their synergistic effects on subclinical atherosclerosis: the atherosclerosis risk in communities study.* Diabetes; 51:3069-76.

[31] Grundy SM, Cleeman JI, Daniels SR, et al. (2005). *Diagnosis and management of the metabolic syndrome: an American Heart Association/National Heart, Lung, and Blood Institute Scientific Statement.* Circulation; 112:2735.

[32] Grundy SM., Brewer HB.Jr., Cleeman JI. et al. (2004). *Definition of Metabolic Syndrome.* Report of the National Heart, Lung, and Blood Institute/American Heart Association Conference on Scientific Issues Related to Definition of Metabolic Syndrome. Circulation; 109: 433-438.

[33] Grundy SM (2006): *Metabolic syndrome: connecting and reconciling cardiovascular and diabetes worlds.* J Am Coll Cardiol 47:1093–1100, 2006.

[34] Grundy SM (2006): *Does the metabolic syndrome exist?* Diabetes Care 29:1689–1692,

[35] Haller H. (1977) "*Epidermiology and associated risk factors of hyperlipoproteinemia.*" Zeitschrift fur die gesamte innere Medizin und ihre Grenzgebiete, 32 (8): 124–8.

[36] Heart Protection Study Collaborative Group (2003), MRC/BHF Heart Protection Study of cholesterol-lowering with simvastatin in 5963 people with diabetes: a randomised placebo-controlled trial. Lancet;361:2005-16

[37] Hu FB, Manson JE, Stampfer MJ, et al (2001). *Diet, lifestyle, and the risk of type 2 diabetes mellitus in women.* N Engl J Med; 345: 790-7

[38] Isomaa B et al. (2001) *Multiple Cardiometabolic Risk (history).* Diabetes Care; 24:683-689

[39] Johnson LW, Weinstock RS. (2006). *The metabolic syndrome: concepts and controversy.* Mayo Clin Proc. Dec;81(12):1615-20.

[40] Julius S., Nesbitt SD (1996) *Sympathetic nervous system as a coronary risk factor in hypertension.* Cardiologia (Rome), Volume: 41, Issue: 4, Pages: 309-317

[41] Kahn R, Buse J, Ferrannini E, et al. (2005). *The metabolic syndrome: time for a critical appraisal: joint statement from the American Diabetes Association and the European Association for the Study of Diabetes. Diabetes Care*; 28(9) :2289-2304.

[42] Kahn R. *Metabolic syndrome – what is the clinical usefulness?* Lancet 371 (9628): 1892–1893.

[43] Kogiso T, Moriyoshi Y, Shimizu S et al. (2009). *High-sensitivity C-reactive protein as a serum predictor of nonalcoholic fatty liver disease based on the Akaike Information Criterion scoring system in the general Japanese population.* J. Gastroenterol. 44 (4): 313–21 ;

[44] Kumada M, Kihara S, Ouchi N et al. (2004) *Adiponectin specifically increased tissue inhibitor of metalloproteinase-1 through interleukin-10 expression in human macrophages.* Circulation;109:2046-9

[45] Lemieux I, Alméras N, Mauriège P, et al. (2002). *Prevalence of "hypertriglyceridemic waist" in men who participated in the Québec Health Survey: Association with atherogenic and diabetogenic metabolic risk factors.* Can J Cardiol;18:725-32.

[46] Lindström J, Louheranta A, Mannelin M. et al. (2003) *The Finnish Diabetes Prevention Study (DPS): Lifestyle intervention and 3-year results on diet and physical activity. Diabetes Care*;26:3230-6.

[47] Matsuzawa Y et al. (2004). *Adiponectin and Metabolic Syndrome.* Arteriosclerosis, Thrombosis and Vascular Biology;24:29-33.

[48] Matsuzawa Y et al. (2002). *Establishing the concept of visceral fat syndrome and clarifying its molecular mechanisms.* JMAJ 45:103-110.

[49] Meigs, JB. (2006). *Metabolic syndrome and the risk for type 2 diabetes.* Expert Rev Endocrin Metab

[50] Meigs JB, Wilson PWF, Nathan DM et al. (2003). *Prevalence and characteristics of the metabolic syndrome in the San Antonio Heart and Framingham Offspring Studies.* Diabetes 52: 2160-2167.

[51] Meigs, JB., D'Agostino, R. B., Sr, Wilson, PW, et al (1997). *Risk variable clustering in the insulin resistance syndrome: the Framingham Offspring Study.* Diabetes 46: 1594–1600.

[52] Miyoshi Y, Funahashi T, Kihara S et al. (2003). *Association of serum adiponectin levels with breast cancer risk.* Clin Cancer Res;9:5699-704

[53] Mulè G, Nardi E, Cottone P, et al. (2005). *Influence of metabolic syndrome on hypertension related to target organ damage.* J Intern Med;257: 503-13

[54] Nakamura T, Tokunga K, Shimomura I et al. (1994). *Contribution of visceral fat accumulation to the development of coronary artery disease in non-obese men. Atherosclerosis*;107:239-46.

[55] Nathan DM, Buse JB, Davidson MB, et al. (2006). *Management of hyperglycemia in type 2 diabetes: A consensus algorithm for the initiation and adjustment of therapy: a consensus statement from the American Diabetes Association and the European Association for the Study of Diabetes.* Diabetes Care;29:1963-72

[56] Nesto RW. (2003) *The relation of insulin resistance syndromes to risk of CVD.* Rev Cardiovasc Med;4(6):S11-S18.

[57] Nicholls SJ, Tuzcu EM, Sipahi I; et al.(2007) *Statins, high-density lipoprotein cholesterol, and regression of coronary atherosclerosis.* JAMA.;297(5):499-508

[58] Palaniappan L, Carnethon MR, Wang Y, et al. (2004) *Predictors of the incident metabolic syndrome in adults: the Insulin Resistance Atherosclerosis Study*. Diabetes Care; 27:788.
[59] Phillips GB. (1978) *Sex hormones, risk factors and cardiovascular disease*. The American Journal of Medicine 1978, 65 (1): 7–11
[60] Praga M. (2002) *Obesity – a neglected culprit in renal disease*. Nephrol Dial Transplant; 17:1157–9
[61] Reaven GM. Banting Lecture 1988. *Role of insulin resistance in human disease*. Diabetes; 37:1595–607.
[62] Ridker PM, Wilson PW, Grundy SM. (2004*) Should C-reactive protein be added to metabolic syndrome and to assessment of global cardiovascular risk?* Circulation Jun 15;109(23):2818-2825.
[63] Robins SJ, Rubins HB, Faas FH et al. (2003) Insulin *resistance and cardiovascular events with low HDL cholesterol*. Diabetes Care;26(5):1513-7.
[64] Robins SJ, Rubins HB, Faas FH et al.(2003) *Insulin resistance and cardiovascular events with low HDL cholesterol (VA-HIT trial)*. Diabetes Care; 26(5):1513-7
[65] Sacks FM for the HDL Expert Group on HDL cholesterol (2002) *The role of high-density lipoprotein (HDL) cholesterol in the prevention and treatment of coronary heart disease: expert group recommendations*. J Cardiol 90:139-143.
[66] Shinozaki K, Ayajiki K, Nishio Y, et al. (2004) *Evidence for a causal role of the renin-angiotensin system in vascular dysfunction associated with insulin resistance*. Hypertension; 43:255–62
[67] Simmons RK, Alberti KG, Gale EA, et al. (2010) *The metabolic syndrome: useful concept or clinical tool?* Report of a WHO Expert Consultation. Diabetologia; 53(4):600-5.
[68] Singer P. (1977) *Diagnosis of primary hyperlipoproteinemias*. Zeitschrift fur die gesamte innere Medizin und ihre Grenzgebiete , 32 (9): 129–33.
[69] Smith SR. (2006) *Importance of Diagnosing and Treating the Metabolic Syndrome in Reducing Cardiovascular Risk*. Obesity 14, 128S–134S
[70] Spellman CW., Chemitiganti R (2010) *Metabolic syndrome: More questions than answers?* JAOA,Vol 110, No 3,suppl 3, , 18-22
[71] *Stedman's Online Medical Dictionary*: http://www.stedmans.com.
[72] Stern M, Williams K, Gonzalez-Villalpando C et al. (2004) *Does the metabolic syndrome improve identification of individuals at risk of type 2 diabetes and/or cardiovascular disease?* Diabetes Care;27(11):2676-81
[73] Sundström J, Vallhagen E, Risérus U, et al. (2006) *Risk associated with the metabolic syndrome versus the sum of its individual components*. Diabetes Care; 29:1673.
[74] The Task Force for the management of dyslipidaemias of the European Society of Cardiology (ESC) and the European Atherosclerosis Society (EAS) ESC/EAS Guidelines for the management of dyslipidaemias European Heart Journal (2011) 32, 1769–1818 doi:10.1093/eurheartj/ehr158
[75] Third report of the National Cholesterol Education Program (NCEP) expert panel on detection, evaluation, and treatment of high blood cholesterol in adults (Adult Treatment Panel III). Final report. Circulation 2002; 106: 3143–3421.
[76] Tuomilehto J, Lindström J, Eriksson JG et al. (2001*) Prevention of Type 2 diabetes mellitus by changes in lifestyle among subjects with impaired glucose tolerance*. NEJM; 344:1343-50
[77] Vague J. (1947) *Sexual differentiation, a factor affecting the forms of obesity*. Presse Méd; 30:339-40.

[78] Watson, Karol (2007) Managing Cardiometabolic Risk: *An Evolving Approach to Patient Care Critical Pathways in Cardiology:* A Journal of Evidence-Based Medicine: March - Volume 6 - Issue 1 - pp 5-14

[79] Weisberg SP, McCann D, Desai M, et al. (2003) *Obesity is associated with macrophage accumulation in adipose tissue.* J Clin Invest; 112:1796–1808.

[80] Weyer C, Funahashi T, Tanaka S et al. (2001) *Hypoadiponectinemia in obesity and type 2 diabetes: close association with insulin resistance and hyperinsulinemia.* J Clin Endocrinol Metab; 86:1930-5

[81] Wilcox I., McNamara SG., Collins FL., et al (1998) *Syndrome Z: the interaction of sleep apnoea, vascular risk factors and heart disease* Thorax; 53:S25-S28

[82] www.idf.org

[83] www.metabolicsyndromeinstitut/informations/screeningdiagnosis/procedures-for-the-measurement-of-the-waist-circumference.php

[84] Zeller M, Steg PG, Ravisy J, et al. (2005) *Prevalence and impact of metabolic syndrome on hospital outcomes in acute myocardial infarction.* Arch Intern Med;165:1192-8

[85] Zimmet P, Alberti KGMM, Shaw J. (2001) Global and societal implications of the diabetes epidemic. Nature; 414:782-7.

12

The Relationship Between AST/ALT Ratio and Metabolic Syndrome in Han Young Adults – AST/ALT Ratio and Metabolic Syndrome

Qiang Lu[1], Xiaoli Liu[1],
Shuhua Liu[2], Changshun Xie[3],
Yali Liu[4] and Chunming Ma[1]
[1]*Department of Endocrinology,*
[2]*Department of Cardiology,*
[3]*Department of Gastroenterology,*
[4]*Medical Examination Center,*
The First Hospital of Qinhuangdao,
Qinhuangdao, Hebei Province,
China

1. Introduction

In previous studies, the relationship between aspartate aminotransferase to alanine aminotransferase ratio(AST/ALT ratio) and liver disease has been evaluated. In viral hepatitis, alcoholic liver disease and primary biliary cirrhosis, AST/ALT ratio has been proven to be an indicator of liver cirrhosis.[1-3] AST/ALT ratio was a potential value in differentiating nonalcoholic steatohepatitis from alcoholic liver disease.The value < 1 suggestted nonalcoholic steatohepatitis, a ratio of ≥ 2 was strongly suggestive of alcoholic liver disease.[4]

Nonalcoholic fatty liver disease(NAFLD) is the most common cause of elevated liver enzymes and also one of the most common forms of liver disease in the world.[5] The AST/ALT ratio of the ultrasound-diagnosed NAFLD patients was lower than controls.[6] AST/ALT ratio < 1 was common NAFLD-related feature.[7] NAFLD is now considered the hepatic manifestation of the metabolic syndrome. When compared with individuals without NAFLD, individuals with NAFLD had significantly higher fasting glucose, insulin, low-density lipoprotein cholesterol, triglycerides, systolic blood pressure and diastolic blood pressure.[8] Recently, NAFLD marker the AST/ALT ratio have attracted great interest as potential novel marker of metabolic syndrome.[9]

Very little information was available about the association of AST/ALT ratio with metabolic syndrome in Han young adults. Thus, this study evaluated the relationship between AST/ALT ratio and metabolic syndrome in Han young adults.

2. Materials and methods

2.1 Subjects

After obtaining the informed consent from all subjects, a cross-sectional, population-based study was conducted. The study population was determined according to 2-stage cluster sampling. In the first stage, a random sample of universities in Qinhuangdao, Hebei Province, China, were obtained; in the second stage, young adults aged 19 to 24 years, randomly selected from these schools, were invited to participate. In the end, 425 Han young adults(males/females 216/209) participated in 2009. Subjects with evidence of alcohol intake, hepatitis B (hepatitis B surface antigen), hepatitis C (hepatitis C antibody), autoimmune hepatitis (antinuclear antibody and anti-smooth muscle antibody) and drug toxicity were excluded. The study protocol was approved and supervised by the ethical committee of the First Hospital of Qinhuangdao.

2.2 Measurements

Anthropometric measurements, including height, weight and waist circumference(WC) were performed when subjects were without shoes and in light clothing. Height and weight were measured to the nearest 0.1 cm and 0.1 kg, respectively. Standing height without shoes was measured three times with a stadiometer, and the three measurements were averaged for analysis. Body mass index (BMI) was defined as weight (kg) divided by height (m) squared. Blood pressure was measured three times with a mercury sphygmomanometer while the subjects were seated after 10 min of rest, and the three measurements were averaged for analysis.

After an overnight fast of 10-12h, blood samples were drawn from an antecubital vein in each subjects into vacutainer tubes. Fasting plasma glucose(FPG) concentration was measured using the glucose oxidase method, serum lipids and alanine aminotransferase (ALT) and aspartate alanine aminotransferase (AST) were measured using enzymatic procedures with an autoanalyzer (Hitachi, Tokyo, Japan). Serum true insulin(TI) was measured using enzyme linked immunosorbent assay(ELISA) with model 680 microplate reader(BIO-RAD, America).The ELISA kits were purchased from USCNLIFE company, America. The following equation for homeostasis model assessment of insulin resistance(HOMA-IR) was used: fasting insulin level (μU/ml) x fasting glucose level (mmol/l)/22.5.

2.3 Definition for metabolic syndrome

Metabolic syndrome was defined as having ≥3 of the 5 factors with the following cut points: abdominal obesity (waist circumference ≥90cm in males and 80 cm in females); high triglycerides(≥1.70mmol/L [150mg/dL]); low high density lipoprotein cholesterol (HDL-C) (<1.03 mmol/L[40mg/dL] for males and <1.30 mmol/L [50 mg/dL] for females); elevated blood pressure (systolic blood pressure≥135mmHg and/or diastolic blood pressure≥85mmHg) and impaired fasting glucose(≥5.6mmol/L[100mg/dL]).[10]

2.4 Statistical analysis

Data are expressed as mean ± standard deviation(SD) or medians with interquartile ranges(IQR).When data was not normally distributed, they were ln transformed for analysis. Continuous variables were analyzed with covariance adjustment for age and sex. To measure the strength of association between 2 variables, partial correlation analysis was used adjustment for age and sex. The χ^2 test was used to test for differences in proportions. To examine the association between AST/ALT ratio and metabolic syndrome, multivariate logistic regression was tested. The results of the logistic regression analysis were expressed as odds ratios with 95% confidence intervals(CI). Analyses were performed with the computer software SPSS version 11.5 software(SPSS Inc., Chicago, IL, U.S.A.). Statistical significance was established at $P<0.05$.

3. Results

3.1 Clinical and laboratory characteristics

In this sample, AST/ALT ratio < 1 was detected in 146 subjects (34.4%). Males had a significantly higher frequency of AST/ALT ratio < 1 than females(48.6% *vs* 19.6%,χ^2 = 39.595,P=0.000). The age was similar in two groups(20.3±0.8 *vs* 20.3±0.8, t=0.057,P=0.955). Table 1 showed clinical and laboratory characteristics in the study subjects. After adjustment for age and sex, young adults with AST/ALT ratio < 1 had higher BMI, WC, SBP, DBP, TG, TI and HOMA-IR than subjects with AST/ALT ratio ≥ 1. Subjects with AST/ALT ratio < 1 also had significantly lower HDL-C than subjects with AST/ALT ratio ≥ 1 ($P<0.05$). The level of FPG was similar between subjects with AST/ALT ratio < 1 and ≥ 1 ($P>0.05$).(Table 1)

Associations of AST/ALT ratio with anthropometric and metabolic variables were presented in Table 2. After adjustment for age and sex, AST/ALT ratio showed positive correlations with HDL-C and negative correlations with BMI, WC, TG, TI and HOMA-IR ($P<0.05$). (Table 2)

3.2 AST/ALT ratio and metabolic syndrome

The prevalence of metabolic syndrome was 2.1% and was similar in males and females(2.3% *vs* 1.9%,χ^2 = 0.082,P= 0.774). Subjects with AST/ALT ratio < 1 had a significantly higher frequency of abdominal obesity, high triglycerides, elevated blood pressure and metabolic syndrome($P<0.05$). (Table 3) After adjustment for age, sex and BMI, the frequency of metabolic syndrome among young adults with AST/ALT ratio < 1 was 6.975(95%CI: 1.430 to 34.019, P=0.016) times compared with young adults with AST/ALT ratio ≥ 1.

4. Discussion

Using Adult Treatment Panel III criteria's definition, we estimated that approximately 2.1% of Han young adults have the metabolic syndrome. The prevalence of metabolic syndrome in this study was lower than previously report from Chinese adults and was similar to Chinese adolescents.[11,12] It was because of a positive effect of age on the prevalence of metabolic syndrome.[13,14] Abdominal obesity, elevated blood pressure and low HDL-C were common components of the metabolic syndrome in this sample. In the insulin resistance atherosclerosis study, NAFLD marker the AST/ALT ratio predict metabolic syndrome independently of potential confounding variables.[15] In this study, we found that the metabolic syndrome was related with a lower AST/ALT ratio in Han young adults. Subjects with AST/ALT ratio < 1 had a significantly higher frequency of abdominal obesity, high triglycerides, elevated blood pressure and metabolic syndrome. The association was not modified by age, sex and BMI.

variable	AST/ALT level ratio≥1 (n=279)	AST/ALT level ratio< 1 (n=146)	*P*
Age(years) mean(SD)	20.3(0.8)	20.3(0.8)	0.955
Sex(male/female)	111/168	105/41	0.000
BMI(kg/m^2) mean(SD)	22.9(3.8)	26.3(4.0)	0.000
WC(cm) mean(SD)	70.8(9.3)	81.4(12.3)	0.000
SBP(mmHg) mean(SD)	109.3(10.7)	115.2(11.5)	0.004
DBP(mmHg) mean (SD)	73.1(8.2)	76.7(9.9)	0.030
FPG(mmol/L) mean (SD)	4.30(0.44)	4.38(0.40)	0.101
TG(mmol/L) mean (SD)	0.69(0.24)	0.83(0.46)	0.000
HDL-C(mmol/L) mean (SD)	1.42(0.22)	1.30(0.24)	0.001
TI(uU/ml) median (IQR)	6.58(3.88)	7.75(4.86)	0.014
HOMA-IR median(IQR)	1.25(0.76)	1.53(1.08)	0.006
ALT(U/L) mean(SD)	10.6(5.0)	30.6(17.3)	0.000
AST(U/L) mean(SD)	17.9(6.0)	20.6(8.5)	0.223

Data are expressed as mean ± standard deviation(SD) or medians with interquartile ranges(IQR). Continuous variables were analyzed with covariance adjustment for age and sex. When data was not normally distributed, they were ln transformed for analysis. ALT: alanine aminotransferase; AST: aspartate aminotransferase; BMI: body mass index; WC: waist circumference; SBP: systolic blood press; DBP: diastolic blood press; FPG: fasting plasma glucose; TG: triglycerides; HDL-C: high density lipoprotein cholesterol; TI: true insulin; HOMA-IR: homeostasis model assessment of insulin resistance; SD: standard deviation; IQR:indicates interquartile range.

Table 1. Clinical and laboratory characteristics of the subjects in different levels of AST/ALT ratio.

variable	*r*	*P**	*r*	*P***
BMI(kg/m^2)	-0.296	0.000	-0.281	0.000
WC(cm)	-0.310	0.000	-0.264	0.000
SBP(mmHg)	-0.141	0.004	-0.072	0.134
DBP(mmHg)	-0.102	0.036	-0.048	0.321
FPG(mmol/L)	-0.051	0.295	-0.039	0.413
TG(mmol/L)	-0.134	0.006	-0.134	0.006
HDL-C(mmol/L)	0.174	0.000	0.125	0.010
TI(uU/ml)	-0.154	0.001	-0.118	0.015
HOMA-IR	-0.158	0.001	-0.121	0.012

*Pearson correlation.**Partial correlation analysis, adjustment for age and sex. ALT: alanine aminotransferase; AST: aspartate aminotransferase; BMI: body mass index; WC: waist circumference; SBP: systolic blood press; DBP: diastolic blood press; FPG: fasting plasma glucose; TG: triglycerides; HDL-C: high density lipoprotein cholesterol; TI: true insulin; HOMA-IR: homeostasis model assessment of insulin resistance.

Table 2 Correlation analysis of AST/ALT ratio with anthropometric and metabolic variables in Han young aduts.

Factor	AST/ALT level ratio≥1 (n=279)	AST/ALT level ratio< 1 (n=146)	*P*
abdominal obesity(%)	9.7	32.2	0.000
high triglycerides(%)	0.0	3.4	0.008
low high density lipoprotein cholesterol(%)	15.1	21.2	0.109
elevated blood pressure(%)	12.9	25.3	0.001
impaired fasting glucose(%)	0.7	0.0	0.548
metabolic syndrome(%)	0.7	4.8	0.016

The χ^2 test was used to test for differences in proportions. ALT: alanine aminotransferase; AST: aspartate aminotransferase.

Table 3 Prevalence of metabolic syndrome in different levels of AST/ALT ratio(%).

In our study, AST/ALT ratio showed negative correlation with HOMA-IR. Insulin resistance is a central feature in the pathogenesis of metabolic syndrome,while insulin resistance is now considered the main link between metabolic disturbances and liver enzymes. Hanley AJ et al.[16] reported that AST/ALT ratio was associated with directly measured insulin sensitivity when conventionally availables were adjusted. This result can be explained by the following possible mechanism. Liver markers were known to be significantly correlated with increased hepatic fat content.[17] Liver fat content was a significant risk factor of HOMA-IR while BMI and waist circumference were not.[18]

In our study, we found that young adults with AST/ALT ratio < 1 had higher TI than subjects with AST/ALT ratio ≥ 1. But the level of FPG was similar between subjects with AST/ALT ratio < 1 and ≥ 1. The liver plays an important role in maintaining normal glucose concentrations during fasting as well as postprandially. The loss of a direct effect of insulin to suppress hepatic glucose production and glycogenolysis in the liver causes an increase in hepatic glucose production.[19] Increased insulin levels with increasing insulin resistance in subjects with AST/ALT ratio < 1 suggested that elevated insulin concentrations reflected increased beta cell output to the elevated insulin concentrations. The hyperinsulinemia can thus be seen as a compensatory mechanism for the preexisting insulin resistance, which represents a mechanism for protection against the development of impaired fasting glucose and diabetes. T2DM will result when there is insufficient insulin secretion to counter preexisting insulin resistance.[20]

Diet habit modifies the relationship of the liver enzymes ratio with metabolic syndrome. For example, Mediterranean diet moderates the association of the liver enzymes ratio with the prevalence of the metabolic syndrome.[9] In China, people's eating habits are quite different in different area. Regrettably, diet habit was not evaluated in our study. This is a limitation of our study.

In conclusion, the prevalence of metabolic syndrome was low in Han young adults. AST/ALT ratio was related with metabolic syndrome in Han young adults.

5. References

[1] Nyblom H, Björnsson E, Simrén M, Aldenborg F, Almer S, Olsson R. The AST/ALT ratio as an indicator of cirrhosis in patients with PBC. Liver Int. 2006;26:840-845.

[2] Giannini E, Risso D, Botta F, Chiarbonello B, Fasoli A, Malfatti F, Romagnoli P, Testa E, Ceppa P, Testa R. Validity and clinical utility of the aspartate aminotransferase-alanine aminotransferase ratio in assessing disease severity and prognosis in patients with hepatitis C virus-related chronic liver disease. Arch Intern Med. 2003;163:218-224.

[3] Nyblom H, Berggren U, Balldin J, Olsson R. High AST/ALT ratio may indicate advanced alcoholic liver disease rather than heavy drinking. Alcohol Alcohol. 2004;39:336-339.

[4] Sorbi D, Boynton J, Lindor KD. The ratio of aspartate aminotransferase to alanine aminotransferase: potential value in differentiating nonalcoholic steatohepatitis from alcoholic liver disease. Am J Gastroenterol. 1999;94:1018-1022.

[5] Kim CH, Younossi ZM. Nonalcoholic fatty liver disease: a manifestation of the metabolic syndrome. Cleve Clin J Med. 2008;75:721-728.

[6] Lee S, Jin Kim Y, Yong Jeon T, Hoi Kim H, Woo Oh S, Park Y, Soo Kim S.Obesity is the only independent factor associated with ultrasound-diagnosed non-alcoholic fatty liver disease: a cross-sectional case-control study. Scand J Gastroenterol. 2006;41:566-572.

[7] Khurram M, Ashraf MM. A clinical and biochemical profile of biopsy-proven non-alcoholic Fatty liver disease subjects. J Coll Physicians Surg Pak. 2007;17:531-534.

[8] Schwimmer JB, Pardee PE, Lavine JE, Blumkin AK, Cook S. Cardiovascular risk factors and the metabolic syndrome in pediatric nonalcoholic fatty liver disease. Circulation. 2008;118:277-283.

[9] Tzima N, Pitsavos C, Panagiotakos DB, Chrysohoou C, Polychronopoulos E, Skoumas J, Stefanadis C. Adherence to the Mediterranean diet moderates the association of aminotransferases with the prevalence of the metabolic syndrome; the ATTICA study. Nutr Metab (Lond). 2009;6:30.

[10] Expert Panel on Detection, Evaluation, and Treatment of High Blood Cholesterol in Adults. Executive Summary of the Third Report of the National Cholesterol Education Program(NCEP) expert panel on detection, evaluation, and treatment of high blood cholesterol in adults(Adult Treatment Panel III) .JAMA. 2001;285:2486-2497.

[11] Gu D, Reynolds K, Wu X, Chen J, Duan X, Reynolds RF, Whelton PK, He J; InterASIA Collaborative Group. Prevalence of the metabolic syndrome and overweight among adults in China. Lancet. 2005;365:1398-1405.

[12] Li Y, Yang X, Zhai F, Kok FJ, Zhao W, Piao J, Zhang J, Cui Z, Ma G. Prevalence of the metabolic syndrome in Chinese adolescents. Br J Nutr. 2008;99:565-570.

[13] Ford ES, Giles WH, Dietz WH. Prevalence of the metabolic syndrome among US adults: findings from the third National Health and Nutrition Examination Survey. JAMA. 2002;287:356-359.

[14] Sharifi F, Mousavinasab SN, Saeini M, Dinmohammadi M. Prevalence of metabolic syndrome in an adult urban population of the west of Iran. Exp Diabetes Res. 2009;2009:136501.

[15] Hanley AJ, Williams K, Festa A, Wagenknecht LE, D'Agostino RB Jr, Haffner SM. Liver markers and development of the metabolic syndrome: the insulin resistance atherosclerosis study. Diabetes. 2005;54:3140-3147.

[16] Hanley AJ, Wagenknecht LE, Festa A, D'Agostino RB Jr, Haffner SM. Alanine aminotransferase and directly measured insulin sensitivity in a multiethnic cohort: the Insulin Resistance Atherosclerosis Study. Diabetes Care. 2007;30:1819-1827.

[17] Browning JD, Szczepaniak LS, Dobbins R, Nuremberg P, Horton JD, Cohen JC, Grundy SM, Hobbs HH. Prevalence of hepatic steatosis in an urban population in the United States: impact of ethnicity. Hepatology. 2004;40:1387-1395.

[18] Yan HM, Gao X, Liu M, Gu Q, Zhang B, Li X. Relationship of liver fat content to insulin resistance and metabolic syndrome.Zhonghua Yi Xue Za Zhi 2008;88:1255-1258.

[19] Michael MD, Kulkarni RN, Postic C, Previs SF, Shulman GI, Magnuson MA, Kahn CR. Loss of insulin signaling in hepatocytes leads to severe insulin resistance and progressive hepatic dysfunction. Mol Cell 2000,6:87–97.
[20] Ten S, Maclaren N. Insulin resistance syndrome in children. J Clin Endocrinol Metab 2004;89:2526-2539.

13

On the Mechanism of Action of Prolylcarboxypeptidase

B. Shariat-Madar[1], M. Taherian[2] and Z. Shariat-Madar[3]
[1]*College of Literature, Science, and the Arts, University of Michigan, Ann Arber, MI,*
[2]*Department of Anesthesia, Massachusetts General Hospital, Harvard Medical School, Boston, MA,*
[3]*School of Pharmacy, Department of Pharmacology, University of Mississippi, University, MS, USA*

1. Introduction

Many mechanisms are involved in the regulation of blood pressure. Among the molecules, hormones, and factors known to be involved in blood pressure regulation, PRCP can generate the most potent inflammatory vasodilator molecules, including nitric oxide (Zhao et al., 2001c), prostaglandins (Kolte et al., 2011), bradykinin (BK)-(Chajkowski et al., 2010) and angiotensin 1-7 (Ang_{1-7})-(Mallela et al., 2008) dependent pathways in the endothelium and astrocytes. Experimental evidence suggest that PRCP appears to metabolize its main substrates, des-Arg^9-bradykinin (des-Arg^9-BK, BK_{1-8})(Chajkowski et al., 2010) and alpha-melanocyte stimulating hormone 1-13 (α-MSH_{1-13})(Wallingford et al., 2009), to prevent the production of prostaglandins and NO, indicating that the enzyme may promote anti-inflammatory effects in cardiovascular and cerebrovascular systems. Evidence shows that *Prcp* gene expression is elevated in the developing murine brain vasculature during the intermediate phase of chick chorio-allantoic membrane (CAM)(Javerzat et al., 2009), suggesting that PRCP has a role during the active phase of vascular remodeling. Interestingly, *Prcp* gene is overexpressed in glioblastoma and it is suggested that PRCP also has a role in tumor angiogenesis(Javerzat et al., 2009). Thus, PRCP plays important roles in response to stress and may be an endothelial gate-keeper regulating blood flow, which tightly regulates endothelial barrier function. The historical perspective of knowledge of PRCP and its roles in physiological and cardiovascular diseases such as inflammation, hypertension, thrombosis, and obesity is tabulated in Table 1.

2. Cardiovascular system function

The cardiovascular system is composed of the heart, blood, and a complex network of blood vessels. Humans have a closed cardiovascular system in which the system allows a complete separation of function and blood loss due to having a relatively low blood volume compared to species with open cardiovascular systems. In a closed cardiovascular system, blood flows rapidly from arteries to capillaries and returns through the venous system. The heart sustains the high pressure necessary for the blood to reach the body's tissues.

Year		References
1971	Human PRCP (EC 3.4.16.2) was found in biological fluids	(Sorrells and Erdos, 1971)
1978	PRCP was purified from human kidney and its potential substrates was reported. The two substrates were angiotensin II, and angiotensin III	(Odya et al., 1978)
1981	A novel and rapid radioassay for PRCP was developed	(Skidgel et al., 1981)
1981	PRCP was found in both inflammatory exudates and in cells that appear at sites of inflammation	(Kumamoto et al., 1981)
1990	Cultured Madin-Darby canine kidney (MDCK) distal tubular cells was found to contain PRCP	(Deddish et al., 1990)
1993	Human PRCP was sequenced and cloned. It was noted that PRCP might have both exopeptidase and endopeptidase activities	(Tan et al., 1993)
1994	PRCP was found to have a modulatory role in the angiotensin II-induced pulmonary vasoconstriction	(Tamaoki et al., 1994)
1995	PRCP was found in monkey kidney	(Suzawa et al., 1995)
1995	PRCP was purified from cell free extracts of Xanthomonas maltophilia, a bacteria species which is normally found in clinical specimens	(Suga et al., 1995)
1995	PRCP was found to be highly active in macrophages	(Jackman et al., 1995)
1997	Watson and associates described localization of *Prcp* gene	(Watson, Jr. et al., 1997)
2002	PRCP was found to be an endothelial cell prekallikrein activator	(Shariat-Madar et al., 2002)
2002	Moreira and associates described the extracellular PRCP that activates prekallikrein	(Moreira et al., 2002)
2005	Overexpression of PRCP on Chinese hamster ovary cells was reported	(Shariat-Madar et al., 2005)
2006	Wang and associates described the functional significance of PRCP in the etiology of preeclampsia	(Wang et al., 2006)
2007	Hooley and associates described a C-terminal extension in the PK serine protease domain as a potential substrate for PRCP.	(Hooley et al., 2007)
2009	Wallingford and associates described that *Prcp*-null mice had elevated levels of alpha-MSH1-13 in the hypothalamus and were leaner and shorter than the wild-type controls on a regular chow diet. *Prcp* null mice were also resistant to high-fat diet-induced obesity	(Wallingford et al., 2009)
2009	Soisson and associates described the crystal structure of human PRCP	(Soisson et al., 2010)
2009	E112D polymorphism in the prolylcarboxypeptidase gene was found to be associated with blood pressure response to benazepril in Chinese hypertensive patients	(ZHANG Yan et al., 2009)
2009	Javerzat and associates described overexpression of PRCP during the intermediate phase of the chick chorio-allantoic membrane	(Javerzat et al., 2009)
2010	Recombinant PRCP (rPRCP) metabolized BK_{1-8} to BK_{1-7}, whereas rPRCP was ineffective in metabolizing BK 1-9	(Chajkowski et al., 2010)
2010	PRCP was found to be active in human cerebrospinal fluid	(Zhao et al., 2010)
2010	Overexpression of angiotensin type 2 (AT2) receptor in mouse coronary artery endothelial cells was found to increase expression of PRCP, which may contribute to kinin release	(Zhu et al., 2010)
2011	PRCP is a 4OHTAM resistance factor in estrogen receptor-positive breast cancer cells	(Duan et al., 2011)
2011	$PRCP^{gt/gt}$ mice were found to be hypertensive and prothrombotic	(Adams et al., 2011)

Table 1. Historical Perspective

To deal with proper delivery of blood to the tissues as well as many types of insults, including chemical and physical damage as well as infection, the cardiovascular system has evolved an intricate multilayer of specialized biochemical pathways. Multiple feedback mechanisms controlling blood flow with contrasting effects regulate normal vascular function, which have either stimulatory or inhibitory effects. These features enable the cardiovascular system to perform its tasks effectively. Of these regulatory feedback machinery, a few have multiple and redundant control mechanisms that tightly uphold cardiovascular functions. Among these regulatory feedback mechanisms within the mammalian cardiovascular system, we review the renin-angiotensin(Savinetskaia et al., 2008; Hayashi et al., 2010), kallikrein-kinin(Bryant and Shariat-Madar, 2009; Saxena et al., 2011), and pro-opiomelanocortin (POMC) (Wang et al., 2008) systems that communicate with each other. Although within each of these systems are surely a network of molecular interactions with other pathways, their interactions are not either compared or reviewed. However, special attention is given to the role of PRCP in health and disease.

2.1 Renin-angiotensin system (RAS)

The systemic RAS is a complex, but fairly well understood pathway(Perret-Guillaume et al., 2009; Molteni, 1982; Brown et al., 1983; Oishi et al., 1996; Renshaw et al., 2001; Hettinger et al., 2002; Volzke et al., 2005; Clerk et al., 2005). Although the physiological importance of the RAS for regulation of blood pressure and water homeostasis has been established(Fukuchi et al., 1973; Bing and Nielsen, 1973), emerging evidence suggests that the components of RAS are important players for maintenance and regulation of many physiological and pathophysiological processes, such as angiogenesis (Abali et al., 2002), inflammation (Akishita et al., 2001), tumorigenesis(Ager et al., 2008), thrombosis (Asselbergs et al., 2008; Asselbergs et al., 2007), vascular hypertrophy (Brede et al., 2001), vascular development (Lasaitiene et al., 2006), and remodeling (Akishita et al., 2000; Alcazar et al., 2009). The molecular mechanisms by which the components of RAS exert their pleiotropic effects are redundant in order to ensure an appropriate balance between the stimulatory and inhibitory signals favoring normal blood delivery. More interestingly, there is also a balance between RAS function and its counter-regulatory hormones, in particular plasma kinins, the main effectors of the plasma Kallikrein-Kinin System (KKS) (Shariat-Madar et al., 2002a). The active metabolites of these two systems regulate each other in an antagonistic manner. In view of the opposing effects of these two systems(Bader, 2001), the complex interplay of RAS and KKS with the local microenvironment of endothelial cells lining blood vessels is responsible for delivering nutrients. The RAS and KKS signaling pathways are also responsible for sustaining the high pressure necessary for the blood to reach all of the tissues of the body while maintaining blood pressure within a narrow range.

The RAS encompasses numerous peptides that act in concert in a cascade triggered by low blood volume or a drop in blood pressure cascades or water-fall(Taquini, Jr. and Taquini, 1961; Nicholls and Robertson, 2000; Shariat-Madar and Schmaier, 2004; Ritz, 2005; Oudart, 2005). These peptides exert their actions, which can be autocrine (Chan and Wong, 1996), paracrine (Haulica et al., 2005), or endocrine(Gohlke et al., 1992), acting through specific cell surface receptors on their target cells to control blood pressure and body fluid homeostasis. In a stepwise enzymatic process, the aspartyl protease renin (a rate-limiting enzyme) cleaves circulating angiotensinogen to the inactive angiotensin I (Ang I) (Helmer, 1965). Subsequently, angiotensin converting enzyme (ACE) cleaves the two C-terminal amino acid residues of Ang I to generate the key effector of RAS, angiotensin II (Ang II, Ang $_{1\text{-}8}$) under physiological conditions (Figure 1)(Peart, 1975). However, the tonin-, cathepsin G-, tissue plasminogen activator- or chymase-induced Ang II generation is apparently important under pathophysiological conditions (Doggrell and Wanstall, 2004; Doggrell and Wanstall, 2003; Leckie, 2005; Belova, 2000). Recent evidence suggests that Ang I can block a downstream protease, PRCP *in vitro* (Mallela et al., 2008). Up to now, the physiological significant role of Ang I in blocking PRCP is uncertain. Ang II primarily exerts its physiological effects by activating angiotensin type 1 (AT1) receptors (Figure 1) (Chassagne et al., 2000). However, angiotensin type 2 (AT2) receptors also appear to mediate Ang II effects (Figure 1)(Anavekar and Solomon, 2005). Activation of this signaling pathway leads to cardioprotection. Both AT1 and AT2 belong to the G-protein couple receptor (GPCR) superfamily(Ali et al., 1997a). While AT1 can couple to two members of the Gα family ($G_{\alpha q/11}$ and $G_{\alpha i}$) and to $G_{\beta\gamma}$ complexes (Okuda et al., 1996), AT2 can couple to $G_{\alpha i}$ and $G_{\alpha s}$ subunits (Kai et al., 1996).

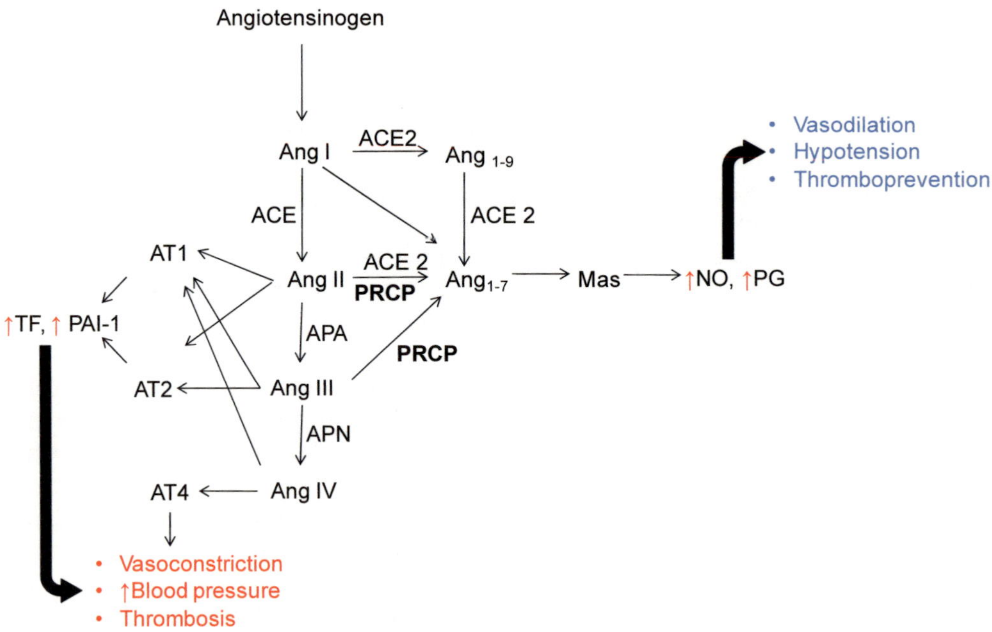

Fig. 1. Metabolites of the renin-angiotensin system influence cardiovascular system.
Ang I; Angiotensin I, **Ang II**; Angiotensin II, **Ang III**; Angiotensin III, **Ang IV**; Angiotensin IV, $Ang_{1\text{-}9}$; Angiotensin 1-9, $Ang_{1\text{-}7}$; Angiotensin 1-7, **ACE;** Angiotensin converting enzyme, **ACE2;** Angiotensin converting enzyme 2, **AT1**; angiotensin type 1, **AT2**; angiotensin type 2, **AT4**; angiotensin type 4, **PAI-1**; plasminogen activator 1, **TF**; tissue activator, **Mas**; $Ang_{1\text{-}7}$ Mas receptor, **NO**; nitric oxide, **PG**; prostaglandin.

Ang II-induced AT1 receptor-dependent vasoconstriction is mediated by activation of $G_{\alpha q/11}$, $G_{\alpha i}$, and $G_{\beta\gamma}$ complexes(Kai et al., 1996). The activation of these heterotrimeric G proteins triggers the activation of phospholipase C (PLC)(Griendling et al., 1997) and phospholipase D (PLD)(Griendling et al., 1997; Ushio-Fukai et al., 1999), leading to an increase in intracellular calcium, actin-myosin interactions, and release of leukotrienes.

Although AT2 appears to be cell-type specific with a low expression pattern in adult tissues, it is the dominate receptor in fetal tissues(Akishita et al., 1999; Guan et al., 2008). Experimental evidence in support of AT2-independent G-protein signaling pathway has been demonstrated (Bottari et al., 1991). AT2 receptors are essential for triggering vasodilation and it can also mediate cell death (Gwathmey et al., 2009). Ang II-induced AT2 receptor-dependent vasodilation is mediated by activation of nitric oxide/cyclic guanosine 3′,5′-monophosphate (cGMP) signaling cascades. On the other hand, AT2 activation by Ang II may lead to the activation of proapoptotic second messengers, MAPK phosphatase 1 (MKP-1)(Horiuchi et al., 1997), SH2 domain-containing phosphatase 1 (SHP-1)(Feng et al., 2002), and protein phosphatase 2A (PP2A)(Huang et al., 1996) and subsequent inactivation of MAPKs(Bedecs et al., 1997; Horiuchi et al., 1997), and ERK1/2(Horiuchi et al., 1997). While identification and characterization of the molecular switch that controls differential activation of distinct downstream signaling pathways by Ang II are poorly understood, our understanding of the downstream events is exponentially mounting.

In the next step of the RAS cascades, angiotensin converting enzyme 2 (ACE2) and PRCP metabolize Ang II (a prothrombotic risk factor) to angiotensin 1-7 (a vasodilator, antithrombotic factor)(Mallela et al., 2008), highlighting the functional significance of these two enzymes. Notably, ACE2 (Gurley et al., 2006) and PRCP (Adams et al., 2011)null mice do not exhibit excessive elevated blood pressure compared to control littermates, suggesting that these enzymes play a critical role in the maintenance of normal vascular physiology, Figure 1. PRCP also metabolizes angiotensin III (Ang III, $Ang_{2\text{-}8}$) to angiotensin 2-7 ($Ang_{2\text{-}7}$)(Mallela et al., 2008). Ang III, like Ang II, is also a pressor agent whose response is mediated by AT_1 receptors (Campbell et al., 1979). Ang III is implicated in cell proliferation and matrix accumulation(Ruiz-Ortega et al., 1998). Ang II- and Ang III-induced AT_1 receptor stimulation mediate vasoconstriction, mitogenic and hypertrophic effects and inflammatory responses (Ishanov et al., 1998; Schluter and Wenzel, 2008; Marshall et al., 2000). Hydrolysis of Ang III by PRCP leads to a decrease in Ang III-mediated effects, further pointing out the importance of PRCP in contributing to regulation of blood pressure.

2.2 RAS and angiogenesis

Ang II is a proangiogenic hormone and AT1 mediates its proangiogenic actions(Wilop et al., 2009). The proangiogenic effect of Ang II leads to upregulation of EGF (Friedlander and Terzi, 2006; Lautrette et al., 2005), βFGF (Liu et al., 2009), PDGF(Blaschke et al., 2002; Li et al., 2005), IGF-1 (Kajstura et al., 2001; Song et al., 2005(Jia et al., 2011), hepatocytes growth factor(Bataller et al., 2003), and NO(Abassi et al., 1997). Ang II-induced AT1 mediated signaling pathway cause an activation of mitogen-activated protein kinases (MAPK) (Guo et al., 2006; Morrell et al., 1999; Taniyama et al., 2004).

The MAPK pathway induces cellular protein synthesis, volume regulation, gene expression, and growth (Morrell et al., 1999). In contrast, activation of AT1-independent G-protein signaling pathway by Ang II can also cause endothelial cell proliferation through non-receptor tyrosine kinase Src-mediated increase of NADP oxidase activation, phosphorylation of extracellular signal-regulated kinases 1 and 2 (ERK1/2), P38 MAP kinase, and a decrease in phosphorylation of Src homology 2 (SH2)-containing inositol phosphatase 2 (SHIP2)(Ali et al., 1997b; Feng et al., 2002; Bedecs et al., 1997). These experimental observations suggest that Ang

II is proangiogenic. However, evidence suggests that Ang II may inhibit angiogenesis under certain conditions by activating AT2-receptors, suggesting that AT1 mediates effects that counteract those mediated by AT2 receptors (Chung et al., 1996).

2.3 RAS in cardiovascular disease

Since Ang II, Ang III, Ang IV, and Ang 1-7 can act systemically and locally to control blood pressure and body fluid homeostasis, components of RAS have become therapeutic targets for diseases such as hypertension(Farmer, 2000), cardiac hypertrophy(Brasier et al., 2000; Billet et al., 2008), congestive heart failure(Volpe and De, 2000; Yang et al., 1998), ischemic heart disease(Burrell et al., 2005), coronary heart disease(Farmer and Torre-Amione, 2001), and renal diseases.

3. Plasma kallikrein kinin system (KKS)

The primary functions of plasma KKS are to 1) assist hemostasis and limit blood loss, 2) increase capillary permeability and dilate arterioles, 3) promote antiatherogenic and antithrombogenic properties of endothelium by maintaining or increasing antiatherogenic agents including nitric oxide, prostaglandins, and tissue plasminogen activator, and 4) induce acute vascular pain. In addition to its hemodynamic actions, antifibrotic and renoprotective effects of kallikrein have been reported (Pawluczyk et al., 2008). Although the expression and activity of components of plasma KKS are known to be age-dependent (Gordon et al., 1980) for three decades, the mechanism underlying this phenomenon is yet to be unravelled.

The components of KKS, also called the contact activation pathway, consist of three serine zymogens (prekallikrein, factor XII, and factor XI) as well as a kinin and antiangiogenic precursor (high molecular weight kininogen)(Figure 2)(Ratnoff and Saito, 1979). Plasma kallikrein, a serine protease, is synthesized in the liver. It is predominantly secreted by hepatocytes as an inactive molecule called prekallikrein (PK) that circulates in plasma as a heterodimer complex bound to high molecular weight kininogen (HK) with 1:1 molar stoichiometry. PK is a single chain α-globulin that is present in the plasma of humans and of other animal species. About 80-90% of PK is normally in complexed with HK.

HK is a single-chained glycoprotein synthesised by liver and secreted into the circulation (Sueyoshi et al., 1987). HK consists of three domains: an amino acid-terminal heavy chain, a carboxyl-terminal light chain, and bradykinin moiety (Figure 3)(Kleniewski et al., 1988). The heavy chain linked to the light chain by a single disulfide bond (Kleniewski et al., 1988). Domain 6 of HK has a PK and FXI-binding site (Reddigari and Kaplan, 1989). HK binding to cell surface proteins or artificial surfaces is vital for activation of the plasma KKS(Pixley et al., 2011; Joseph et al., 2001; Zhao et al., 2001). The procoagulant activity of HK is dependent on whether it is in complexed with PK or FXI (Gailani and Broze, Jr., 1991). The proteolytic cleavage of HK by kallikrein results in the production of BK and cleaved HK (HKa). HK could be metabolized by activated factor XI into three peptide fragments, yet its physiological significance has been unclear. HK is involved in angiogenesis and in cell adhesion and the matrix of various endothelial cells (Motta et al., 2001).

Unlike PK, factor XI (FXI) is involved in normal hemostasis *in vivo*. FXI synthesis is primarily in the liver. Factor XI activity is age-dependent (Andrew et al., 1987). While its activity is low at birth, FXI levels are reached to normal adult plasma levels by six months of age. FXI circulates in the plasma as a disulfide bond-linked dimer complexed with HK. It is important for propagation of blood coagulation(Walsh and Griffin, 1981). FXI can be activated to activated FXI (FXIa) by FXIIa-mediated activation on the negatively charged surfaces or thrombin-mediated activation on the platelet surface(Baglia et al., 2004), Figure 2. FXIa augments thrombin generation via interaction with a coagulation factor of the extrinsic pathway, factor IX(Baglia and Walsh, 1998; Taketomi et al., 2008). It appears that FXI along with activated platelet are a prerequisite for optimum thrombin generation in which the procoagulant activity of KKS is so just below the threshold point (Keularts et al., 2001).

Plasma KKS activation has been demonstrated under physiological conditions and in numerous inflammatory human diseases. Under pathological conditions, conversion of plasma factor XII (FXII) to its active form (FXIIa) is concomitant with the appearance of hematologic responses including coagulation, fibrinolytic, and inflammation. FXIIa initiates propagation of the intrinsic pathway (IP) of blood coagulation via factor XI activation, Fig. **2** (1; Pathway 1). In the presence of HK, FXIIa converts plasma prekallikrein (PK) to kallikrein, Fig. **2** (2; Pathway 2). In a reciprocal feedback mechanism, kallikrein accelerates FXII activation. Kallikrein causes the release of tissue plasminogen activator (tPA) via a bradykinin-dependent pathway.

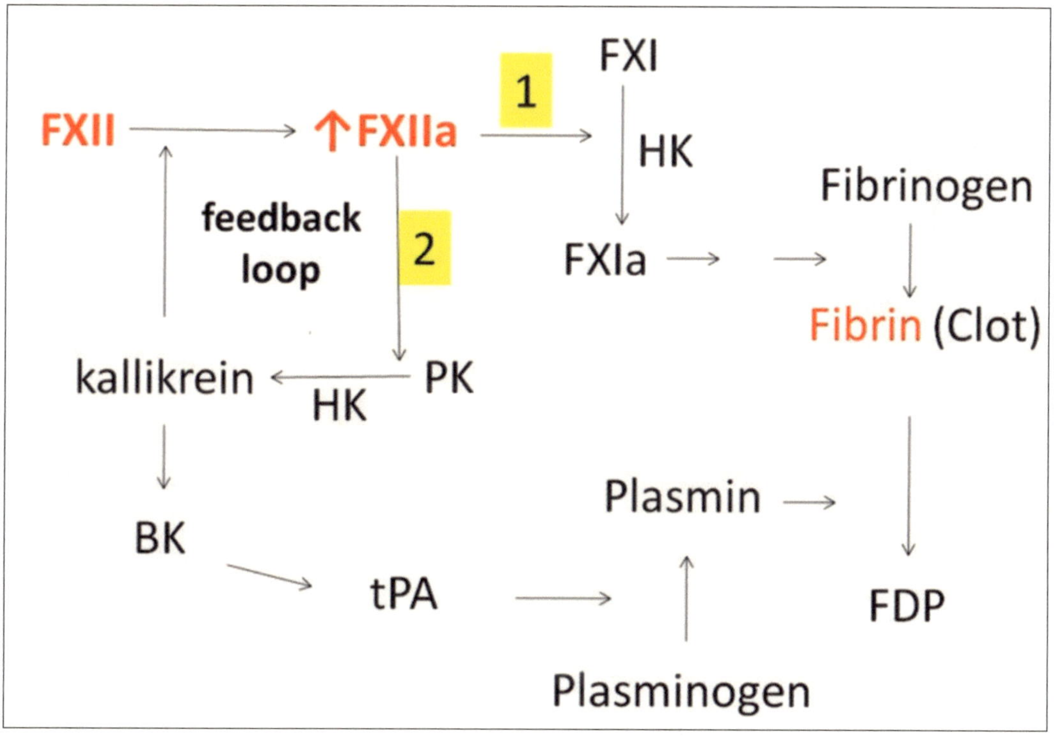

Fig. 2. A schematic representation of factor XII (FXII) activation during pathological plasma proteolytic states. **FXIIa;** activated factor XII, 1; pathway 1, **FXI;** factor XI, **FXIa;** activated factor XI, 2; pathway 2, **HK;** high molecular weight kininogen, **PK;** prekallikrein, **BK;** bradykinin, **tPA;** tissue plasminogen activator, **FDP**; Fibrin degradation Products.

Fibrinolysis is the process by which plasmin digests fibrin, Fig. **2**. This aids in thrombus (clot) dissolution and limits the promotion of coagulation (clot formation). tPA converts plasma plasminogen to plasmin, which in turn remodels the thrombus. Plasmin breaks down the clot fibrin to fibrin degradation products (FDP). Consequently, FDP blocks thrombin-induced fibrin (clot) formation, Figure 2. Notably, plasmin triggers a positive feedback amplification by accelerating conversion of PK to kallikrein.

Kallikrein acts on HK to generate HKa (cleaved HK) and bradykinin (BK), Figure 3. BK-induced activation of the B2 (B_2) receptor leads to the formation of tissue plasminogen activator (tPA, a potent fibrinolytic molecule)(Czokalo-Plichta et al., 2001), Fig. **3**. BK upon activation of its constitutive B_2 receptors on endothelial cells leads to an increase in intracellular Ca^{2+} levels and subsequent production of nitric oxide (NO, a vasodilator) and prostacyclin (PGI_2, a platelet activation inhibitor), ultimately leading to vasodilation, increased vascular permeability and edema (Zhao et al., 2001b; Hong, 1980; Palmer et al., 1987). Whereas B_2 receptors are constitutively expressed, the expression of bradykinin B 1 (B_1) receptors is induced during inflammation (Marceau, 1995). Metabolism of BK by carboxypeptidase N (CPN) in plasma or carboxypeptidase M (CPM) on endothelial cells yields des-Arg^9-BK which interacts with B_1 receptors to potentiate and/or perpetuate the inflammatory response (Figure 3)(Marceau et al., 1981).

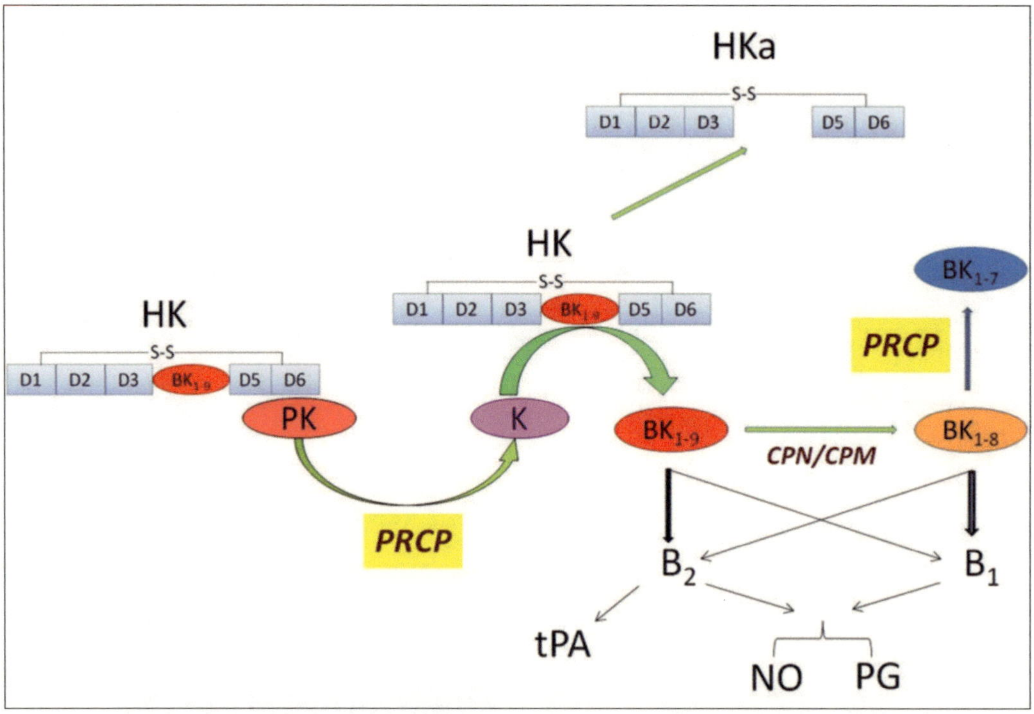

Fig. 3. A schematic representation of PRCP-dependent prekallikrein activation. **HK**; high molecular weight kininogen, **PK;** prekallikrein, **PRCP**; prolylcarboxypeptidase, **K**; kallikrein, **BK_{1-9}**; bradykinin, **HKa**; cleaved HK, **BK**; bradykinin, **NO**; nitric oxide, **PGI2**; prostacyclin, **tPA**; tissue plasminogen activator, **CPN**; carbox peptidase N, **CPM**; Carboxypeptidase M, **BK_{1-8}**; bradykinin 1-8 (des-Arg^9-bradykinin), **BK_{1-7}**; bradykinin 1-7.

Under physiological conditions, PK bound to HK on endothelial cells can lead to PK activation through a FXIIa-independent mechanism, which in turn leads to BK generation. While assembly and activation of the plasma KKS is regulated by PRCP on several cultured cell lines, heat shock protein 90 (HSP90) is the main activator of the plasma PK in mesothelium-derived cell lines (Varano, V et al., 2011). Thus, the plasma KKS participates in both surface-dependent activation of blood clotting and inflammatory process. Further, PRCP participates in cell surface - dependent activation of PK and its dependent pathways. The question remains how PRCP-dependent PK signaling pathway is assembled, activated, and regulated in response to plasma levels of Ang II and/or Ang III. However, in an elegant study, the authors find evidence for a cross-talk among the kinin, PRCP, and angiotensin signaling pathways(Zhu et al., 2010).

3.1 The plasma KKS and cardiovascular diseases

Whereas the normally functioning KKS can successfully counteract blood pressure, promote smooth blood flow, modulates neovascularisation and eliminates pathogens by promoting the recruitment of neutrophils to the site of injury, inappropriate responses can lead to extensive tissue damage. KKS has been implicated in the pathogenesis of inflammation, hypertension, endotoxemia, and coagulopathy. Increased BK levels is a hallmark in all of these cases. In some cases, the persistent production of BK due to the deficiency of the blood protein C1-inhibitor, which controls kallikrein and activated FXII, is detrimental to the survival of the patients with hereditary angioedema (HAE). In others, the inability of angiotensin converting enzyme (ACE) to degrade BK leads to elevated BK levels and edema in patients on ACE inhibitors.

3.2 The importance of KKS for angiogenesis

Various cancers exhibit upregulation of either epidermal growth factor or urokinase receptor or both, which leads to poor prognosis. On studies done on human prostate cancer cells (DU145) the cleaved fragment of HK, HKa and also domain 5 prevented colocalization of uPAR and EGFR, decreased downstream extracellular signal-regulated kinase (ERK) and AKT-mediated signal transduction at EGFR(Wuepper and Cochrane, 1972). This indicates therapeutic potential of HKa and D5 to inhibit metastasis involving migration and invasion of human prostate cancer cells.

Both HK and LK are proangiogenic as demonstrated by induction of vascularization on chorioallantoic membrane. Monoclonal antibody directed against HK has been shown to inhibit HK-induced neovascularization on chorioallatoic membrane as well as HK-induced fibrosarcoma formation. Domain 5 of HK, also called kininostatin, is antiangiogenic(Colman et al., 2000). There are reports that peptides derived from domain 3 and domain 5 inhibit angiogenesis in Zn^{2+} independent and dependent manner (Zhang et al., 2002). Antibody directed against domain 5 also prevents neovascularization(Song et al., 2004).

Like HK, BK also is proangiogenic and a reduction in its levels may be associated with impaired neovascularization(Krankel et al., 2008). But HKa is antiangiogenic as it prevents VEGF and FGF2 induced vascularization. HKa through its D5 domain has been shown to inhibit sphingosine 1-phosphate (S1P) and vascular endothelial growth factor (VEGF) mediated endothelial cell migration by modifying PI3 kinase-Akt signaling (Katkade et al.,

2005). HKa acting through uPAR can also bring about apoptosis in endothelial cells, which is due to inhibition of uPA binding to uPAR thus preventing subsequent uPAR internalization and regeneration to the cell surface (Cao et al., 2004). This results in interference with all aspects of angiogenesis such as cell migration, proliferation, and survival.

Histidine proline rich glycoprotein (HPRG) is present in plasma abundantly and might be the predecessor of HK(Koide and Odani, 1987). HPRG is similar in sequence and function to HKa and is shown to bind to tropomyosin and inhibit angiogenesis through apoptosis (Donate et al., 2004).

4. Pro-opiomelanocortin (POMC)

POMC is expressed in numerous mammalian tissues (Tatro et al., 1992; Tatro and Reichlin, 1987). It undergoes extensive posttranslational modification by a family of serine proteases and the prohormone convertases (PCs). The metabolism of POMC results in the generation of alpha-melanocyte stimulating hormone (α-MSH, α-MSH_{1-13}) along with β-MSH, γ-MSH, and β-endorphin (Shariat-Madar et al., 2010). Although all four of these hormones are important, only α-MSH_{1-13} will be discussed here. The synthesis of α-MSH_{1-13} from POMC involves numerous specific enzymes in addition to PC1 and PC2. It appears that PRCP plays an important role in regulating α-MSH.

5. The interactions among KKS, RAS, and POMC

The participation of the components of the plasma kallikrein-kinin system in some pathological processes like hypertension and cardiovascular diseases is still a matter of controversy. The availability of transgenic and knock-out mice for B2 and B1 receptors and angiotensinogen and angiotensin II receptors have advanced our understanding about the roles of KKS and specifically these receptors in cardiovascular regulation and inflammatory processes.

Bradykinin (BK) is the natural hypotensive agent that causes vasodilatation by stimulation of endothelial B2 receptors of arteries and arterioles, and the subsequent endothelial release of nitric oxide and prostaglandins(Sharma, 2009). BK influences the kidneys to produce diuresis and natriuresis (Katori and Majima, 2008; Katori and Majima, 2003). The diuretic effect of the exogenous BK administered by the renal artery is by B_2 receptors (Boric et al., 1998; Croxatto et al., 1999), whereas the BK–induced natriuresis and increase in renal blood flow are due to both B_1 and B_2, Figure 3 (Lortie et al., 1992). Tissue injury such as myocardial ischemia and inflammation can cause the expression of B1 receptors on their surfaces (Foucart et al., 1997b; Foucart et al., 1997a). In addition, elevated concentrations of BK have been observed in ischemic myocardium(Burch and DePasquale, 1962; Burch and DePasquale, 1963). Occlusion of the proximal left anterior coronary artery causes a change in BK(Hashimoto et al., 1979; Kimura et al., 1973; Hashimoto et al., 1977). Exposure of the epicardium of anesthetized dogs to BK leads to stimulation of sympathetic afferent fibers protruding into the left ventricle(Uchida and Murao, 1974). Inhibition of the B_2 receptor inhibitor resulted in increased kallikrein activity, but not kallikrein mRNA levels, in kidney of adult rats. There is a direct correlation between increased renal interstitial BK levels in dogs in low-sodium balance and the presence of B_2 receptors(Siragy et al., 1997). There is also evidence that kinin or B_2-receptor inhibitor administration increases renin secretion or decrease plasma renin levels in anesthetized rabbits, respectively(Chiu and Reid, 1997). This data plus the location of B_2 receptors in different parts of the kidney and vascular endothelium suggests a role for the plasma KKS in the cardiovascular system (Schricker et al., 1995).

There have been numerous suggestions that kallikrein converts prorenin to renin and a few results suggest that RAS and KKS are interdependent and KKS regulates RAS activity (Sealey et al., 1979). In this report, the plasma prorenin was activated to renin *in vitro* by kallikrein when plasma acidity increased (Sealey et al., 1979). Later, Purdon and colleagues evaluated the effect of kallikrein converting prorenin to renin in plasma deficient in C1 inhibitor (hereditary angioedema) at neutral pH(Purdon et al., 1985). Although PK was completely activated to kallikrein and despite normal prorenin concentration, prorenin was not converted to an active enzyme. Regardless of kallikrein metabolic capability in converting prorenin to renin, studies suggest the presence of a crosstalk between the vasoconstricting RAS and the vasodilating KKS(Yokosawa et al., 1979).

In summary, the increased activity of RAS could be responsible both for arterial wall constriction and KKS activation and subsequent BK production to relief vasoconstriction. This explains the previous finding when the pressure is raised in the perfused heart muscle and brain, the flow can be held constant independently of any external neurogenic control(Mosher et al., 1964). The regulation of tissue flow as perfusion pressure changes can be affected by the rate of delivery or removal of BK and Ang II to the perfused region, influencing the state of contraction of the smooth muscle cells of the blocked vessels directly. This signifies the importance of the feedback mechanism between KKS and RAS. These systems may serve as a "on-off" biological switch impacting the risk of thrombosis/bleeding and those of low/high blood pressure.

6. Prolylcarboxypeptidase or angiotensinase C

PRCP has a subtle role in preserving the blood flow through the endothelial lining of blood vessels so that the tissues can maintain cellular function. PRCP exerts this effect through regulation of local levels of autocrine-paracrine hormones such as angiotensin II (Ang II), angiotensin III (Ang III), and bradykinin generation via kallikrein-kinin pathway. Subsequently, the modification of these vasoactive substances influences the secretion or expression of a diverse group of endothelium mediators that are involved in the contraction and relaxation of smooth muscles, regulating blood flow, blood clotting, inhibition of platelet aggregation, and electrolyte homeostasis. It is well-established that dysfunction of endothelium significantly contributes to the development of thrombosis.

6.1 Physiology

PRCP is a serine peptidase that cleaves peptides at C-terminal amino acids linked to a proline residue. The first evidence that PRCP might play a role in the cardiovascular system was provided by catalytic activity analysis, which showed the metabolism of angiotensin II (Ang II) to angiotensin 1-7 (Ang 1-7)(Odya et al., 1978b). The mere inactivation of Ang II results in two events that broaden the functional spectrum of PRCP. First, it is a negative regulator of the pressor actions of the renin-angiotensin system (RAS). Second, PRCP activity provides a measure of endothelium relaxation due to its ability to initiate nitric oxide generation through Mas receptor activation (Silva et al., 2007). PRCP metabolizes angiotensin III (Ang III) to angiotensin 2-7 (Ang 2-7)(Odya et al., 1978c). Ang III is a pressor agent whose response, like that of Ang II, is mediated by AT_1 receptors(Felix et al., 1991a; Gammelgaard et al., 2006b). We described that when the complex of high molecular weight kininogen (HK) and prekallikrein (PK, Fletcher factor) binds to endothelium membrane, PK is rapidly converted to kallikrein by PRCP, Figure 3(Shariat-Madar et al., 2002b). The formed kallikrein then cleaves HK to liberate bradykinin (BK), which leads to vasodilation and subsequent nitric oxide and PGI2 formation by activating constitutive bradykinin B_2 and inducible bradykinin B_1 receptors (Zhao et al., 2001a; Colman and Schmaier, 1997). BK also causes release of tissue plasminogen activator (tPA, a profibrinolytic factor) to convert plasminogen to plasmin, which inhibits platelet aggregation, thrombus formation and promotes fibrinolysis, Figure 2(Pawluczyk et al., 2006). Thus, PRCP locally regulates nitric oxide-dependent vasodilation and indirectly modulates fibrinolysis within the vascular wall.

6.2 Protein structure and molecular biology

The human *Prcp* gene has been mapped to 11q14 and the gene is more than 147 kb in length and has 9 exons (Watson, Jr. et al., 1997). More recently, a new *Prcp*-like gene (*Prcp*2) has been discovered. The human Prcp gene family contains at least 2 genes. Both genes share important similarities including significant homology at the nucleotide level. Both genes encode for putative serine proteases. However, the functional role of *Prcp2* gene has not been characterized.

PRCP belongs to the single chain serine peptidase S28 family. It is derived from a larger precursor, prepro-PRCP, whose primary nucleotide structure was first described in a human cDNA clone by Tan et al., 1993. It appears that the precursor is homodimer polypeptides containing a secretory signal sequence. PRCP regulates the activity of bradykinin, Ang II, Ang III, prekallikrein, and α-MSH(Odya et al., 1978a; Shariat-Madar et al., 2002c; Moreira et al., 2002; Wallingford et al., 2009), suggesting that PRCP has versatile roles in influencing cardiovascular system. The enzyme is ubiquitously present in all major areas of the vascular bed as well as in the kidney, heart, placenta, and hypothalamus (Jackman et al., 1995b; Skidgel et al., 1981; Rosenblum and Kozarich, 2003; Schmaier, 2003; Shariat-Madar et al., 2010). However, PRCP is highly produced in endothelial cells, which is one cell type involved in the release of vasodilators and antithrombotic mediators.

6.3 PRCP in cardiovascular diseases

PRCP and angiotensin converting enzyme 2 (ACE2) are exopeptidases, which convert Ang II to Ang 1-7. ACE2 metabolizes AngII at a much faster rate than PRCP (Rice et al., 2004), suggesting that Ang II is a poor substrate for PRCP. Clinical studies have provided reliable evidence that ACE2 is an essential regulator of angiotensin I (Ang I), Ang II and angiotensin-induced cardiac hypertrophy (Huentelman et al., 2005). Increased myocardial levels of Ang II concomitant with a significant decrease in Ang 1-7 in ACE2 deficient hearts has been reported (Kassiri et al., 2009). These data suggest that PRCP may indeed be important in metabolizing Ang II in the absence of ACE2. These observations suggest that PRCP is a redundant catalyst contributing to alternate pathways for Ang II metabolism.

Over thirty years ago, Odya et al (Odya et al., 1978d) showed that PRCP can metabolize Ang III to Ang 2-7. Evidence indicates that Ang 2-7 excites some neurons in the paraventricular nuclease (Ambuhl et al., 1992). Differential regulation of Ang 2-7 during ACE inhibitor treatment suggests a cardiovascular role for this peptide (Campbell et al., 1991). Because of the significance of Ang 2-7, AngIII regulation and metabolism are important. Results from several studies show that Ang III is a pressor agent. It exerts its hypertensive effects via AT_1 receptors (Felix et al., 1991b; Gammelgaard et al., 2006a). Ang III can enhance renal disease through the overproduction of aldosterone and subsequent development of arterial hypertension and/or to atrial fibrillation (Al-Aloul et al., 2006). Aldosterone which is produced by adrenal cortex maintains blood volume, pressure, and electrolyte balance. It is tightly regulated by renin, an enzyme produced in the juxtaglomerular apparatus of the kidneys. Renin production is elevated by low blood pressure, decreased blood flow to the kidneys or sodium deficiency. In theory, inactivation of Ang III by PRCP might lead to a decrease in blood pressure. However, further studies are needed before claims can be made of a beneficial effect of PRCP on hypertension.

It is well known that cells produce and secrete a large variety of proteases either as proenzymes or activated proteases. Although PRCP can be viewed as a proenzyme based on its primary structure, its post-translational regulation has not been characterized. PRCP is distributed throughout endothelial cells, including lysosome, cytoplasm, and plasma membrane. The membrane bound PRCP activates plasma PK to kallikrein in endothelial cells. The activation of PK is characterized by elevated kallikrein expression along with increased local BK production. Kallikrein-induced BK production causes endothelial cells to produce proinflammatory prostaglandins and vasodilatory nitric oxide (Ngo et al., 2009). Thus, the PRCP-dependent PK activation pathway might be considered as an additional mechanism to counteract the hypertensive activities of both Ang II and Ang III.

Local skeletal muscle ischemia and acidosis are shown to increase the generation of BK and prostaglandins, the two circulating end-products of the PRCP-dependent pathways, Figure 3 (Piepoli et al., 2001). The increased acidotic response during exercise and inflammatory mediators such as BK and prostacyclin have been shown to cause the abnormal exercise-related symptoms and autonomic responses in congestive heart failure syndrome (Scott et al., 2003). Emerging evidence suggest that the long-term elevated concentrations of NO and prostacyclin may be detrimental and eventually responsible for cardiovascular diseases such as congestive heart disease (Kai C.Wollert and Helmut Drexler, 2004). Needless to say, the reduction of endogenous PGI2 synthesis is associated with the occurrence of cyclic reduction of coronary flow(Tada et al., 1984). Thus, PRCP-dependent Ang_{1-7} and PRCP-dependent BK pathways have important biological activities. Altered PRCP expression levels mediates pathophysiological changes in the cardiovascular system.

PK is markedly elevated during pregnancy(Maki and Soga, 1981). Among proteases that metabolize neuropeptide Y 3-36 (NPY_{3-36}, anorexigenic hormone), plasma kallikrein metabolizes NPY_{3-36} to NPY_{3-35}(Abid et al., 2009). In addition, specific inhibitor of plasma kallikrein prevents the production of NPY_{3-35}. We find these studies intriguing because elevation of kallikrein should provoke anorectic effect via accelerated inactivation of NPY_{3-36}. Recent evidence suggests that there is a link between severe prekallikrein deficiency and pregnancy loss (Dasanu and Alexandrescu, 2009). As mentioned earlier, PRCP activates PK to kallikrein. If PRCP is inhibited/down-regulated, kallikrein levels are lower. Thus, disruption of PRCP-dependent PK activation may be a risk factor for pregnancy losses. The inhibitors of both kallikrein and PRCP may be contraindicated during pregnancy. However, further investigations are required to define the safety of these inhibitors.

The activation of POMC is characterized by elevated α-MSH_{1-13} production. α-MSH_{1-13} regulates inflammation and food intake, suggesting that it may contribute to tissue damage production. Recently, experimental evidence indicated that PRCP metabolizes α-MSH_{1-13} to α-MSH_{1-12} (Wallingford et al., 2009). Mice deficient for PRCP present high blood pressure (Adams G.N et al., 2009), a sustained long-term reduction in food intake, and increased energy expenditure (Wallingford et al., 2009). In humans, hypertension is considered to be a multifactorial disorder. *Prcp* gene and its variants contribute to hypertension (Wang et al., 2006c; Zhang et al., 2009; Zhu et al., 2010). Rutaecarpine stimulates expression of PRCP in the circulation and small arteries in renovascular hypertensive rats (Qin et al., 2009). Since PRCP variant promotes disease progression (Zhang et al., 2009) in Chinese hypertensive patients and risk of preeclampsia in black and non-black women (Wang et al., 2006b), it is a candidate for pharmacological intervention.

7. Conclusions and future directions

In conclusion, PRCP is one of the conserved proteases throughout evolution in vertebrates. In-vitro and in-vivo studies of PRCP, this enzyme serves to generate nitric oxide and prostaglandins. Notably, bradykinin and bradykinin 1-8 are important mediators of pain (Argent et al., 1954) and endotoxin-induced vascular permeability {Ueno, 1995 783 /id}. BK production is increased in ischemic myocardial tissue (Dell'Italia and Oparil, 1999). They are involved in the control of local blood flow. Although PRCP is less efficient than ACE2-induced NO and prostaglandin generation under pathophysiological conditions, this redundant mechanism has presumably evolved for ischemic remodeling and smooth blood flow (Figure 1 and Figure 3). Overactivation of this mechanism may contribute to myocardial tissue damage or endothelial dysfunction. It inactivates BK_{1-8}, suggesting that PRCP may also reduce marked inflammatory response. It appears that PRCP is fine-tuned to discriminate between physiological and pathophysiological changes. Since cardiomyocytes are unable to proliferate (Lagrand et al., 2000), inactivation of BK_{1-8} by PRCP may contribute to prevention of tissue damage. Further studies are warranted to evaluate the role of PRCP in cardiovascular system, in particular the heart.

8. Acknowledgment

This work was supported by National Institute of Health [NCRR/NIH P20RR021929] to ZSM.

9. References

Adams, G.N., LaRusch, G.A., Stavrou, E., Zhou, Y., Nieman, M.T., Jacobs, G.H., Cui, Y., Lu, Y., Jain, M.K., Mahdi, F., Shariat-Madar, Z., Okada, Y., D'Alecy, L.G., and Schmaier, A.H. (2011). Murine prolylcarboxypeptidase depletion induces vascular dysfunction with hypertension and faster arterial thrombosis. Blood *117*, 3929-3937.

Baglia, F.A., Shrimpton, C.N., Emsley, J., Kitagawa, K., Ruggeri, Z.M., Lopez, J.A., and Walsh, P.N. (2004). Factor XI interacts with the leucine-rich repeats of glycoprotein Ibalpha on the activated platelet. J. Biol. Chem. *279*, 49323-49329.

Baglia, F.A. and Walsh, P.N. (1998). Prothrombin is a cofactor for the binding of factor XI to the platelet surface and for platelet-mediated factor XI activation by thrombin. Biochemistry *37*, 2271-2281.

Billet, S., Aguilar, F., Baudry, C., and Clauser, E. (2008). Role of angiotensin II AT1 receptor activation in cardiovascular diseases. Kidney Int. *74*, 1379-1384.

Boric, M.P., Croxatto, H.R., Moreno, J.M., Silva, R., Hernandez, C., and Roblero, J.S. (1998). Kinins mediate the inhibition of atrial natriuretic peptide diuretic effect induced by pepsanurin. Biol. Res. *31*, 33-48.

Brasier, A.R., Jamaluddin, M., Han, Y., Patterson, C., and Runge, M.S. (2000). Angiotensin II induces gene transcription through cell-type-dependent effects on the nuclear factor-kappaB (NF-kappaB) transcription factor. Mol. Cell Biochem. *212*, 155-169.

Brown, J.J., Fraser, R., Lever, A.F., and Robertson, J.I. (1983). The renin-angiotensin system in congestive cardiac failure: a selective review. Eur. Heart J. *4 Suppl A*, 85-87.

Bryant, J.W. and Shariat-Madar, Z. (2009). Human plasma kallikrein-kinin system: physiological and biochemical parameters. Cardiovasc. Hematol. Agents Med. Chem. *7*, 234-250.

Burch, G.E. and DePasquale, N.P. (1962). Bradykinin, digital blood flow, and the arteriovenous anastomoses. Circ. Res. *10*, 105-115.

Burch, G.E. and DePasquale, N.P. (1963). Bradykinin. Am. Heart J *65*, 116-123.

Burrell, L.M., Risvanis, J., Kubota, E., Dean, R.G., MacDonald, P.S., Lu, S., Tikellis, C., Grant, S.L., Lew, R.A., Smith, A.I., Cooper, M.E., and Johnston, C.I. (2005). Myocardial infarction increases ACE2 expression in rat and humans. Eur. Heart J. *26*, 369-375.

Chajkowski, S.M., Mallela, J., Watson, D.E., Wang, J., McCurdy, C.R., Rimoldi, J.M., and Shariat-Madar, Z. (2010). Highly selective hydrolysis of kinins by recombinant prolylcarboxypeptidase. Biochem. Biophys. Res. Commun.

Chiu, N. and Reid, I.A. (1997). Role of kinins in basal and furosemide-stimulated renin secretion. J Hypertens. *15*, 517-521.

Clerk, A., Cullingford, T.E., Kemp, T.J., Kennedy, R.A., and Sugden, P.H. (2005). Regulation of gene and protein expression in cardiac myocyte hypertrophy and apoptosis. Adv. Enzyme Regul. *45*, 94-111.

Croxatto, H.R., Figueroa, X.F., Roblero, J., and Boric, M.P. (1999). Kinin B2 receptors mediate blockade of atrial natriuretic peptide natriuresis induced by glucose or feeding in fasted rats. Hypertension *34*, 826-831.

Czokalo-Plichta, M., Skibinska, E., Kosiorek, P., and Musial, W.J. (2001). Kallikrein-kinin system activation and its interactions with other plasma haemostatic components in the coronary artery disease. Rocz. Akad. Med. Bialymst. *46*, 209-224.

Deddish, P.A., Skidgel, R.A., Kriho, V.B., Li, X.Y., Becker, R.P., and Erdos, E.G. (1990). Carboxypeptidase M in Madin-Darby canine kidney cells. Evidence that carboxypeptidase M has a phosphatidylinositol glycan anchor. J Biol. Chem. *265*, 15083-15089.

Duan, L., Motchoulski, N., Danzer, B., Davidovich, I., Shariat-Madar, Z., and Levenson, V.V. (2011). Prolylcarboxypeptidase regulates proliferation, autophagy, and resistance to 4-hydroxytamoxifen-induced cytotoxicity in estrogen receptor-positive breast cancer cells. J Biol. Chem. *286*, 2864-2876.

Farmer, J.A. (2000). Renin angiotensin system and ASCVD. Curr. Opin. Cardiol. *15*, 141-150.

Farmer, J.A. and Torre-Amione, G. (2001). The renin angiotensin system as a risk factor for coronary artery disease. Curr. Atheroscler. Rep. *3*, 117-124.

Foucart, S., Grondin, L., Couture, R., and Nadeau, R. (1997a). Modulation of noradrenaline release by B1 and B2 kinin receptors during metabolic anoxia in the rat isolated atria. Can. J Physiol Pharmacol. *75*, 639-645.

Foucart, S., Grondin, L., Couture, R., and Nadeau, R. (1997b). Paradoxical action of desipramine on the modulatory effect of bradykinin on noradrenaline release in a model of metabolic anoxia in rat isolated atria. Can. J Physiol Pharmacol. *75*, 646-651.

Gailani, D. and Broze, G.J., Jr. (1991). Factor XI activation in a revised model of blood coagulation. Science *253*, 909-912.

Gordon, E.M., Ratnoff, O.D., Saito, H., Gross, S., and Jones, P.K. (1980). Studies on some coagulation factors (Hageman factor, plasma prekallikrein, and high molecular weight kininogen) in the normal newborn. Am. J Pediatr. Hematol. Oncol. *2*, 213-216.

Gurley, S.B., Allred, A., Le, T.H., Griffiths, R., Mao, L., Philip, N., Haystead, T.A., Donoghue, M., Breitbart, R.E., Acton, S.L., Rockman, H.A., and Coffman, T.M. (2006). Altered blood pressure responses and normal cardiac phenotype in ACE2-null mice. J. Clin. Invest *116*, 2218-2225.

Hashimoto, K., Hirose, M., Furukawa, S., Hayakawa, H., and Kimura, E. (1977). Changes in hemodynamics and bradykinin concentration in coronary sinus blood in experimental coronary artery occlusion. Jpn. Heart J *18*, 679-689.

Hashimoto, K., Mitamura, H., Honda, Y., Kawasumi, S., Takano, T., Kimura, E., and Tsunoo, M. (1979). Changes in blood level of kininogen, prostaglandin E and hemodynamics during experimental acute myocardial ischemia with and without FOY-007. Adv. Exp. Med. Biol. *120B*, 403-411.

Hayashi, T., Takai, S., and Yamashita, C. (2010). Impact of the Renin-Angiotensin-Aldosterone-System on Cardiovascular and Renal Complications in Diabetes Mellitus. Curr. Vasc. Pharmacol.

Hettinger, U., Lukasova, M., Lewicka, S., and Hilgenfeldt, U. (2002). Regulatory effects of salt diet on renal renin-angiotensin-aldosterone, and kallikrein-kinin systems. Int. Immunopharmacol. *2*, 1975-1980.

Hooley, E., McEwan, P.A., and Emsley, J. (2007). Molecular modeling of the prekallikrein structure provides insights into high-molecular-weight kininogen binding and zymogen activation. J Thromb. Haemost. *5*, 2461-2466.

Jackman, H.L., Tan, F., Schraufnagel, D., Dragovic, T., Dezso, B., Becker, R.P., and Erdos, E.G. (1995). Plasma membrane-bound and lysosomal peptidases in human alveolar macrophages. Am. J Respir. Cell Mol. Biol. *13*, 196-204.

Javerzat, S., Franco, M., Herbert, J., Platonova, N., Peille, A.L., Pantesco, V., De, V.J., Assou, S., Bicknell, R., Bikfalvi, A., and Hagedorn, M. (2009). Correlating global gene regulation to angiogenesis in the developing chick extra-embryonic vascular system. PLoS One *4*, e7856.

Jia, G., Aggarwal, A., Yohannes, A., Gangahar, D.M., and Agrawal, D.K. (2011). Cross-talk between angiotensin II and IGF-1-induced connexin 43 expression in human saphenous vein smooth muscle cells. J Cell Mol. Med *15*, 1695-1702.

Joseph, K., Shibayama, Y., Ghebrehiwet, B., and Kaplan, A.P. (2001). Factor XII-dependent contact activation on endothelial cells and binding proteins gC1qR and cytokeratin 1. Thromb. Haemost. *85*, 119-124.

Kai, H., Fukui, T., Lassegue, B., Shah, A., Minieri, C.A., and Griendling, K.K. (1996). Prolonged exposure to agonist results in a reduction in the levels of the Gq/G11 alpha subunits in cultured vascular smooth muscle cells. Mol. Pharmacol. *49*, 96-104.

Katori, M. and Majima, M. (2003). The renal kallikrein-kinin system: its role as a safety valve for excess sodium intake, and its attenuation as a possible etiologic factor in salt-sensitive hypertension. Crit Rev. Clin. Lab Sci. *40*, 43-115.

Katori, M. and Majima, M. (2008). Are all individuals equally sensitive in the blood pressure to high salt intake? (Review article). Acta Physiol Hung. *95*, 247-265.

Keularts, I.M., Zivelin, A., Seligsohn, U., Hemker, H.C., and Beguin, S. (2001). The role of factor XI in thrombin generation induced by low concentrations of tissue factor. Thromb. Haemost. *85*, 1060-1065.

Kimura, E., Hashimoto, K., Furukawa, S., and Hayakawa, H. (1973). Changes in bradykinin level in coronary sinus blood after the experimental occlusion of a coronary artery. Am. Heart J *85*, 635-647.

Kleniewski, J., Dingle, S., and Donaldson, V.H. (1988). Comparison of properties of monoclonal and polyclonal antibodies against the light chain of human high molecular weight kininogen. J. Lab Clin. Med. *111*, 93-103.

Koide, T. and Odani, S. (1987). Histidine-rich glycoprotein is evolutionarily related to the cystatin superfamily. Presence of two cystatin domains in the N-terminal region. FEBS Lett. *216*, 17-21.

Krankel, N., Katare, R.G., Siragusa, M., Barcelos, L.S., Campagnolo, P., Mangialardi, G., Fortunato, O., Spinetti, G., Tran, N., Zacharowski, K., Wojakowski, W., Mroz, I., Herman, A., Manning Fox, J.E., MacDonald, P.E., Schanstra, J.P., Bascands, J.L., Ascione, R., Angelini, G., Emanueli, C., and Madeddu, P. (2008). Role of kinin B2 receptor signaling in the recruitment of circulating progenitor cells with neovascularization potential. Circ. Res. *103*, 1335-1343.

Kumamoto, K., Stewart, T.A., Johnson, A.R., and Erdos, E.G. (1981). Prolylcarboxypeptidase (angiotensinase C) in human lung and cultured cells. J. Clin. Invest *67*, 210-215.

Lortie, M., Regoli, D., Rhaleb, N.E., and Plante, G.E. (1992). The role of B1- and B2-kinin receptors in the renal tubular and hemodynamic response to bradykinin. Am. J Physiol *262*, R72-R76.

Marceau, F., Gendreau, M., Barabe, J., St-Pierre, S., and Regoli, D. (1981). The degradation of bradykinin (BK) and of des-Arg9-BK in plasma. Can. J. Physiol Pharmacol. *59*, 131-138.

Molteni, A. (1982). Considerations of the renin-angiotensin aldosterone system in the pathogenesis of hypertension in infancy. Ann. Clin. Lab Sci. *12*, 492-499.

Moreira, C.R., Schmaier, A.H., Mahdi, F., da, M.G., Nader, H.B., and Shariat-Madar, Z. (2002). Identification of prolylcarboxypeptidase as the cell matrix-associated prekallikrein activator. FEBS Lett. *523*, 167-170.

Mosher, P., Ross, J., Jr., McFate, P.A., and Shaw, R.F. (1964). Control of coronary blood flow by an autoregulatory mechansim. Circ. Res. *14*, 250-259.

Motta, G., Shariat-Madar, Z., Mahdi, F., Sampaio, C.A., and Schmaier, A.H. (2001). Assembly of high molecular weight kininogen and activation of prekallikrein on cell matrix. Thromb. Haemost. *86*, 840-847.

Nicholls, M.G. and Robertson, J.I. (2000). The renin-angiotensin system in the year 2000. J. Hum. Hypertens. *14*, 649-666.

Odya, C.E., Marinkovic, D.V., Hammon, K.J., Stewart, T.A., and Erdos, E.G. (1978). Purification and properties of prolylcarboxypeptidase (angiotensinase C) from human kidney. J. Biol. Chem. *253*, 5927-5931.

Oishi, T., Ogura, T., Yamauchi, T., Harada, K., and Ota, Z. (1996). Effect of renin-angiotensin inhibition on glomerular injuries in DOCA-salt hypertensive rats. Regul. Pept. *62*, 89-95.

Oudart, N. (2005). [The renin-angiotensin system: current data]. Ann. Pharm. Fr. *63*, 144-153.

Pawluczyk, I.Z., Tan, E.K., Lodwick, D., and Harris, K.P. (2008). Kallikrein gene 'knock-down' by small interfering RNA transfection induces a profibrotic phenotype in rat mesangial cells. J. Hypertens. *26*, 93-101.

Perret-Guillaume, C., Joly, L., Jankowski, P., and Benetos, A. (2009). Benefits of the RAS blockade: clinical evidence before the ONTARGET study. J. Hypertens. *27 Suppl 2*, S3-S7.

Pixley, R.A., Espinola, R.G., Ghebrehiwet, B., Joseph, K., Kao, A., Bdeir, K., Cines, D.B., and Colman, R.W. (2011). Interaction of high-molecular-weight kininogen with endothelial cell binding proteins suPAR, gC1qR and cytokeratin 1 determined by Surface Plasmon Resonance (BiaCore). Thromb. Haemost. *105*.

Purdon, A.D., Schapira, M., De, A.A., and Colman, R.W. (1985). Plasma kallikrein and prorenin in patients with hereditary angioedema. J. Lab Clin. Med. *105*, 694-699.

Ratnoff, O.D. and Saito, H. (1979). Surface-mediated reactions. Curr. Top. Hematol. *2*, 1-57.

Reddigari, S.R. and Kaplan, A.P. (1989). Monoclonal antibody to human high-molecular-weight kininogen recognizes its prekallikrein binding site and inhibits its coagulant activity. Blood *74*, 695-702.

Renshaw, M.A., Ellingsen, D., Costner, B., Benson, J., Heit, J.A., and Hooper, W.C. (2001). Fluorescent multiplex polymerase chain reaction analysis of four genes associated with inpaired fibrinolysis and myocardial infarction. Blood Coagul. Fibrinolysis *12*, 245-251.

Ritz, E. (2005). The role of the kidney in cardiovascular medicine. Eur. J. Intern. Med. *16*, 321-327.

Savinetskaia, G.A., Golubeva, A.A., Pogoda, T.V., and Generozov, E.V. (2008). [Contribution of rennin-angiotensin-aldosterone system genes and NO synthase gene to the development of arterial hypertension]. Klin. Med. (Mosk) *86*, 12-17.

Saxena, P., Thompson, P., d'Udekem, Y., and Konstantinov, I.E. (2011). Kallikrein-kinin system: a surgical perspective in post-aprotinin era. J Surg. Res. *167*, 70-77.

Schricker, K., Hegyi, I., Hamann, M., Kaissling, B., and Kurtz, A. (1995). Tonic stimulation of renin gene expression by nitric oxide is counteracted by tonic inhibition through angiotensin II. Proc. Natl. Acad. Sci. U. S. A *92*, 8006-8010.

Sealey, J.E., Atlas, S.A., Laragh, J.H., Silverberg, M., and Kaplan, A.P. (1979). Initiation of plasma prorenin activation by Hageman factor-dependent conversion of plasma prekallikrein to kallikrein. Proc. Natl. Acad. Sci. U. S. A *76*, 5914-5918.

Shariat-Madar, B., Kolte, D., Verlangieri, A., and Shariat-Madar, Z. (2010). Prolylcarboxypeptidase (PRCP) as a new target for obesity treatment. Diabetes Metab Syndr. Obes. *3*, 67-78.

Shariat-Madar, Z., Mahdi, F., and Schmaier, A.H. (2002). Identification and characterization of prolylcarboxypeptidase as an endothelial cell prekallikrein activator. J Biol. Chem. *277*, 17962-17969.

Shariat-Madar, Z., Rahimy, E., Mahdi, F., and Schmaier, A.H. (2005). Overexpression of prolylcarboxypeptidase enhances plasma prekallikrein activation on Chinese hamster ovary cells. Am. J. Physiol Heart Circ. Physiol *289*, H2697-H2703.

Shariat-Madar, Z. and Schmaier, A.H. (2004). The plasma kallikrein/kinin and renin angiotensin systems in blood pressure regulation in sepsis. J. Endotoxin. Res. *10*, 3-13.

Sharma, J.N. (2009). Hypertension and the bradykinin system. Curr. Hypertens. Rep. *11*, 178-181.

Siragy, H.M., Jaffa, A.A., and Margolius, H.S. (1997). Bradykinin B2 receptor modulates renal prostaglandin E2 and nitric oxide. Hypertension *29*, 757-762.

Skidgel, R.A., Wickstrom, E., Kumamoto, K., and Erdos, E.G. (1981). Rapid radioassay for prolylcarboxypeptidase (angiotensinase C). Anal. Biochem. *118*, 113-119.

Soisson, S.M., Patel, S.B., Abeywickrema, P.D., Byrne, N.J., Diehl, R.E., Hall, D.L., Ford, R.E., Reid, J.C., Rickert, K.W., Shipman, J.M., Sharma, S., and Lumb, K.J. (2010). Structural definition and substrate specificity of the S28 protease family: the crystal structure of human prolylcarboxypeptidase. BMC Struct. Biol. *10*, 16.

Sorrells, K. and Erdos, E.G. (1971). Prolylcarboxypeptidase in biological fluids. Adv. Exp. Med. Biol. *23*, 393-397.

Sueyoshi, T., Miyata, T., Hashimoto, N., Kato, H., Hayashida, H., Miyata, T., and Iwanaga, S. (1987). Bovine high molecular weight kininogen. The amino acid sequence, positions of carbohydrate chains and disulfide bridges in the heavy chain portion. J. Biol. Chem. *262*, 2768-2779.

Suga, K., Ito, K., Tsuru, D., and Yoshimoto, T. (1995). Prolylcarboxypeptidase (angiotensinase C): purification and characterization of the enzyme from Xanthomanas maltophilia. Biosci. Biotechnol. Biochem. *59*, 298-301.

Suzawa, Y., Hiraoka, B.Y., Harada, M., and Deguchi, T. (1995). High-performance liquid chromatographic determination of prolylcarboxypeptidase activity in monkey kidney. J. Chromatogr. B Biomed. Appl. *670*, 152-156.

Tada, M., Esumi, K., Yamagishi, M., Kuzuya, T., Matsuda, H., Abe, H., Uchida, Y., and Murao, S. (1984). Reduction of prostacyclin synthesis as a possible cause of transient flow reduction in a partially constricted canine coronary artery. J Mol. Cell Cardiol. *16*, 1137-1149.

Taketomi, T., Szlam, F., Bader, S.O., Sheppard, C.A., Levy, J.H., and Tanaka, K.A. (2008). Effects of recombinant activated factor VII on thrombin-mediated feedback activation of coagulation. Blood Coagul. Fibrinolysis *19*, 135-141.

Tamaoki, J., Sugimoto, F., Tagaya, E., Isono, K., Chiyotani, A., and Konno, K. (1994). Angiotensin II 1 receptor-mediated contraction of pulmonary artery and its modulation by prolylcarboxypeptidase. J. Appl. Physiol *76*, 1439-1444.

Tan, F., Morris, P.W., Skidgel, R.A., and Erdos, E.G. (1993). Sequencing and cloning of human prolylcarboxypeptidase (angiotensinase C). Similarity to both serine carboxypeptidase and prolylendopeptidase families. J. Biol. Chem. *268*, 16631-16638.

Taquini, A.C., Jr. and Taquini, A.C. (1961). The renin-angiotensin system in hypertension. Am. Heart J. *62*, 558-564.

Tatro, J.B. and Reichlin, S. (1987). Specific receptors for alpha-melanocyte-stimulating hormone are widely distributed in tissues of rodents. Endocrinology *121*, 1900-1907.

Tatro, J.B., Wen, Z., Entwistle, M.L., Atkins, M.B., Smith, T.J., Reichlin, S., and Murphy, J.R. (1992). Interaction of an alpha-melanocyte-stimulating hormone-diphtheria toxin fusion protein with melanotropin receptors in human melanoma metastases. Cancer Res. *52*, 2545-2548.

Uchida, Y. and Murao, S. (1974). Bradykinin-induced excitation of afferent cardiac sympathetic nerve fibers. Jpn. Heart J *15*, 84-91.

Varano, D., V, Lansley, S., Tan, A.L., Creaney, J., Lee, Y.C., and Stewart, G.A. (2011). Mesothelial cells activate the plasma kallikrein-kinin system during pleural inflammation. Biol. Chem. *392*, 633-642.

Volpe, M. and De, P.P. (2000). Angiotensin II AT2 subtype receptors: an emerging target for cardiovascular therapy. Ital. Heart J. *1*, 96-103.

Volzke, H., Kleine, V., Robinson, D.M., Grimm, R., Hertwig, S., Schwahn, C., Eckel, L., and Rettig, R. (2005). Renin-angiotensin system and haemostasis gene polymorphisms and outcome after coronary artery bypass graft surgery. Int. J. Cardiol. *98*, 133-139.

Wallingford, N., Perroud, B., Gao, Q., Coppola, A., Gyengesi, E., Liu, Z.W., Gao, X.B., Diament, A., Haus, K.A., Shariat-Madar, Z., Mahdi, F., Wardlaw, S.L., Schmaier, A.H., Warden, C.H., and Diano, S. (2009). Prolylcarboxypeptidase regulates food intake by inactivating alpha-MSH in rodents. J. Clin. Invest *119*, 2291-2303.

Walsh, P.N. and Griffin, J.H. (1981). Platelet-coagulant protein interactions in contact activation. Ann. N. Y. Acad. Sci. *370*, 241-252.

Wang, L., Feng, Y., Zhang, Y., Zhou, H., Jiang, S., Niu, T., Wei, L.J., Xu, X., Xu, X., and Wang, X. (2006). Prolylcarboxypeptidase gene, chronic hypertension, and risk of preeclampsia. Am. J. Obstet. Gynecol. *195*, 162-171.

Wang, S.X., Fan, Z.C., and Tao, Y.X. (2008). Functions of acidic transmembrane residues in human melanocortin-3 receptor binding and activation. Biochem. Pharmacol. *76*, 520-530.

Watson, B., Jr., Nowak, N.J., Myracle, A.D., Shows, T.B., and Warnock, D.G. (1997). The human angiotensinase C gene (HUMPCP) maps to 11q14 within 700 kb of D11S901: a candidate gene for essential hypertension. Genomics *44*, 365-367.

Wilop, S., von, H.S., Crysandt, M., Esser, A., Osieka, R., and Jost, E. (2009). Impact of angiotensin I converting enzyme inhibitors and angiotensin II type 1 receptor blockers on survival in patients with advanced non-small-cell lung cancer undergoing first-line platinum-based chemotherapy. J. Cancer Res. Clin. Oncol. *135*, 1429-1435.

Yang, B., Li, D., Phillips, M.I., Mehta, P., and Mehta, J.L. (1998). Myocardial angiotensin II receptor expression and ischemia-reperfusion injury. Vasc. Med. *3*, 121-130.

Yokosawa, N., Takahashi, N., Inagami, T., and Page, D.L. (1979). Isolation of completely inactive plasma prorenin and its activation by kallikreins. A possible new link between renin and kallikrein. Biochim. Biophys. Acta *569*, 211-219.

Zhang Yan, Hong Xiu-mei, Hou-xun, Li Jian-ping, Huo Yong, and Xu Xi-ping (2009). E112D polymorphism in the prolylcarboxypeptidase gene is associated with blood pressure response to benazepril in Chinese hypertensive patients. Chinese Medical Journal *122*, 2461-2465.

Zhao, X., Southwick, K., Cardasis, H.L., Du, Y., Lassman, M.E., Xie, D., El-Sherbeini, M., Geissler, W.M., Pryor, K.D., Verras, A., Garcia-Calvo, M., Shen, D.M., Yates, N.A., Pinto, S., and Hendrickon, R.C. (2010). Peptidomic profiling of human cerebrospinal fluid identifies YPRPIHPA as a novel substrate for prolylcarboxypeptidase. Proteomics.

Zhao, Y., Qiu, Q., Mahdi, F., Shariat-Madar, Z., Rojkjaer, R., and Schmaier, A.H. (2001). Assembly and activation of HK-PK complex on endothelial cells results in bradykinin liberation and NO formation. Am. J. Physiol Heart Circ. Physiol *280*, H1821-H1829.

Zhu, L., Carretero, O.A., Liao, T.D., Harding, P., Li, H., Sumners, C., and Yang, X.P. (2010). Role of prolylcarboxypeptidase in angiotensin II type 2 receptor-mediated bradykinin release in mouse coronary artery endothelial cells. Hypertension *56*, 384-390.

14

Adolescent Obesity Predicts Cardiovascular Risk

Jarosław Derejczyk[1], Barbara Kłapcińska[2], Ewa Sadowska-Krępa[2], Olga Stępień-Wyrobiec[1], Elżbieta Kimsa[2] and Katarzyna Kempa[2]
[1]John Paul II Geriatric Hospital in Katowice,
[2]Department of Physiological and Medical Sciences, Academy of Physical Education in Katowice
Poland

1. Introduction

Rapid increase in the prevalence of obesity among children and adolescents has become a major worldwide health issue. Several large epidemiological studies have demonstrated that childhood and adolescent obesity is a significant independent predictor of metabolic disorders, such as hypertension, dyslipidemia and insulin resistance, which have a major impact on the premature development of atherosclerosis and cardiovascular morbidity and mortality in adulthood (Bibbins-Domingo et al., 2007; Dietz & Robinson, 2005; Franks et al., 2010). The cluster of metabolic disorders including abdominal obesity, insulin resistance, dyslipidemia and elevated blood pressure has been defined as metabolic syndrome (Alberti et al., 2006; Aggoun, 2007, Han & Lean, 2006). It is now generally accepted that overweight or obese children and adolescents are at increased risk for some or all of the metabolic syndrome (MS) features (Carnethon et al., 2004; Franks et al., 2010; Magnussen et al., 2010; Zimmet et al., 2007). The data from the Third National Health and Nutrition Examination Survey (NHANESIII, 1988-1994) have demonstrated that about 4 % of the whole population and almost 30% of the overweight or obese 12 to 19-y-old adolescents met the criteria of MS (Cook et al., 2003). The early occurrence of the MS in childhood and at the pubertal age was also found to have a major impact on the development of atherosclerosis, a life-time risk of cardiovascular disease (Aggoun, 2007), and an increased rate of premature death (Franks et al., 2010; Nieto, 1992). Excessive body weight in childhood and adolescence is considered a strong predictor of adult obesity (Wang et al. 2008) and obesity-related health consequences including diabetes and heart disease (Carnethon et al., 2004; Must et al., 1992; Morrison et al. 2007) regardless of whether the parents were obese. Notably, parental obesity was found to double the risk of being obese in adulthood (Shengxu et al., 2003; Whitaker et al., 1997).

The main reason for undertaking the present study was to evaluate the prevalence of obesity among 15-y-old adolescents and to estimate the risk for adverse health outcomes in this population sample. Another goal was to find out relatively simple biochemical markers that could be suitable for the early diagnosis of metabolic disorders and cardiovascular risk, and would help to implement prevention programs targeted at risk groups.

2. Methods

2.1 Population sample

The data were obtained from 505 adolescents, middle school pupils (264 boys and 241 girls) aged 15 years, who were enrolled into a cross- sectional health screening study undertaken by the municipal health care authorities of Katowice (Poland) - in collaboration with our group. In the morning, after an overnight fast, the participants reported to the hospital to undergo a brief general medical examination, including assessment of anthropometric parameters, measurement of blood pressure, and collection of venous blood samples for biochemical analyses. The participants, boys and girls separately, were classified into one of the four groups, according to their Body Mass Index (BMI) score, using the age and gender-specific cut-off points of the BMI percentiles established for 15-years old Polish youth by Palczewska & Niedźwiecka (2002): group A of the underweight (<25 c), group B of the normal weight (25-75c), group C of the overweight (75-97 c), and group D of the obese (>97 c) individuals (Table 1). Criterion for diagnosis of obesity at BMI≥ 97th percentile was consistent with the WHO references for children 5 to 19 years old (available at http://www.who.growthref). Informed consent was obtained from all adolescents and their parents prior to participation in the study, the protocol of which was approved by the local Ethics Committee.

Gender	Variable	Percentile ranges (c)			
		Underweight (<25 c) X±SD	Normal weight (25-75 c) X±SD	Marginally overweight (75-90 c) and overweight (90-97 c) X±SD	Obese (>97 c) X±SD
Boys	No. of cases	N=55	N=98	N=54	N=57
	Body height, m	1.65*±0.08	1.71±0.07	1.69±0.09	1.70±0.08
	Body mass, kg	45.9***±5.2	57.7±6.0	70.3***±7.93	82.7***±11.6
	BMI	16.7***±0.9	19.7±1.1	24.6***±0.9	28.6***±3.4
	SBP, mm Hg	118.8±10.6	124.9±14.3	132.8*±14.8	135.7**±15.2
	DBP, mm Hg	71.3±8.5	71.6±11.1	73.4±9.2	73.7±10.2
Girls	No. of cases	N=58	N=81	N=46	N=56
	Body height, m	1.65±0.08	1.66±0.08	1.65±0.09	1.64±0.08
	Body mass, kg	46.1***±5.1	54.1±6.5	67.2***±7.8	79.4***±11.8
	BMI	17,0***±0.9	19.6±1.2	24.7***±0.8	29.3***±3.2
	SBP, mm Hg	118.7±12.9	124.8±12.4	124.7±15.7	132.5*±15.3
	DBP, mm Hg	69.4±0.08	74.4±9.2	72.9±11.1	74.8±11.1

Table 1. Anthropometric characteristics, and systolic (SBP) and diastolic (DBP) blood pressure of 15-year-old Polish adolescents. Significance of differences *vs.* normal weight individuals: *p<0.05, *** p<0.001

2.2 Analytical procedures

Concentrations of serum glucose, total cholesterol (TC), HDL-cholesterol (HDL-C), triglycerides (TG) were assessed by the enzymatic methods using commercially available diagnostic kits (BioMaxima cat.no. 1-033-0400, 1-023-0400, 1-029-0200, 1-053-0400, respectively). Concentrations of low-density lipoprotein cholesterol (LDL-C) were calculated from TC, HDL-C, and TG using the Friedewald formula (Friedewald et al., 1972). Serum insulin was measured by the immunoradiometric method (Insulin IRMA IM3210, Immunotech SA, France), sensitivity was 2.0 mIU/ml, and autoantibodies against oxidized LDL (oLAb) in serum samples were evaluated using ELISA assay (oLAb-ELISA, BI-20032; Biomedica GmbH, Wien, Austria) according to Tatzber & Esterbauer (1995).

To evaluate risk for vascular disease , the lipid ratios (TC/HDL-C, LDL-C/HDL-C, TG/HDL-C) and atherogenic index of plasma [AIP= log_{10}(TG/HDL-C) with TG and HDL-C expressed in molar concentrations] (Dobiášová & Frohlich, 2001, 2004, 2011) were calculated. The homeostatic model assessment (HOMA) was used to estimate insulin resistance according to the method described by Matthews (1998). Insulin resistance score (HOMA-IR) was computed using the following formula: HOMA-IR=glucose (mmol/L)*insulin (mIU/L)/22.5, with the cut-off point for adolescents less than or equal to 3.16 , as suggested by Keskin et al. (2005). Moreover, in 231 individuals (121 boys and 110 girls) serum adiponectin was measured by an immunoenzymatic method (Human Adiponectin ELISA, BioVendor, cat. no. RD195023100), and serum insulin-like growth factor (IGF-1) was evaluated in 80 adolescents (40 boys and 40 girls) using a commercially available diagnostic kit (IGF-I ELISA, Immunodiagnostic Systems GmbH, sensitivity 3.1 µg/L, reference range for 12 to 15 y old subjects 142-525 µg/L).

2.3 Statistics

All statistical analyses were performed with STATISTICA 7.1 software (StatSoft, Tulsa, OK, USA). The data reported as means ± SD were tested for homogeneity of variances by using the Levene test, then two-way ANOVA was performed to analyze the effect of gender and the degree of overweight/obesity on the studied variables, followed where appropriate, by the Tukey post-hoc comparisons. Spearman's rank order correlation analysis was performed to assess relationships between selected variables. Additionally, Pearson's Chi-square test of independence was used to evaluate the impact of the degree of overweight/obesity on SBP, serum triglycerides and surrogate markers of insulin resistance (HOMA-IR, TG/HDL-C). To predict the relative contribution of selected metabolic variables to prevalence of over normal SBP, insulin resistance (as assessed by HOMA-IR) and atherogenic potential of plasma (as assessed by AIP) a stepwise multiple regression analysis was applied. The level of significance of $P<0.05$ was chosen for all statistical comparisons.

3. Results

Physical characteristics of individual groups of the participants are presented in Table 1. In the evaluation of between-group differences, the data obtained in 113 adolescents (55 boys and 58 girls) with underweight, in 100 individuals (54 boys and 46 girls) with a tendency to overweight or overweight, and in 113 obese subjects (57 boys and 56 girls) were compared to the data obtained in 179 adolescents (98 boys and 81 girls) with normal weight. Mean values and percentiles of BMI were similar among the groups of boys and girls with various degree of overweight, while the mean values of BMI in both groups of normal-weight teens were very close to the 50 percentile of BMI distribution for 15 year old boys and girls (Palczewska & Niedźwiecka, 2001; WHO Growth reference data for 5 to 19 years, available at http://www.who.growthref).

The readings of systolic and diastolic blood pressure (SBP and DBP) in all groups of adolescents, stratified according to gender and degree of overweight, were compared with the data of the updated blood pressure charts for children and adolescents according to the child's age and height percentile. For the purposes of this study, the following criteria were adopted. The adolescents were classified as normotensive if their systolic BP was <90th percentile, i.e. <130 mm Hg. The measured SBP >90th percentile, which could indicate prehypertension or hypertension, was classified as "over normal". These criteria were conform to the recommendations of the National High Blood Pressure Education Program The Fourth Report on the Diagnosis, Evaluation and Treatment of High Blood Pressure in Children and Adolescents, (2004), and to the guidelines of the IDF 2007 Consensus Statement (Zimmet et al., 2007; Alberti et al.,2006, 2007). There were numerous cases, in particular in overweight or obese boys and in obese girls, when SBP exceeded 136 mm Hg, the level suggesting occurrence of significant hypertension according to blood pressure criteria established by the Task Force report (Blood pressure charts for children and adolescents by age and height percentile, 2005; Update on the 1987 Task Force Report on High Blood Pressure in Children and Adolescents. A Working Group report from the National High Blood Pressure Education Program, 1996). Notably, more than a half of obese teens, especially girls, had over normal systolic BP.

Results of biochemical tests obtained in all groups stratified by gender and the degree of overweight are presented in Table 2. Except for a very limited number of cases, fasting blood glucose level, in all groups of boys and girls, did not exceed the upper limit of the normal range (100 mg/dL), while fasting insulin concentration tended toward higher values with growing degree of overweight to reach, in several cases, levels exceeding the upper limit of the reference range of the method used (2,6 – 22 μU/mL) (Table 2, Fig.1). As expected, the prevalence of insulin resistance, as assessed by the HOMA-IR index, increased significantly with the degree of overweight as measured by BMI. In the prevailing number of cases, the fasting serum levels of total cholesterol, HDL-C, LDL-C and calculated lipid ratios (TC /HDL-C, LDL-C / HDL-C) were within the specific reference ranges, while the concentration of TG and the TG/HDL-C ratio were found to reach the markedly higher values only in both groups of obese individuals (Table 2, Fig.1). Except for serum HDL-C, which was higher ($p<0.05$) in girls, there were no significant inter-gender differences for the remaining tested variables. There was a clear tendency toward higher levels of SBP, insulin, HOMA-IR , triglycerides, and TG/HDL-C ratio with increased degree of overweight (Fig.1) in adolescent boys and girls, and most of these measures were affected significantly by the degree of overweight (Table 2). It is also worth to note that the degree of overweight/obesity significantly affected the atherogenic index of plasma (AIP), which adopted the lowest (most favorable) levels in the underweight groups, and then increased progressively with rising body mass index (Table 2, Fig.1). No between-group differences were found in titers of autoantibodies against oxidized LDL (oLAb), while individual oLAb titers were very variable, reaching over normal levels (>600 mU/mL) (Pincemail et al., 2000) in several subjects from each group. Similarly, no between-group differences were observed

Gender	Variables	Percentile ranges (c) Underweight (<25 c) X±SD	Normal weight (25-75 c) X±SD	Marginally overweight (75-90 c) and overweight (90-97 c) X±SD	Obese (>97 c) X±SD	Main effect: degree of overweight P value
Boys	No. of cases	N=55	N=98	N=54	N=57	N=264
	Cholesterol (TC), mg/dL	169.4±25.3	167.2±26.0	170.5±25.1	174.1±24.3	P<0.05
	HDL-C, mg/ dL	54.5±5.3	53.5±5.3	54.8±6.1	54.9±4.8	NS
	LDL-C, mg/ dL	93.3±22.9	92.1±22.0	93.2±22.8	93.0±24.6	NS
	oLAb, mU/mL	921.6±817.8	947.6±726.9	845.3±849.8	821.1±672.4	NS
	TG, mg/ dL	108.0±27.3	108.0±22.9	112.3±29.0	130.7**±50.0	P<0.005
	TC/HDL-C	3.12±0.44	3.13±0.41	3.12±0.40	3.18±0.42	NS
	LDL-C/HDL-C	1.72±0.41	1.72±0.38	1.71±0.40	1.70±0.44	NS
	TG/HDL-C	2.00±0.55	2.02±0.42	2.07±0.59	2.41*±0.98	P<0.005
	AIP	-0.074±0.114	-0.063±0.090	-0.059±0.111	-0.007*±0.117	P<0.01
	Glucose, mg/ dL	84.2±11.9	82.2±11.8	83.7±11.8	81.5±10.2	NS
	Insulin, mIU/L	9.4±7.8	11.6±8.0	13.7±12.3	16.1*±9.5	P<0.005
	HOMA-IR	1.97±1.61	2.38±1.80	2.89±2.82	3.24±1.94	P<0.05
	Adiponectin, ng/mL (N=121)	14.3**±19.9	9.5±7.7	9.9±6.4	9.4±5.3	P<0.005
	IGF-1, ng/mL (N=40)	287.8±118.6	500.3±261.4	432.8±127.6	420.8±123.3	NS
Girls	No. of cases	N=58	N=81	N=46	N=56	N=241
	Cholesterol (TC), mg/dL	173.7±23.2	167.0±26.1	175.5±23.9	171.4±22.5	NS
	HDL-C, mg/dL	56.7±6.1	55.03±5.486.3	55.23±5.14	55.65±5.91	NS
	LDL-C, mg/dL	95.8±20.9	89.1±23.4	96.8±20.0	89.5±20.7	NS
	oLAb, mU/mL	877.3±800.0	790.5±688.7	980.5±800.8	787.5±705.2	NS
	TG, mg/dL	106.0±25.2	114.7±29.0	117.3±25.4	131.6*±51.6	P<0.05
	TC/HDL-C	3.08±0.44	3.05±0.46	3.18±0.34	3.10±0.44	NS
	LDL-C/HDL-C	1.71±0.39	1.63±0.43	1.75±0.32	1.62±0.39	NS
	TG/HDL-C	1.89±0.51	2.10±0.54	2.13±0.44	2.41±1.07	P<0.005
	AIP	-0.097±0.110	-0.051±0.105	-0.041±0.089	-0.009±0.151	P<0.01
	Glucose, mg/ dL	81.2±9.7	80.8±10.4	83.7±12.6	83.3±10.8	NS
	Insulin, mIU/L	8.4±4.2	12.6±12.9	15.5±13.3	18.3±15.1 P=0.06	P<0.005
	HOMA-IR	1.69±0.90	2.65±2.86	3.29±3.08	3.74±3.11	P<0.05
	Adiponectin, ng/mL (N=110)	14.2**±10.1	8.3±4.7	9.0±4.5	11.3±5.5	P<0.01
	IGF-1, ng/mL (N=40)	385.0±76.5	387.5±170.5	398.0±98.5	388.3±60.8	NS

Table 2. Serum biochemical parameters in 15-year-old Polish adolescents. Significance of differences *vs.* normal weight individuals: *p<0.05, ** p<0.005, NS-non significant

in serum IGF-1, there was only a slight tendency toward higher IGF-1 levels in boys and the lowest values in underweight individuals, although both effects did not reach statistical significance. Serum adiponectin in both groups of overweight or obese individuals was close to the levels recorded in normal weight teens, but the highest concentrations of this adipokine, significantly (p<0.05) different from the values recorded in normal weight individuals, were found in the underweight groups (Table 2, Fig1).

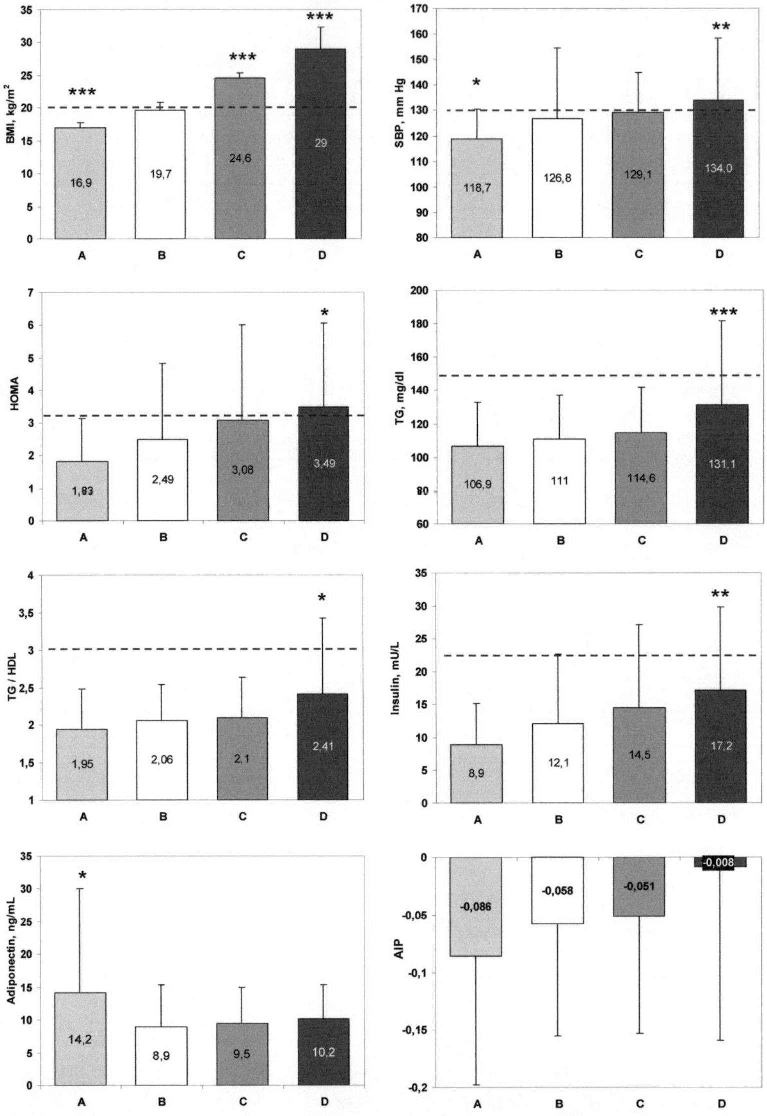

Fig. 1. The impact of the degree of overweight/obesity on systolic blood pressure (SBP), HOMA-IR, serum concentration of triglycerides (TG), TG/HDL ratio, insulin and adiponectin levels, and atherogenic index of plasma (AIP) in 15-year-old Polish adolescents with underweight (A), normal weight (B), overweight (C) and obesity (D). Significance of differences *vs.* individuals with normal weight: *p<0.05,** p<0.01, ***p<0.001

The analysis carried out to assess the prevalence (%) of adolescents with over normal values of SBP (>130 mm Hg), serum triglycerides (> 150 mg/dL) (Zimmet et al., 2007), HOMA-IR (>3.16) (Keskin et al., 2005), and TG/HDL-C ratio (>3.0) (McLaughlin et al., 2003; Hannon et al., 2006) revealed a rising number of individuals fulfilling these criteria with an increasing degree of overweight (Table 3). Noteworthy, Pearson's chi-square test showed significant increases in the prevalence (%) of individuals with over normal levels of these parameters with raising BMI.

Prevalence (%) of individuals with over normal values of SBP, HOMA-IR, TG, and TG/HDL-C ratio							Pearson's Chi-square (df=3)	
Group: Boys (B) and/or girls (G)			Underweight (<25 c)	Normal weight (25-75 c)	Marginally overweight (75-90 c) and overweight (90-97 c)	Obese (>97c)	X^2	P value
SBP >130 mmHg	B+G	34.5	13.4	31.1	40.0	56.9	48.5	$<10^{-5}$
	B	36.2	13.0	32.3	50.0	52.8	24.1	$<10^{-4}$
	G	32.8	13.8	29.6	28.3	60.7	30.1	$<10^{-5}$
HOMA-IR >3,16	B+G	22.5	8.0	19.6	25.5	39.3	33.2	$<10^{-5}$
	B	21.7	10.9	20.1	22.6	33.3	8.4	<0.05
	G	23.4	5.2	18.5	28.9	45.5	27.5	$<10^{-5}$
TG >150 mg/dL	B+G	10.7	6.2	6.7	7.0	24.8	30.3	$<10^{-5}$
	B	9.5	7.3	3.1	7.4	24.6	20.4	<0.0005
	G	12.0	5.2	11.1	6.5	25.0	12.9	<0.005
TG/HDL-C > 3.0	B+G	6.3	4.4	3.4	5.0	14.2	15.3	<0.005
	B	7.2	5.5	2.1	7.4	17.5	13.3	<0.005
	G	5.4	3.5	5.0	2.2	10.7	4.5	NS

Table 3. Prevalence (%) of 15 year-old boys (B) and girls (G) with over normal values of systolic blood pressure (SBP), HOMA-IR, triglycerides (TG), and TG/HDL-C.

In order to assess the impact of the degree of overweight on selected biochemical parameters and biomarkers of atherogenic risk, the Spearman rank correlation coefficients were computed, and selected statistically significant associations are summarized in Tables 4 and 5. As expected, the BMI and serum triglycerides correlated positively with systolic and diastolic blood pressure, insulin, and HOMA-IR. Serum adiponectin correlated negatively with lipid ratios (TG/HDL-C, TC/HDL-C, LDL-C/HDL-C), while it was positively associated with HDL-C. The oLAb titers correlated positively with serum LDL-C and LDL-C/HDL-C ratio (Table 4).

The important finding was that the atherogenic index of plasma (AIP) was positively correlated with the BMI, systolic and diastolic blood pressure, TG, total cholesterol, common lipid ratios (LDL-C/HDL-C, TC/HDL-C), insulin, HOMA-IR, but negatively associated with HDL-C and adiponectin (Table 5). Although these relationships do not infer casual dependence between the variables studied, they may suggest that there is a cluster of metabolically linked risk factors that, along with the hypertension and degree of obesity, determines the risk of atherosclerotic vascular disease. This hypothesis was fully supported by our results of a stepwise multivariate regression analyses that have shown that the main predictors of insulin resistance, as assessed by HOMA-IR, were concentrations of insulin and TG or TG/HDL-C ratio (R^2=0.96, p<0.0001), while concentrations of TG, LDL-C and of total cholesterol (TC) accounted for 95% (R^2=0.95, p<0.0001) of atherogenic potential of plasma (AIP) variance, and the most important predictors of systolic blood pressure (SBP) were BMI, TG and LDL/HDL ratio (R^2=0.16, p<0.001).

Variables	N	R	p
BMI & SBP	498	0.332	$P<10^{-6}$
BMI & DBP	498	0.128	P<0.005
BMI & insulin	502	0.377	$P<10^{-6}$
BMI & HOMA-IR	502	0.360	$P<10^{-6}$
BMI & TG	505	0.189	$P<10^{-4}$
BMI & TG/HDL-C	505	0.174	$P<10^{-4}$
TG & SBP	498	0.184	$P<10^{-4}$
TG & DBP	498	0.170	p<0.0005
TG & insulin	502	0.272	$P<10^{-6}$
TG & cholesterol	505	0.343	$P<10^{-6}$
TG & HOMA-IR	502	0.266	$P<10^{-6}$
TG/HDL-C & HOMA-IR	502	0.262	$P<10^{-6}$
Adiponectin & HDL-C	231	0.308	$P<10^{-4}$
Adiponectin & TG/HDL-C	231	-0.194	P<0.005
Adiponeectin & TC/HDL-C	231	-0.208	P<0.005
Adiponectin &LDL/HDL-C	231	-0.198	P<0.005
Adiponectin & oLAb	231	-0.169	P<0.05
oLAb & LDL-C	438	0.106	P<0.05
oLAb & LDL-C/HDL-C	438	0.129	P<0.01

Table 4. Spearman's rank order correlation coefficients between selected anthropometric and biochemical variables in 15-year- old Polish adolescents.

Variables	N	R	p
AIP & BMI	505	0.174	P<0.0001
AIP & SBP	498	0.139	P<0.005
AIP & DBP	498	0.104	p<0.05
AIP & TG	505	0.907	$P<10^{-6}$
AIP & HDL-C	505	-0.297	$P<10^{-6}$
AIP & INS	502	0.272	$P<10^{-6}$
AIP & HOMA-IR	502	0.262	$P<10^{-6}$
AIP & adiponectin	231	-0.194	P<0.005

Table 5. Spearman's rank order correlation coefficients between atherogenic index of plasma (AIP) and selected physical and biochemical variables in 15-year- old Polish adolescents.

4. Discussion

Multiple studies (Aggoun, 2007; Carnethon et al., 2004; Davis et al., 2001; Dietz, 1998; Dietz & Robinson, 2005; Franks et al., 2010; Han & Lean, 2006; Magnussen et al., 2010; Morrison et al., 2007; Must et al., 1992; Shengxu et al., 2003; Wang et al., 2008; Whitaker et al., 1997) have demonstrated that obesity at the developmental age poses an important risk factor for the development of cardiovascular diseases in youth and adulthood. The main objective of this cross-sectional study was screening for cardiovascular risk factors in a locally living urban population of 15-year old adolescents that could be easily applied in the early diagnosis of metabolic disorders in overweight and obese youth. The following independent risk factors were taken into consideration : degree of overweight/obesity, over normal blood pressure, insulin resistance, dyslipidemia, and adiponectin level (Aggoun, 2007; McLaughlin et al., 2003; Hannon et al., 2006; Kaelber & Pickett, 2009; McNiece et al., 2007;The Fourth report on the Diagnosis, Evaluation, and Treatment of High Blood Pressure in Children and Adolescents, 2004).

The important finding of this study is that over normal SBP and DBP values were strongly associated with body mass index (BMI). Namely, the prevalence of over normal SBP (i.e.>130 mmHg) was twice as high in the obese, compared with normal-weight teens, and four times higher in the obese than in the underweight groups, but there was no significant difference in the prevalence of over normal SBP between the two sexes. The marked increase of prevalence of over normal SBP with the degree of overweight in the participants of our study strongly supports the view that obesity is becoming a significant health issue in the young Polish population. Our observations fully support previous studies among various ethnic and racial groups that have shown the higher prevalence of abnormally high blood pressure in obese, compared with non-obese children and adolescents (Mc Niece et al. , 2007; Sorof &Daniels, 2002; Verma et al., 1994; Macedo et al., 1997).

Obesity-related elevated blood pressure in adolescence, is known to increase the risk of hypertension in adulthood (Cook et al., 2003; The Fourth Report on the Diagnosis, Evaluation and Treatment of High Blood Pressure in Children and Adolescents, 2004; Williams et al., 2002). Increased blood pressure is also considered the independent predictor of atherosclerosis, hyperplasia and hypertrophy of vascular smooth muscle, the factors affecting arterial stiffness (Aggoun, 2007).

There is a large body of evidence that obesity is associated with metabolic pathology such as impaired glucose tolerance, insulin resistance, and dyslipidemia. Studies using specimens collected at autopsy (McGill, 1997; Berenson et al., 1998), or using non-invasive assessment of carotid intima-media thickness (IMT) by ultrasonography (Berenson, 2002; Davis et al., 2001; Raitakari et al., 2003; Shengxu et al., 2003) demonstrated that the atherosclerotic process begins in childhood and adolescence and may track into adulthood. In this regard, the occurrence of highly statistically significant positive correlations between body mass index (BMI) and serum levels of triglycerides and insulin, or surrogate markers of insulin resistance (HOMA-IR and TG/HDL-C) fully confirmed the view that obesity occurring during developmental age raises the risk of developing type 2 diabetes and cardiovascular disease in the young .

In the present study, the assessment of risk for CVD and insulin resistance in 15-year old subjects was based on the analysis of serum biomarkers, such as total cholesterol (TC) and its lipoprotein fractions (LDL-C and HDL-C), triglycerides (TG), insulin, and glucose. Interestingly, no between group differences in serum concentrations of total cholesterol, LDL- and HDL cholesterol, lipid ratios (TC/HDL-C and LDL-C/HDL-C) and glucose were found. The mean values of these variables did not exceed the cut-off points recommended by the American Heart Association (Kavey et al., 2003) set at 170 mg/dL for TC, 110 mg/dL for LDL-C and 35 mg/dL for HDL-C. In this respect, the results of the present study are consistent with those previously reported by Lee at al. (2009), who found that the BMI percentiles do not provide effective discrimination for distinguishing children with abnormal TC and LDL-C levels. On the contrary, compared with the control groups of normal weight teens, the mean concentration of serum TG was significantly higher in the obese boys and girls, although it did not exceed the borderline level (150 mg/dL) as defined by the IDF guidelines (Alberti et al., 2006, 2007; Zimmet et al. , 2007). A similar trend was observed for TG/HDL-C ratio, considered a simple metabolic marker for identification of overweight individuals who are insulin resistant (McLaughlin et al., 2003; Hannon et al., 2006; Brehm et al., 2004).

The usefulness of the TG/HDL-C ratio as a marker of insulin resistance was additionally supported by its significant correlation with HOMA-IR. It should be stressed, however, that not all overweight and obese teens could be diagnosed as insulin resistant. Noteworthy, the prevalence of individuals with HOMA-IR exceeding the cut-off point (3.16) for adolescents (Keskin et al., 2005) rose with degree of overweight, and reached the highest levels in the obese groups, but only in about 40% of obese teens it exceeded the borderline level. Noteworthy is that the risk of becoming insulin resistant was higher among obese girls than among obese boys. Less marked increases were observed for TG or TG/HDL-C levels, as only in about 25% or 15 % of obese individuals they exceeded the respective cutoff points. Significantly higher serum levels of TG in obese individuals may indicate increased risk for atherosclerosis and obesity-related insulin resistance. This hypothesis is strongly supported by our finding of significant correlations between TG and atherogenic index of plasma (AIP), total cholesterol (TC), insulin, and HOMA-IR. Existing evidence suggests that serum TG is a strong predictor of CVD (Gotto, 1998), although it was found that TG can regulate lipoprotein interactions, but is not an independent risk factor.

This opinion is supported by the evidence that hypertriglyceridemia is associated with predominance of more atherogenic small dense LDL particles (sdLDL) (Packard, 1996). The increased risk may be related to easier penetration of sdLDL into the sub-endothelial space, their lower binding affinity to the LDL receptor and a higher susceptibility to oxidation. Although various techniques are available for direct measurement of LDL particle size distribution (Superko, 1996) , an indirect (surrogate) method may be used for evaluation of the atherogenicity of plasma lipoproteins based on the assessment of the Atherogenic Index of Plasma (AIP), calculated as log(TG/HDL-C) (with TG and HDL-C expressed in molar concentrations) (Dobiášová & Frohlich , 2001). It is well documented that changes in AIP may predict LDL particle size, and provide reliable information about the atherogenicity of plasma (Dobiášová & Frohlich, 2001; Dobiášová, 2004; Dobiášová et al., 2011; Onat et al., 2010). One of the most important findings of the present study is that there was a statistically significant trend toward higher values of AIP with raising degree of overweight, which supports the view that obesity is the main predictor of the CVD risk, and that atherogenic index of plasma (AIP) is a suitable tool to evaluate the risk.

It has been suggested that accelerated atherosclerosis in diabetes may be due to an enhanced oxidative modification of LDL, and of sdLDL in particular (Uusitupa et al., 1996). It was also suggested that LDL modified by glycation, as it may occur in diabetic patients, may be more susceptible to oxidation (Jenkins et al., 2004). Oxidatively modified LDL (oxLDL) that are strongly atherogenic may induce the immune response associated with enhanced production of specific autoantibodies against oxLDL (oLAb) (Steinerová et al., 2001; Shoenfeld et al., 2004). In the present study, the oLAb titers, the mean values of which were within the reference range set by Pincemail et al. (2000) for the method used in our study, appeared to be independent of the degree of obesity and HOMA-IR estimated insulin resistance but, as could be predicted, they were correlated with serum LDL-C and the LDL-C/HDL-C ratio. These results are fully consistent with those reported by Uusitupa et al (1996) and Jenkins et al. (2004) who found that autoantibodies against oxLDL indicate the presence of oxidatively modified LDL *in vivo*, but their titers do not seem to predict cardiovascular morbidity or carotid IMT.

Research into the mechanisms and mediators of obesity-related pathologies also called attention to the involvement of the adipose tissue in the regulation of energy balance by a number of adipose tissue -derived peptide hormones (adipocytokines), such as leptin, adiponectin and resistin, all seem to be involved in insulin resistance associated with obesity. We focused our attention on adiponectin, and we found that the highest circulating levels of this adipocytokine were found in the underweight groups of teens. This observation is consistent with the previously described effects of weight-loss on increases in serum adiponectin (Elloumi et al., 2009). Interestingly, high levels of serum adiponectin have been reported in anorectic patients (Nedvidkova et al., 2005; Pannacciulli et al., 2003). Adiponectin is recognized for its beneficial antiatherogenic, antidiabetogenic, and anti inflammatory action, mainly due to its ability to improve insulin sensitivity (Körner et al., 2007; Cruz et al., 2004; Nedvidková et al., 2005), to inhibit TNF-α mediated adherence of monocytes, to reduce their phagocytic activity, to suppress the accumulation of modified lipoproteins in the vascular wall , and to stimulate endothelial NO production (Ekmekci & Elmekci, 2006). Statistically significant positive correlation between serum adiponectin and HDL-cholesterol, and the negative associations with common lipid ratios (TC/HDL-C and LDL-C/HDL-C) and AIP seem to confirm the beneficial antiatherogenic effect of this hormone, and suggest low risk of dyslipidemia in adolescents with low body weight. Of note, the associations of adiponectin with HOMA-IR, LDL-cholesterol, triglycerides and insulin were also negative, but they did not reach statistical significance, most likely due to the limited number (N=231) of adiponectin data.

In the present study we have also made a preliminary attempt to investigate the association between serum IGF-1 and obesity-related insulin resistance in adolescent subjects. The data from the literature suggest that IGF-1 may have beneficial effect on glucose homeostasis, due to its glucose lowering and insulin sensitizing actions (Kabir et al., 2010). Adult studies suggest that lower IGF-1 level in childhood predict increased risk for developing insulin resistance and type 2 diabetes (Dunger et al., 2003). Moreover, previous studies reported that circulating fasting free IGF-1 were higher in obese subjects compared with normal weight controls, whereas total IGF-1 were not significantly different between the groups (Nam et al., 1997). Our results on obesity- related changes in serum total IGF-1, that found neither between group differences nor significant associations between total IGF-1 and selected indices of insulin resistance, are consistent with the latter findings.

The main limitation of this cross-sectional study was that it did not allow to validate the hypothesis of tracking the obesity-related cardiovascular risk into adulthood . Therefore, a follow up study of adolescent subjects diagnosed as being at higher risk for CVD would be necessary. However, given a large body of evidence provided by numerous previously mentioned prospective studies substantiating this assumption, early detection and awareness of CVD risk in adolescent subjects may allow the implementation of preventive strategies at a stage when intervention, such as personal advice for lifestyle improvement or well targeted drug therapy, may reverse damage.

4.1 Conclusions

We seem to be authorized to conclude that:

1. Overweight and obesity in adolescents strongly predispose them to a range of adverse health outcomes, including insulin resistance, hypertension and cardiovascular morbidities, despite the absence of evident symptoms of impaired glucose tolerance or dyslipidemia, as they are rarely reported for this age group.
2. Obese adolescents are at significant risk for becoming obese adults.
3. The most suitable metabolic markers and predictors of cardiovascular disease risk during adolescence and adulthood are HOMA-IR , TG/HDL-C ratio, and atherogenic index of plasma (AIP).
4. High serum adiponectin concentration and low HOMA-IR or TG/HDL-C ratio are good prognostic markers of low risk for insulin resistance and atherosclerotic vascular disease.

5. Acknowledgment

A preliminary report of this work was presented in the poster session of the conference "Nutrition and physical activity in inhibiting the aging process" in Wroclaw (4-6 November, 2010). This study was partially supported by statutory funding from the Academy of Physical Education, Katowice, Poland.

6. References

Aggoun, Y. (2007) Obesity, metabolic syndrome, and cardiovascular disease. *Pediatric Res* 61: 653-659

Alberti, K.G.M.M,. Zimmet, P., Shaw, J. (2006) Metabolic syndrome-a new world-wide definition . A Consensus Statement from the International Diabetes Federation. *Diabet Med* 23:469-480

Alberti, K.G.M.M., Zimmet, P. & Shaw, J. (2007) International Diabetes Federation: a consensus on Type 2 diabetes prevention. *Diabet Med* 24:451-463

Berenson, G.S. (2002) Childhood risk factors predict adult risk associated with subclinical cardiovascular disease. The Bogalusa Heart Study. *Am J Cardiol* 90 (suppl):3L-7L

Berenson, G.S., Srinivasan, S.R., Bao, W., Newman III,W.P., Tracy, R.E. & Wattigney, W.A. (1998) Association between multiple cardiovascular risk factors and atherosclerosis in children and young adults. *N Engl J Med* 338:1650-1656

Bibbins-Domingo, K., Coxson, P., Pletcher, M.J., Lightwood, J. & Goldman, L. (2007) Adolescent overweight and future adult coronary heart disease. *N Engl J Med* 357: 2371-2379

Blood pressure charts for children and adolescents by age and height percentile (in Polish) (2005) *Endokrynologia* 1 (1): 34-40

Brehm ,A., Pfeiler, G., Pacini, G., Vierhapper, H. & Roden, M. (2004) Relationship between serum lipoprotein ratios and insulin resistance in obesity *Clin Chem* 50:2316-2322

Carnethon, M.R., Loria, C.M., Hill, J.O., Sidney, S., Savage P.J. & Liu, K. (2004) Risk factors for Metabolic Syndrome. The Coronary Artery Risk Development in Young Adults (CARDIA) study, 1885-2001. *Diabetes Care* 27: 2707-2715

Cook, S., Weitzman,M., Auinger, P., Nguyen, M. & Dietz, W.H. (2003) Prevalence of a metabolic syndrome phenotype in adolescents: findings from the Third National Health and Nutrition Examination Survey, 1988–1994. *Arch Pediatr Adolesc Med* 157: 821–827

Cruz, M., Garcia-Macedo. R., Garcia-Valerio, Y. , Gutierez,M., Medina-Navarro, R., Duran, G., Wacher, N. & Kumate,J. (2004) Low adiponectin levels predict type 2 diabetes in Mexican children. *Diabetes Care* 27: 1451-1453

Davis, P.H., Dawson, J.D., Riley,W.A. & Lauer, RM. (2001) Carotid intimal-medial thickness is related to cardiovascular risk factors measured from childhood through middle age: the Muscatine Study. *Circulation* 104:2815-2819

Dietz W.H. & Robinson T.N. (2005) Overweight children and adolescents. *N Engl J Med* 352:2100-2109

Dietz W.H. (1998) Health consequences of obesity in youth: childhood predictors of adult disease. *Pediatrics* 101: 518-525

Dobiášová, M. & Frohlich, J. (2001) The plasma parameter log(TG/HDL-C) as an atherogenic index: correlation with lipoprotein particle size and esterification rate in apoB-lipoprotein-depleted plasma (FER_{HDL}). *Clin Biochem* 34:583-588.

Dobiášová, M. (2004) Atherogenic index of plasma [Log(triglyceride/HDL-Cholesterol)]: theoretical and practical implications. *Clin Chem* 50:1113-1115

Dobiášová, M., Frohlich, J., Šedová, M., Cheung, M.C. & Brown, B.G. (2011) Cholesterol esterification and atherogenic index of plasma correlate with lipoprotein size and findings on coronary angiography. J *Lipid Res* 52: 566-571

Dunger, D.B., Ong, K.K.L. & Sandhu, M.S. (2003) Serum insulin-like growth factor -1 levels and potential risk of type 2 diabetes. *Horm Res* 60:131-135

Ekmekci, H. & Ekmekci O.B. (2006) The role of adiponectin in atherosclerosis and thrombosis. *Clin Appl Thrombosis/Hemostasis* 12:163-168

Elloumi, M., Ben Ounis, O., Makni, E., Van Praagh, E., Tabka,Z. & Lac G. (2009) Effect of individualized weight-loss programmes on adiponectin, leptin and resistin levels in obese adolescent boys. *Acta Pædiatrica* 98:1487-1493

Franks, P.W., Hanson, R.L., Knowler, W.C., Siebers, M.L., Bennett, P.H. & Hooker H.C. (2010) Childhood obesity, other cardiovascular risk factors and premature death. *N Engl J Med* 162: 485-493

Friedewald, W.T., Levy, R.I. & Fredrickson, D.S. (1972) Estimation of the concentration of low-density lipoprotein cholesterol in plasma, without use of the preparative ultracentrifuge. *Clin Chem* 18: 499-502

Gotto, A.M. Triglyceride. (1998) The forgotten risk factor. *Circulation* 97:1027-1028

Han, T.S . & Lean, M.E. (2006) Metabolic syndrome. *Medicine* 34 (12): 536-542

Hannon, T.S., Bacha, F., Lee, S.J., Janosky, J., Arsalanian,S.A.. (2006) Use of markers of dyslipidemia to identify overweight youth with insulin resistance. *Pediatric Diabetes* 7: 260-266

Jenkins, A.J., Thorpe, S.R., Anderson, N.L., Hermayer, K.L., Lyons, T.J., Kong LP, Chassereau ,C.N. & Klein, R.L. (2004) In vivo glycated low-density lipoprotein in not more susceptible to oxidation than nonglycated low-density lipoprotein in type 1 diabetes. *Metabolism- Clinical and Experimental* 53:969-976

Kabir, G., Hossain, M., Faruque, M.O., Hassan, N,. Hassan, Z., Nahar,Q., Shefin, S.M., Alauddin, M. & Ali, L. (2010) Associations of serum free IGF-1 and IGFBP-1 with insulin sensitivity in impaired glucose tolerance (IGT). *Int J Diab Mellitus* 2:144-147

Kaelber, D.C. & Pickett, F. (2009) Simple table to identify children and adolescents needing further evaluation of blood pressure. *Pediatrics* 123:e972-e974].

Kavey, W.E.W., Daniels, S.E., Lauer, R.M., Atkins ,D.L., Hayman, L. & Taubert K. (2003) AHA Scientific Statement American Heart Association Guidelines for Primary Prevention of Atherosclerotic Cardiovascular Disease Beginning in Childhood. *Circulation* 107:1562-1566

Keskin, M., Kurtoglu, S., Kendirci, M., Atabek, M.E. & Yazici,C. (2005) Homeostasis Model Assessment Is More Reliable Than the Fasting Glucose/Insulin Ratio and Quantitative Insulin Sensitivity Check Index for Assessing Insulin Resistance Among Obese Children and Adolescents. *Pediatrics* 115: e500-e503

Körner, A., Kratzsch, J., Gausche, R., Schaab, M., Erbs, S. & Kiess, W. (2007) New predictors of the metabolic syndrome in children-Role of adipocytokines. *Pediatr Res* 61:640-645

Lee, J.M., Gebremariam, A., Card-Higginson, P., Shaw, J.L., Thompson, J.W. & Davis MM. (2009) Poor performance of body mass index as a marker for hypercholesterolemia in children and adolescents. *Arch Pediatr Adolesc Med* 163: 716-723

Macedo, M.E., Trigueiros, D. & De Freitas, F. (1997) Prevalence of high blood pressure in children and adolescents. Influence of obesity. *Rev Port Cardiol* 16:27-28

Magnussen, C.G., Koskinen, J., Chen, W. , Thomson, R., Schmidt, M.D., Srinivasan, S.R. et al. (2010) Pediatric Metabolic Syndrome predicts adulthood Metabolic Syndrome, subclinical atherosclerosis, and type 2 diabetes mellitus but is no better than Body Mass Index alone. The Bogalusa heart study and the cardiovascular risk in young Finns study. *Circulation* 122: 1604-1611

Matthews, D.R., Hosker, J.P., Rudenski ,A.S., Naylor, B.A,, Treacher, D.F. & Turner, R.C. (1995) Homeostasis model assessment: insulin resistance and β-cell function from fasting plasma glucose and insulin concentrations in man. *Diabetologia* 28: 412-419

McGill, H.C.Jr, McMahan, C.A., Malcolm, G.T., Oalmann, M.C. & Strong, J.P. (1997) Effects of serum lipoproteins and smoking on atherosclerosis in young men and women: the Pathobiological Determinants of Atherosclerosis in Youth (PDAY) Research Group. *Arterioscler Thromb Vasc Biol* 17:95-106;

McLaughlin, T., Abbasi,F., Chel, K., Chu, J., Lamendola, C.& Reaven, G. (2003) Use of metabolic markers to identify overweight individuals who are insulin resistant. *Ann Intern Med* 139: 802-809

McNiece, K.L., Poffenbarger, T.S., Turner, J.L., Franco, K.D., Sorof, J.M.& Portman, R.J. (2007) Prevalence of hypertension and pre-hypertension among adolescents. *J Pediatr* 150, 640-644.e1

Morrison, J.A., Friedman, L.A.& Gray-McGuire, C. (2007) Metabolic syndrome in childhood predicts adult cardiovascular disease 25 years later: the Princeton Lipid Research Clinics follow-up study. *Pediatrics* 120: 340-345

Must, A., Jacques, P.F., Dallal, G.E., Bajema, C.J.& Dietz W.H. (1992) Long-term morbidity and mortality of overweight adolescents. *N Engl J Med* 327: 1350-1355

Nam, S.Y., Lee, E.J., Kim, K.R., Cha, B.S., Song, Y.D., Lim, S.K., Lee, H.C. & Huh, K.B. (1997) Effect of obesity on total and free insulin-like growth factor (IGF)-1, and their relationship to IGF-binding (BP)-1, IGFBP-2, IGFBP-3, insulin, and growth hormone. *Int J Obes Relat Metab Disord* 21: 355-359.

Nedvidková, J., Smitka, K., Kopský, V. & Hainer, V. (2005) Adiponectin, an adipocyte-derived protein. *Physiol Res* 54: 133-140

Nieto, F.J.: (1992) Childhood weight and growth rate as predictors of adult mortality. *Am J Epidemiol* 136: 201:213

Onat, A., Can, G., Kaya, H. & Hergenç, G. (2010) "Atherogenic index of plasma" (log_{10}triglyceride/high-density lipoprotein-cholesterol) predicts high blood pressure, diabetes, and vascular events. *J Clin Lipid* 4: 89-98

Packard, C.J. (1996) LDL subfractions and atherogenicity: an hypothesis from the University of Glasgow. *Curr Med Res Opin* 13:379-390

Palczewska, I., Niedźwiecka, Z. (2001) Somatic development indices in children and youth of Warsaw(in Polish), *Med. Wieku Rozwoj* 5 (2 Suppl 1):18-118

Pannacciulli, N., Vettor, R., Milan, G., Granzotto, M., Catucci, A., Federspil,G., De Giacomo,P., Giorgino, R. &De Pergola, G. (2003) Anorexia nervosa is characterized by increased adiponectin plasma levels and reduced nonoxidative glucose metabolism. *J Clin Endocrinol Metab* 88: 1748-1752

Pincemail , J., Siquet, J., Chapelle, J.P., Cheramy-Bien, J.P., Paulissen, G., Chantillon, A.M., Christiaens, G., Gielen, J., Limet, R. & Defraigne, J.O. (2000) Determination of concentrations of antioxidants, antibodies against oxidized LDL, and homocysteine in a population sample from Liège. *Ann Biol Clin (Paris)* (in French) 58: 177-185

Raitakari, O.T., Juonala, M., Kähönen, M, Taittonen, L., Laitinen, T., Maki-Torkko, N., Järvisalo, M.J., Uhari, M., Jokinen, E., Rönnemaa, T, Åkerblom, H.K. & Viikari, J.S.A. (2003) Cardiovascular risk factors in childhood and carotid artery intima-media thickness in adulthood. The cardiovascular risk in young Finns study. *JAMA* 290:2277-2283

Shengxu, L., Chen, W., Srinivasan, S.R., Bond, M.G., Tang ,R., Urbina, E.M. & Berenson, G.S. (2003) Childhood cardiovascular risk factors and carotid vascular changes in adulthood. The Bogalusa Heart Study. *JAMA* 290:2271-2276

Shoenfeld, Y., Wu, R., Dearing, L.D. & Matsuura, E. (2004) Are anti-oxidized low-density lipoprotein antibodies pathogenic or protective? *Circulation* 110:2552-2558

Sorof, J. & Daniels,S. (2002) Obesity hypertension in children. A problem of epidemic proportions. *Hypertension* 40: 441-447

Steinerová, A., Racek, J., Stožický, F., Zima, T., Fialová, L. & Lapin, A. (2001) Antibodies against oxidized LDL - theory and clinical use. *Physiol Rev* 50: 131-141

Superko, H.R. (1996) Beyond LDL cholesterol reduction. *Circulation* 94:2351-2354

Tatzber, F. & Esterbauer, H. Autoantibodies to oxidized low-density lipoprotein. In: Free Radicals IX, Bellomo G., Finardi E., Maggi E., Rice-Evans C. (eds) Richelieu Press, London 1995; pp.245-262

The fourth report on the diagnosis, evaluation, and treatment of high blood pressure in children and adolescents. National High Blood Pressure Education Program Working Group on High Blood Pressure in Children and Adolescents (2004) *Pediatrics* 114:555-576

Update on the 1987 Task Force Report on High Blood Pressure in Children and Adolescents. A Working Group report from the National High Blood Pressure Education Program. (1996) *Pediatrics* 98: 649–657

Uusitupa, M.I.J., Niskanen, L., Luoma, J., Vilja, P., Mercouri, M., Rauramaa, R. & Yla-Herttuala, S. (1996) Autoantibodies against oxidized LDL do not predict atherosclerotic vascular disease in non-insulin –dependent diabetes mellitus. *Arteriosclerosis, Thrombosis, and Vascular Biology* 16: 1236-1242

Verma, M., Chhatwal, J. & George, S.M. (1994) Obesity and hypertension in children. *Indian Pediatr* 31:1065-1069

Wang, L.Y., Chyen, D., Lee, S. &Lowry R. (2008) The association between body mass index in adolescence and obesity in adulthood. *J Adolesc Health* 42: 512-518

Whitaker, R.C., Wright, J.A., Pepe, M.S., Seidel, K.D. & Dietz, W.H. (1997) Predicting obesity in young adulthood from childhood and parental obesity. *N Eng J Med* 337:869-873

WHO. Growth reference data for 5 to 19 years (available at http://www.who.growthref)

Williams, C.L., Hayman, L.L., Daniels, S.R., Robinson, T.N., Steinberger, J, Paridon, S. & Bazzarre, T. (2002) Cardiovascular health in childhood: a statement for health professionals from the Committee on Atherosclerosis, Hypertension, and Obesity in the Young (AHOY) of the Council on Cardiovascular Disease in the Young, American Heart Association. *Circulation* 106:143–160

Zimmet, P., Alberti ,K.,G., Kaufman, F., Tajima ,N., Silink, M., Arslanian, S., Wong, G., Bennett ,P.& Shaw, J., Caprio, S. (2007) IDF Consensus Group. The metabolic syndrome in children and adolescents - an IDF consensus report. *Pediatric Diabetes* 8: 299-306

15

Peculiarities of Coronary Artery Disease in Athletes

Halna du Fretay Xavier[1,2], Akoudad Hafid[3],
Hamadou Ouceyni[2] and Benhamer Hakim[2,4,5]
[1]*Centre Hospitalier Universitaire Bichat Claude Bernard, Paris,*
[2]*Hopital Foch, Suresnes*
[3]*Centre Hospitalier Universitaire Hassan II, Fez*
[4]*Hôpital Européen de Paris la Roseraie, Aubervilliers*
[5]*Institut Cardiovasculaire Paris Sud, Massy*
[1,2,4,5]*France*
[3]*Maroc*

1. Introduction

Intense physical activity increases the risk of acute coronary syndrome but regular physical training is a cardio vascular protective factor (Shepard & Balady, 1999).

Sport related myocardial infarctions (SMI) are rare but serious. They present angiographic features that explain some clinical characteristics, the limits of the detection of coronary disease in this population and encourage decision making in order to have a better regulation of sport such as rules of good practice and dissemination of defibrillators on sports sites.

However, athletes could be asymptomatic despite tight coronary stenosis as in the three clinical cases presented. The reasons for the asymptomatic nature of these coronary diseases are probably due to cardiovascular adaptation to regular training. These athletes are at risk of major cardiac events and the place of stress testing remains important in this population.

2. Sport related myocardial infarctions

2.1 Clinical cases

2.1.1 Methods

We report a retrospective study of twelve cases of SMI. All patients had myocardial infarction (MI) defined as ischemic symptoms and ST segment elevation on ECG. MI was considered to be related to sport if it occurred during sport with vigorous exertions (METs > or = 6) or within 2 hours afterward according to the definition of Von Klot et al (Von Klot et al, 2008). All patients had emergent coronary angiography.

2.1.2 Results

A total of twelve patients are studied, all men. The mean age is 47.7 years (24 to 64). Eight of these patients considered themselves as insufficiently trained. Chest pain is the most common presentation (11/12) with initial collapse in one case (case 12). SMI occur after exercise in 3 cases and during in 9 cases with unusual very vigorous exertion in 5 cases. One patient returned to sport after a year off (case 12). In this series, the most common sport was running (33%). The clinical characteristics of patients are presented on table 1.

Only two patients had multivessel diseases. Primary coronary intervention (PCI) was performed in nine patients, fibrinolysis in two patients (cases 1 and 4). The last patient (case 7) had normal coronary angiography just after relief of chest pain but elevated markers of myocardial necrosis. Coronary angiographic findings are presented on table 2.

N°	Age (years)	Sex	Risk factors	Sports	Symptoms	Circumstances
1	40	M	S, FC	Swimming	Chest pain	After sport
2	51	M	0	Running	Syncope	During sport
3	52	F	H, FC	Running	Chest pain	During sport
4	45	M	0	Triathlon	Chest pain	During sport
5	40	M	FC	Running	Chest pain	During sport
6	24	M	S, FC	Football	Chest pain	After sport
7	39	M	0	Rugby	Chest pain	During sport
8	63	M	0	Cycling	Chest pain	During sport
9	48	M	S, FC	Karate	Chest pain	During sport
10	64	M	H, FC	Running	Chest Pain	After sport
11	50	M	D, FC	Tennis	Chest Pain	During sport
12	33	M	D	Football	Chest pain	During sport

Table 1. M: male; F: Female; S: cigarette smoking; FC: family history of coronary artery disease; D: dyslipidemia; H: hypertension; 0 : no risk factor

N°	Ter	CA	TIMI flow	Collaterals	Thrombus	AL
1	Ant	LAD	3	0	0	0
2	Ant	LAD	2	0	0	0
3	Ant	LAD	2	0	+	0
4	Ant	LAD	3	0	+	0
5	Ant	LAD	2	0	+	0
6	Glob	LM	2	0	+	CD
7	Inf	0	3	0	0	0
8	Inf	RCA	1	0	+	0
9	Inf	RCA	2	0	+	0
10	Inf	RCA	0	0	+	LAD
11	Inf	RCA	2	0	+	0
12	Inf	RCA	0	+	+	Mg *

Table 2. Ter: territory ; Ant: anterior wall ; Inf: inferior wall, Glob: global; CA: culprit artery; LM: left main; LAD: left anterior descending artery; RCA : right coronary artery; Mg: marginal branch of circumflex artery; AL: associated lesion, * lesion < 70 %

Thus the most common angiographic presentation is a single-vessel disease with thrombus as case N°11.

This patient had inferior SMI. Chest pain occurred during tennis training and he arrived in our cath lab three hours after symptom onset. Cardiac catheterization was performed using a 6 French sheath via right radial artery access. Pharmacotherapy included 70 U/Kg unfractionated heparin and 250 mg aspirin intravenous and clopidogrel 600 mg loading dose. The left coronary artery was normal (figure 1). The right was occluded, flow TIMI 0 (Figure 2). PCI was performed with use of a thrombus aspiration catheter. Fresh clots were retrieved from the filtered aspirated blood (Figure 3).

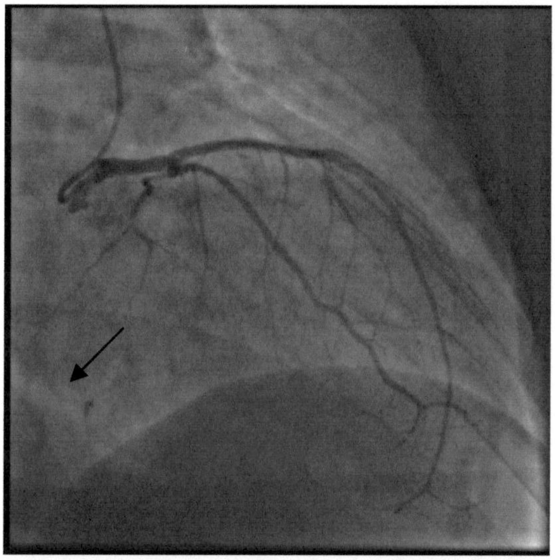

Fig. 1. Left coronary artery with collateral flow in the right coronary artery (black arrow)

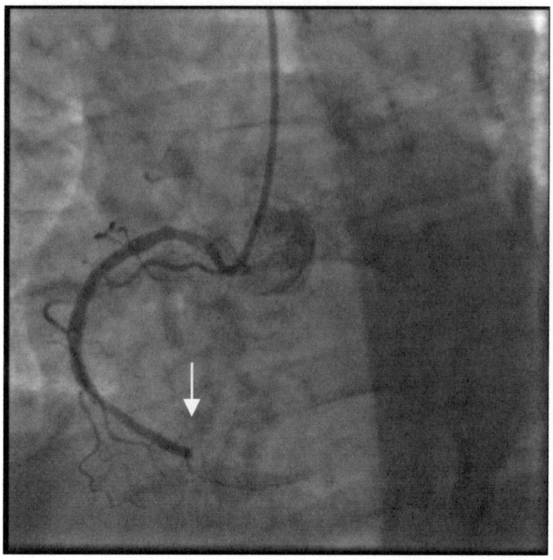

Fig. 2. Right coronary artery with thrombus (white arrow)

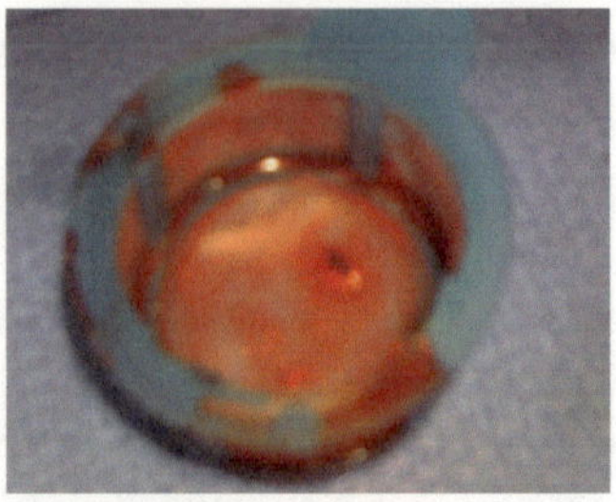

Fig. 3. Fresh clot removed by aspiration

Although after thromboaspiration only a limited stenosis remained (figure 4) a bare metal stent was placed to optimize the result (Figure 5).

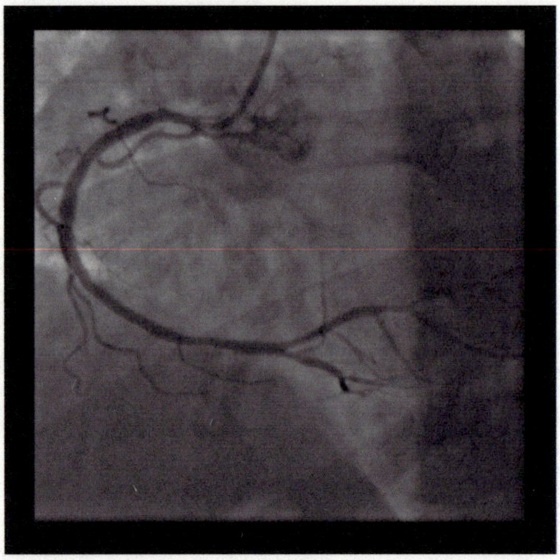

Fig. 4. Result after thrombus aspiration

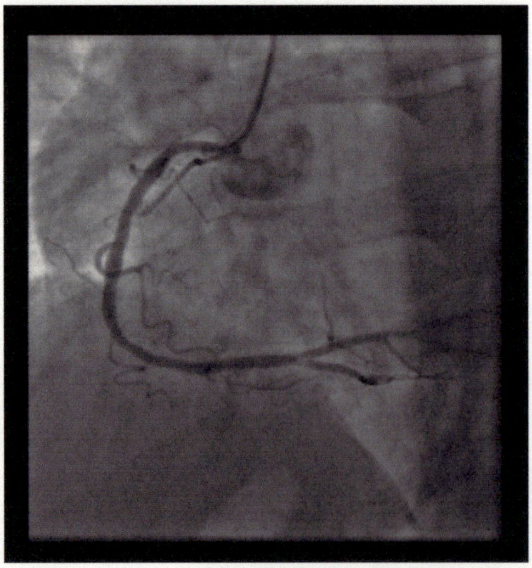

Fig. 5. Final result

2.2 Discussion and literature review

2.2.1 Prevalence of SMI

It is well reported that MI risk is increased during and after vigorous exercise (Gibson et al, 1980; Mittelman et al, 1993; Willich et al, 1993; Von Klot et al 2008). Ciampriccotti and Taverne reported even one case of MI twice during sporting activities (Ciampriccotti and Taverne, 1992). Mittelman et al reported that 4.4 % of MI were related to exercise which would represent more than 5000 MI per year in France. In addition, the majority of sport-related sudden deaths (SSD) are due to coronary artery disease and mainly MI.

The prevalence of SSD is more often evaluated, in retrospective studies (Maron et al, 1996; Peddoe, 2007), that of SMI. The SSD rates are between 1/50000 to 1/80000 athletes in these studies. SSD are most commonly related to coronary disease in the general population contrary to young competitive athletes (Marijon et al 2011).

Chevallier et al reported in a prospective study a yearly SMI incidence of 2.6/100000 persons. (50 SMI, lethal in 3 cases) (Chevallier et al, 2009).

So, SMI are rare but occur in a supposedly healthy population and shock the public opinion and the medical profession especially as the clinical presentation can be severe particularly when it comes to a sudden death.

2.2.2 Which athletes and which sports?

Running is the most commonly practiced sport in our study, reflecting European trends. Indeed the number of runners who completed the Paris Marathon has increased from 9000 to 30000 from 1990 to 2010. We have previously reported data for European studies about the type of sport during SMI (figure 6). The most commonly practiced sports in Europe are present. The number of runner is low as this is old data.

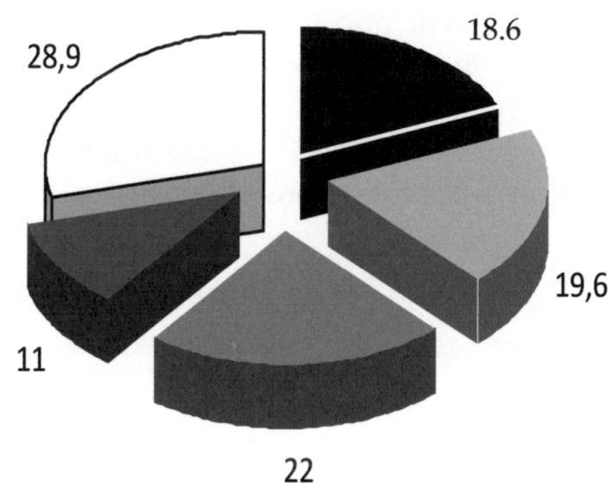

Fig. 6. Sports practiced during SMI : Tennis : ■; Cycling: ■; Football : ■ ; Running : ■; Other : □. (Halna du Fretay and Gerardin, 2008)

Recently, Marijon et al reported that cycling (30.6 %), running (21.3 % and football (13 %) were the most common sports related to sudden death (Marijon et al, 2011).

Hiltgen et al reported that SMI occurred most commonly after exertion and that the recovery period was particularly at high risk of SMI (Hiltgen et al 1989). The vagal stimulation may be the cause of coronary spasm, especially if the athlete smokes at this time. On the contrary, among runners, cardiac events occur in one third of cases at the end or after exercise and the rest during exercise (Robert and Maron, 2005; Pedoe, 2007; Gerardin, 2009). Gerardin reported even one case of SSD just at the start of the Paris Marathon.

SMI concern most often men aged over 35 years as in our study (10/12 patients) and is previously well reported (Roberts & Maron, 2005; Chevallier et al, 2009). Giri et al reported that patients with an exertion-related MI were more likely to have risk factors including male sex, hyperlipidemia, hypertension and current cigarette smoking (59 % versus 37 % in non exertion-related MI) but in a population of which had known coronary artery disease and older than that of our study (Giri et al 1999). There were 28 cigarette smokers in a population of 42 patients in one study on unstable angina, SMI and SSD related to sport (Ciampricotti et al, 1990). We find in our study, with a small number of patients, few risk factors in this population but often family history of coronary disease and 4/12 patients without risk factor. This is similar to those who suffer MI at young age (Kanitz et al 1996; Bajaj et al, 2011).

High frequency of exertion is a protection factor against SMI as reported by Giri and Mittelmann. The latter showed that the risk of MI during exertion or within one hour afterward was elevated 107 times for subjects who usually exercise less than one a week and only 2.4 times for those having more than 5 times (Mittelman et al, 1993). So the subject most at risk of SMI is an untrained man over 35 years, current smoker and SMI can occur throughout or after exercise.

2.2.3 Clinical characteristics

The existence of prodromata before SMI or SSD is variable in studies. Chest pain is most commonly reported in high cardiac risk population or in case of known ischemic heart disease (Opie, 1975; Northcote et al, 1986). Several studies reported the existence of symptoms neglected before SMI (Droniou et al, 1987; François et al, 1989). In the study of Droniou and all, symptoms were present in 45 % of cases particularly after the age of 40 years with angina in 11/20 cases. The prevalence of risk factor was high in this study.

In a population with few or no (23.8 % of patients) coronary risk factor, Ciampriccotti et al reported only 3 patients with prodromata in their study of 42 cases of SSD, SMI or unstable angina related to sport (Ciampriccotti et al, 1990). Pedoe and Gerardin reported very few or no symptom in cases of SSD most commonly due to ischemic heart diseases (Pedoe, 2007; Gerardin, 2009).

Giri and all found ventricular fibrillation in 20 % of exertion-related MI and 11 % in non exertion-related MI (Giri and all, 1999).

Thus SSD appears to be a common mode of SMI or unstable angina related to sport presentation, as reported by Ciampriccotti (28 % of cases), Gerardin (all cases) (Ciampriccotti et al, 1900; Gerardin, 2009). We find in our study just one case of possible ventricular arrhythmia. It may be due to the small number of patients and the fact that SMI occurred during trainings. Mental stress caused by a competitive situation leads to an greater increase in the heart rate during exertion (Lindholm et al, 2006;) and Viru et al reported that competitive conditions increase the cortisol response to exercise, suggesting that sympatho-adrenal system activation occur in such situations (Viru et al, 2010). Such complications are probably explained by high heart oxygen consumption during exertion at the time of SMI, the activation of the sympathoadrenergic system with increase of plasma nor epinephrine and epinephrine (Strobel et al, 1999), the absence of myocardial preconditioning due to the features of coronary disease in SMI wich could promote malignant ventricular arrhythmias.

2.2.4 Angiographic characteristics

In our study, 1 patient had normal coronary angiography, 8 patients had single vessel disease, and 3 multivessel disease. We had previously reported data from European studies showing the prevalence of single-vessel disease (Figure 7).

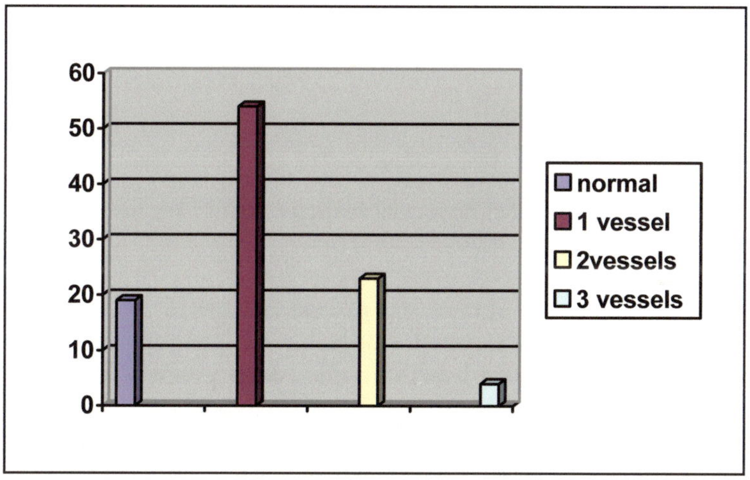

Fig. 7. Angiographic characteristics of SMI in European studies, percentage value of 97 patients, Halna du Fretay and Gerardin, 2008.

These angiographic characteristics are similar to those of MI in the young (Kanitz et al, 1996; Bajaj et al, 2011) despite a mean age of 45.7 years in our study.

Giri et al reported in their study 50 % of single-vessel disease in case of MI related to exertion and 28 % in case of MI none related to exertion. Three vessels disease was finding respectively in 8 % and 41 % of cases. Nevertheless, in the first group the population was more likely to have risk factors but was also more likely regular exertions with its probable beneficial effect (Giri et all 1999).

Most of the studies on SMI, usually with a younger population, show in more than 50 % of cases single vessel disease. Ambrose et al reported that MI frequently develops from previously non severe lesions (Ambrose et al, 1988). It is recognized that plaque rupture is the most common substrate for coronary thrombosis and occurs in case of vulnerable plaques as thin-caps fibroatheroma (Fuster et all, 2005). During exertion several phenomena occur as increased coronary flow, adrenergic activity, blood pressure and heart rate causing a shearing effect of the coronary arteries and favouring plaque rupture, intimal haemorrhage. Platelets are also implicated in the participation of acute coronary syndromes particularly in exercise (Hilberg et al, 2003) and strenuous exercise is associated with a transient hypercoagulability state (Lippi and Maffulli, 2009). In vivo platelet activation is reported in marathon runners (Kratz et al, 2006). Exertion can be the trigger of a vulnerable plaque rupture and thrombosis promoted by modifications of haemostasis. Another possible pathophysiological mechanism is the occurrence of spam (Hiltgen et al, 1989) and could explain the case N° 7 of our study. Few cases of spontaneous coronary dissection (Kalaga et al, 2007) and congenital coronary artery anomalies (Corrado et al, 1998) are also reported but concern young athletes with a different pathophysiological mechanism.

We can suppose that most of these patients with single-vessel disease had no severe coronary stenosis before SMI and that would explain the limits of stress testing to prevent SMI. Gerardin reported in their study 3 SMI with negative stress testing a few months before in 2 cases (Gerardin, 2009).

The patient of case N° 11 is a typical example of the probable pathophysiological mechanism of SMI.

2.2.5 Which specific treatment?

There is no specific treatment of SMI but some features should be noticed.

2.2.5.1 Prevention rules

Smoking is not only a risk factor of coronary disease but has also deleterious effects in the short term as an increased level of carboxyhemoglobin reducing the amount of haemoglobin available to carry oxygen, increased heart rate and blood pressure but with a decrease in coronary blood flow. It follows in an increase in myocardial consumption but a decreased supply. Smoking is also associated with an increased risk of vasospastic angina (Caralis et al, 1992). This can be mediated by increased catecholamines or during the recovery phase by acetylcholine release with vasospastic paradoxical effect in case of endothelial dysfunction. Chevallier et al reported that 73 % of young athletes smoke a cigarette in the last hour or two hours after a strenuous exercising (Chevallier et al, 2005). So educational measures against smoking are a priority.

Because of platelet activation during exercise aspirin use was discussed by some authors (Mittelman et al, 1993, Burtscher et al, 2007) but criticized by other and not recommended in case of exertion in hot weather (Fred, 1981) or with risk of body collision. Its use should be clarified by further studies, especially in athletes at risk of SMI.

2.2.5.2 Reperfusion therapy

Reperfusion strategies in SMI must be consistent with the recommendations of ESC for the treatment of STEMI but although the use of manual catheter thrombus aspiration during PCI is only class II a in the recent guidelines on myocardial revascularization (The Task Force on Myocardial Revascularization of ESC/EACTS, 2010), the advantage of this technique seems to be especially great in case of SMI.

2.2.5.3 Management of complications

We have previously emphasized the risk of sudden death or serious ventricular arrhythmias in SMI. Roberts and Maron reported nine cardiac events occurring during marathons, with SD (5 cases) and non fatal cardiac arrest (NFCA) (4 cases) from 1976 to 2004. Seven of the nine runners had underlying atherosclerotic coronary disease. The four patients with NFCA had external defibrillation performed promptly within 5 min. These authors observed a decrease in mortality since 1995, which was largely attributable to the expanded access to external defibrillators (figure 8).

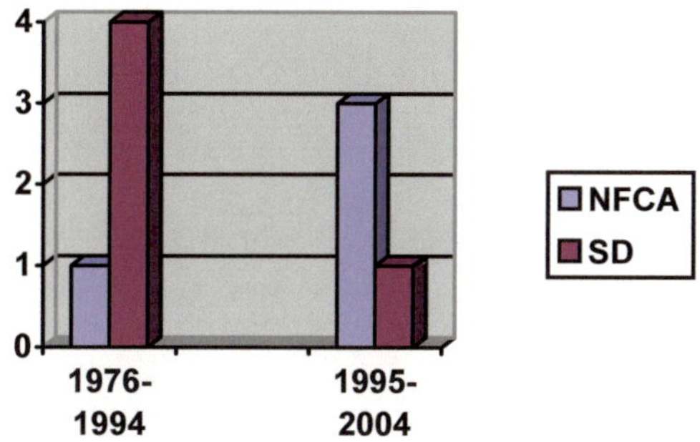

Fig. 8. Cardiac events occurring during marathons from 1976 to 2004, (Roberts and Maron, 2005)

Gerardin reported four cardiac arrests related to sport, with proven coronary diseases and no deaths. Sport events were marathons or running races of 20 km with a medical supervision by mobile intensive care units (ambulances). These four athletes had external defibrillation for ventricular fibrillation (SMI in 3 cases) (Gerardin, 2009).

So for these competitions the organization of medical teams including physicians, paramedics and emergency medical technicians trained to use defibrillators is saving-life.

3. Unrecognized coronary disease among athletes

In France 75 % of people aged 40 to 60 years report taking part in sporting competitions or recreational sport. A proportion of these people will have coronary artery disease either known or unknown. These athletes with unknown ischemic heart disease, sometimes asymptomatic, should be screened.

3.1 Case reports

Case N°1: A 43-year-old man presented with discomfort after running to catch his train. His risk factors were smoking and dyslipidemia. He was a well trained athletes, previous professional basketball player, and tennis player at a regional level with training at least three times per week. He was examined in emergency department a few hours later with a normal examination including ECG and troponin. The diagnosis was a vagal discomfort and consultation from a cardiologist was requested. ECG showed negative T waves in leads II,

III and aVF. Conventional ECG exercise testing showed late but profound ST segment depression in leads V1- V4, asymptomatic and coronary angiography was performed showing two vessel disease (figures 9, 10 and 11).

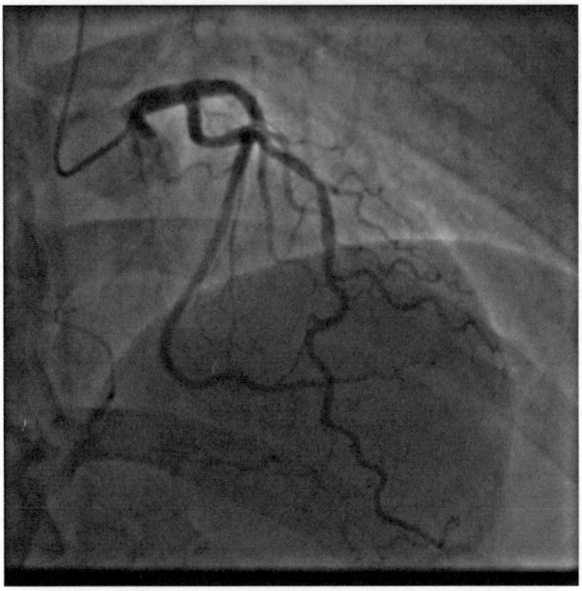

Fig. 9. Left coronary artery with short stenosis of LAD

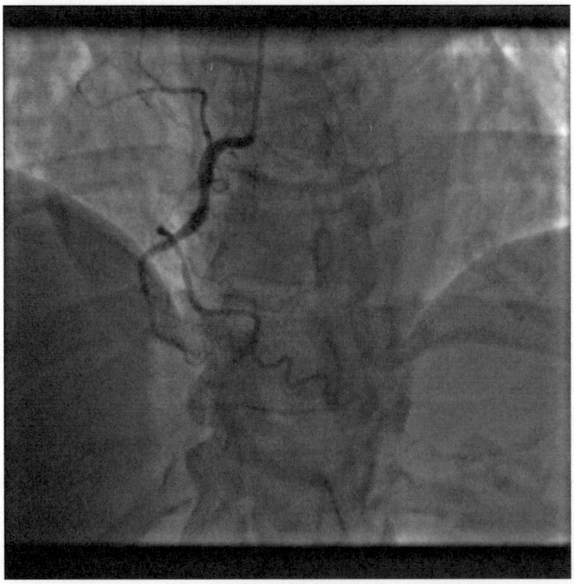

Fig. 10. RCA occlusion

This athlete was able to play tennis in competition despite at least one chronic lesion (occlusion of the RC may be recent and the cause of the discomfort). Coronary artery bypass grafting was performed in this patient who seeks now to return the competitive sport.

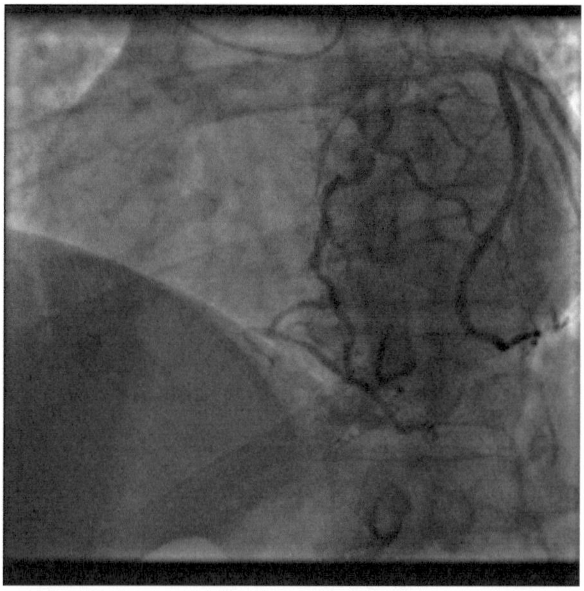

Fig. 11. Distal RCA perfused by collaterals from LAD

Case N° 2: A 54-year-old man had myocardial perfusion scintigraphy for the exploration of abnormal routine ECG. He had FC and dyslipidemia as risk factor and had stopped smoking 10 years before. He ran 10 km twice a week and had completed several marathons and a 100 km race. He was asymptomatic but myocardial perfusion sintigraphy showed defect in the anterior wall. Coronary angiography was performed showing 2 vessel disease (figures 12 and 13).

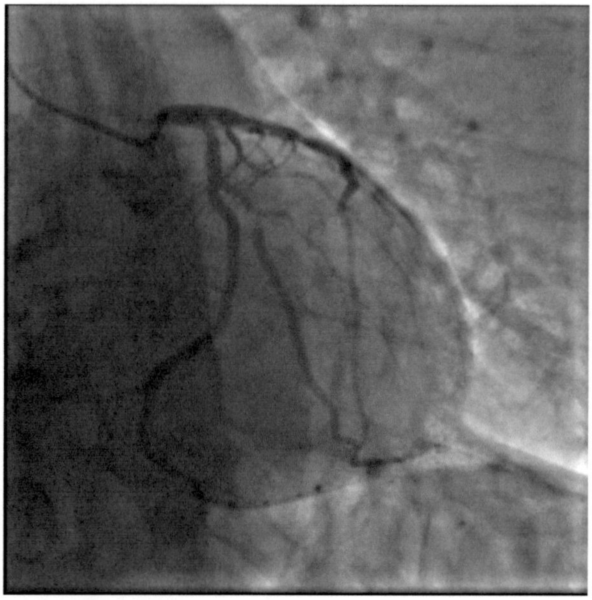

Fig. 12. Very tight lesion of marginal branch

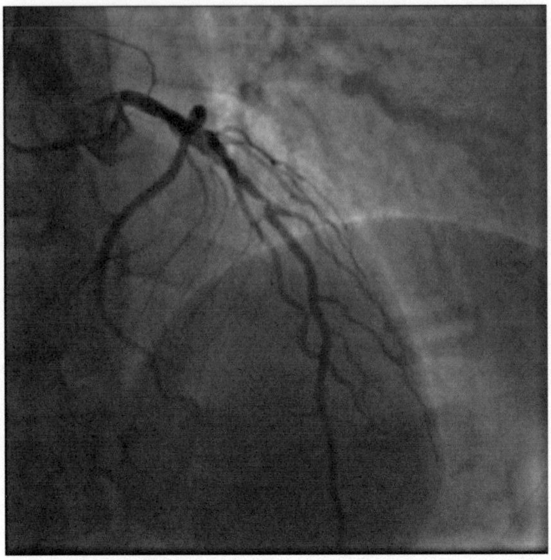

Fig. 13. LAD stenosis including septal a diagonal branches

Coronary angioplasty was performed to LAD and Mg with a good result. This athlete returns to recreational sport and remains asymptomatic.

Case N ° 3: A 50-year-old man presented inaugural anterior STMI revealed by sever chest pain at rest. His risk factors were smoking and dyslipidemia. He was a well trained runner and had performed the Paris marathon two weeks before. Pre-hospital treatment included unfractionated heparin and GPIIb/IIIa antagonist. Coronary angiography was performed 90 mn after onset symptoms via right radial artery access showing 3 vessel disease (Figures 14, 15 and 16).

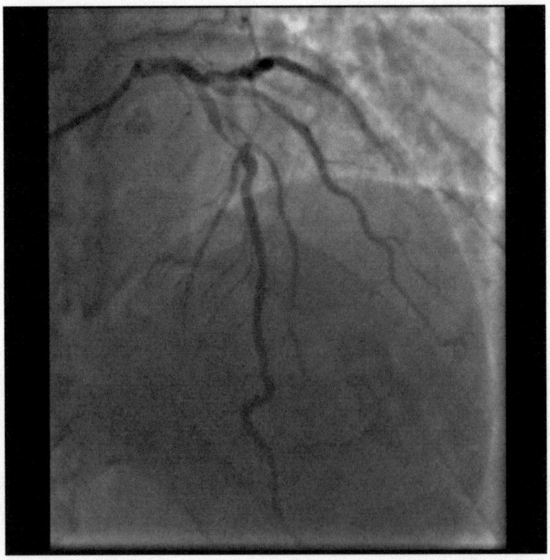

Fig. 14. Stenosis on proximal LAD

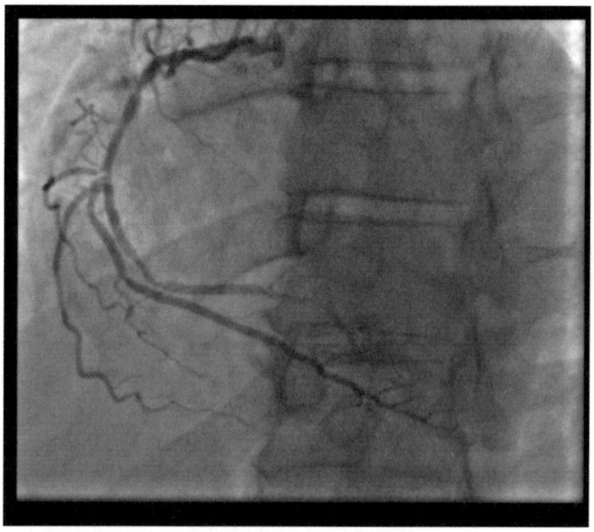

Fig. 15. Stenosis on mild RCA and occlusion of distal RCA

PCI was performed to the LAD requiring predilatation. Angioplasty of RCA and Mg was performed few days later.

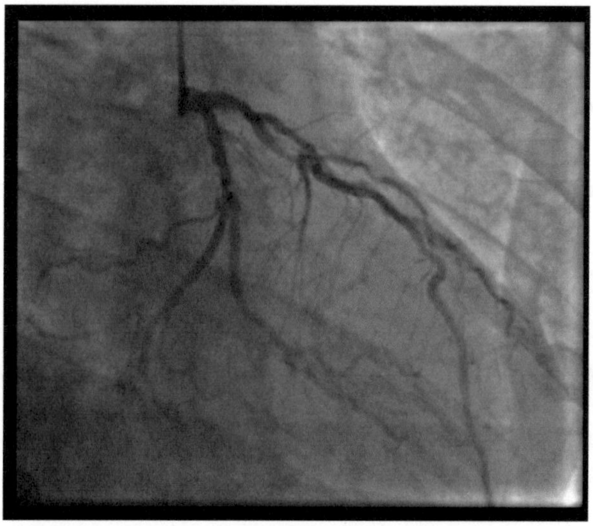

Fig. 16. Stenosis on Cx

In this case lesions of LAD, Mg and mild RCA seemed to be chronics, were very tight and had not stopped this athlete completing a marathon. The real culprit lesion was probably the distal occlusion of the RCA reperfused previously the LAD below of the tight stenosis.

In these three different cases of patients with chronic coronary lesions, strenuous exercise was possible without symptom even in competition. Cardiovascular adaptation to regular exercise may explain this fact but these patients have high risk of major cardiac events and should be screened.

3.2 Discussion

3.2.1 Why a lack of symptom in these three athletes?

Firstly, the athletes appear casual in their approach to possibily cardiac symptoms (Chevallier et al 2005). Secondly, silent ischemia in chronic ischemic heart disease has been commonly reported but is usually associated with angina (Rogers et al, 1995). At last, exercise training improves clinical symptoms of patients with stable coronary artery disease and increase maximal exercise tolerance (Wannamethee et al, 2000; Hambrecht et al, 2004). Explanation could be that moderate exercise training improve left ventricular function du to a decrease of blood pressure and an increase in myocardial contractile response to beta adrenergic stimulation. It also promotes coronary collateral development (Belardinelli et al, 1998) and improves peripheral endothelial function (Gokce et al, 2002). However, in these three cases the patients made frequent strenuous exertions. Zinden et al reported a direct demonstration of coronary collateral flow by intense physical endurance exercise. The subject was a 46 year old healthy cardiologist who had performed long distance running. This invasive study including coronary angiography with measurement of coronary flow reserve showed increase of collateral flow index after regular training and one ultra marathon run (Zbinden et al 2004).

So the lack of symptoms in these patients could be du to cardiovascular adaptation to regular training and a development of coronary collateral particularly important.

3.2.2 What consequences?

It is recognized that ischaemia is a factor of poor prognosis even if it is silent (Rogers, 1995). Secondly although the major acute coronary syndromes occur more on moderate coronary stenosis, small luminal area is a predictor of events at lesion site (Stone et al, 2011). It can be assumed that these patients were at risk of serious cardiac events either acute coronary syndrome through occlusion of tight sténosis or plaque rupture but also severe ischemic arrhythmias related to strenuous exercises (6 or more metabolic equivalents as in practice of football, running, cycling, tennis). However increasing levels of habitual physical activity is associated with progressively lower relative risks os SMI.

Finally, these patients should not have been allowed to practice sports in competition (exept low-moderate dynamic and low static sports, I A, B as bowling, golf, table tennis, doubles tennis, volleyball) and could be screened as recommended by ESC because of their risk factors (Pelliccia et al, 2005). Indeed these three athletes are men over 40 years with at least two risk factors.

4. Conclusions

SMI are rare but can have a severe clinical presentation and are the primary cause of SD in athletes over 35 years. The probable pathophysiological mechanism of SMI is a rupture and thrombosis of a vulnerable plaque often in a patient with single vessel coronary disease. These features may have some therapeutic consequences such as the use manual catheter thrombus aspiration during PCI and may explain the limits of the effectiveness of stress testing for the prevention of these events. This prompts us to determine rules of good practice, including information on the risks of smoking and promote equipment defibrillator on sports sites.

However some athletes have unknown severe coronary disease probably detectable by a stress test and should be screened. So athletes with multiple risk factors could benefit from screening for coronary artery disease, must respect rules of good practices and be advised of the possibility of SMI despite a negative stress test.

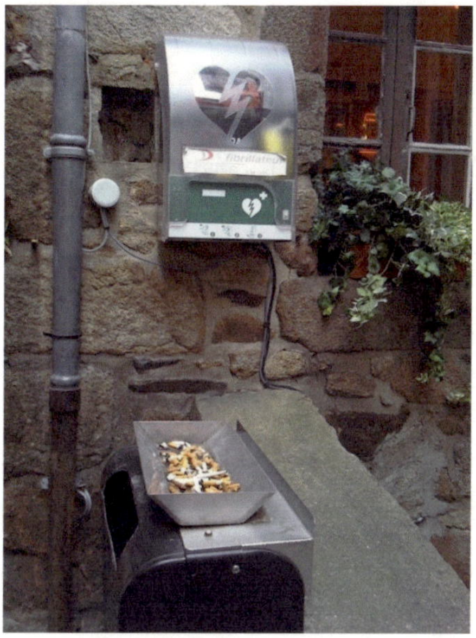

Fig. 17. Personal photo in the famous Mont Saint Michel which is held every year a marathon

5. References

Ambrose, JA; Tannenbaum, MA; Alexopoulos, D; Hjemdahl-Monsen, CE; Leavy, J; Weiss, M; Borrico, S; Gorlin, R & Fuster,V. (1988). Angiographic progression of coronary artery disease and the development of myocardial infarction. *Am Coll Cardiol,* Vol. 12, N°. 1, (July 1988), pp. 56-62, ISSN 0735-1097

Bajaj, S; Shamoon, F,; Gupta, N; Parikh, R; Debari ,VA; Hamdan, A & Bikkina, M.. (June 2011). Acute ST segment élévation myocardial infarction in young adults: who is at risk? *Coron Artery Dis,* Vol.22, N°.4, (June 2011), pp 238-244, ISSN 0954-6928

Belardinelli, R; Georgiou, D; Ginzton, L; Cianci, G & Purcaro, A. (1998). Effects of moderate exercise training on thallium uptake and contractile response to low-dose dobutamine of dysfunctional myocardium in patients with ischémie cardiomyopathy. Circulation. 1998 Feb 17;Vol. 97, N°.6, (Februar 1998), pp. 553-561, ISSN 0009-7322

Burtscher, M; Pachinger, O; Schocke, MF & Ulmer, H. (2007). Risk factor profile for sudden cardiac death during mountain hiking. *Int J Sports Med,* Vol. 28, N°.7, (July 2007), pp. 621-624, ISSN 0943-917X.

Caralis, DG; Deligonul, U; Kern, MJ & and Cohen, JD. (1992). Smoking is a risk factor for coronary spasm in young women. *Circulation,* Vol. 85, N°3, (March 1992), pp. 905-909, ISSN: 0009-7322

Chevalier, L ; Douard, H ; Laporte, T ; Hajar, M ; Baudot, C ; Genson, F ; Labanere, C ; Merle, F &Vincent, MP. (2005). Survey of cardiovascular risk assessment and the behaviour of a sporting population. *Arch mal Cœur Vaiss,* Vol.98, N°.2, (February 2005), pp.109-114, ISSN 0003-9683

Chevalier, L; Hajjar, M; Douard, H; Cherief, A; Dindard, JM; Sedze, F; Ricard, R; Vincent, MP; Corneloup, L; Gencel, L & Carre, F. (2009). Sports-related acute cardiovascular events in a général population: a French prospective study. *Eur] Cardiovasc Prev Rehabil,* Vol. 16, N°. 3 (June 2009), pp. 365-370, ISSN 1741-8267

Ciampricotti, R; El-Gamal, M; Relik, T; Taverne, R; Panis, J; de Swart, J; van Gelder, B & Relik-Van Wely, L. (1990).

Clinical characteristics and coronary angiographie findings of patients with unstable angina, acute myocardial infarction, and survivors of sudden ischémie death occurring during and after sport. *Am Heart /.* Vol. 120, N°.6 Pt 1, (December 1990), pp. 1267-1278, ISSN 0002-8703

Ciampricotti ,R & Taverne, R. (1992). Récurrent acute myocardial infarction during sport. (1992). *Int J Cardiol.* Vol.37, N°l, (October 1992), pp. 120-122, ISNN 0167-5273

Droniou, J ; Brion, R ; Quatre, JM ; de Bourayne, J &, Ollivier, JP. (1987). Acute myocardial infarct during sports practice: a préventive approach based on 40 cases with a non-fatal outcome in a military environment. *Ann Med Interne,* Vol. 138, N°.7, (1987), pp.506-511, ISSN 0003-410X

François, G & Monpere, C. (1989). Myocardial infarction related to thé practice of sports. Clinical and coronary angiography apropos of 35 cases. *Arch Mal Coeur Vaiss,* Vol 82, N°.2, (August 1989), pp.73-78, ISSN: 0003-9683

Fred HL. (1980). The 100-mile run: préparation, performance, and recovery. A case report. *Am] Sports Med,* Vol. 9, N°.4, (July-August 1981), pp.258-61, ISSN 1040-2446

Fuster, V; Moreno, PR; Fayad, ZA; Corti, R & Badimon, JJ. (2005). Atherothrombosis and High-Risk Plaque: Part I: Evolving Concepts. *J Am. Coll. Cardiol,* Vol.46, N° 6, (September 2005), pp. 937-954, ISSN 0735-1097

Gerardin, B. (2009). Etude RACcE. *GRCI 16° Réunion Nationale,* December 3-4, 2009, Paris

Gibbson, LW; Cooper, KH; Meyer, B & Ellison RC. (1980). The Acute Cardiac Risk of Strenuous Exercise. *JAMA,* Vol.244, N°.16, (October 1980), pp.1799-1801, ISSN 0098-7484

Giri, S; Thompson, PD; Kiernan, FJ; Clive J; Fram, DB; Mitchel JF, Hirst JA, McKay, RG & Waters, DD. (1998). Clinical and angiographic characteristics of exertion-related acute myocardial infarction. *JAMA,* Vol.282, N°.18, (November 1999), pp.1731-1736, ISSN 0098-7484

Gokce, N; Vita, JA; Bader, DS; Sherman, DL; Hunter, LM; Holbrook, M; O'Malley, C; Keaney, JF Jr & Balady, GJ. (2002). Effect of exercise on upper and lower extremity endothelial function in patients with coronary artery disease. *Am J Cardiol,* Vol. 90, N°. 2(July 2002), pp. 124-127, ISSN 0002-9149

Halna du Fretay, X & Gerardin, B. Sportman's myocardial infarction. (2008). *Ann Cardiol Angiol,* Vol.57, N°.6, (December 2008), pp. 335-340, ISSN 0003-3928

Hambrecht, R ;Walther, C ; Mobius-Winkler, S ; Gielen, S ; Linke, A ; Conradi, K ; Erbs, S ; Kluge, R ; Kendziorra,

K ; Sabri,O ; Sick, P & Schuler, G. (2004). Percutaneous Coronary Angioplasty Compared With Exercise Training in Patients With Stable Coronary Artery Disease : A Randomized Trial. *Circulation,* Vol.109, N° 11, (March 2004), pp. 1371-1378, ISSN: 0009-7322

Hilberg, T;Gla, D; Schmidt, V; Losche, W; Franke, G; Schneider, K & Gabriel, HH. (2003). Short-term exercise andplatelet activity, sensitivity to agonist, and platelet-leukocyte conjugate formation. *Platelets,* Vol. 14, N°. 2, (March 2003), pp. 67-74, ISSN 0953-7104

Hiltgen, M ; Guérin, Y ; Lefevre, T ; Saudemont, JP ; Gallet, B & Pruvot, H. (1989). Myocardial infarction during or after exertion related to sports. Clinical and coronary angiographic analysis of 10 cases. *Arch Mal Coeur Vaiss,* Vol.82, N°. 2, (August 1989), pp. 83-87, ISNN 0003-9683

Kalaga, RV; Malik, A & Thompson, PD. (2007). Exercise-related spontaneous coronary artery dissection: case report and literature review. *Med Sci Sports Exerc.,* Vol. 39, N°. 8, (August 2007), pp. 1218-1220, ISSN 0195-9131

Kanitz, MG ; Giovannucci, SJ ; Jones, JS & Mott, M. (1996). Myocardial infarction in young adults: risk factors and Clinical features. *J Emerg Med.,* Vol.14, N°2, (March-April 1996), pp.139-145, ISSN 0969-9546.

Kratz, A; Wood, MJ; Siegel, AJ; Hiers, JR & Van Cott, EM. (2006). Effects of marathon running on platelet activation markers : direct evidence for in vivo platelet activation. *Am J Clin Pathol,* Vol. 125, N. 2, (February 2006), pp. 296-300, ISSN 0002-9173

Lindholm, P ; Nordh, J& Gennser, M. (2006). The heart rate of breath-hold divers during static apnea: effects of compétitive stress. *Undersea Hyperb Med,* Vol. 33, N°2, (March 2006), pp. 119-124, ISSN 1066-2936

Lippi, G & Maffulli, N. (2009). Biological influence of physical exercise on hemostasis. *Semin Thromb Hemost.,* Vol. 35, N°. 3, (April 2009), pp. 269-276, ISSN 0094-6176

Marijon ; E, Tafflet, M ; Celermajer, DS ; Dumas, F ; Perier, MC ; Mustafic ,H ; Toussaint, JF ; Desnos, M ; Rieu, M ;

Benameur, N ; Le Heuzey, JY ; Empana, JP & Jouven, X.. (2011). Sports-Related Sudden Death in thé General Population. *Circulation,* Vol.124, N°.6, (August 2011), pp. 672-681, ISSN 0009-7322

Maron, BJ; Polliac, LC & Roberts, WO. (1996). Risk for Sudden Cardiac Death Associated With Marathon Running. *J Am Coll Cardiol,* Vol. 28, N°.2, (August 1996), pp. 428-431, ISSN 0735-1097

Mittelman, M; Maclure, M; Tofler, GH; Sherwood, JB; Goldberg, RJ & Muller, JE. (1993). Triggering of acute myocardial infarction by heavy physical exertion. Protection against triggering by regular exertion. Determinants of Myocardial Infarction Onset Study Investigators.*N Engl J Med,* Vol. 329, N°.23, (Décembre 1993), pp. 1677-83, ISSN 0028-4793

Northcote, RJ; Flannigan, C & Ballantyne, D (1986). Sudden death and vigorous exercise - a study of 60 deaths associated with squash. *Br Heart J,* Vol 55, N°. 2, (Februar 1986), pp. 198-203, ISSN 0007-0769

Opie LH. (1975). Sudden death and sport. *Lancet,* Vol. 1, N°. 7901, (February 1975), pp.263-266, ISSN 0140-6736

Pelliccia, A ; Fagard, R ; Bjornstad, HH ; Anastassakis, A ; Arbustini, E; Assanelli, D ; Biffi, A; Borjesson, M ; Carre, F ; Corrado, D ; Delise, P ; Dorwarth, U ; Hirth, A ; Heidbuchel, H ; Hoffmann, E ; Mellwig, KP ; Panhuyzen- Goedkoop, N ; Pisani, A ; Solberg, EE ; van-Buuren, F ; Vanhees, L; Blomstrom-Lundqvist, C ; Deligiannis, A;Dugmore, D; Glikson, M; Hoff, PI ; Hoffmann, A ; Hoffmann, E; Horstkotte, D; Nordrehaug, JE ; Oudhof, J; McKenna, WJ; Penco, M; Priori, S; Reybrouck, T; Senden, J; Spataro, A & Thiene, G. (2005). Recommendations for competitive sports participation in athlètes with cardiovascular disease : a consensus document from the Study Group of Sports Cardiology of the Working Group of Cardiac Réhabilitation and Exercise Physiology and the Working Group of Myocardial and

Pericardial Diseases of the European Society of Cardiology. *Eur Heart J,* Vol.26, N°.14, (Jully 2005), pp. 1422-1445, ISSN 1520-765X

Pedoe, T. (2007). Marathon cardiac deaths : thé london expérience. *Sports Med,* Vol.37, N°. 4-5, (2005), pp. 448-50, ISSN 0112-1642

Roberts, WO & Maron, BJ. (2005). Evidence for decreasing occurrence of sudden cardiac death associated with thé marathon. (2005). *J Am Coll Cardiol,* vol..46, N°. 7, (October 2005), pp. 1373-1374, ISSN 0735-1097

Rogers, WJ; Bourassa, MG; Andrews, TC; Bertolet, BD; Blumenthal, RS ; Chaitman, BR; Forman, SA; Geller, NL;

Goldberg, AD; Habib, GB; Masters, RG; Moisa, RB; Mueller, H; Pearce, DJ; Pepine, CJ; Sopko, G; Steingart, R; Stone, PH; Knatterud, GL & Conti, R for the ACIP Investigators. (1995). Asymptomatic Cardiac Ischemia Pilot (ACIP) Study: Outcome at 1 Year for Patients With Asymptomatic Cardiac Ischemia Randomized to Médical Therapy or Revascularization. *JAm Coll Cardiol,* Vol.26, N°.3, (September 1995), pp. 594-605, ISSN 0735-1097

Stone, GW; Maehara, A; Lansky, AJ; de Bruyne, B; Cristea ,E; Mintz, GS; Mehran, R; McPherson, J; Farhat, N; Marso, SP; Parise, H; Templin, B; White, R; Zhang, Z & Serruys, PW; PROSPECT Investigators. (2011). A prospective natural-history study of coronary atherosclerosis. N *Engl J Med.,* Vol. 364, N°. 3, (January 2011), pp.226-235, ISSN : 0028-4793

The Task Force on Myocardial Revascularization of the Européen Society of Cardiology (ESC) and the European Association for Cardio-Thoracic Surgery (EACTS). (2010). Guidelines on myocardial revascularization *European Heart Journal,* Vol 31, N°.20 (October 2010), pp.2501-2555, ISSN 0195-668x

Shephard, RJ & Balady, GJ (1999). Exercise as cardiovascular therapy.*Circulation,* Vol.99, N°.7 (February 1999), pp. 963-972, ISSN 0009-7322

Strobel, G; Friedmann ,B; Siebold, R & Bartsch, P. (1999). Effect of severe exercise on plasma catecholamines in differently trained athlètes. *Med Sci Sports Exerc.* Vol. 31, N°. 4, (April 1999); pp. 560-565, ISSN 0195-9131

Viru, M ; Hackney, AC ; Karelson, K ; Janson, T ; Kuus, M & Viru, A. (2010). Compétition effects on physiological responses to exercise: performance, cardiorespiratory and hormonal factors. *Acte Physiol Hung,* Vol.97, N°.l, (March 2010), pp. 22-30, ISSN 0231-124X

Wannamethee, SG; Shaper, AG & Walker, M. (2000). Physical activity and mortality in older men with diagnosed coronary heart disease. *Circulation,*Vol. l02, N°.12(September 2000), pp.1358-1363, ISNN 0009-7322

Willich, SN; Lewis, M; Lowel, H; Arntz, HR; Schubert, F & Schroder, R. (1993). Physical exertion as a trigger of acute myocardial infarction. Triggers and Mechanisms of Myocardial Infarction Study Group *N Engl J Med,* Vol. 329, N°. 23, (December 1993), pp. 1684-1690, ISSN 0028-4793

Winniford, MD; Wheelan, KR; Kremers, MS; Ugolini, V; Van den Berg, E Jr; Niggemann, EH; Jansen, DE & Hillis LD.(1986). Smoking-induced coronary vasoconstriction in patients with atherosclerotic coronary artery disease : évidence for adrenergically mediated altérations in coronary artery tone. *Circulation,* Vol. 73, N°. 4, (April 1986), pp. 662-667, ISNN ISNN 0009-7322

Zbinden, R; Zbinden, S; Windecker, S; Meier, B & Seiler, C. (2004). Direct démonstration of coronary collatéral growth by physical endurance exercise in a healthy marathon runner. *Heart,* Vol.90, N°. 11, (November 2004), pp.1350-1351, ISSN 1355-6037

16

Blood Pressure Regulation During Bathing: Is There a Cardiovascular Risk?

Takeshi Otsuki and Yasuko Okuda
Ryutsu Keizai University & Hiroshima Bunka Gakuen University, Japan

1. Introduction

Water immersion-induced augmentations of external hydrostatic pressure increase central venous and atrial volume and pressure (Arborelius et al., 1972; Gabrielsen et al., 1993; Onodera et al., 2001). The increased left ventricular preload results in the elevation of stroke volume and cardiac output (Arborelius et al., 1972; Ueno et al., 2005). In Poiseuille's law, an elevated stroke volume should increase blood pressure. Therefore, it is reasonable to predict that blood pressure increases during bathing. However, previous studies have reported contradictory results. Ohnaka et al. (1995) have demonstrated that 10-min bathing (40 °C) decreased systolic blood pressure (SBP) in young and middle-aged subjects. Additionally, Nagasawa et al. (2001) have reported that SBP decreased during hot-water immersion (40 °C, 10 min) in young subjects, but increased at the onset of immersion and recovered during the latter phase of immersion in older subjects. Furthermore, Allison & Reger (1998) have reported that SBP in young and middle-aged men showed initial decrease, followed by a gradual increase back toward the baseline during 21-min bathing (40.0 °C). Taken together, the vasopressor effects of bathing are less likely to be marked. Blood pressure during bathing may be maintained by some facilitated regulatory mechanisms.

Blood pressure is regulated mainly by autonomic nervous, endocrine, and renal body-fluid modulation systems. Particularly, the autonomic nervous system rapidly responds to changes in blood pressure. The cardiovagal baroreflex is one of the autonomic functions that regulate blood pressure. Arterial baroreceptors, stretch receptors in the carotid arterial and aortic bodies, detect any blood pressure-associated strain of arterial walls and send afferent signal to increase or decrease heart rate (HR). In this way, the cardiovagal baroreflex regulates blood pressure. Since the baroreceptor firing rate is proportional to changes in arterial circumference at a physiological blood pressure (Aars, 1969), cardiovagal baroreflex sensitivity (BRS) is considered to be affected by carotid arterial or aortic stiffness (Kingwell et al., 1995; Monahan et al., 2001; Rowe, 1987). Additionally, *in vitro* diameter-pressure curves at different temperatures, illustrated using harvested human common carotid arteries, have suggested that hyperthermia may have softening effects on the carotid artery (Guinea et al., 2005). Therefore, bathing-induced hyperthermia may reduce carotid arterial stiffness and consequently increase cardiovagal BRS. Evidence demonstrating that short-term heat stress (5 min, 46.0-48.0 °C) increases skeletal muscle sympathetic BRS (Keller et al., 2006), may support this hypothesis. However, it has remained unclear whether cardiovagal BRS increases during bathing.

We hypothesized that cardiovagal BRS increases during bathing to attenuate bathing-induced blood pressure changes. To test this hypothesis, cardiovagal BRS and hemodynamics in women were measured before, during, and after bathing. Cardiovagal BRS was evaluated using the sequence method (Bertinieri et al., 1988; Hayashi et al., 2006). As a control experiment, a showering session was performed according to the protocol for the bathing session. Body temperature before and after showering/bathing and carotid arterial pulse wave velocity (PWV; an index of arterial stiffness) at rest were also investigated.

2. Methods

2.1 Subjects

Twelve women [age, 35.5±6.6 (19-69) years; height, 157±2 (147-169) cm; weight, 52.4±2.1 (39.3-62.7) kg; and BMI, 21.2±0.7 (16.2-25.4) kg/m^2] volunteered to participate in this study. All subjects were free of signs and symptoms of cardiac diseases, diabetes, and hypertension. None of the participants were currently taking any medications. Premenopausal women were tested at least 3 days before or 3 days after menses. All subjects provided written informed consent before inclusion in the study. This study conformed to the principles outlined in the Helsinki Declaration.

2.2 Experimental protocol

Two testing sessions, showering and bathing sessions, were performed in a randomized order on the same day, at least 2 h apart, in a quiet and temperature-controlled room. First, carotid arterial PWV was measured at supine position after a rest period (formPWV/ABI; Omron Colin, Tokyo, Japan). Second, radial arterial pulse waveforms were continuously recorded for 5 min by applanation tonometry in a seated position (BP-508SD, Omron Colin). At the onset of waveforms recording, brachial arterial pressure was measured by oscillometry (BP-508SD, Omron Colin). Skin temperature was measure at the end of the rest period using an electronic axillary thermometer (CT513, Citizen Systems, Tokyo, Japan). Also, tympanic temperature was measured via an infrared ear thermometer (CT820, Citizen Systems). Third, subjects were showered with hot water (40 °C, 12.5 L/min) or immersed in hot water (40 °C) up to the axillae for 10 min in a sitting position. The radial arterial waveforms and brachial blood pressure waveforms were investigated as previously mentioned. Finally, subjects underwent a 10-min recovery period after the cessation of showering/bathing in the same position as in the pre-showering/bathing period. Again, radial pressure waveforms, brachial blood pressure, and body temperatures were measured in this period.

2.3 Carotid arterial PWV

Carotid arterial PWV was measured using a device to investigate PWV (formPWV/ABI; Omron Colin), as previously described with minor modifications (Kimoto et al., 2003; Kobayashi et al., 2004). Briefly, subjects assumed a supine position with a cardiac sound microphone placed at the right sternal margin at the second intercostal level, with an applanation tonometer on the common carotid artery. The pulse wave transit time between the aortic valve and carotid artery was determined based on the time delay between the beginning of the second heart sound and notch of the carotid artery pulse wave. The distance traveled by the pulse waves was estimated according to the height of subjects using the following equation: 0.2437 x height - 18.999 (Kimoto et al., 2003; Kobayashi et al., 2004). Carotid arterial PWV was calculated as the distance divided by the transit time.

2.4 Cardiovagal BRS

Cardiovagal BRS was assessed according to previous studies with minor modifications (Bertinieri et al., 1988; Hayashi et al., 2006). Under all recording conditions, an applanation tonometer (BP-508SD, Omron Colin) was placed at the forth intercostal level. The applanation tonometer sampled the radial arterial pressure waveforms and stored data in a computer. HR was calculated from pulse intervals. We identified baroreflex sequences (three or more beats relating to pulse intervals and progressively and spontaneously changing SBP at the same detection points). Next, we determined the slope of the linear relationship between the pulse intervals and SBP at these points. The minimum changes observed were 1 mmHg for SBP and 1 ms for the pulse interval. Linear regressions relating SBP to the pulse interval were plotted for each sequence; only those sequences with linear r values > 0.85 were accepted. For the latter 5-min of respective period, the results were averaged to provide a single data set.

2.5 Statistical analysis

Data are expressed as means±SE. Statistical analysis was carried out using repeated-measures two-way ANOVA followed by Scheffe's test for multiple comparisons. Linear correlation analysis was used to examine the relationship between carotid arterial PWV and cardiovagal BRS. $P<0.05$ was regarded as significant.

3. Results

Respective temperatures of shower/bath water were 40.6±0.2/40.6±0.1 °C. Bathroom temperature in showering and bathing sessions was 27.3±0.1 and 27.8±0.1 °C, and room humidity was 66.7±0.9 and 62.3±1.7 %, respectively.

Cardiovagal BRS before, during, and after showering/bathing is indicated in Fig. 1. Two-way ANOVA revealed an interaction between session (showering or bathing) and time in cardiovagal BRS. In multiple comparisons, cardiovagal BRS did not change during showering but increased during bathing compared to the baseline. Also, cardiovagal BRS was greater during bathing than during showering. The elevated cardiovagal BRS recovered to the baseline after the cessation of bathing.

Hemodynamics during sessions are summarized in Table 1. We did not identify interactions (session x time) in all measures. Again, there were no main effects of session in all indices. Main effects of time were detected in SBP, mean blood pressure (MBP), HR, and double-product (DP, *i.e.*, product of SBP and HR). In details, SBP was higher during and after showering and bathing than the baseline. MBP increased after showering and bathing compared to at rest. HR was higher during showering and bathing in comparison to before showering and bathing. Increased DP was observed during and after showering and bathing. Time was not associated with diastolic blood pressure and pulse pressure.

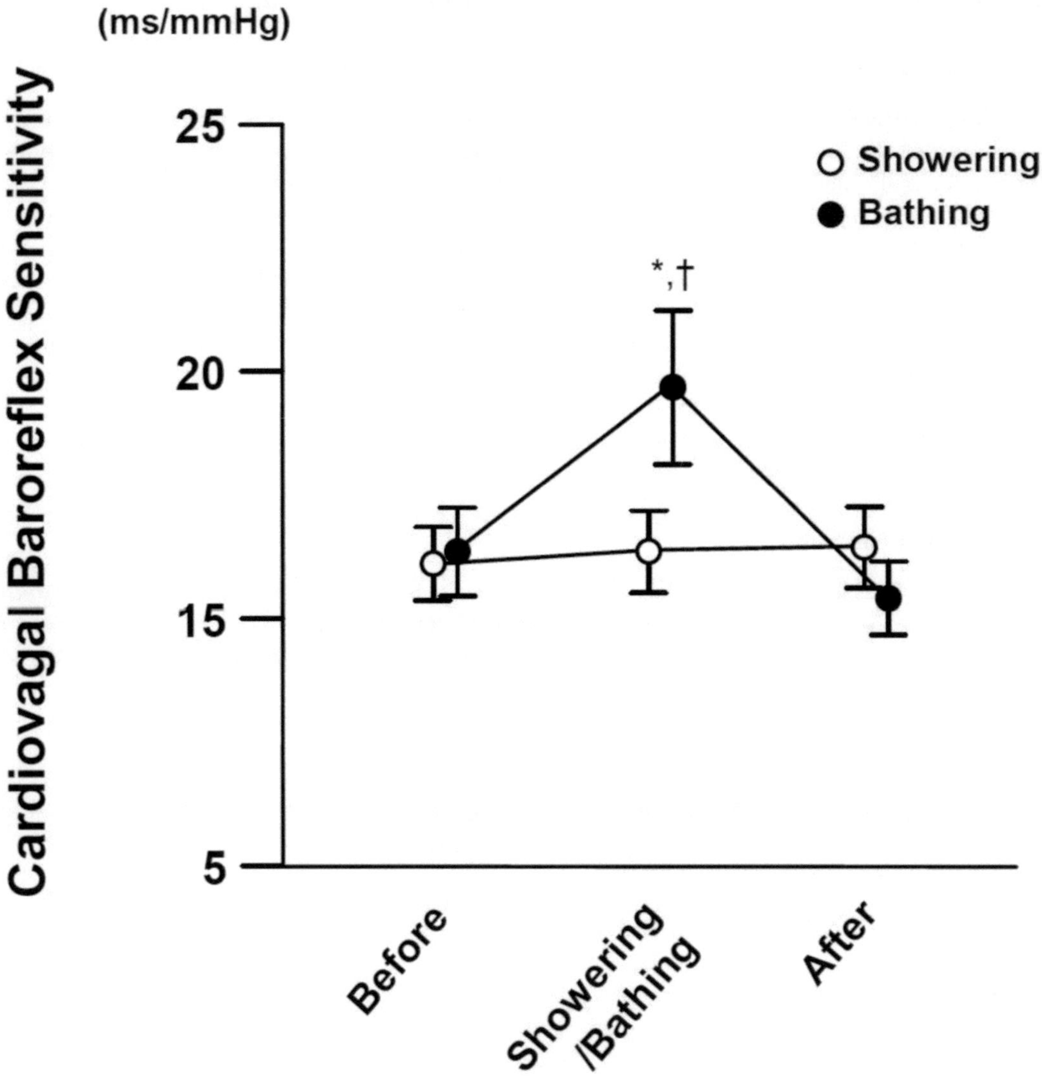

Fig. 1. Cardiovagal baroreflex sensitivity (BRS) before, during, and after showering/bathing. Data are expressed as means±SE. Repeated-measures two-way ANOVA (session x time) revealed an interaction in cardiovagal BRS (F=6.4, P<0.01). On multiple comparisons, showering was not associated with cardiovagal BRS, but bathing increased it compared to the baseline. The increased BRS during bathing recovered to the baseline after the cessation of bathing. *P<0.05 vs. before bathing; †P<0.05 vs. showering.

		Before			Showering /Bathing			After			Interaction
SBP, mmHg	Showering	100	±	2	103	±	2	105	±	2	*F*=0.3
	Bathing	99	±	3	103	±	2	102	±	3	*P*=0.73
MBP, mmHg	Showering	67	±	2	71	±	2	73	±	3	*F*=0.7
	Bathing	70	±	2	71	±	2	72	±	2	*P*=0.49
DBP, mmHg	Showering	55	±	2	55	±	2	56	±	2	*F*=1.3
	Bathing	52	±	3	56	±	4	58	±	3	*P*=0.28
PP, mmHg	Showering	45	±	2	48	±	2	49	±	3	*F*=1.4
	Bathing	46	±	2	47	±	4	44	±	2	*P*=0.27
HR, bpm	Showering	68	±	1	70	±	2	68	±	2	*F*=2.2
	Bathing	68	±	2	72	±	3	71	±	2	*P*=0.12
DP, AU	Showering	68.4	±	1.7	71.5	±	1.6	71.3	±	1.4	*F*=1.6
	Bathing	66.5	±	2.7	73.7	±	3.3	72.0	±	3.0	*P*=0.20

Table 1. Hemodynamics before, during, and after showering/bathing. Values are means±SE. SBP, systolic blood pressure; MBP, mean blood pressure; DBP, diastolic blood pressure; PP, pulse pressure; HR, heart rate; DP, double product; AU, arbitrary unit.

The relationship between carotid arterial PWV and cardiovagal BRS at rest is demonstrated in Fig. 2. Carotid arterial PWV was correlated with cardiovagal BRS.

Table 2 shows body temperatures before and after showering/bathing. There was no interaction between session and time in skin temperature. However, two-way ANOVA identified the main effect of time; skin temperature increased after showering and bathing. No differences in skin temperature between showering and bathing were present. On the other hand, we observed an interaction (session x time) in tympanic temperature. In multiple comparisons, showering did not change tympanic temperature but bathing increased it.

4. Discussion

Spontaneous cardiovagal BRS, hemodynamics, and body temperature in women were measured before, during, and after showering/bathing. Carotid arterial PWV, an index of arterial stiffness, was also measured at rest. We demonstrated for the first time that spontaneous cardiovagal BRS increased during bathing compared to the baseline. There were no differences in the changes from the baseline in blood pressure, HR, and DP between showering and bathing sessions. Tympanic temperature did not change after showering but increased after bathing in comparison to the baseline. Cardiovagal BRS was negatively correlated with carotid arterial PWV. We concluded that cardiovagal BRS increases during bathing. Increased cardiovagal BRS may attenuate the blood pressure changes during bathing, resulting in comparable hemodynamics responses between showering and bathing. We would like to propose that it may be unreasonable to withhold bathing by reason of cardiovascular risk. Taking into consideration the slight but significant hyperthermic effects, bathing may be more beneficial to humans in comparison to showering, although caution may be required for humans with stiffened carotid arteries.

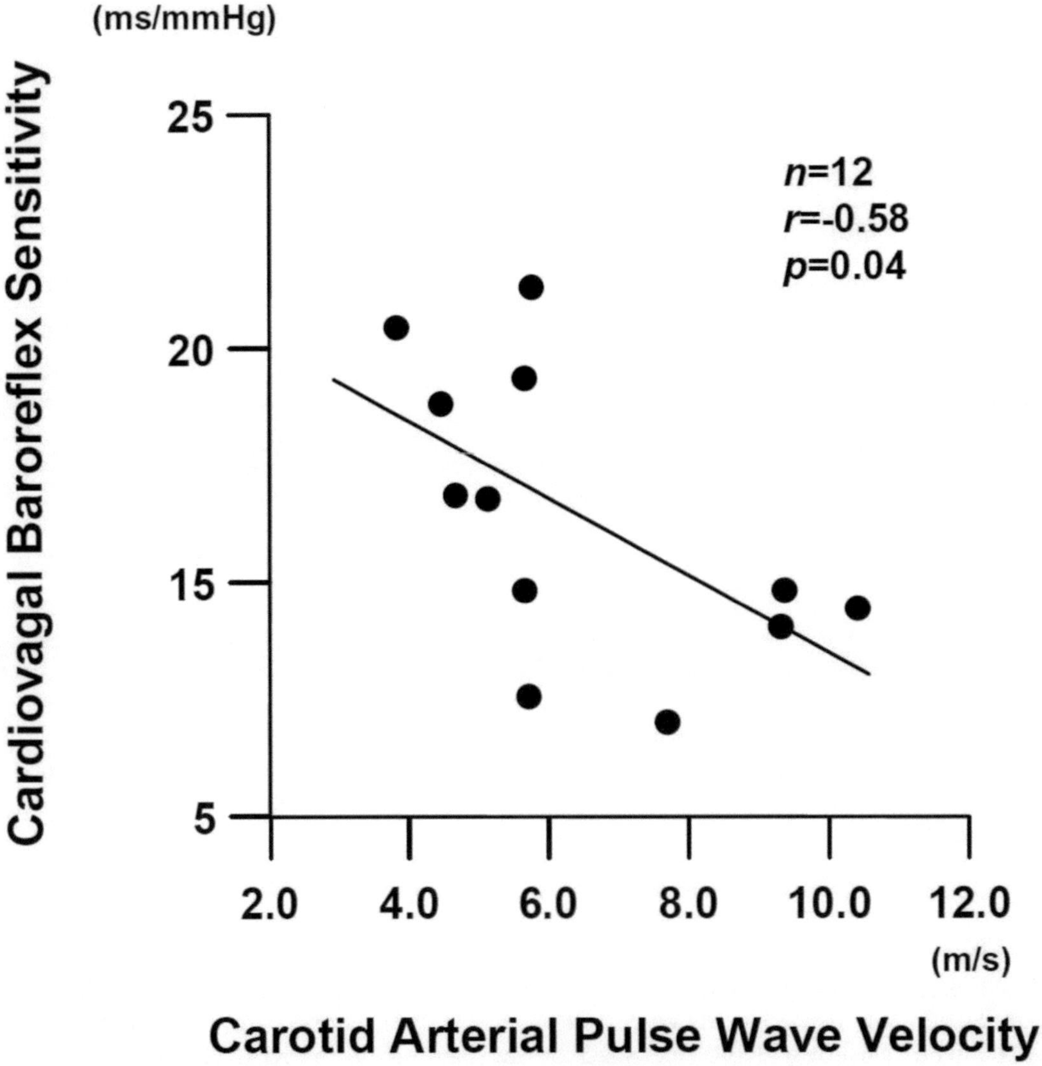

Fig. 2. Relationship between carotid arterial pulse wave velocity (PWV), an index of arterial stiffness, and cardiovagal baroreflex sensitivity (BRS) at rest. Carotid arterial PWV was correlated with cardiovagal BRS.

		Before			After			Interaction
Skin temperature, °C	Showering	36.4	±	0.1	36.6	±	0.2	F=0.3
	Bathing	36.3	±	0.2	36.6	±	0.1	P=0.57
Tympanic temperature, °C	Showering	37.0	±	0.1	36.9	±	0.1	F=7.4
	Bathing	37.0	±	0.1	37.1	±	0.1*	P=0.01

Values are means±SE. *P<0.05 vs.

Table 2. Body temperature before and after showering/bathing.

Water immersion increases venous return and ventricular preload (Arborelius et al., 1972; Gabrielsen et al., 1993; Onodera et al., 2001). Consequently, stroke volume and cardiac output increases in the water-immersed subjects (Arborelius et al., 1972; Ueno et al., 2005). Therefore, theoretically, arterial SBP and pulse pressure are speculated to be elevated during bathing. However, the reported effects of bathing on blood pressure are not consistent (Allison & Reger, 1998; Nagasawa et al., 2001; Ohnaka et al., 1995). Also in this study, we did not observe differences in blood pressure changes between showering and bathing periods. It is reasonable to consider that the effects of bathing on blood pressure are not marked. The mechanisms underlying the paradox (*i.e.*, bathing increases blood flow but not arterial blood pressure) have, up to now, remained unclear. This study demonstrated that cardiovagal BRS increases during bathing. This enhanced cardiovagal BRS may participate in the regulation of blood pressure and reduce cardiovascular risks during bathing.

Cardiovagal BRS is regulated via arterial baroreceptors, stretch receptors in arterial tissue. The baroreceptors are located in carotid arterial and aortic bodies. Baroreceptors sense arterial wall strain caused by blood pressure changes and send afferent signals corresponding to the strain level to the cardiovascular center. The stiffness of baroreceptor-containing arteries such as the carotid artery has been hypothesized to be one of the key factors determining cardiovagal BRS (Kingwell et al., 1995; Monahan et al., 2001; Rowe, 1987). Indeed, Monahan et al. (2001) have demonstrated that age-related carotid arterial stiffening, evaluated using echo tracking, was closely associated with decreased cardiovagal BRS, investigated using the Oxford technique. Again, we demonstrated a linear relationship between carotid arterial PWV and cardiovagal BRS. It is well-established that arterial stiffness increases with advancing age (Avolio et al., 1985; Otsuki et al., 2006a; Otsuki et al., 2006b; Vaitkevicius et al., 1993). Central arterial stiffness are also associated with daily physical activities (Iemitsu et al., 2006; Sugawara et al., 2006). Although the present subjects did not experience a marked blood pressure increase during bathing [*e.g.*, maximal SBP increase was 16 mmHg (from 98 at rest to 114 mmHg)], humans with markedly stiff arteries may need to take precautions.

Body temperature was measured before and after showering/bathing at two sites. The skin temperature increased after both showering and bathing. On the other hand, the effects on tympanic temperature were different between showering and bathing. Showering did not change the tympanic temperature, bathing slightly but significantly increased it. The tympanic temperature is closer to the core temperature than skin temperature. It is possible that bathing elevated not only the surface but also internal temperature. At least, the hyperthermic effects are likely to be greater in bathing compared to showering.

We showed that cardiovagal BRS increased on short-term (*i.e.*, 10 min, 40.6 °C) bathing. Also, Keller et al. (2006) have demonstrated that skeletal muscle sympathetic BRS is enhanced by short-term heat stress (5 min, 46.0-48.0 °C). On the other hand, prolonged bathing may be counterproductive. Lee et al. (2003) have reported that hot-water (44.0 °C) immersion of the lower legs for 30 min reduced spontaneous cardiovagal BRS. Prolonged hot-water bathing should be refrained from.

The mechanisms responsible for bathing-induced increases in cardiovagal BRS remain unclear. One explanation for this response may be hyperthermia-related reduction of arterial stiffness. Guinea et al. (2005) have reported that hyperthermia shifts the carotid arterial diameter-pressure curve to the right, suggesting that hyperthermia reduces carotid arterial stiffness. Carotid arterial baroreceptors are stretch receptors. A compliant carotid artery is easily stretched and would be sensitive to changes in blood pressure. Indeed, the present and previous (Monahan et al., 2001) studies have showed a negative relation between cardiovagal BRS and carotid arterial stiffness. We observed that showering increased only the skin temperature, but bathing increased both the skin and tympanic temperature. Collectively, it may be possible that a hyperthermia-induced reduction of carotid arterial stiffness is associated with increased cardiovagal BRS during bathing. Another possible explanation for the changes in cardiovagal BRS is the direct effect of an elevated core temperature on central baroreflex pathways. Previous findings have demonstrated that an increased temperature enhances the neuronal firing rate of thermosensitive neurons (Boulant, 1998). While these findings were limited to the hypothalamic region of the brain, it is a possibility that neurons involved in the pathways of baroreflex control are also thermosensitive and are responsible for the changes in cardiovagal BRS with bathing.

In conclusion, cardiovagal BRS appears to increase during bathing. It may attenuate the bathing-induced blood pressure changes.

5. References

Aars, H. (1969). Relationship between aortic diameter and aortic baroreceptor activity in normal and hypertensive rabbits, *Acta Physiol Scand* 75 (3):406-414.

Allison, T. G. & Reger, W. E. (1998). Comparison of responses of men to immersion in circulating water at 40.0 and 41.5 degrees c, *Aviat Space Environ Med* 69 (9):845-850.

Arborelius, M., Jr., Ballidin, U. I., Lilja, B. & Lundgren, C. E. (1972). Hemodynamic changes in man during immersion with the head above water, *Aerosp Med* 43 (6):592-598.

Avolio, A. P., Deng, F. Q., Li, W. Q., Luo, Y. F., Huang, Z. D., Xing, L. F. & O'Rourke, M. F. (1985). Effects of aging on arterial distensibility in populations with high and low prevalence of hypertension: Comparison between urban and rural communities in china, *Circulation* 71 (2):202-210.

Bertinieri, G., Di Rienzo, M., Cavallazzi, A., Ferrari, A. U., Pedotti, A. & Mancia, G. (1988). Evaluation of baroreceptor reflex by blood pressure monitoring in unanesthetized cats, *Am J Physiol* 254 (2 Pt 2):H377-383.

Boulant, J. A. (1998). Cellular mechanisms of temperature sensitivity in hypothalamic neurons, *Prog Brain Res* 115: 3-8.

Gabrielsen, A., Johansen, L. B. & Norsk, P. (1993). Central cardiovascular pressures during graded water immersion in humans, *J Appl Physiol* 75 (2):581-585.

Guinea, G. V., Atienza, J. M., Elices, M., Aragoncillo, P. & Hayashi, K. (2005). Thermomechanical behavior of human carotid arteries in the passive state, *Am J Physiol Heart Circ Physiol* 288 (6):H2940-2945.

Hayashi, K., Miyachi, M., Seno, N., Takahashi, K., Yamazaki, K., Sugawara, J., Yokoi, T., Onodera, S. & Mesaki, N. (2006). Fluctuations in carotid arterial distensibility during the menstrual cycle do not influence cardiovagal baroreflex sensitivity, *Acta Physiol* 186 (2):103-110.

Iemitsu, M., Maeda, S., Otsuki, T., Sugawara, J., Tanabe, T., Jesmin, S., Kuno, S., Ajisaka, R., Miyauchi, T. & Matsuda, M. (2006). Polymorphism in endothelin-related genes limits exercise-induced decreases in arterial stiffness in older subjects, *Hypertension* 47 (5):928-936.

Keller, D. M., Cui, J., Davis, S. L., Low, D. A. & Crandall, C. G. (2006). Heat stress enhances arterial baroreflex control of muscle sympathetic nerve activity via increased sensitivity of burst gating, not burst area, in humans, *J Physiol* 573 (Pt 2):445-451.

Kimoto, E., Shoji, T., Shinohara, K., Inaba, M., Okuno, Y., Miki, T., Koyama, H., Emoto, M. & Nishizawa, Y. (2003). Preferential stiffening of central over peripheral arteries in type 2 diabetes, *Diabetes* 52 (2):448-452.

Kingwell, B. A., Cameron, J. D., Gillies, K. J., Jennings, G. L. & Dart, A. M. (1995). Arterial compliance may influence baroreflex function in athletes and hypertensives, *Am J Physiol* 268 (1 Pt 2):H411-418.

Kobayashi, K., Akishita, M., Yu, W., Hashimoto, M., Ohni, M. & Toba, K. (2004). Interrelationship between non-invasive measurements of atherosclerosis: Flow-mediated dilation of brachial artery, carotid intima-media thickness and pulse wave velocity, *Atherosclerosis* 173 (1):13-18.

Lee, K., Jackson, D. N., Cordero, D. L., Nishiyasu, T., Peters, J. K. & Mack, G. W. (2003). Change in spontaneous baroreflex control of pulse interval during heat stress in humans, *J Appl Physiol* 95 (5):1789-1798.

Monahan, K. D., Tanaka, H., Dinenno, F. A. & Seals, D. R. (2001). Central arterial compliance is associated with age- and habitual exercise-related differences in cardiovagal baroreflex sensitivity, *Circulation* 104 (14):1627-1632.

Nagasawa, Y., Komori, S., Sato, M., Tsuboi, Y., Umetani, K., Watanabe, Y. & Tamura, K. (2001). Effects of hot bath immersion on autonomic activity and hemodynamics: Comparison of the elderly patient and the healthy young, *Jpn Circ J* 65 (7):587-592.

Ohnaka, T., Tochihara, Y., Kubo, M. & Yamaguchi, C. (1995). Physiological and subjective responses to standing showers, sitting showers, and sink baths, *Appl Human Sci* 14 (5):235-239.

Onodera, S., Miyachi, M., Nishimura, M., Yamamoto, K., Yamaguchi, H., Takahashi, K., In, J. Y., Amaoka, H., Yoshioka, A., Matsui, T. & Hara, H. (2001). Effects of water depth on abdominal [correction of abdominails] aorta and inferior vena cava during standing in water, *J Gravit Physiol* 8 (1):P59-60.

Otsuki, T., Maeda, S., Kesen, Y., Yokoyama, N., Tanabe, T., Sugawara, J., Miyauchi, T., Kuno, S., Ajisaka, R. & Matsuda, M. (2006a). Age-related reduction of systemic arterial compliance induces excessive myocardial oxygen consumption during sub-maximal exercise, *Hypertens Res* 29 (2):65-73.

Otsuki, T., Maeda, S., Sugawara, J., Kesen, Y., Murakami, H., Tanabe, T., Miyauchi, T., Kuno, S., Ajisaka, R. & Matsuda, M. (2006b). Age-related reduction of systemic arterial compliance relates to decreased aerobic capacity during sub-maximal exercise, *Hypertens Res* 29 (10):759-765.

Rowe, J. W. (1987). Clinical consequences of age-related impairments in vascular compliance, *Am J Cardiol* 60 (12):68G-71G.

Sugawara, J., Otsuki, T., Tanabe, T., Hayashi, K., Maeda, S. & Matsuda, M. (2006). Physical activity duration, intensity, and arterial stiffening in postmenopausal women, *Am J Hypertens* 19 (10):1032-1036.

Ueno, L. M., Miyachi, M., Matsui, T., Takahashi, K., Yamazaki, K., Hayashi, K., Onodera, S. & Moritani, T. (2005). Effect of aging on carotid artery stiffness and baroreflex sensitivity during head-out water immersion in man, *Braz J Med Biol Res* 38 (4):629-637.

Vaitkevicius, P. V., Fleg, J. L., Engel, J. H., O'Connor, F. C., Wright, J. G., Lakatta, L. E., Yin, F. C. & Lakatta, E. G. (1993). Effects of age and aerobic capacity on arterial stiffness in healthy adults, *Circulation* 88 (4 Pt 1):1456-1462.

17

Sagittal Abdominal Diameter as the Anthropometric Measure of Cardiovascular Risk

Edita Stokić[1], Biljana Srdić[2], Vladimir Brtka[3] and Dragana Tomić-Naglić[1]
[1]*Department of Endocrinology, Institute of Internal Disease, Clinical Centre Vojvodina, Novi Sad,*
[2]*Department of Anatomy, Medical Faculty, Novi Sad, Medical Faculty Novi Sad,*
[3]*Technical Faculty "Mihajlo Pupin" Zrenjanin, Serbia*

1. Introduction

Obesity has a profound impact on the cardiovascular disease development, and is associated with a reduced overall survival. There is a strong correlation between the central (abdominal) type of obesity and the cardiovascular and metabolic diseases. Among a variety of anthropometric measurements of the abdominal fat size, sagittal abdominal diameter has been proposed as the valid measurement of the visceral fat mass and cardiometabolic risk level. Many studies have analyzed the relationship between sagittal abdominal diameter (SAD), visceral fat area, and different markers of cardiometabolic disturbances with respect to age, gender and ethnicity. Some of them have offered the cut-off values that could be useful in clinical practice, in identifying individuals who are at higher risk of comorbidities of the obesity. Using the principles of rough set theory, based on producing *If-Then* rules, we have developed a model that allows better applicability of SAD in identifying patients at higher cardiovascular risk. In this chapter, we describe the basic principles of the proposed model. Furthermore, we give a broad overview of the main concerns regarding the significance of SAD and its use in diagnosing the abdominal obesity and predicting the adverse cardiometabolic outcomes.

2. Obesity as a cardiovascular risk factor

The prevalence of obesity has increased dramatically worldwide during the past few decades. Obesity is recognized as an independent factor for the development of the cardiovascular diseases. It also predisposes to the development of other cardiovascular risk factors.

Obesity implies increased body weight due to the enlargement of the adipose tissue to the extent that impairs health. Regional obesity appears to be an important indicator of the risk level. Thus, the diagnosis of obesity depends on three main aspects: relative weight (total body mass with relation to body height), total body fat, and fat distribution.

Body mass index (BMI) has been widely accepted as a simple and the most practical measure of fatness in clinical and epidemiological surveys, eventhough it doesn't distinguish fat from lean body mass. In fact, it is an indicator of the nutritional status, not a measure of body fat mass. It has been shown that BMI≥25 kg/m^2 is associated with increased morbidity, while BMI≥30 kg/m^2 carries increased risk for both morbidity and mortality, primarily from diabetes and cardiovascular diseases (Irribaren et al., 1995). However, recent studies showed that BMI can be a reliable predictor of cardiovascular mortality only in severe obesity (Romero-Corral et al., 2006). The category of overweight people (BMI: 25-29.9 kg/m^2) seems to be the most confusing, especially from the aspect of the therapeutic approach.

BMI doesn't provide sufficient information about fat mass. Therefore, body composition assessment is necessary for the diagnosis of obesity and prediction of its comorbidities. It discriminates individuals with true excess body fat from those with "normal weight obesity", as well as from overweight individuals with normal body fat mass. Using a cut-off value of 30% body fat, Marques-Vidal et al. (2008) reported prevalence of "normal weight obesity" of 10.1% in women, and 3.2% in men, with increasing prevalence with aging.

Specific fat distribution determines the risk level more accurately than the total body fatness *per se*. Excess adipose tissue in the abdominal region is more hazardous than the overall obesity, due to higher visceral fat deposition. Furthermore, it is associated with greater risk of cardiovascular diseases, metabolic disorders and type 2 diabetes mellitus (Després et al., 1990; Molarius & Seidell, 1998). Central or abdominal obesity (firstly assigned as android type of obesity) has been identified as a risk factor for the cardiovascular diseases, as well as a symptom of metabolic syndrome. Normal weight subjects with higher visceral fat mass are at a higher risk (metabolically obese normal weight subjects). In addition, obese subjects with normal visceral fat mass can present with normal metabolic profile (metabolically healthy obese subjects) (Ruderman et al., 1998; Sims, 2001).

2.1 Abdominal obesity

It is well known that the risk of cardiovascular and metabolic abnormalities is determined by specific distribution of the adipose tissue. Abdominal (central) obesity is associated with dyslipidemia, impaired fasting glucose, insulin resistance and hypertension, which result in increased risk of cardio- and cerebrovascular diseases, and consequently premature death (Guzzaloni, 2009).

Adverse effects of the abdominal obesity have been supported by many studies of the metabolism and endocrine activity of adipocytes from different regions of the abdominal adipose tissue. Abdominal fat includes two morphologically and functionally different depots: subcutaneous (superficial) and deep, visceral (intraabdominal). The latter is located in the abdominal cavity and includes intraperitoneal (omental and mesenterial) adipose tissue, which makes 80% of the intraabdominal fat mass, and retroperitoneal adipose tissue, which makes 20% of the intraabdominal fat mass (Misra&Vikram, 2003). Abdominal obesity can reflect expansion of either subcutaneous or visceral depot, or a combination of excess fat in both depots. However, visceral adipose tissue compartment has been considered more important in pathogenesis of the obesity complications. It is responsible for the development of insulin resistance, glucose intolerance and type 2 diabetes mellitus. According to Brochu et al. (2000), visceral fat depot explains 10% of variability of insulin resistance and 16% of blood glucose. Visceral adipose tissue enlargement is mainly associated with lower values of HDL-cholesterol, elevated tryglicerides, apolipoprotein B (Couillard et al., 1996), as well as with elevated atherogenic lipoprotein subfractions and reduced concentration of HDL particles (Nakata et al., 2010). It positivly correlates with glucose intolerance and hyperinsulinemia (Wajchenberg, 2000), as well as the markers of the proinflammatory and prothrombotic state.

Visceral adipose tissue function plays a crucial role in the development of metabolic abnormalities and insulin resistance, mainly due to the direct access of intraperitoneal adipose tissue to the liver through the portal circulation (Matsuzawa et al. 1995, Bosello & Zamboni, 2000). In comparison to the subcutaneous adipose tissue, visceral adipose tissue contains higher number of adipocytes per unit mass, higher number of endothelial cells in the stromal vascular fraction, higher β_3-adrenoreceptor and α_2-adrenergic receptor sensitivity, and it is better vascularized (Misra & Vikram, 2003; van Harmelen et al., 2004). Visceral adipocytes are more metabolically active, have higher lipolytic activity when stimulated by catecholamines, and are poorly responsive to the antilipolythic action of insulin. In addition, they secrete more proinflammatory (interleukin-6, interleukin-8, interleukin-1β) and prothrombotic (plasminogen-acivator inhibitor-1) adipokines. Obesity is characterized by an increased number of β_3- and decreased number of α_2-adrenergic receptors, decreased insulin activity, increased activity of lipoprotein-lipase and acylation-stimulating protein, with higher upload of triglycerides and lower postprandial suppression of lipolysis (Wajchenberg, 2000; van Herpen & Schrauwen-Hinderling, 2008). All of the above mentioned changes in the visceral adipose tissue provide increased release of free fatty acids and their flux towards the liver, where they induce gluconeogenesis, synthesis of triglycerides and apolipoprotein-B rich lipoproteins, as well as impairment of insulin action (Lonnquist et al., 1995, Freedland, 2004). Free fatty acids also exhibit proarrhythmic properties which explains association between the visceral fat and sudden death (Empana et al. 2004). On the other hand, obese adipose tissue is characterized by impairment of blood flow, development of hypoxia and local inflammation, infiltration by macrophages, and by disturbances in secretion of adipokines, which all together result in insulin resistance and systemic inflammation (Berg & Scherer, 2005; Coppack, 2005; Goossens, 2008).

Computerized tomography (CT) and magnetic resonance imaging (MRI), performed at the L_4-L_5 level, are the most reliable anatomical methods for abdominal fat assessment, since they discriminate between the subcutaneous and the visceral fat depots (van der Kooy et al., 1993). However, these methods are expensive, not feasible and unportable, which makes their use in clinical and epidemiological practice limited. Anthropometric parameters are more suitable as they are inexpensive, non-invasive and simple. Besides, most of them show a strong correlation with visceral abdominal fat size.

2.1.1 Anthropometric parameters of abdominal obesity

Several anthropometric indicators of abdominal obesity have been developed to measure abdominal adipose tissue mass. Some of them are presented in the form of ratios, especially the ones that incorporate body height, which gives more realistic picture of body proportions. On the other hand, it is difficult to interpret them biologically (Bouchard et al., 1990). Many studies have compared them in order to demonstrate advantages of a particular parameter in predicting the risk and visceral fat mass. As a rule, an ideal anthropometric measure of abdominal adiposity should predict individual cardiometabolic risk and clearly show effects of different preventative and therapeutic approaches.

Waist-to-hip and waist-to-thigh ratios (WHR and WTR, respectively) were originally proposed as the key determinants of android and gynoid obesity (Krotkiewski et al., 1983; Molarius & Seidell, 1998). WHR has been most commonly used in identifying abdominal fat distribution. Waist circumference alone has received more attention in management of obesity since it requires only one measurement. It showed to be a better predictor of visceral fat volume and related cardiovascular risk profile than WHR (Després et al., 1991; Pouilot et al., 1994; Vissher et al., 2001; Wajchenberg, 2000; Logfren et al., 2004). Moreover, changes in waist circumference better reflect changes in cardiovascular risk factors. It is widely accepted as a surrogat marker of abdominal fat. On the other hand, waist circumference has been criticized for measuring both visceral and subcutaneous adipose tissues (Molarius & Seidell, 1998). Other studies suggest waist-to-height ratio (WHTR) as the better marker because it correlates highly with cardiometabolic risk factors (Hsieh & Yoshinaga, 1995; Ashwell, 2005). Conicity index, which is based on cylindrical shape of the body, has also been introduced as a potentially useful measure of abdominal adiposity (Valdez, 1991). However, it is considered to be very complex because it requires calculations from several different anhropometric values (Molarius & Seidell, 1998).

Sagittal abdominal diameter (SAD), or abdominal height was first demonstrated by Kvist et al. (1988) to be a good correlate of visceral adipose tissue volume, observed by CT. Sjöstrom et al. (1994) proposed the use of sagittal abdominal diameter in the assessment of visceral fat mass. Soon after, Richelsen and Pedersen (1995) confirmed its value in assessing the abdominal fatness and prediction of the metabolic risk profile.

3. Sagittal abdominal diameter – Visceral fat measure and cardiovascular risk predictor

First measures of SAD were done on CT images and showed good predictive values in the assessment of visceral adipose tissue volume (Kvist et al., 1988). SAD, thus, may be a reliable represent of the visceral fat size. Moreover, two recent studies confirmed that SAD was a stronger predictor of metabolic syndrome than the whole visceral fat area (Valsamakis et al., 2008; Hoenig, 2010), which could pointed to functionally different adipose tissue in the midline.

External, anthropometric measurement of SAD is usually done using Holtain-Kahn abdominal caliper, at the level of the iliac crest, which approximates to the L_4-L_5 interspace (Figure 1). Since it has been proposed, SAD has been considered as more closely related to visceral fat mass than the other anthropometric measures beacuse it is measured in a supine position, when a subcutaneous fat is moved to the sides of the waist (van der Kooy et al., 1993; Mukunddem-Petersen, 2006; Sampaio et al., 2007). Measuring SAD in that position reflects the width of intraabdominal fat in the antero-posterior plane, like on CT or MRI images. At the same value of SAD, an increase of waist circumference may reflect increase of subcutaneous adipose tissue size.

Many studies confirmed strong association between anthropometrically assessed SAD and visceral adipose tissue area. Anjana et al. (2004), Sampaio et al. (2007) and Yim et al. (2010)

reported stronger correlation between SAD and visceral fat area, comparing to waist circumference. Zamboni et al. (1998) found better association between SAD and visceral fat area in lean and moderately overweight subjects than in the obese. Regarding to gender, some studies have found better correlation in men, ranged between 0.61 and 0.82 (van der Kooy et al., 1993; Zamboni et al., 1998), while others have reported stronger relationship in women, with the range between 0.52 and 0.87 (Pouilot et al., 1994, Sampaio et al., 2007). Some studies demonstrated that SAD is a better predictor of visceral fat than waist circumference in men (Després et al., 1991; van der Kooy et al., 1993), while others gave opposite results in women (Sampaio et al., 2007). In the MRI study, van der Kooy et al. (1993) showed that SAD was superior to waist circumference and WHR in assessing visceral fat mass changes in men, while waist circumference and WHR were better measures in women.

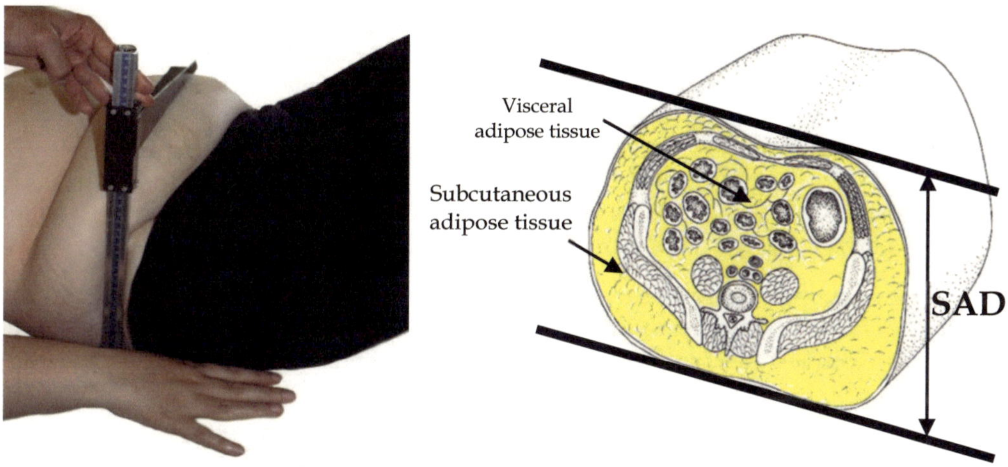

Fig. 1. Measurement of sagittal abdominal diameter (horizontal section of abdomen)

Comparing to other anthropometric measures, like waist circumference or WHR, SAD has been showed to have better correlation with biochemical and hemodynamic parameters associated with cardiovascular diseases and metabolic syndrome in both, lean and obese subjects:

- Higher values of SAD correlate with **atherogenic lipid profile** including elevated triglycerides, reduced HDL-cholesterol, elevated apolipoprotein B levels, and atherogenic lipoprotein subfractions (Pouilot et al., 1994; Sjöstrom, 1994; Richelsen & Pedersen, 1995; Öhrvall et al., 2000; Turcato et al., 2000; Sampaio et al., 2007; Petersson et al., 2007; Nakata et al., 2010).
- SAD is an important factor in prediction of **glucose intolerance and insulin resistance** (Pouliot et al., 1994; Öhrvall et al., 2000; Gustat et al., 2000; Risérus et al., 2004; Mazzali et al., 2006; Vasques et al., 2009a). Risérus et al. (2004) found that SAD was a strong predictor of hyperproinsulinemia, higher values of C-peptide and lower levels of insulin-like growth factor (IGF) binding protein-1.
- SAD highly correlates with **inflammatory and prothrombotic markers**, like CRP (Mazzali et al., 2006; Petersson et al. 2007; Nakata et al., 2010) or PAI-1 (Öhrvall et al., 2000). According to Petersson et al. (2007), every one-centimetre increase in SAD is followed by an increase of C-reactive protein (CRP) by 0.41 mg/L. The same authors

suggested that SAD may carry information concerning inflammatory status and possibly insulin resistance beyond that of other measures of obesity and fat distribution.

- SAD is associated with **blood pressure** and predicts hypertension (Öhrvall et al., 2000; Strazzulo et al., 2001). Gustat et al. (2000) highlight that SAD can predict blood pressure when other measures cannot.
- Among **adipokines**, SAD correlates with leptin and adiponectin blood levels (Mazzali et al., 2006); it also correlates with 11β-hydroxysteroid dehydrogenase-type 1 (11β-HSD-1) mRNA expression in visceral adipose tissue, which is known to be associated with features of metabolic syndrome (Desbriere et al., 2006).

Our previous results showed significantly higher values of SAD in obese women who displayed lipid and lipoprotein disturbances and hyperinsulinemia, comparing to healthy normal-weight women (Stokić et al, 1996, Stokić & Ivković-Lazar, 1996). According to our unpublished results (a group of 1090 men and 1231 women of different BMI-values, aged 18-79 years), SAD showed a significant correlation with sistolic and diastolic blood pressure and glycaemia in both genders, and with total cholesterol and triglycerides in men. In both, men and women, SAD showed best correlation with diastolic blood pressure (men: $r=0.340$, women:$r=0.198$). By discriminative analysis we determined range of SAD that correspond with lowest risk (men: 20.12-24.97 cm; women: 19.85-24.75 cm), while extremely high values were in the following ranges: 32.58-34.65 cm (men) and 29.87-31.80 cm (women).

In the large longitudinal study, Iribarren et al. (2006) confirmed utility of SAD in prediction of cardiovascular risk, independently of body mass index. Reed et al. (2003) found association between SAD and carotid artery intima-media thickness.

Empana et al. (2004) established that age-adjusted risk of sudden death increases linearly with SAD increasement in both, normal-weight and overweight men. SAD has been shown to be an independent risk factor for death and morbidity in patients in the intensive care unit (Paolini et al., 2010).

There are also two indexes derived from SAD:

- SAD-to-body height ratio (SAD/H) has been showed as slightly better predictor than SAD alone. Kumlin et al. (1997) reported that SAD/H is a strong predictor of Framingham coronary risk score.
- SAD to mid-thigh circumference ratio, or abdominal diameter index (ADI), has been proposed by Kahn (1993) as even better predictor of cardiovascular risk, which was confirmed by Smith et al. (2005).

3.1 Application of sagittal abdominal diameter in elderly

Aging process is characterized by body composition changes that could not be captured by standard anthropometric measures like BMI. Increasing of total body fat occurs in both genders, which is followed by decreasing of muscle mass (sarcopenic obesity) and body fat redistribution in terms of changes from peripheral to central (abdominal) pattern (Prentice & Jebb, 2001; Greenlund & Nair, 2003; Davidson & Getz, 2004). In women, menopause plays important role in transitioning from a premenopausal gynoid (gluteo-femoral) to a postmenopausal central (visceral) pattern of body fat distribution and increase in total body fat (Movsesyan et al., 2003). Even in early menopause women have a 49% greater visceral fat mass comparing with premenopausal women (Toth et al., 2000). Together with other physiological and life style changes caused by aging, age-associated central fat distribution contributes to cardiovascular morbidity and mortality. That is why is highly recommended to assess central adiposity in older persons (Dorner & Rieder, 2011).

Some evidences pointed to better predictive value of SAD in younger individuals (Iribarren et al., 2006, Mukuddem-Petersen et al., 2004). However, SAD could be also very useful indicator in the elderly. According to Turcato et al. (2000), SAD and waist circumference are the anthropometric parameters which are the most closely related to cardiovascular risk factors in women and men aged from 67 to 78 years, independently of BMI. Harris et al. (2000) and Snijder et al. (2002) found that SAD was even better predictor of visceral fat area in subjects older than 70 years, comparing to waist circumference, while Mukuddem-Petersen et al. (2004) indicated that SAD had no advantages over simpler and more commonly used anthropometric measures such as waist circumference, regarding to their associations with components of the metabolic syndrome in older subjects.

3.2 Gender and ethnic specific usage of sagittal abdominal diameter

Men and women have different adipose tissue topography. Fat deposition is gluteo-femoral region is more typical for women, while men show preferential abdominal fat accumulation. Within abdominal region, visceral fat compartment is more predominant in men, while women have higher size of subcutaneous fat compartment (Anjana et al., 2004). Men and women also have different dynamics of losing visceral and subcutaneous fat during weight loss - men lose more visceral, and women lose more subcutaneous fat (van der Kooy et al., 1993).

It is assumed that SAD has a stronger capacity to predict visceral fat area, insulin resistance, and cardiometabolic risk in men, because they have higher visceral fat mass (Risérus et al., 2004). Vasques et al. (2009b) confirmed its greater ability to identify insulin resistance in men. However, according to the results given by Mukuddem-Petersen et al. (2004) SAD is a stronger predictor of cardiovascular risk in women, while Duarte-Pimentel et al. (2010) recommend SAD as a marker of central adiposity preferentially in women.

Some ethnic groups show different pattern of body fat distribution and different susceptibility to insulin resistance. For example, Asian Indians have greater abdominal fat mass than Europeans of the same nutrition level (Anjana et al., 2004), while middle-aged and older African-American men and women have lower visceral fat than Hispanic and white men and women (Carroll et al., 2008). There are race and ethnical differences in the relationship between body fat distribution and health risk factors; thus, anthropometric measures could differ regarding the predictive capacity of cardiovascular risk factors. However, according to the results of several studies, SAD seems to be an excellent marker of metabolic and cardiovascular risk factors, irrespectively of national origin or ethnic background (Hwu et al., 2003; Valsamakis et al., 2004; Petersson et al., 2007, Iribarren et al., 2006).

3.3 Treshold values for sagittal abdominal diameter – Reflection of critical visceral fat mass or cardiometabolic risk

In spite of many evidences that SAD is very good in capturing the cardiometabolic risk, its use in clinical practice is limited due to a lack of specific cut-offs. Some authors have proposed cut-off values for SAD using different criteria, usually its correlation with cardiometabolic parameters and visceral fat area (Table 1). These results were mostly obtained using Receiver Operating Characteristics (ROC) curves, or linear regression analysis, and vary from 19.3 cm (Sampaio et al., 2007) to 27.6 cm (Valsamakis et al., 2004). Our results were obtained using the principles of rough set theory that will be described below. They were derived from evaluation of relationship between SAD and cardiovascular risk factors.

We produced "transparent", semantic model which can be easily analyzed. The most important information which can be extracted from semantic models is concerned with the meaning and importance of its elements, as well as with the relations between them. Data were represented in the form of a table with rows containing the objects and columns containing the attributes, and model was produced in the multiple sets containing *If – Then* rules.

SAD (cut-offs)	Population	Criterion	Author
≥25 cm	Men/Women	Association with multiple metabolic disorders	Pouliot et al., 1994
≥22.8 cm ≥25.2 cm	Men Women	Corresponds to 130 cm^2 of visceral fat area	Lemieux et al., 1996
≥27.6 cm	Men	Predictive value for metabolic syndrome	Valsamakis et al., 2004
≥23 cm	Men	Predictive value for sudden death	Empana et al., 2004
≥20.5 cm ≥19.3 cm	Men Women	Corresponds to 100 cm^2 of visceral area	Sampaio et al., 2007
≥20 cm	Men	Predictive value for insulin resistance	Vasques et al., 2009a
≥22.2 cm ≥20.1 cm	Men Women	Predictive value for an elevated cardiometabolic risk score	Risérus et al., 2010
≥23.1 cm ≥20.1 cm	Men Women	Corresponds to altered waist circumference (>102 cm for men and >88 cm for women)	Duarte Pimentel et al., 2010
≥24.3 cm	Men/Women	Corresponds to increased cardiovascular risk in overweight and obese individuals	Stokić et al., 2010

Table 1. Recommended cut-off values for SAD

4. Model for the better applicability of SAD in identifying patients at higher cardiovascular risk

Modern healthcare and computer science are fields that are interlaced to form the field of medical informatics. As mentioned by Øhrn (1999), Blois and Shortliffe define medical informatics as "the rapidly developing scientific field that deals with the storage, retrieval and optimal use of biomedical information, data, and knowledge for problem solving and decision making." In its broadest sense, medical informatics can be said to concern itself with the management of information in the context of modern healthcare. According to Øhrn (1999) current research in the field of medical informatics covers a wide array of topics, including:

- **Data acquisition:** Capturing and recording of the medical data usually include things that are not easily recorded or precisely defined.
- **Medical vocabularies:** Medical data has to be represented in machine-readable form.
- **Electronic medical records:** An electronic medical record has to be searchable. Its content should be structured internally.
- **Decision support systems:** These are computer programs that help clinicians make clinical decisions.
- **Deployment barriers:** The barriers of deployment may be technical, operational, organizational and legal nature. Often, systems that may prove successful in research settings do not make it into clinical use.
- **Confidentiality issues:** Medical information is often sensitive and with a potential for misuse by third-parties.

Obviously, as a main prerequisite there is a existence of medical dataset or database. Medical datasets are often described as incomplete, sparse, vague, fuzzy, etc. According to Greco et al. (1998), the rough sets theory has often proved to be an excellent mathematical tool for the analysis of a vague description of objects.

On the base of the table-organized data it is possible to produce semantic model which provides information about meaning and importance of its elements, as well as the relationship between them (Brtka et al., 2008; Stokić et al., 2010). In order to investigate relationship between SAD and anthropometric and cardiovascular risk factors, we used methodology based on rough set theory (Pawlak et al, 1995, Pawlak & Skowron, 2007) applied to table–organized data with producing decision rules in the *If -Then* form.

Our study included 1334 subjects (700 women and 634 men), aged 43.49±10.43 years. Following parameters were analyzed: age (years), body mass index (kg/m^2), SAD (cm), body fat mass (%), systolic and diastolic blood pressure (mmHg), total-, LDL- and HDL-cholesterol (mmol/L), triglycerides (mmol/L), fasting plasma glucose (mmol/L), fibrinogen (g/L), uric acid (μmol/L), and 10-year Framingham Risk Score. The experiments were conducted by software system *Rosetta - A Rough Set Toolkit for Analysis of Data*. All numerical attributes were discretized using a simple "equal frequency binning" technique. The attribute SAD was chosen to be the decision attribute while all remaining attributes were chosen to form the set of condition attributes and the set of rules containing rules in the *If – Then* form was generated. The decision attributes (SAD) were classified into three classes:

- 13.00-24.2 cm,
- 24.3-31.6 cm and
- 31.7-36.2 cm.

4.1 Rough-set theory principles

As the mathematical basis of the rough set theory there is the indiscernibility relation. Every object of the universe is described by certain amount of information expressed by means of some attributes used for that object description. The objects characterized by the same information are indiscernible in view of the available information about them.

As in Greco et al. (1998), Øhrn (1999) and Pawlak & Skowron (2007), let U be a universe (finite set of objects), $Q=\{q_1,q_2,...,q_m\}$ is a finite set of attributes, V_q is the domain of attribute q (attribute values) and V is the union of V_q for every $q \in Q$. An information system is the 4-tuple $S=(U,Q,V,f)$ where f is a function such that $f(x,q) \in V_q$ for each $q \in Q$, $x \in U$, called information function.

Let $x,y \in U$ (x and y are two objects e.g. patients), f is an information function and $q \in Q$. Every non-empty subset of attributes P determines an indiscernibility relation on U, denoted by

$$I_P = \{(x,y) \in U \times U : f(x,q) = f(y,q), \forall q \in P\} \quad (1)$$

The I_P is an equivalence relation. The family of all the equivalence classes of the I_P is denoted by U/I_P and the equivalence class containing an element x by $I_P(x)$.

Let us consider a simple example of an information system based on the example from Greco et al. (1998), see Table 2.

Object	Age	Body Mass (BM)	Systolic blood pressure	SAD
x_1	young	good	low	low
x_2	middle-age	medium	low	high
x_3	middle-age	medium	low	low
x_4	old	medium	low	high
x_5	middle-age	good	high	high
x_6	young	medium	high	low

Table 2. Simple example of an information system

In the given table, there is a universe of six objects $U=\{x_1,...,x_6\}$ and each object is described by means of four attributes: *Age*, *Body Mass*, *Systolic Blood Pressure (SBP)* and *SAD*.

If $P=\{Age,BM,SBP\}$ then, by (1), we have: $I_P=\{(x_1,x_1), (x_2,x_2), (x_2,x_3), (x_3,x_2), (x_3,x_3), (x_4,x_4), (x_5,x_5)$ $(x_6,x_6)\}$, $U/I_P=\{\{x_1\}, \{x_2,x_3\}, \{x_4\}, \{x_5\}, \{x_6\}\}$.

4.1.1 The definition of the rough set

The rough set theory proved to be an excellent mathematical tool for the analysis of data in various domains. The information about the real world is given in a form of a decision system. The next definitions are based on Pawlak et al. (1995), Greco et al. (1998), Øhrn (1999) and Pawlak & Skowron (2007).

Let $C \subset Q$ and $D \subset Q$ so that $C \cap D = \emptyset$, where Q is a set of attributes. The attributes from C are called the condition attributes and the attributes from D are called the decision attributes. An information system where the set of condition attributes and the set of decision attributes are defined is called the decision system.

In most cases there is usually one binary decision attribute, while the other attributes are the condition attributes. In the previous example P might be the set of the condition attributes, and the set of decision attributes contains one element: $D=\{SAD\}$.

Let X be a non-empty subset of U and $\emptyset \neq P \subseteq Q$. The set X is approximated by means of P-lower (2) and P-upper (3) approximations of X:

$$\underline{P}(X) = \{x \in U : I_P(x) \subseteq X\} \tag{2}$$

$$\overline{P}(X) = \bigcup_{x \in X} I_P(x) \tag{3}$$

The P-boundary region $Bn(X)$ of X is defined by:

$$Bn(X) = \overline{P}(X) - \underline{P}(X) \tag{4}$$

For example, let us consider a case when the set X contains only those elements where the value of the decision attribute SAD is low: $X=\{x_1,x_3,x_6\}$ (Table 2). Now, we can approximate the set X using only the information contained in P by constructing the P-lower (2) and P-upper (3) approximations of X:

$$\underline{P}(X) = \{x_1, x_6\},$$

$$\overline{P}(X) = \{x_1, x_2, x_3, x_6\}.$$

The P-boundary region (4) of X is:

$$Bn(X) = \{x_2, x_3\}.$$

The reader may notice that the objects x_2 and x_3 have exactly the same values of the condition attributes but different value of the decision attribute. So, they constitute boundary region. We can say that the rough sets can be defined as follows (Pawlak et al., 1995; Pawlak & Skowron, 2007):

The set X is rough (inexact) with respect to I_P, if the boundary region of X is nonempty. The set X is crisp (exact) with respect to I_P, if the boundary region of X is empty.

4.1.2 Data reduction

If we manage to identify equivalence classes then some savings (reductions) are to be made since only one element of the equivalence class is needed to represent the entire equivalence class. An issue of practical importance in reduction is to keep only those attributes that preserve the indiscernibility relation and consequently, the set approximation. The rejected attributes are redundant (superfluous) since their removal cannot worsen the classification (Greco et al., 1998).

Let $\varnothing \neq P \subseteq Q$ and $a \in P$. Attribute a is superfluous in P if $I_P = I_{P-\{a\}}$.

For example, if *R*= {*Age*, *BM*}, *S*= {*Age*, *SBP*}, and *T*= {*BM*, *SBP*} (Table 2), then it is obvious that $I_R = I_P$ and $I_S = I_P$ while $I_T \neq I_P$. This means that *R* and *S* are reducts of *P*, while *T* is not. The attribute *Age* is indispensable, but the attributes *BM* and *SBP* may be mutually exchanged. This means that it is enough to use reduct {*Age*, *BM*} to estimate the value of the decision attribute *SAD*. In the analog case we can use the reduct {*Age*, *SBP*} to estimate the value of decision attribute *SAD*, but we can not use the reduct {*BM*, *SBP*}.

The calculation of all reducts is very complex but in many practical applications it is not necessary to calculate all the reducts, but only some of them.

4.1.3 Discretization

If we want numerical attributes to be properly incorporated into the classification rules, we should to discretize them. This enables the numerical attributes to be treated as categorical ones, and several algorithms for this purpose are available (Greco et al., 1998; Øhrn, 1999). The goal of the discretization process is to search for intervals or bins, where all cases that fall within the same interval are grouped together. This process can be also seen as the process of classification of the attributes' value set to some classes. The discretization is not specific to the rough set approach but is a pre - required step and is often performed implicitly, behind the scene, using human expert knowledge.

4.1.4 Decision rules

The expression $a = v$, where a is an attribute and v is an attribute value is called the descriptor. Now, it is possible to investigate the rules of the form: *If* α *Then* β. Here α denotes a conjunction (AND logical operator) of descriptors that only involve attributes of some reduct (rule's antecedent) and β (rule's consequent) denote a descriptor $d = v$, where d is a decision attribute and v is the allowed decision value.

For example, if we use the reduct *R={Age, BM}* from Table 2 and *SAD* as a decision attribute, then it is possible to generate the rules with two descriptors in the antecedent part and one descriptor in the consequent part of the rule. It is important to notice that a shorter reduct set means shorter decision rules in the rule set generated from that reduct.

4.2 Application of rough-set theory in identification of patients at higher cardiovascular risk using SAD

Our results showed that SAD could be a clinically useful marker for identification of combination and structure of risk factors by applying different rules in individuals of different BMI-categories.

Lower values of SAD in normal-weight individuals younger than 50 years always corresponded with Framingham risk score <9. However, in normal-weight subjects older than 50 years, SAD couldn't identify those at lower risk. SAD values between 24.3 and 31.6 cm, or even lower, between 13.0 and 24.2 cm, corresponded with Framingham risk score between 9 and 14 (Table 3). It is in agreement with observations which indicate a centralization of adipose tissue with aging, irrespective of BMI. This would represent a category of metabolically obese normal weight individuals.

According to these results, measurement of SAD is not enough for identification of cardiovascular risk in normal-weight individuals. In that regard, it is necessary to include other methods of fat mass assessment, like CT or MRI.

IF												THEN SAD (cm)
Age (years)	Body fat mass (%)	Systolic blood pressure (mmHg)	Diastolic blood pressure (mmHg)	Total cholesterol (mmol/L)	Triglycerides (mmol/L)	LDL-cholesterol (mmol/L)	HDL-cholesterol (mmol/L)	Glycaemia (mmol/L)	Fibrinogen (g/L)	Acidum uricum (μmol/L)	Framingham risk score	
<41	<28.92	<123	>88	<5.37	1.4-2.19	<3.24	1.01-1.21	<4.7	3.06-3.76	273-344	<9	
	<28.92	123-141	>88	>6.51	<1.4	<3.24	<1.01	4.7-5.4	>3.76	<273	<9	
41-50	<28.92	<123	78-88	<5.37	<1.4	3.24-4.0	<1.01	<4.7	<3.06	<273	<9	13.0-24.2
	<28.92	123-141	>88	<5.37	>2.19	<3.24	<1.01	4.7-5.4	>3.76	<273	<9	
	<28.92	<123	78-88	>6.51	1.4-2.19	>4.00	>1.21	>5.4	3.06-3.76	<273	<9	
>50	<28.93	123-141	>88	>6.51	>2.19	3.24-4.0	>1.21	4.7-5.4	3.06-3.76	273-344	9-14	13.0-24.2 OR 24.3-31.6

Table 3. Obtained rules for normal-weight subjects (BMI<26.43 kg/m^2)

By examining the decision rules, SAD could point out a group of overweight patients with high level of visceral fat with different combination and composition of cardiovascular risk factors (Table 4). Thus, in overweight individuals aged 41-50 years, with higher fat mass, and SAD between 24.3 and 31.6 cm, we could expect higher values of diastolic blood pressure, total- and LDL-cholesterol, triglycerides, uric acid, as well as Framingham risk score over 14. The same range of SAD in older overweight individuals (>50 years) with higher fat mass, include higher systolic blood pressure, fasting plasma glucose and fibrinogen. On the other side, in younger overweight subjects with lower SAD (<24.3 cm) we could expect lower values of all atherogenic parameters, higher values of HDL-cholesterol and Framingham risk score <9, even if they have higher fat mass.

It means that SAD could identify metabolically healthy overweight individuals.

IF												THEN SAD (cm)
Age (years)	Body fat mass (%)	Systolic blood pressure (mmHg)	Diastolic blood pressure (mmHg)	Total cholesterol (mmol/L)	Triglycerides (mmol/L)	LDL-cholesterol (mmol/L)	HDL-cholesterol (mmol/L)	Glycaemia (mmol/L)	Fibrinogen (g/L)	Acidum uricum (μmol/L)	Framingham risk score	
<41	>39.71	<123	<78	<5.37	<1.4	<3.24	>1.21	4.7-5.4	>3.76	>344	<9	13.0-24.2
41-50	>39.71	<123	>88	>6.51	>2.19	<3.24	1.01-1.21	>5.4	>3.76	>344	9-14	13.0-24.2 OR 24.3-31.6
	28.92-39.71	<123	>88	>6.51	<1.4	>4.0	1.01-1.21	<4.7	>3.76	>344	9-14	
>50	<28.92	123-141	>88	5.37-6.51	>2.19	<3.24	>1.21	4.7-5.4	>3.76	<273	9-14	
	<28.92	<123	78-88	>6.51	1.4-2.19	>4.00	1.01-1.21	>5.4	>3.76	273-344	9-14	
<41	<28.92	123-141	78-88	<5.37	<1.4	<3.24	>1.21	4.7-5.4	3.06-3.76	>344	<9	24.3-31.6
41-50	28.92-39.71	<123	>88	>6.51	>2.19	>4.00	1.01-1.21	4.7-5.4	<3.06	>344	>14	
	>39.71	123-141	>88	>6.51	<1.4	>4.00	>1.21	<4.7	3.06-3.76	<273	9-14	
>50	28.92-39.71	>141	>88	>6.51	>2.19	>3.24	1.01-1.21	>5.4	3.06-3.76	273-344	9-14	
	28.92-39.71	>141	>88	>6.51	>2.19	>4.00	>1.21	<4.7	<3.06	<273	9-14	

Table 4. Obtained rules for overweight subjects (BMI: 26.43-32.52 kg/m^2)

As it is displayed in the Table 5, SAD values above 31.7 cm in obese subjects always correspond to Framingham risk score >14. Younger obese individuals (<41 years) with lower values of SAD usually are at the lower cardiovascular risk (metabolically healthy obese individuals).

IF												THEN SAD (cm)
Age (years)	Body fat mass (%)	Systolic blood pressure (mmHg)	Diastolic blood pressure (mmHg)	Total cholesterol (mmol/L)	Triglycerides (mmol/L)	LDL-cholesterol (mmol/L)	HDL-cholesterol (mmol/L)	Glycaemia (mmol/L)	Fibrinogen (g/L)	Acidum uricum (μmol/L)	Framingham risk score	
<41	>39.71	<123	<78	<5.37	>2.19	<3.24	1.01-1.21	4.7-5.4	3.06-3.76	<273	<9	13.0-24.2
	>39.71	<123	>88	<5.37	<1.4	3.24-4.00	1.01-1.21	<4.7	3.06-3.76	>344		
	28.92-39.71	123-141	>88	>6.51	1.4-2.19	>4.00	>1.21	>5.4	>3.76	>344	>14	
41-50	>39.71	123-141	>88	>6.51	>2.19	3.24-4.00	>1.21	4.7-5.4	<3.06	>344	9-14	
<41	>39.71	<123	78-88	5.37-6.51	<1.4	>4.00	>1.21	4.7-5.4	>3.76	>344	<9	24.3-31.6
	>39.71	<123	<78	<5.37	<1.4	<3.24	<1.01	<4.7	3.06-3.76	<273		
	>39.71	123-141	>88	<5.37	<1.4	<3.24	>1.21	4.7-5.4	3.06-3.76	>344		
	>39.71	<123	<78	<5.37	<1.4	<3.24	<1.01	<4.7	3.06-3.76	<273		
	>39.71	123-141	>88	>6.51	1.4-2.19	3.24-4.00	<1.01	4.7-5.4	3.06-3.76	273-344	9-14	
>50	>39.71	123-141	78-88	5.37-6.51	1.4-2.19	<3.24	1.01-1.21	4.7-5.4	3.06-3.76	>344	>14	
41-50	>39.71	>141	>88	5.37-6.51	>2.19	3.24-4.00	<1.01	>5.4	3.06-3.76	273-344	>14	24.3-31.6 OR 31.7-36.2
>50	28.92-39.71	123-141	>88	>6.51	<1.4	3.24-4.00	>1.21	>5.4	>3.76	273-344	9-14	
<41	>39.71	123-141	78-88	>6.51	>2.19	3.24-4.00	<1.01	>5.4	>3.76	>344	>14	31.7-36.2
>50	>39.71	>141	>88	>6.51	>2.19	>4.00	>1.21	>5.4	>3.76	>344	>14	

Table 5. Obtained rules for obese subjects (BMI>32.52 kg/m^2)

5. Conclusion

Many studies have proved that SAD is a good predictor of abdominal, especially visceral, fat mass, as well as of cardiometabolic risk. Several authors have suggested specific cut-off values for SAD that corresponded with cardiovascular and metabolic risk or with visceral fat area obtained by CT. Using the concept of a rough set, proved as a formal tool for modeling and processing information systems, we developed a useful model for identification of individuals with multiple cardiovascular risk factors using SAD.

Our results revealed connection between SAD and cardiovascular risk factors which showed dependence on age and nutrition level. We primarily recommend application of SAD in the assessment of the cardiovascular risk in overweight and obese individuals. SAD values ≥24.3 cm in overweight and obese subjects older than 41 years should correspond to increased risk, while values <24.3 cm in overweight subjects younger than 41 years could point to healthy metabolic profile.

6. References

Anjana, M.; Sandeep, S.; Deepa, R.; Vimaleswaran K.S.; Farooq, S. & Mohan, V. (2004). Visceral and central abdominal fat and anthropometry in relation to diabetes in Asian Indians. *Diabetes Care*, Vol.27, No.12, pp. 2948-2953

Ashwell, M. (2005). Waist to height ratio and the Ashwell shape chart could predict the health risks of obesity in adults and children in all ethnic groups. *Nutrition&Food Science*, Vol.35, No.5, pp. 359-64

Berg, A.H. & Scherer, P.E. (2005). Adipose tissue, inflammation, and cardiovascular disease. *Circulation Research*, Vol.96, pp. 939-949

Bosello, O. & Zamboni, M. (2000). Visceral obesity and metabolic syndrome. *Obesity Reviews*, Vol.1, pp. 47-56

Bouchard, C.; Bray, G.A. & Hubbard, V.S. (1990). Basic and clinical aspects of regional fat distribution. *American Journal of Clinical Nutrition*, Vol.52, pp.946-950

Brochu, M.; Starling, R.D.; Tchernof, A.; Matthews, D.E.; Garcia-Rubi, E. & Poehlman, E.T. (2000). Visceral adipose tissue is an independent correlate of glucose disposal in older obese postmenopausal women. *The Journal of Clinical Endocrinology & Metabolism*, Vol.85, pp. 2378-2384

Brtka, V.; Stokić, E. & Srdić, B. (2008). Automated extraction of decision rules for leptin dynamics--a rough sets approach, *Journal of Biomedical Informatics*, Vol.41, No.4, pp. 667-674

Carroll, J.F.; Chiapa, A.L.; Rodriquez, M.; Phelps, D.R.; Cardarelli, K.M.; Vishwanatha, J.K.; Bae, S. & Cardarelli, R. (2008). Visceral fat, waist circumference, and BMI: impact of race/ethnicity. *Obesity*, Vol.16, No.3, pp. 600–607

Coppack, S.W. (2005). Adipose tissue changes in obesity. *Biochemical Society Transactions*, Vol.33, pp. 1049-1052

Couillard, C.; Lamarche, B.; Tchernof, A.; Prud'homme, D.; Tremblay, A.; Bouchard, C.; Moorjani, S.; Nadeau, A.; Lupien, P.J. & Després J-P. (1996). Plasma high-density lipoprotein cholesterol but not apolipoproetin A-I is a good correlate of the visceral obesity-insulin resistance dyslipidemic syndrome. *Metabolism*, Vol.45, pp.882-888

Davidson, J. & Getz, M. (2004). Nutritional risk and body composition in free-living elderly participating in congregate meal-site programs. *Journal of Nutrition for the Elderly*, Vol.24, No.1, pp. 53-68

Desbriere, R.; Vuaroqueaux, V.; Achard, V.; Boullu-Ciocca, S. Labuhn, M.; Dutour, A. & Grino, M. (2006). 11β-Hydroxysteroid Dehydrogenase Type 1 mRNA is Increased in Both Visceral and Subcutaneous Adipose Tissue of Obese Patients. *Obesity*, Vol.14, pp. 794–798

Després, J-P.; Moorjani, S.; Lupien, P.J.; Tremblay, A.; Nadeau, A. & Bouchard C. (1990). Regional distribution of body fat, plasma lipoproteins, and cardiovascular disease. *Arteriosclerosis*, Vol.10, No.4, pp. 497-511

Després, J-P.; Prud'homme, D.; Pouiliot, M.C.; Tremblay, A. & Bouchard C. (1991). Estimation of deep abdominal adipose-tissue accumulation from simple anthropometric measurements in men. *American Journal of Clinical Nutrition*, Vol.54, pp. 471-477

Dorner, T.E. & Rieder, A. (2011). Obesity paradox in elderly patients with cardiovascular diseases. *International Journal of Cardiology*, doi: 10.1016/j.ijcard.2011.01.076

Duarte Pimentel, G.; Portero-McLellan, K.C.; Maestá, N.; Corrente, J.E. & Burini, R.C. (2010). Accuracy of SAD as predictor of abdominal fat among Brazilian adults: a comparation with waist circumference. *Nutrición hospitalaria*, Vol.25, No.4, pp. 656-661

Empana, J.P.; Ducimetiere, P.; Charles, M.A. & Jouven, X. (2004). SAD and risk of sudden death in asymptomatic middle-aged men - the Paris prospective study. *Circulation*, Vol.110, pp. 2781-2785

Freedland, E.S. (2004). Role of a critical visceral adipose tissue threshold (CVATT) in metabolic syndrome: implications for controlling dietary carbohydrates: a review. *Nutrition&Metabolism*, Vol.1, (November 2004), doi: 10.1 186/1743-7075-1-12

Goossens, G.H. (2008). The role of adipose tissue dysfunction in the pathogenesis of obesity-related insulin resistance. *Physiology&Behaviour*, Vol.94, pp. 206-218

Greco, M.; Benedetto, R.; Slowinski, R. (1998). New developments in the rough set approach to multi-attribute decision analysis, *Proceedings of 16th European Conference on Operational Research*, Brussels, July 1998

Greenlund, LJ.S. & Nair K.S. (2003). Sarcopenia - consequences, mechanisms, and potential therapies. *Mechanisms of Aging and Development*, Vol.124, pp. 287-299

Gustat, J., Elkasabany, A., Srinivasan, S. & Berenson, G.S. (2000). Relation of abdominal height to cardiovascular risk factors in young adults. *American Journal of Epidemiology*, Vol.151, No.9, pp. 885-891

Guzzaloni, G.; Minocci, A.; Marzullo, P. & Liuzzi, A. (2009). SAD is more predictive of cardiovascular risk than abdominal fat compartments in severe obesity. *International Journal of Obesity*, Vol.33, pp. 233-238

Harris, T.B.; Visser, M.; Everhart, J.; Cauley, J.; Tylavsky, F.; Fuerst, T.; Zamboni, M.; Taaffe, D.; Resnick, H.E.; Scherzinger, A. & Nevitt, M. (2000). Waist circumference and sagittal diameter reflect total body fat better than visceral fat in older men and women. The Health, Aging and Body Composition Study. *Annals of the New York Academy of Sciences*, Vol.904, pp. 462-473

Hoenig, M.R. (2010). MRI sagittal diameter is a stronger predictor of metabolic syndrome than visceral fat area or waist circumference in a high-risk vascular cohort. *Vascular Health and Risk Management*, Vol.6, pp. 629-633.

Hsieh, S.D. & Yoshinaga, H. (1995). Abdominal fat distribution and coronary heart disease risk factors in men - waist/height ratio as a simple and useful predictor. *International Journal of Obesity and Related Metabolic Disorders*, Vol.19, pp. 585-589

Hwu, C.M.; Hsiao, C.F.; Sheu, W.H.H.; Pei, D.; Tai, T.Y.; Quertermous, T.; Rodriguez, B.; Pratt, R.; Chen, Y.DI, Ho, L.T. (2003). SAD is associated with insulin sensitivity in Chinese hypertensive patients and their siblings. *Journal of Human Hypertension*, Vol.17, pp. 193-198

Iribarren, C.; Darbinian, J.A.; Lo, J.C.; Fireman, B.H. & Go, A.S. (2006). Value of the SAD in coronary heart disease risk assessment: cohort study in a large, multiethnic population. *American Journal of Epidemiology*, Vol.164, No.12, pp. 1150–1159

Iribarren, C.; Sharp, D.S.; Burchfiel, D.M. & Petrovich, H. (1995). Association of weight loss and weight fluctuation with mortality among Japanese men. *New England Journal of Medicine*, Vol.333, pp. 686-692

Kahn, H.S. (1993). Choosing an index for abdominal obesity: an opportunity for epidemilogical clarification. *Journal of Clinical Epidemiology*, Vol.46, pp. 491-494

Krotkiewski, M.; Björntorp, P.; Sjöström, L. & Smith, U. (1983). Impact of obesity on metabolism in men and women. Importance of regional adipose tissue distribution. *Journal of Clinical Investigation*, Vol.72, pp. 1150-1162

Kumlin, L.; Dimberg, L. & Mårin, P. (1997). Ratio of abdominal sagittal diameter to heigh is strong indicator of coronary risk (letter). *British Medical Journal*, Vol.314, p. 830

Kvist, H.; Chowdhury, B.; Grangard, U.; Tylen, U. & Sjostrom L. (1988). Total and visceral-adipose tissue volumes derived from measurements with computed tomography in adults man and women: predictive equations. *American Journal of Clinical Nutrition*, Vol.48, No.6, pp. 1351-1361

Lemieux, S.; Prud'homme, D.; Bouchard, C.; Tremblay, A. & Despres, A. (1996). A single threshold value of waist girth identifies normal-weight and overweight subjects with excess visceral adipose tissue. *American Journal of Clinical Nutrition*, Vol.64, pp.685-693

Lofgren, I.; Herron, K.; Zern, T.; West, K.; Partalay, M.; Shachter, N.S.; Koo, S.I. & Fernandez, M.L. (2004). Waist circumference is a better predictor than body mass index of coronary heart disease risk in overweight premenopausal women. *Journal of Nutrition*, Vol.134, pp. 1071–1076

Lonnqvist, F.; Thorne, A.; Large, V. & Arner, P. (1995). Sex differences in visceral fat lipolysis and metabolic complications of obesity. *Atherosclerosis, Thrombosis, and Vascular Biology*, Vol.17, No.7, pp. 1472-1480

Marques-Vidal, P.; Chiolero, A. & Paccaud, F. (2008). Large differences in the prevalence of normal weight obesity using various cut-offsfor excess body fat. *e-SPAN, the European e-Journal of Clinical Nutrition and Metabolism*, Vol.3, pp. e159-e162

Matsuzawa, Y.; Shimomura, I.; Nakamura, T.; Keno, Y.; Kotani, K. & Tokunaga, K. (1995). Pathophysiology and pathogenesis of visceral fat obesity. *Obesity Research*, Vol.3, No.2, pp.187-194S.

Mazzali, G.; Di Francesco, V.; Zoico, E.; Fantin, F.; Zamboni, G.; Benati, C.; Bambara, V.; Negri, M.; Bosello, O. & Zamboni M. (2006). Interrelations between fat distribution, muscle lipid content, adipocytokines, and insulin resistance: effect of moderate weight loss in older women. *American Journal of Clinical Nutrition*, Vol.84, No.5, pp. 1193-1199

Misra, A. & Vikram, N.K. (2003). Clinical and patophysiological consequences of abdominal adiposity and abdominal adipose tissue depots. *Nutrition*, Vol.19, pp. 457-66

Molarius, A. & Seidell, J.C. (1998). Selection of anthropometric indicators for classification of abdominal fatness: A critical review. *International Journal of Obesity and Related Metabolic Disorders*, Vol.22, No.8, pp. 719-727

Movsesyan, L.; Tanko, L.B.; Larsen, P.J.; Christiansen, C. & Svendsen, O.L. (2003). Variations in percentage of body fat within different BMI groups in young, middle-aged and old women. *Clinical Physiology and Funcional Imaging*, Vol.23, pp.130-133

Mukuddem-Petersen, J.; Snijder, M.B.; van Dam, R.B.; Dekker, J.M.; Bouter, L.M.; Stehouwer, C.D.A.; Heine, R.J.; Nijpels, G. & Seidell, J.C. (2004). SAD: no advantage compared with other anthropometric measures as a correlate of components of the metabolic syndrome in elderly from the Hoorn Study. *American Journal of Clinical Nutrition*, Vol.84, pp.995-1002

Nakata, K.; Choo, J.; Hopson, M.S.J.; Ueshima, H.; Curb, D.; Shin, C.; Evans, R.W.; Kadowaki, T.; Otake, T.; Kadota, A.; Kadowaki, S.; Miura, K.; El-Saed, A.; Edmudowicz, D.; Sutton-Tyrell, K.; Kuller, L.H. & Sekikawa, A. (2010). Stronger associations of SAD with atherogenic lipoprotein subfractions than waist circumference in middle-aged US white and Japanese men. *Metabolism Clinical and Experimental*, Vol.59, pp.1742-1751

Øhrn, A. (1999). Discernibility and Rough Sets in Medicine: Tools and Applications. PhD thesis. Department of Computer and Information Science (Norwegian University of Science and Technology, Trondheim, Norway)

Öhrvall, M.; Berglund, L. & Vessby, B. (2000). SAD compared with other anthropometric measurements in relation to cardiovasular risk. *International Journal of Obesity and Related Metabolic Disorders*, Vol.24, No.4, pp.497-501.

Paolini, J.B.; Mancini, J.; Genestal, M.; Gonzalez, H.; McKay, R.E.; Samii, K. & Fourcade, O.A. (2010). Predictive value of abdominal obesity vs. body mass index for determining risk of intensive care unit mortality. *Critical Care Medicine*, Vol.38, No. 5, pp. 1308-1314

Pawlak, Z. & Skowron, A. (2007). Rudiments of rough sets. *An International Journal of Information Sciences*, Vol.177, pp. 3–27

Pawlak, Z.; Grzymala-Busse, J.; Slowinski, R. & Ziarko, W. (1995). Rough sets. *Communications of the ACM*, Vol.38, No.11, pp. 89–95R.

Petersson, H.; Daryani, A. & Risérus, U. (2007). SAD as a marker of inflammation and insulin resistance among immigrant women from the Middle East and native Swedish women: a cross-sectional study. *Cardiovascular Diabetology*, Vol.6, pp. 10.

Pouliot, M.C.; Despres, J.P.; Lemieux, S.; Moorjani, S.; Bouchard, C. & Tremblay, A. (1994). Waist circumference and abdominal sagittal diameter: best simple anthropometric indexes of abdominal visceral adipose tissue accumulation and related cardiovascular risk in men and women. *American Journal of Cardiology*, Vol.73, No.7, pp. 460-468

Prentice, A.M. & Jebb, S.A. (2001). Beyond body mass index. Obesity Reviews, *Vol.2, No.3, pp. 141-147*

Reed, D.; Dwyer, K.M. & Dwyer, J.H.; (2003). Abdominal obesity and carotid artery wall thickness. The Los Angeles Atherosclerosis Study. *International Journal of Obesity and Related Metabolic Disorders*, Vol.27, pp. 1546-1551

Richelsen, B. & Pedersen, S.B. (1995). Associations between different anthropometric measurements of fatness and metabolic risk parameters in non-obese, healthy, middle-aged men. *International Journal of Obesity*, Vol.19, No.3, pp. 169-174

Risérus, U.; Ärnlöv, J.; Brismar, K.; Zethelius, B.; Berglund, L. & Vessby, B. (2004). SAD is a strong anthropometric marker of insulin resistance and hyperinsulinemia in obese men. *Diabetes Care*, Vol.27, No.8, pp. 2041-2046

Risérus, U.; de Faire, U.; Berglund, L. & Hellénius, M.L. (2010). SAD as a screening tool in clinical research: cutoffs for cardiometabolic risk. *Journal of Obesity*, doi:10.1155/2010/757939

Romero-Corral, A.; Montori, V.M.; Somers, V.K.; Korinek, J.; Thomas, R.J.; Allison, T.G.; Mookadam, F. & Lopez-Jimenez, F. (2006). Association of bodyweight with total mortality and with cardiovascular events in coronary artery disease: a systematic review of cohort studies. *Lancet*, Vol.368, No.9536, pp.666-678

Ruderman, N.; Chisholm, D., Pi-Sunyer, X. & Schenider, S. (1998). The metabolically obese, normal-weight individual revisited. *Diabetes*, Vol.47, pp.699-713

Sampaio, L.R.; Simões, E.J.; Assis, A.M.O. & Ramos, L.R. (2007). Validity and reliability of the SAD as a predictor of visceral abdominal fat. *Arquivos Brasileiros de Endocrinologia & Metabologia*, Vol.51, No.6, pp. 980-986

Sims, E.A. (2001). Are there persons who are obese, but metabolically healthy? *Metabolism*, Vol.50, pp. 1499-1504

Sjöstrom, L. (1994). The sagittal diameter is valid marker of visceral adipose tissue. *International Journal of Obesity*, Vol.18, No.2, pp. 46-52

Smith, D.A.; Ness, E.M.; Herbert, R.; Schechter, C.B.; Phillips, R.A.; Diamond, J.A. & Landrigan, P.J. (2005). Abdominal diameter index: a more powerful anthropometric measure for prevalent coronary heart disease risk in adult males. *Diabetes, Obesity and Metabolism*, Vol.7, pp.370-380.

Snijder, M.B.; Visser, M.; Dekker, J.M.; Seidell, J.C.; Fuerst, T.; Tylavsky, F.; Cauley, J.; Lang, T.; Nevitt, M. & Harris, T.B. (2002). The prediction of visceral fat by dual-energy X-ray absorptiometry in the elderly: a comparison with computed tomography and anthropometry. *International Journal of Obesity*, Vol.26, pp. 984-993

Stokić, E. & Ivković-Lazar, T. (1996). Relation between the abdominal sagittal diameter, fat tissue distribution and metabolic complications. *Medicinski Pregled*, Vol.49, No. 9-10, pp. 365-368

Stokić, E.; Brtka, V. & Srdić, B. (2010). The synthesis of the rough set model for the better applicability of SAD in identifying high risk patients. *Computers in Biology and Medicine*, Vol. 40, pp. 786-90

Stokić, E.; Đureković-Katona, A. & Ivković-Lazar, T. (1996). The role and significance of SAD in the determination of adipose tissue distribution. *Medicinski Pregled*, Vol.49, No.5-6, pp. 217-220

Strazzullo, P.; Barba, G.; Cappuccio, F.P.; Siani, A.; Trevisan, M.; Farinaro, E.; Pagano, E.; Barbato, A.; Iacone, R. & Galletti, F. (2001). Altered renal sodium handling in men with abdominal adiposity: a link to hypertension. *Journal of Hypertension*, Vol.19, No.12, pp. 2157-2164.

Toth, M.J.; Tchernof, A.; Sites, C.K. & Poehlman, E.T. (2000). Effect of menopausal status on body composition and abdominal fat distribution. *International Journal of Obesity*, Vol.24, pp. 226-231

Turcato, E.; Bosello, O.; Di Francesco, V.; Harris, T.B.; Zoico, E.; Bissolo, L; Fracassi, E. & Zamboni, M. (2000). Waist circumference and abdominal sagittal diameter as surogates of body fat distribution in the elderly: their relation with cardiovascular risk factors. *International Journal of Obesity*, Vol.24, pp. 1005-1010

Valdez, R. (1991). A simple model-based index of abdominal adiposity. *Journal of Clinical Epidemiology*, Vol.44, pp. 955-956

Valsamakis, G.; Chetty, R.; Anwart, A.; Banerjee, A.K.; Barnett, A. & Kumar, S. (2004). Association of simple anthropometric measures of obesity with visceral fat and the metabolic syndrome in male Caucasion and Indo-Asian subjects. *Diabetic Medicine*, Vol.21, pp. 1339-1345

Valsamakis, G.; Jones, A.; Chetty, R.; McTernan,P.G.; Boutsiadis, A.; Barnett, A.H.; Banerjee, A.K. & Kumar, S. (2008). MRI total SAD as a predictor of metabolic syndrome compared to visceral fat at L4-L5 level. *Current Medical Research&Opinion*, Vol.28, pp. 1853-1860

van der Kooy, K.; Leenen, R.; Seidell, J.C.; Deurenberg, P. & Visser M. (1993). Abdominal diameters as indicators of visceral fat: comparison between magnetic resonance imaging and anthropometry. *British Journal of Nutrition*, Vol.70, No.1, pp. 47-58

van Harmelen, V.; Röhrig, K. & Hauner, H. (2004). Comparison of proliferation and differentation capacity of human adipocyte precursor cells from the omental and subcutaneous adipose tissue depot of obese subjects. *Metabolism*, Vol.53, No.5, pp.632-7

van Herpen, N.A, & Schrauwen-Hinderling, V.B. (2008). Lipid accumulation in non-adipose tissue and lipotoxicity. *Physiology&Behaviour*, Vol.94, pp. 231-41

Vasques, A.C.; Rosado, L.E.; Rosado, G.P.; Ribeiro R. de C.; Franceschini S. do C.; Geloneze, B.; Priore, S.E. & Oliveira, D.R. (2009a). Predictive ability of anthropometric and body composition indicators in the identification of insulin resistance. *Arquivos Brasileiros de Endocrinologia & Metabologia*, Vol.53, No.1, pp.72-79

Vasques, A.C.; Rosado, L.E.; Rosado, G.P.; Ribeiro R. de C.; Franceschini, S. do C.; Geloneze, B.; Priore, S.E. & Oliveira, D.R. (2009b). Different measurements of the SAD and waist perimeter in the prediction of HOMA-IR. *Arquivos Brasileiros de Endocrinologia & Metabologia*, Vol.93, No.5, pp. 511-518

Visscher, T.L.; Seidell, J.C.; Molarius, A.; van der Kuip, D.; Hofman, A. & Witteman, J.C. (2001). A comparison of body mass index, waist-hip ratio and waist circumference as predictors of all-cause mortality among the elderly: the Rotterdam study. *International Journal of Obesity and Related Metabolic Disorders*, Vol.25, No.11, pp. 1730–1735

Wajchenberg, B.L. (2000). Subcutaneous and visceral adipose tissue: their relation to the metabolic syndrome. *Endocrine Reviews*, Vol.21, No.6, pp. 697-738

Yim, J.Y.; Kim, D.; Lim, S.H.; Park, M.J.; Choi, S.H.; Lee, C.H.; Kim, S.S. & Cho, S.H. (2010). SAD is a strong anthropometric measure of visceral adipose tissue in the Asian general population. *Diabetes Care*, Vol.33, No.12, pp. 2665-2670

Zamboni, M.; Turcato, E.; Armellini, F.; Kahn, H.S.; Zivelonghi, A.; Santana, H.; Bergamo-Andreis, I.A. & Bosello, O. (1998). SAD as a practical predictor of visceral fat. *Interantional Journal of Obesity*, Vol.22, pp. 655-660

18

The Use of Reynolds Risk Score in Cardiovascular Risk Assessment in Apparently Healthy Bosnian Men and Women: Cross-Sectional Study

Asija Začiragić
Department of Physiology, School of Medicine, University of Sarajevo, Bosnia and Herzegovina

1. Introduction

Cardiovascular diseases (CVD) remain a major burden for public health worldwide. Pivotal concern of primary prevention is identification of individuals that are at risk for developing cardiovascular disease. The use of different algorithms for an assessment of cardiovascular risk allows physicians to identify and treat in a simple and cost-effective manner individuals that may be at high long-term cardiovascular risk.

A cardiovascular risk factor represents a condition that is related to increased risk for the development of cardiovascular disease. This relation is used in statistical terms. If certain individual has particular risk factor he/she has increased probability for the development of CVD. However, not all individual with cardiovascular risk will develop CVD and sometimes coronary events may occur in the absence of major risk factors (Ridker et al, JAMA 2007). Identification of individuals at cardiovascular risk results in a cost-effective prevention. Significant efforts are made to ensure most reliable tools in cardiovascular risk assessment. For a risk factor to be useful in routine clinical diagnostics, following criteria must be fulfilled: its analysis must be easy and available, there must be pathophysiological evidence that confirms causal link of risk factor with the disease, and also there must be certain knowledge on treatment options for patients with established high values of a certain risk factor (Thomas et al, 2009).

Cardiovascular risk factors are divided into three main categories: non-modifiable (age, gender, heredity); modifiable (increased blood pressure, dyslipidemia, fibrinogen, obesity, glucose intolerance, diabetes, left ventricular hypertrophy, cocaine, behavioral factors); and protective factors (HDL-cholesterol, exercise, estrogen, moderate alcohol intake). It is important to emphasize that treatment of certain modifiable cardiovascular risk factor will not result in total elimination of probability in CVD development, but the possibility of CVD development will be reduced.

As for non-modifiable cardiovascular risk factors, many epidemiological studies have reported age as one of the strongest predictors of CVD. Furthermore, investigations have shown that men are more prone to CVD development then women for reason yet not completely understood. In most societies, development of cardiovascular risk factors begins in younger age, and manifests itself in middle age. Almost 85% of all deaths due to CVD occur in people 65 years of age or older. It has been reported that mortality rate for men before the age of 50 with no pre-existing myocardial infarction or stroke was 20%, which increased up to 80 % in those older then 70 years of age (Wannamethee et al, 1995).

Inherited likelihood for the development of CVD has been well documented. In some cases, such as familial hypercholesterolemia ways of inheritance are well defined. However, for other cardiovascular risk factors pattern of inheritance is still unknown. According to current assumptions, role of heredity in the development of CVD is multifactorial with genetic, environmental, and behavioral component (Phillips et al, 1988). Studies have shown that risk of developing premature CVD was increased more then threefold when any first-degree relative was affected and about sixfold when at least two first-degree relatives had a history of CVD (Eaton et al, 1996).

Of all the modifiable cardiovascular risk factors, hypertension is best investigated. Both systolic and diastolic blood pressures are important in the assessment of individual's risk. However, majority of complications of hypertension are attributed to systolic blood pressure. Studies have indicated that the risk of a cardiac event increases by 1.6 in men and 2.5 in women when blood pressure rises from an optimal (<120/80 mmHg) to high normal (130-139/85-89 mmHg) level (Vasan et al, 2000). Although hypertension is an independent cardiovascular risk factor, data have shown its strong relations with other risk factors, such as age, sex, race and hypercholesterolemia.

Increased levels of serum lipids are another common modifiable cardiovascular risk factor. According to current guidelines fasting lipoprotein profile (total cholesterol, triglycerides, LDL-cholesterol and HDL- cholesterol) should be preformed every five years in all adults age 20 years and older. Level of total cholesterol is strong predictor of CVD and to a lesser degree of stroke. Close linear relationship exists between cholesterol level and the mortality rate. Studies have shown that low-density cholesterol (LDL-C) and high-density cholesterol (HDL-C) and their relationship may have even more significant prognostic value in the prediction of CVD then total cholesterol. Men aged 45 to 65 years with total serum cholesterol level < 240 mg/dL and/or LDL-cholesterol > 160 mg/dL are considered to be at an increased risk for CVD (Wilson et al, 1998). Reduction of increased levels of total cholesterol and LDL-cholesterol is accompanied with the decline of cardiovascular risk. Earlier studies failed to demonstrate predictive value of triglycerides, but results of novel studies point to possible importance of triglycerides in the prediction of cardiovascular risk, especially in women and patients with diabetes. HDL-cholesterol attenuates atherogenicity of LDL-cholesterol. High levels of HDL-cholesterol have protective properties, while its low levels represent a major risk for CVD (P.W. Wilson, 1990; Schafer et al, 1994).

Recent data report on possible role of fibrinogen as cardiovascular risk factors. Even though mechanisms by which fibrinogen fulfills this role are still not completely known, it is believed that individuals with raised fibrinogen are more susceptible to the development of clots in arteries, and thereby have increased risk of heart attack or stroke. Evidences have shown that fibrinogen levels have tendency to rise with advancing age and in that sense fibrinogen does not represent modifiable cardiovascular risk factor. However, it has been proven that smoking cessation reduces fibrinogen levels which make fibrinogen a cardiovascular risk factor that can be controlled. In a 13-year longitudinal CARDIA study (D. Green et al, 2010) higher levels of fibrinogen during young adulthood were positively associated with incidence of subclinical atherosclerosis and coronary artery calcification in middle-age. However, study has shown that this association declines with advancing age.

A major contributor to CVD is cigarette smoking. It is estimated that out of approximately 500.000 deaths from coronary heart disease, 30-40% can be attributed to smoking. Studies have shown that risk of sudden death increases more then tenfold in men and almost fivefold in women who smoke. Smoking is associated with accelerated atherosclerosis and inflammatory processes. Smoking cessation and reduced tobacco exposure result in decrease of inflammatory component of CVD and this decrease is reversible (Bakhru & Erlinger, 2005; Tracy et al, 1997; Dobson et al, 1991).

Obese individuals (more then 30% over ideal body weight) are more likely to develop CVD, even in absence of other cardiovascular risk factors. A strong association has been found between overweight that begins in childhood and the development of other risk factors over time, such as hypertension and diabetes. The cause of overweight and obesity in majority of cases is excessive food intake and sedentary lifestyle. A study among middle-aged men has shown that risk of developing fatal and non-fatal CVD increased up to 72% if their body mass index (BMI) increased from less then 23 to the range of 25-29 (Rimm et al, 1995). For all of these reasons obese individuals tend to be at high risk for CVD, and weight management is extremely important lifestyle intervention that can lead to significant reduction of cardiovascular risk.

Individuals with glucose intolerance and diabetes mellitus have increased risk for CVD. These two conditions are often accompanied with raised levels of insulin that in this setting increases blood pressure and aids in plaque deposition. As a result of these insulin actions, atherosclerosis and its complications will develop. Data have reported that there is a liner association between glucose levels and CVD mortality (Balkaue et al, 1999). It is of note that influence of diabetes mellitus on the development of CVD differs among ethnic groups. A prospective study in individuals of African-American origin has shown that 27% of women and 8% of men had CVD that could be attributed to diabetes mellitus. In individuals of Caucasian origin, 15% of men and 12% of women had CVD that could also be attributed to diabetes mellitus (Folsom et al, 1997)

Even though certain authors disagree, many others find behavioral risk factors such as type A personality and stress as important risk factors for CVD. Type A or coronary-prone personality is an individual that is always in hurry, under pressure by time, becomes upset often with no objective reason, has chronic impatience and sometimes overwhelming hostility. Results from GAZEL French prospective study have demonstrated that neurotic hostility, coronary-prone personality and antisocial personality are all predictive of mortality outcomes (Nabi et al, 2008).

Left ventricular hypertrophy (LVHT) is a major independent risk factor for cardiovascular mortality. Studies have shown that individuals with LVHT are more susceptible to arrhythmias, heart failure and sudden death and this condition is often accompanied with hypertension. Appropriate treatment of these conditions reduces cardiovascular risk. Novel findings suggest that there are racial and ethnic differences in cardiovascular mortality related to LVHT. It has been demonstrated that LVHT contributes more to the risk of cardiovascular mortality in African American then it does in White individuals (Havranek et al, 2008).

Cocaine is a sympathomimetic agent that can cause hypertension, arrhythmias, angina and sudden death. Cocaine is also a risk for congenital heart disease. Main mechanism of cocaine action is that it constricts coronary blood vessels and reduces oxygen supply to the heart. It has been reported that concomitant use of cigarettes exacerbates the deleterious effects of cocaine on myocardial oxygen supply and demand (Lange et al, 2004).

Alongside with non-modifiable and modifiable cardiovascular risk factors, there are also some proven protective factors that in fact protect from the development of CVD. Sedentary life-style is associated with the development of obesity, metabolic risk factors, insulin resistance, and early onset of diabetes mellitus type 2. Regular exercise is one of those protective factors that helps in weight management, increases HDL-cholesterol concentration, enhances utility of insulin in organism, reduces stress and decreases blood pressure. There are convincing data that it also reduces chances for having a myocardial infarction. Significant changes in classical cardiovascular risk factors are preceded by reductions of vascular functions. Important guidelines for primary and secondary prevention settings should be based on the encouragement of regular physical activity that has been shown to have many beneficial effects on the vascular wall (D.J. Green et al, 2008). Studies have found that increased physical activity leads to the decline of CVD mortality (Blair et al, 1995). Results of a meta-analysis reported that physical activity was inversely associated to the development of CVD, with a relative increased risk of 1.9 in people with sedentary lifestyle compared to physically active individuals (Berlin et al, 1990).

Another protective factor against CVD is estrogen. It reduces likelihood of heart attack by increase in HDL-cholesterol levels. However, once women reach an age of menopause this protective action of estrogen diminishes, and women are at same cardiovascular risk as men. According to recent findings, estrogen decreases production of reactive oxygen species in mitochondria. Studies have shown that estrogen promotes angiogenesis, enhances endothelial vasodilator function and modulates autonomic function (Miller et al, 2008).

Moderate alcohol consumption is proven to have protective effects against atherosclerosis and coronary heart disease. Mechanisms by which these effects are achieved are still not completely understood, but it seems that consumption of one or two drinks a day increases levels of HDL-cholesterol. A systematic review of literature and meta-analysis on association between alcohol consumption and overall mortality from CVD, incidence of and mortality from coronary heart disease, and incidence of and mortality from stroke has observed that light to moderate alcohol consumption is associated with reduced risk of multiple cardiovascular outcomes (Ronksley et al, 2011). However, consumption of alcohol in larger amounts increases blood pressure and risk of CVD.

Prevalence of cardiovascular risk factors differs around the globe. Data from USA indicate that nearly 70% of adult Americans are overweight or obese. Less than 15% of adults or children exercise sufficiently, and over 60% do not engage in vigorous activity. Among adult population, 11%–13% have diabetes, 34% have hypertension, 36% have prehypertension, 36% have prediabetes, and 12% have both prediabetes and prehypertension, At least one cardiovascular risk factor is present in 50% of adults. Furthermore, almost 65% of patients do not have their traditional cardiovascular risk biomarkers under control (Kones, 2011).

Another study in US population (Danaei et al, 2009) aimed to assess the number of disease-specific deaths attributable to all non-optimal levels of risk factors exposure, by age and sex. Results have shown that in year 2005, cigarette smoking was responsible for an estimated 467.000 deaths and high blood pressure for 395.000 deaths in US adults. Overweight-obesity, physical inactivity, and high blood glucose caused 8%-9% of all deaths in same population. Other dietary risk factors also caused significant number of deaths in the US.

A comprehensive, population-based study compared cardiovascular risk profiles among individuals of white, South Asian, Chinese and black ethnic groups living in Canada (Chiu et al, 2010). Results have shown that there is a considerable variation in the prevalence of smoking, hypertension, obesity, and diabetes mellitus among four ethnic groups included in the study. Authors concluded that these results may lead to the development of CVD prevention programs for specific ethnic groups.

Prediction of risk for future cardiovascular events or stratification of healthy individuals into risk categories by different algorithms has been widely used in clinical practice. Important issue is critical appraisal of implemented prediction models. Even though validity of models can be evaluated by different means, calibration and discrimination represent two most important measures of accurate models assessment. Calibration is a measure of how well predicted probabilities agree with actual observed risk, whereas calibration is a measure of how well the model can separate those who do and do not have the disease of interest. A measure of discrimination that is broadly used is *c* statistics, also known as the area under the Receiver Operating Characteristic (ROC) curve, or *c* index. Results of a Women Health Study have shown that use of *c* statistics can be advocated because of its specificity and sensitivity in differentiating between those who do and those who do not have a certain disease. Also, its use may contribute to more exact reclassification of large proportion of patients into higher- risk or lower-risk categories. However, it seems unlikely that it can be used in the evaluation of algorithms that predicts future risk or stratify individuals into risk categories. Another conclusion of this study was that use of *c* statistics as the only measure of the possible usefulness of traditional or novel risk factors could not be advised (Cook N, 2007). Finally, decision on inclusion of novel risk marker in prediction algorithms should be based on the knowledge whether measurement of potential risk marker will result in different treatment options, and whether it has perspectives in disease prevention.

Etiology of CVD is multifactorial. In order to better assess cardiovascular risk, new biomarkers have been introduced as part of global cardiovascular risk assessment. Novel findings suggest that important role in atherosclerosis has inflammation. These conclusions led to the measurement of numerous markers of inflammatory processes to better identify individuals that are at the increased risk. C-reactive protein (CRP) is currently most studies and best validated biomarker of inflammatory processes. It is an acute phase protein, which is primarily synthesized in the liver and it represents a marker of systemic, non-specific, inflammation. CRP production is stimulated by cytokines (in particular interleukin-6, interleukin-1, and tumor necrosis factor-alpha) in response to systemic or local infection or inflammation by variety of cells, including adipocytes (Pepys & Hirschfield, 2003).

The Centers for Disease Control and Prevention and the American Heart Association published a statement in 2003 in which measurement of CRP is given at the discretion of physicians to be used in clinical practice as part of global risk assessment in adults (Pearson et al, 2003). According to existing guidelines, individuals with CRP values < 1 mg/L are considered to be in low, those with CRP values 1-3 mg/L in moderate and those with CRP values > 3 mg/L in high cardiovascular risk (Packard et al, 2008).

Current main goal in CRP testing is to identify individuals that can benefit from lipid-lowering treatment in order to prevent first cardiovascular event, especially for those individuals that have CRP > 3mg/L, and are in intermediate risk (10-20% 10-year predicted risk). However, it is of critical importance in any interpretation of CRP values to differentiate modest increase of CRP baseline values from its major rise that occurs in conditions such as tissue necrosis, sepsis and acute trauma. Furthermore, because of its completely unspecific nature, it is not possible or clinically appropriate to interpret CRP values without full medical information of individual, including history, physical examination, and results of all investigations (Casas et al, 2008). Although more sophisticated inflammatory biomarkers (such as interleukin-6, intercellular adhesion molecule-1, macrophage inhibitory cytokine-1, and CD40 ligand) have been shown to be predictive of cardiovascular disease, their use in routine clinical evaluation is highly unlikely because of short half-lives of these proteins (Katrinchak &Fritz, 2007).

Findings of many clinical, experimental, prospective epidemiological and cohort studies have demonstrated that CRP may play role in atherogenesis, since it was found in endothelial atherosclerotic lesions, and raise in CRP concentrations is linked with the increased prevalence of myocardial infarction, peripheral vascular disease, and stroke. Furthermore, CRP provides additional information for the prevention of cardiovascular disease, has a prognostic value of incident cardiovascular events in those with and without preexisting CVD, the increased risk associated with high CRP is independent of other established risk factors, and CRP is biologically stable over time and assays for its measurements are standardized (de Ferranti et al, 2007). For all of the stated properties, certain authors believe that CRP represents not only a marker but as well a mediator of cardiovascular disease (Ridker et al, 2004). Conversely, there are studies that reported that CRP is only a relatively modest predictor of coronary heart disease, and suggest that its use in the prediction of coronary heart disease development should be revised (Danesh et al, 2004).

Data have shown that conventional cardiovascular risk factors fail to predict development of coronary heart disease in 25-50% of cases. Certain authors believe that possible explanation of observed discrepancy may be endothelial dysfunction that may be a missing link between atherosclerotic disease and cardiac risk factors (Reriani et al, 2010). According to relatively recent hypothesis endothelial dysfunction has significant impact on the development and progression of atherosclerosis and atherothrombosis. One of the currently mostly used markers of endothelial dysfunction is asymmetric dimethylarginine (ADMA). ADMA is a endogenous inhibitor of all three isoforms of the enzyme nitric oxide synthase (NOS) and causes endothelial dysfunction by inhibiting production of nitric oxide (one of the major endothelium-derived vasoactive mediators). Prospective clinical studies have shown that elevated levels of ADMA are related to increased incidence of cardiovascular events, as well as with overall mortality (Anderssohn et al, 2010). Large multicentric CARDIAC study has found that elevated ADMA concentration significantly increases the risk of coronary heart disease (Landim et al, 2009). These findings point to the important role of functional vascular status in cardiovascular prognosis. However, it remains unclear whether increased values of ADMA represent only a marker of endothelial dysfunction that may be used in cardiovascular risk assessment or elevated ADMA concentration itself predispose the development of CVD.

Alongside with conventional biomarkers for the prediction of incident cardiovascular events, there are also some other novel biomarkers that are tested for their possible usefulness in cardiovascular risk assessment. Recent Swedish study assessed a panel of contemporary biomarkers, such as mid-regional-pro-atrial natriuretic peptide, N-terminal pro-B-type natriuretic peptide (N-BNP), mid-regional-pro-adrenomedullin (MRproADM), lipoprotein-associated phospholipase-2, and cystatin C in prediction of future cardiovascular events. Results have shown that 10-year incidence of coronary events was 4.4%. Another important finding of the study was that selected biomarkers may be used in the prediction of future cardiovascular events, but benefits over traditional risk factors are minimal. Furthermore, their use did not reclassify a substantial proportion of individuals to higher or lower risk categories (Melander et al, 2009).

A study in Hispanic population used standard risk assessment tools and the B-type natriuretic peptide biomarker to assess coronary heart disease risk (Macabasco-O'Connell et al, 2011). Based on their findings, authors concluded that the inclusion of B-type natriuretic peptide to the traditional risk scores may be helpful in cardiovascular risk prediction.

One of the most frequently used cardiac risk prediction model in clinical practice is Framingham Risk Score. Its use started in the 1980s and based on its implementation in cardiovascular risk assessment, individuals can be divided in those at low (less then 5%), intermediated (6-20%) and high (>20%) cardiovascular risk (Ridker et al, 2004). However, over time, Framingham Risk Score showed certain limitations. Evidences have shown that cardiovascular events occur in every fifth individual in whom classical risk factors have not been recognized. Furthermore, there is a limitation in specificity of conventional risk factors and it has been shown that overall cardiovascular risk differs across populations. It has also been concluded that intermediate risk category is broad and that there is a necessity for better risk stratification of that risk category. For all of the above reasons, there was a need for new and more comprehensive cardiovascular risk prediction tools.

So far, several other risk prediction models have been proposed to be used in every-day clinical practice for cardiovascular risk assessment, such as: Adult Treatment Panel III, ASSIGN (Assessing Cardiovascular Risk to Scottish Intercollegiate Guidelines Network), QRISK (QRESEARCH Cardiovascular Risk Algorithm), and SCORE (Systematic Coronary Risk Evaluation) project (Berger et al, 2010).

Majority of the studies so far evaluated risk of CVD in a 10-year or shorter time period. Contrary to these studies, there is a study in which individuals, free of conditions at baseline, were followed-up for 30-years and in that period incidence of CVD and death was ascertained. Results of this study demonstrated that standard risk factors remain highly predictive of cardiovascular risk over 30-years follow-up period and their impact is significant even if levels are not updated (Pencina et al, 2009).

A global vascular risk score was recently designed and validated that combines conventional risk factors with behavioral (alcohol consumption and physical activity) and anthropometric risk factors in African-American and Hispanic individuals at risk for vascular disease (Sacco et al, 2009). The use of this risk prediction model demonstrated an improvement in the prediction of global vascular risk.

Reynolds Risk Score (RRS) represents risk prediction algorithm that was designed, validated and used in the prediction of 10-year cardiovascular risk in initially healthy men and women. It is based on two separate large prospective studies that included more then 20.000 women, 45 years of age and older, with median follow-up period of 10.2 years and more the 10.000 men, 50 years of age and older, that were followed up over a median period of 10.8 years for incident myocardial infarction, stroke, coronary revascularization, or cardiovascular death (Ridker 2007, 2008). The main aim of these two studies was to compare predictive value of traditional risk prediction model based on age, blood pressure, smoking status, total cholesterol and high-density lipoprotein cholesterol and RRS in which alongside with traditional risk markers, hsCRP and parental history of cardiovascular diseases are included. Results have confirmed significant predictive value of traditional risk factors as well as of hsCRP and parental history. Furthermore, both of the studies have shown that RRS had better predictive value in the prediction of incident cardiovascular events in women and in men compared to traditional cardiovascular risk prediction model. Study in initially healthy female subjects have also demonstrated that use of RRS improved risk stratification in a sense that 40-50% of women that were previously categorized to be at intermediate risk could be reclassified into higher or lower risk categories. Study in initially healthy male subjects showed that up to 20% of men previously categorized to be at intermediate risk could be reclassified into higher or lower risk categories. Conclusion derived from both of the studies was that use of RRS can serve in primary prevention settings to better targeting of treatments in order to increase benefits and reduce toxicity. RRS comprises of four 10-year risk categories: 0% to less then 5% - low risk category, 5% to less then 10% - low to medium risk category, 10% to less then 20% - medium to high risk category, and > 20% – high risk category (Ridker et al, 2004; Cook et al, 2006).

To date, no data exist on use of RRS in cardiovascular risk assessment among apparently healthy Bosnian men and women. To address this issue, we used Reynolds Risk Score calculator (http://www.reynoldsriskscore.org) to ascertain 10-year cardiovascular risk with the use of traditional factors such as age, smoking status, systolic blood pressure, blood levels of total cholesterol, HDL-cholesterol, as well as hcCRP and parental history of myocardial infarction and stroke before the age 60 in our study sample.

2. Methods

2.1 Subjects

Between February and March 2011, 230 of men and 270 women visited Family Medicine Out-Patient Clinic "Visnjik", Sarajevo, Bosnia and Herzegovina, for general health screening. Among them, 200 of men and 250 women signed informed consent. Excluding subjects with history of cardiovascular disease, malignancy, liver disease, alcohol abuse, use of antidiabetic, antihypertensive, or lipid-lowering drugs, or CRP values > 10 mg/L, and those aged < 45 years, the resulting 76 men and 120 women comprised the subjects in the present study. The study was approved by the Ethics Committee of the Medical Faculty University of Sarajevo. Written informed consent was obtained from all subjects included in the study. Participants underwent a medical history, physical examination and laboratory assessment. Investigations were carried out in accordance with the Declaration of Helsinki as revised in 2000.

2.2 Blood sampling

Blood was collected in the morning after an overnight fast and after a 30-minutes rest in a semi-recumbent position. Sampling was done without stasis, using the vacutainer technique.

2.3 Blood chemistry analysis

High sensitivity CRP was determined by means of particle enhanced immunonephelometry (BN Systems, Dade Behring, Marburg, Germany). The lower limit of detection of this assay was 0.18 mg/L. Levels of hs-CRP >10mg/L were excluded from the analysis, as they are likely related to infections or other acute inflammatory processes. Total cholesterol, HDL - cholesterol, triglycerides were measured by direct colorimetric reflectance spectrophotometry using Dimension clinical chemistry system (Dade Behring, Marburg, Germany). LDL - cholesterol was calculated by means of Friedwald formula.

2.4 Blood pressure measurements

Three supine blood pressure recordings were made after a 5-minutes rest using an Omron 705c oscillometric device. The mean of the second and third readings was used. Hypertension was defined as systolic blood pressure ≥140 mmHg, diastolic pressure ≥90 mmHg, or self-reported high blood pressure with use of anti-hypertensive medications. Prehypertension was defined as systolic blood pressure of 120–140 mmHg or diastolic blood pressure of 80–90 mmHg.

None of the included subjects was pregnant or had a history of intercurrent diseases. Parental history of myocardial infarction or stroke before the age 60 (genetic factor) was defined as family history of heart disease or stroke. Smoking status and genetic factor were assessed by self-administrated questioner.

Statistical analysis. The Kolmogorov-Smirnov test of normality was used to test the distribution of variables. Normally distributed data are presented as mean ± SEM and skewed variables as median and interquartile ranges. An unpaired Student t-test or Mann-Whitney U-test was used to compare the difference between two groups, as appropriate. Frequencies were tested by Chi-square test. In order to determine the factors associated with absolute 10-year Reynolds Risk Score, multiple regression analysis was performed. A p value of less then 0.05 was considered statistically significant. The software used was SPSS for Windows (version 17.0; SPSS, Chicago, IL, USA).

3. Results

Variables	Men (n=76)	Women (n=120)	p<
Age (yrs)	58.64±2.12	57.06±1.67	NS
Smoking (yes/no)	(29/47)	(36/84)	NS
SBP (mmHg)	136.43±2.13	130.92±1.71	0.05

Variables	Men (n=76)	Women (n=120)	p<
TC (mmol/L)	5.48±0.13	6.01±0.12	0.001
HDL (mmol/L)	1.22±0.04	1.39±0.03	0.001
hsCRP (mg/L)	1.33(0.78-3.92)	1.71(0.80-3.92)	NS
GF (yes/no)	(17/59)	(11/109)	0.05
Absolute RRS (%)	19.37±1.67	9.76±1.03	0.0001

Data are presented as mean ± SEM, median and inter-quartile range, or in total count. SBP: systolic blood pressure; TC: total cholesterol; HDL-cholesterol: high density lipoprotein - cholesterol; hsCRP: high sensitivity C-reactive protein; GF: genetic factor; Absolute RRS: absolute Reynolds Risk Score, n: number of subject.

Table 1. The values of Reynolds Risk Score factors in apparently healthy male and female subjects. Subjects did not differ in age, smoking status and CRP values. Statistically significant difference was observed in systolic blood pressure, total cholesterol, HDL-cholesterol, genetic factor presence and in absolute Reynolds risk score values between men and women.

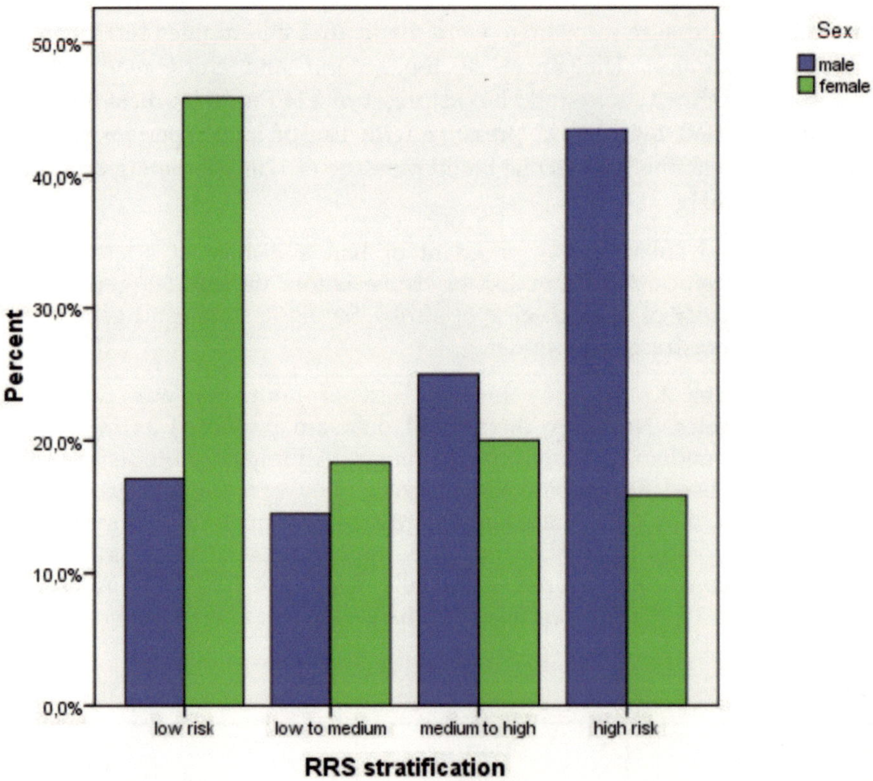

Fig. 1. Frequency of Reynolds Risk Score categories by gender. Results have shown that 6.63% of men and 28.6% of women were in low risk category, 5.6% of men and 11.2% of women in low to medium risk category, 9.7% of men and 12.2% of women in medium to high risk category, and 16.8% of men and 9.7% of women in high risk category.

Independent Variables	ß coefficient	t value	p<
Age (yrs)	0.553	7.753	0.0001
Smoking (yes/no)	0.023	0.359	NS
SBP (mmHg)	0.420	5.905	0.0001
TC (mmol/L)	0.095	1.422	NS
HDL (mmol/L)	-0.016	-0.244	NS
hsCRP (mg/L)	-0.005	-0.073	NS
GF (yes/no)	-0.143	-2.244	0.05

Table 2. Results of multiple regression analysis for absolute 10-year Reynolds Risk Score as dependent variable in men. Multiple regression analysis revealed that in male subjects most predictive value in cardiovascular risk assessment had age followed by systolic blood pressure and genetic factor, respectively.

Independent Variables	ß coefficient	t value	p<
Age (yrs)	0.287	4.394	0.0001
Smoking (yes/no)	-0.230	-4.265	0.0001
SBP (mmHg)	0.561	8.647	0.0001
TC (mmol/L)	0.093	1.701	0.092
HDL (mmol/L)	0.012	0.222	0.825
hsCRP (mg/L)	0.075	1.367	0.174
GF (yes/no)	-0.044	-0.804	0.423

Table 3. Results of multiple regression analysis for absolute 10-year Reynolds Risk Score as dependent variable in women. In female subjects most predictive value in cardiovascular risk assessment had systolic blood pressure, followed by age and smoking, respectively.

4. Discussion

CVD is one of the leading causes of death worldwide. It is estimated that for individuals at age of 50 years, the lifetime risk of CVD is, on average, for men 52% and 39% for women (Berger et al, 2010).

To the best of our knowledge, we are the first to report high prevalence of cardiovascular risk factors in apparently healthy Bosnian men and women with the use of Reynolds Risk Score calculator. Results have shown that in a total study sample, 34.7% of subjects were in low, 16.8% in low to medium, 21.9% in medium to high, and 26.5% of subjects were in high cardiovascular risk category. Our results are consistent with previous report (Cushman et al, 2009). Majority of women in both studies belonged to low and low to medium risk category group, and majority of men belonged to medium to high and high risk category group. The mean absolute 10-year cardiovascular risk determined with RRS calculator in men included in our study was 19.37%, and 9.97% in women. Our observations are not in accordance with the study among commercial pilots in UK that revealed that 9.7% of all male pilots were at high cardiovascular risk and that the mean 10-year cardiovascular risk for the entire pilot population was 8.41% (Houston et al, 2010).

Data on prevalence of cardiovascular risk factors in less developed countries are not abundant. In urban Tanzania, prevalence of cardiovascular risk factors was high, especially in women. The age-adjusted prevalence of obesity in men was 13%, and 35% in women. In men, BMI and waist circumference (WC) were significantly correlated with blood pressure, triglycerides, total cholesterol, LDL- cholesterol, and HDL-cholesterol (BMI only), and fasting glucose. Conversely, in women only blood pressure was positively associated with BMI and WC (Njelekela et al, 2009).

Study in urban Asian Indian subjects observed low prevalence of smoking, hypertension, dyslipidemia, metabolic syndrome and diabetes in adolescents, with rapid escalation of these risk factors by age of 30-39 years (Gupta et al, 2009).

Results of a first nationwide survey on cardiovascular risk factors in Grand-Duchy of Luxembourg have shown the most predominant cardiovascular risk factors was dyslipidemia (69.9%), followed with hypertension (34.5%), smoking (22.3%), and obesity (20.9%), while diabetes was present in 4.4% of study population. Furthermore, only 14.7% of men and 23.1% of women were free of any cardiovascular risk factor (Alkerwi et al, 2010).

Studies have demonstrated that incidence and prevalence of CVD increase with advancing age. However, the predictive value of classic risk factors diminishes with age. The mean value of age of male participants in our study was 58.64 years, and of female participants 57.06 years. There was no significant difference in age between these two groups. Population based observational cohort study in very old people (aged 85 years) with no history of CVD aimed to assess classic risk factors and some new biomarkers (homocysteine, folic acid, CRP, interleukin- 6) as predictors of cardiovascular mortality in this age group. Their results have shown that homocysteine alone accurately identified individuals at high cardiovascular risk, whereas classic risk factors included in the Framingham risk score did not (de Ruijter et al, 2008).

A study that investigated age relations of blood pressure, anthropometric indexes, serum lipids, and hemostatic variables in a population of Papua New Guinea (Lindberg et al., 1997) has found that diastolic blood pressure was not associated with age, while systolic blood pressure linearly increased after 50 years of age in both sexes. BMI decreased with age in both sexes. Serum total cholesterol, triglycerides, LDL-cholesterol increased in males between 20 and 50 years of age, whereas HDL-cholesterol decreased. Authors concluded that some of the relations of age with other cardiovascular risk factors represent effects of biological aging.

Results from EURIKA study (Guallar et al, 2011), which involved participants from 12 European countries with at least one cardiovascular risk, but without CVD reported that the average 10-year risk of CVD death in study participants was 8.2%. Hypertension was responsible for 32.7%, hyperlipidemia for 15.1%, smoking for 10.4%, and diabetes for 16.4% of CVD risk. The four risk factors accounted for 57.7% of CVD risk, representing a 10-year excess risk of CVD death of 5.66%. Study also demonstrated that lack of control of these cardiovascular risk factors was responsible for almost 30% of the risk of CVD death.

Besides age, hypertension, smoking, diabetes, and hyperlipidemia, risk factors for CVD also include obesity, physical inactivity and insulin resistance. A study conducted among adults seeking primary care in Germany reported high prevalence of overweight and obese individuals. Furthermore, a high waist to hip ratio (WHR) was associated with an increased prevalence of high triglycerides, a high blood pressure, an increased fasting glucose, and the presence of diabetes mellitus. On the other hand, a family history of myocardial infarction was not more frequent in patients with high WC compared to patients with normal WC. The prevalence of smoking was significantly lower in overweight men with an elevated and high WC, but not in women (Hauner et al, 2008).

According to Seventh Report of the Joint National Committee on Prevention, Detection, Evaluation, and Treatment of High Blood Pressure, systolic blood pressures of 120-139 mmHg and/or diastolic blood pressures of 80-89 mmHg are classified as prehypertension. Individuals with this condition are thought to be at increased risk of CVD. Results from a cross-sectional study in Jamaica have shown that the prevalence of prehypertension among Jamaicans was 30%. Prehypertension was found in 35% of male subjects, and 25 % of female subjects. Almost 46% of study participants were overweight; 19.7% were obese; 14.6% had hypercholesterolemia; 7.2% had diabetes mellituss, and 17.8% smoked cigarettes. With the exception of cigarette smoking and low physical activity, all the CVD risk factors had significantly higher prevalence in the prehypertensive and hypertensive groups compared to the normotensive group (Ferguson et al, 2008). Results of our study have shown that mean value of systolic blood pressure both in men and in women was bellow 140 mm/Hg. Men had significantly higher values of systolic blood pressure compared to women. Another observation of our study was that there was no significant difference in smoking status between men and women.

Diets high in fat, especially saturated fat, are frequently associated with hypercholesterolemia, hypertension and obesity. Resent findings have reported significant increase in the prevalence of obesity in all age groups, including children, adolescents and adults. A study conducted among physically active college students reported that 45% of participants were overweight or obese. Furthermore, positive association between grain consumption, alcohol intake and BMI was observed. Another finding of this study was that high percentage of subjects had high WHR, elevated systolic and diastolic blood pressure, blood glucose and total cholesterol levels (Sharma et al, 2008). The average value of total cholesterol level both in men and women in our study was above referent limits. On the contrary, average values of HDL-cholesterol in both groups were within normal range. However, since we did not conduct a survey on dietary habits of our participants, we are in no position to draw any conclusions whether there is an association between total cholesterol and HDL-cholesterol values and dietary habits of our study sample. Future studies should address this issue, among population of Bosnia and Herzegovina, since it has been well documented that caloric intake differs between ethnicities, age and socioeconomic groups.

The growing evidence supports the hypothesis that there is ethnic variation in CRP levels. Results of a large population-based study in Black and White men and women in the United States have shown that increased CRP values were more common among women than men, blacks than whites, and in the stroke belt compared to the rest of the U.S. Results of a same study also demonstrated that the use of RRS reclassified population to a different 10-year vascular risk level than the new Framingham Vascular Score (Cushman et al, 2009)). Our results did not show significant difference in CRP values between men and women included in our study. Thus, we were not able to confirm previous findings that gender influences CRP levels. However, this could be due to a limited size of our study sample.

Earlier results have demonstrated that inclusion of CRP in global risk prediction model improves risk classification in women (Cook et al, 2006). On the contrary, critical appraisal of literature on CRP measurement for the prediction of coronary heart disease event (Shah et al, 2009) have revealed that benefits of addition of CRP to models based on traditional risk factors are small and are only slightly resulting in better improvement in risk classification and reclassification.

It is of interest to note that in the present study CRP did not show significant predictive value in cardiovascular risk assessment both in men and in women. Thus, data on possible use of CRP in cardiovascular risk assessment remain conflicting and inconsistent. Possible explanation for the observed inconsistency may be a fact that normal functions of CRP as well as its possible roles in diseases are yet incompletely defined (Casas et al, 2008). The reason for this is that so far no deficiency or structural polymorphism of human CRP have been reported nor is any therapeutic intervention available which specifically inhibits CRP in vivo. Consequently, until today the effects of absence, lack of function or inhibition of human CRP have not been tested.

A large prospective study in Chinese male adults has demonstrated that hypertension and cigarette smoking were the leading predictive parameter for CVD (Ji et al, 2011). Our study had similar observations. We established that in male subjects most predictive value in cardiovascular risk assessment had age followed by systolic blood pressure and genetic factor, respectively. In female subjects, most predictive value in cardiovascular risk assessment had systolic blood pressure followed by age and smoking, respectively.

Limitations of our study merit careful considerations. Importantly, present study was cross-sectional and we did not include prediction of cardiovascular events. Subjects were not a general population but visitors to a Family Medicine Out-patient Clinic in capital city of an urban region in Bosnia and Herzegovina. Longitudinal studies and in larger populations are warranted to test present findings. Another limitation is that this study relied on self- reported smoking history and parental history of myocardial infarction which could bias the validity of findings. However, this potential limitation is extremely unlikely, because self-reported risk factors are commonly used in studies with reasonable accuracy (Sesso et al, 2001).

5. Conclusion

In conclusion, results of this cross-sectional study showed that significant proportion of our study sample belong to medium to high and high cardiovascular risk category. Significant reduction in cardiovascular risk can be achieved by scheduled cardiovascular risk assessment accompanied with appropriate interventions. One of the purposes of the present study was to inform physicians, especially in Bosnia and Herzegovina, about advantages of possible use of web-based RRS calculator in cardiovascular risk assessment of patients they treat in their everyday practice.

The advantage of RRS is that it includes traditional cardiovascular risks accompanied with blood-based biomarkers and parental history of cardiovascular disease that results in better risk assessment and is easily accessible and cost-effective in primary prevention. With the use of RRS, we were able to identify individuals who may require more comprehensive risk stratification. Moreover, findings of the present study suggest that use of RRS may serve in better targeting of treatments in primary prevention settings.

RRS calculator provides information not only on total cardiovascular risk but also how control of certain cardiovascular risk can lead to the reduction of absolute cardiovascular risk in percentages. The use of RRS in cardiovascular risk assessment may result in a better compliance of patients and physicians in their joint efforts to achieve better control of cardiovascular risks.

Based on the results of present study, physicians are strongly encouraged to promote and to intensify well established interventions such as blood pressure control, lipid reduction, smoking cessation, heart-healthy diet, physical activity and weight reduction. One can not foreseen that CVD will be eliminated in a near future, but education, screening, monitoring, and appropriate treatment will certainly lead to the decrease of the morbidity and mortality of these diseases.

6. References

Alkerwi, A., Sauvageot, N., Donneau, A-F., Lair, M-L., Couffignal, S., Beissel, J., Delagardelle, C., Wagener, Y., Albert, A., Guillaume, M. (2010) First nationwide survey on cardiovascular risk factors in Grand-Duchy of Luxembourg (ORISCAV-LUX). *BMC Public Health* 10:468.

Anderssohn, M., Schwedhelm, E., Lüneburg, N., Vasan, RS., Böger, RH. (2010) Asymmetric dimethylarginine as a mediator of vascular dysfunction and a marker of cardiovascular disease and mortality: an intriguing interaction with diabetes mellitus. *Diab Vasc Dis Res.* 7(2):105-18.

Bakhru, A., Erlinger, TP. (2005) Smoking Cessation and Cardiovascular Disease Risk Factors: Results from the Third National Health and Nutrition Examination Survey. *PLoS Med* 2(6): e160.

Balkau, B., Bertrais, S., Ducimetiere, P., Eschwege, E. (1999) Is there a glycemic threshold for mortality risk? *Diabetes Care* 22:696-699.

Berger, JS., Jordan, CO., Lloyd-Jones, D., Blumenthal, RS. (2010) Screening for cardiovascular risk in asymptomatic patients. *J Am Coll Cardiol.* 55(12):1169-77.

Berlin, JA., Colditz, GA. (1990) A meta-analysis of physical activity in the prevention of coronary heart disease. *Am J Epidemiol* 132:612-628.

Blair, SN., Kohl, HW III., Barlow, CE., Paffenbarger, RS Jr., Gibbons, LW., Macera, CA. (1995) Changes in physical fitness and all-cause mortality: a prospective study of healthy and unhealthy men. *JAMA* 273: 1093-1098.

Casas, JP., Shah, T., Hingorani, AD., Danesh, J., Pepys. MB. (2008) C-reactive protein and coronary heart disease: a critical review. *J Intern Med* 264:295-314.

Chiu, M., Austin, PC., Manuel, DG., Tu, JV. (2010) Comparison of cardiovascular risk profiles among ethnic groups using population health surveys between 1996 and 2007. *CMAJ* 182(8):301-310.

Cook, NR., Buring, JE., Ridker, PM. (2006) The effect of including C-reactive protein in cardiovascular risk prediction models for women. *Ann Intern Med.* 145(1):21-29.

Cook, NR. (2007) Use and Misuse of the Receiver Operating Characteristic Curve in Risk Prediction. *Circulation* 115;928-935.

Cushman, M., McClure, LA., Howard, VJ., Jenny, NS., Lakoski, SG., Howard G. (2009) Implications of Elevated C-reactive Protein for Cardiovascular Risk Stratification in Black and White Men and Women in the United States. *Clin Chem.* 55(9): 1627–1636.

Danaei, G., Ding, EL., Mozaffarian, D., Taylor, B., Rehm, J., Murray, CJL., Ezzati M. (2009) The Preventable Causes of Death in the United States: Comparative Risk Assessment of Dietary, Lifestyle, and Metabolic Risk Factors. *PLoS Med* 6(4): e1000058.

Danesh, J., Ch, B., Phil, D., Wheeler, JG., Hirschfield, GM., Eda, S., Eiriksdottir, G., Rumley, A., Lowe, GDO., Pepys, MB., Gudnason V. (2004) C-reactive protein and other circulating markers of inflammation in the prediction of coronary heart disease. *N Engl J Med* 350:1387-1397.

de Ferranti, SD., Rifai, N. (2007) C-reactive protein: a nontraditional serum marker of cardiovascular risk. *Cardiovasc Pathol.* 16:14-21.

de Ruijter, W., Westendorp, RGJ., Assendelft, WJJ., den Elzen, WPJ., de Craen, AJM., le Cessie, S., Gussekloo, J. (2008) Use of Framinghamrisk score andnewbiomarkers to predict cardiovascular mortality in older people: population based observational cohort study. *BMJ* 337:a3083.

Dobson, AJ., Alexander, HM., Heller, RF., Lloyd, DM. (1991) How soon after quitting smoking does risk of heart attack decline? *J Clin Epidemiol* 44:1247–1253.

Eaton, CB., Bostom, AG., Yanek, L. (1996) Family history and premature heart disease. *J Am Board Fam Pract* 9:312-318.

Ferguson, TS., Younger, NOM., Tulloch-Reid, MK., Wright, MBL., Ward, EM., Ashley, DE., Wilks, RJ. (2008) Prevalence of prehypertension and its relationship to risk factors for cardiovascular disease in Jamaica: Analysis from a cross-sectional survey. *BMC Cardiovascular Disorders* 8:20.

Folsom, AR., Szklo, M., Stevens, J., Liao, F., Smith, R., Eckfeldt, JH. (1997) A prospective study of coronary heart disease in relation to fasting insulin, glucose, and diabetes: the Atherosclerosis Risk in Communities (ARIC) Study. *Diabetes Care* 20:935-942.

Green, DJ., O'Driscoll, G., Joyner, MJ., Cable, NT. (2008) Exercise and cardiovascular risk reduction: Time to update the rationale for exercise? *J Appl Physiol.* 105(2):766-768.

Green, D., Chan, C., Kang, J., Lin, K., Schreiner, P., Jenny, N., Tracy, RP. (2010) Longitudinal assessment of fibrinogen in relation to subclinical cardiovascular diseases: the CARDIA study. *J Thromb Haemost* 8(3):489-495.

Guallar, E., Banegas, JR., Blasco-Colmenares, E., Jiménez, FJ., Dallongeville, J., Halcox, JP., Borghi, C., Massó-González, EL., Tafalla, M., Perk, J., Backer, GD., Steg, PG., Rodríguez-Artalejo, F. (2011) Excess risk attributable to traditional cardiovascular risk factors in clinical practice settings across Europe - The EURIKA Study. *BMC Public Health* 11:704.

Gupta, R., Misra, A., Vikram, NK., Kondal, D., Gupta, SS., Agrawal, A., Pandey, RM. (2009) Younger age of escalation of cardiovascular risk factors in Asian Indian subjects. *BMC Cardiovascular Disorders* 9:28.

Havranek, EP., Froshang, DB., Emserman, CDB., Hanratty, R., Krantz, MJ., Masoudi, FA., Dickinson, LM., Steiner, JF. (2008) Left ventricular hypertrophy and cardiovascular mortality by race and ethnicity. *Am J Med.* 121(10):870-875.

Hauner, H., Bramlage, P., Lösch, C., Steinhagen-Thiessen, E., Schunkert, H., Wasem, J., Jöckel, K-H., Moebus, S. (2008) Prevalence of obesity in primary care using different anthropometric measures - Results of the German Metabolic and Cardiovascular Risk Project (GEMCAS). *BMC Public Health* 8:282.

Houston, S., Mitchell, S., Evans, S. (2010) Application of a cardiovascular disease risk prediction model among commercial pilots. *Aviat Space Environ Med.* 81(8):768-73.

Ji, J., Pan, E., Li, J., Chen, J., Cao, J., Sun, D., Lu, X., Chen, S., Gu, D., Duan, X., Wu, X., Huang, J. (2011) Classical risk factors of cardiovascular disease among Chinese male steel workers: a prospective cohort study for 20 years. *BMC Public Health* 11:497.

Katrinchak, C., Fritz, K. (2007) Clinical implications of C-reactive protein as a predictor of vascular risk. *J Am Acad Nurse Pract.* 19:335-340.

Kones, R. (2011) Primary prevention of coronary heart disease: integration of new data, evolving views, revised goals, and role of rosuvastatin in management. A comprehensive survey. *Drug Des, Devel Ther.* 5: 325–380.

Landim, MB., Casella-Filho, A., Chagas, AC. (2009) Asymmetric dimethylarginine (ADMA) and endothelial dysfunction: implications for atherogenesis. *Clinics (Sao Paulo).* 64(5):471-478.

Lange, RA., Cigarroa, JE., Hillis, LD. (2004) Theodore e. Woodward award: cardiovascular complications of cocaine abuse. *Trans Am Clin Climatol Assoc.* 115:99-114.

Lindberg, S., Berntrop, E., Nilsson-Ehle, P., Terent, A., Vessby, B. (1997) Age relations of cardiovascular risk factors in traditional Melanesian society: the Kitava Study. *Am J Clin Nutr.* 66:845-852.

Macabasco-O'Connell, A., Danwalder, S., Sinha, K. (2011) Cardiac risk scores in high-risk Hispanics and the predictive value of BNP. *J Clin Nurs.* (epub ahead of print)

Melander, O., Newton-Cheh, C., Almgren, P., Hedblad, B., Berglund, G., Engström, G., Persson, M., Smith, JG., Magnusson, M., Christensson, A., Struck, J., Morgenthaler, NG., Bergmann, A., Pencina, M., Wang, TJ. (2009) Novel and conventional biomarkers for the prediction of incident cardiovascular events in the community. *JAMA* 302(1):49–57.

Miller, VM., Duckles, SP. (2008) Vascular actions of estrogens: functional implications. *Pharmacol Rev.* 60(2): 210-241.

Nebi, H., Kivimaki, M., Zins, M., Elovainiio, M., Conseli, SM., Cordier, S., Ducimetiere, P., Goldberg, M., Singf-Manoux, A. (2008) Does personality predict mortality? *Int J Epidemiol.* 37(2):386-396.

Njelekela, MA., Mpembeni, R., Muhihi, A., Mligiliche, NL., Spiegelman, D., Hertzmark, E., Liu, E., Finkelstein, JL., Fawzi, WW., Willett, WC., Mtabaji, J. (2009) Gender-related differences in the prevalence of cardiovascular disease risk factors and their correlates in urban Tanzania. *BMC Cardiovascular Disorders* 9:30.

Packard, RRS., Libby, P. (2008) Inflammation in atherosclerosis: from vascular biology to biomarker discovery and risk prediction. *Clin Chem.* 54(1):24-38.

Pearson, TA., Mensah, GA., Alexander, RW., Anderson, JL., Cannon, RO., Criqui, M. (2003) Markers of inflammation and cardiovascular disease: application to clinical and public health practice: A statement for healthcare professionals from the Centers for Disease Control and Prevention and the American Heart Association. *Circulation* 107:499–511.

Pencina, MJ., D'Agostino, Sr. RB., Larson, MG., Massaro, JM., Vasan, RS. (2009) Predicting the Thirty-year Risk of Cardiovascular Disease: The Framingham Heart Study. *Circulation* 119(24): 3078–3084.

Pepys, M., Hirschfield, G. (2003) C-reactive protein: a critical update. *J Clin.Invest.* 111:1805-1812.

Phillips, AN., Shaper, AG., Pocock, SJ., Walker, M. (1988) Parental death from heart disease and risk of heart attack. *Eur Heart J* 9:243-251.

Reriani, MK., Lerman, LO., Lerman, A. (2010) Endothelial function as a functional expression of cardiovascular risk factors. *Biomark Med.* 4(3):351–360.

Ridker, PM., Wilson, PWF., Grundy, SM. (2004) Should C-reactive protein be added to metabolic syndrome and to assessment of global cardiovascular risk? *Circulation* 109(23):2818-2825.

Ridker, PM., Buring, JE., Rifai, N., Cook, NR. (2007) Development and validation of improved algorithms for the assessment of global cardiovascular risk in women: The Reynolds Risk Score. *JAMA* 297(6):611-619.

Ridker, PM., Paynter, NP., Rifai, N., Gaziano, JM., Cook, NR. (2008) C-Reactive Protein and Parental History Improve Global Cardiovascular Risk Prediction: The Reynolds Risk Score for Men. *Circulation* 118;2243-2251.

Rimm, EB., Stampfer, MJ., Giovannuci, E. (1995) Body size and fat distribution as predictors of coronary heart disease among middle-age and older U.S. men. *Am J Epidemiol* 141:1117-1127.

Ronksley, PE., Brien, SE., Turner, BJ., Mukamai, KJ., Ghali, WA. (2011) Assocaition of alcohol consumption with selected cardiovascular diseases outcomes: a systematic review and meta-analysis. *BMJ* 342:d671.

Sacco, RL., Khatri, M., Rundek, T., Xu, O., Gardener, H., Boden-Albala, B., Di Tullio MR., Homma, S., Mitchell SVE., Paik, MC. (2009) Improving Global Vascular Risk Prediction with Behavioral and Anthropometric Factors: The Multi-ethnic Northern Manhattan Cohort Study. *J Am Coll Cardiol.* 54(24): 2303–2311.

Schaefer, EJ., Lamon-Fava, S., Ordovas, JM. (1994) Factors associated with low and elevated plasma high density lipoprotein cholesterol and apolipoprotein A-I levels in the Framingham offspring study. *J Lipid Res* 35:871-882.

Sesso, HD., Lee, IM., Gaziano, JM., Rexrode, KM., Glynn, RJ., Buring, JE. (2001) Maternal and paternal history of myocardial infarction and risk of cardiovascular disease in men and women. *Circulation* 104:393-398.

Shah, T., Casas, JP., Cooper, JA., Tzoulaki, I., Sofat, R., McCormack, V., Smeeth, L., Deanfield, JE., Lowe, GD., Rumley, A., Fowkes, GR., Humphries, SE., Hingorani, AD. (2009) Critical appraisal of CRP measurement for the prediction of coronary heart disease events: new data and systematic review of 31 prospective cohorts. *Int J Epidemiol.* 38:217–231.

Sharma, SV., Bush, JA., Lorino, AJ., Knoblauch, M., Abuamer, D., Blog,G., Bertman D. (2008) Diet and Cardiovascular Risk in University Marching Band, Dance Team and Cheer Squad Members: a cross-sectional study. J Int Soc Sports Nutr. 5:9.

Thomas, JC., Vohra, RS., Beer, S., Bhatti, K., Ponnambalam, S., Homer-Vanniasinkam, S. (2009) Biomarkers in peripheral arterial disease. *Trends Cardiovasc Med.* 19(5):147-151.

Tracy, RP., Psaty, BM., Macy, E., Bovill, EG., Cushman, M. (1997) Lifetime smoking exposure affects the association of C-reactive protein with cardiovascular disease risk factors and subclinical disease in healthy elderly subjects. *Arterioscler Thromb Vasc Biol* 17: 2167–2176.

Vasan, RS., Larson, MG., Kannel, WB., Levy, D. (2000) Evolution of hypertension from non-hypertensive blood pressure levels: rates of progression in the Framingham Heart Study (abstract 869-2). *J Am Coll Cardiol* 35:292A.

Wannamethee, G., Whincup, PH., Shaper, AG., Walker, M., MacFarlane, PW. (1995) Factors determining case fatality in myocardial infarction "who dies in a heart attack?" *Brit Heart J* 74:324-331.

Wilson, PF., D'Agostino, RB., Levy, D., Belanger, AM., Silbershatz, H., Kannel, WB. (1998) Prediction of coronary heart disease using risk factor categories. *Circulation* 97:1837-1847.

Wilson, PW. (1990) High-density lipoprotein, low-density lipoprotein, and coronary artery disease. *Am J Cardiol* 66:7A-10A.

19

The Assessment of Prevalence of Hypertension as Cardiovascular Risk Factors Among Adult Population

Aida Pilav
Federal Ministry of Health,
Faculty of Health Studies, University of Sarajevo,
Bosnia and Herzegovina

1. Introduction

Significant increase in noncommunicable diseases, in particular cardiovascular disease, in the past few decades worldwide represents one of the major health challenges in the overall global and social development of society. Cardiovascular conditions have the highest impact on lost years of life, lost quality of life, but also on the differences in longevity in different population groups. Global statistics show that cardiovascular conditions are responsible for one third of global deaths, while coronary heart conditions are the leading cause of death worldwide. (1,2) Many population research studies corroborated that high blood pressure is an independent and significant risk factor of cardiovascular disease and coronary heart disease and most significant determinant of morbidity and mortality in developed countries. (2,3)

Constant increase in morbidity and mortality caused by cardiovascular disease, in particular high blood pressure as one of the most significant public health problem, evaluation of prevalence of high blood pressure and evaluation of control of high blood pressure in the population, including the distribution of cardiovascular risk factors altogether represent the basis for the modeling of an integrated risk and disease prevention program - an integrated management of hypertension in the community (4), which is effectively a step further in providing efficient, effective and high-quality health care.

Globally health care is becoming more complex and more expensive and countries are now faced with various problems that need to be addressed in order to ensure sustainability of their health care systems. With the advance in technology, clinical treatment is also becoming more complex and more expensive so that countries are now more and more focused on preventive programs and controls of conditions which entail less direct costs. Key argument for introduction of preventive public health programs is that such programs have much bigger potential for long-term improvement of the population's health status and also involve much lower costs than clinical medicine. (1,3)

2. Cardiovascular diseases and leading risk factors

A number of research studies clearly showed that cardiovascular disease can be attributed to unhealthy life styles and poor social and physical environment. Unhealthy diet, smoking, physical inactivity and psychosocial stress are the leading risk factors for cardiovascular disease, as well as consequential manifestations of such life styles: hypertension, glucose intolerance and hyperlipidemia. These risk factors also reflect major preventable health problems. (5-12))

In the world the issue of cardiovascular disease became very pressing in early 1970s. At that time many health intervention program were planned at the level of the community and their purpose was to promote health and reduce detrimental life style changes. The basic starting premise was that the use of measures to reduce risk factors in population with clinically identified risk factors has only a limited effect on prevention of cardiovascular risk factor at the national level; on the other hand, global public health actions have more effects altogether.

The first implemented program that was based on these ideas was the North Karelia Project carried out in Finland in 1972. This project achieved significant results, in particularly through the hypertension control programs. It started off as a pilot but after significant net reductions in both risk factors and cardiovascular disease-caused mortality rate, the project was rolled out to the national level. Over the next 25 years, smoking prevalence in men was significantly reduced and so was serum cholesterol and blood pressure levels. Over this period, mortality rate caused by cardiovascular disease in men aged 35-64 years dropped by 68%, coronary heart disease mortality rate by 73%, cancer mortality rate by 44%, and mortality rate for all samples effectively dropped by 49%. (13-15)

Building on this success, many projects have been implemented since then in the form of demonstrational projects under different WHO programs: CINDI (WHO/EURO), CARMEN (WHO/AMRO), and INTERHEALTH (WHO/HQ). Apart from clinical trials, all these projects involved different design, intervention approach, method, intensity, goals in reducing the risk factors, evaluation measurements and timeline. Major role of projects implemented in community is to demonstrate and stimulate health policies of non-contagious disease prevention. (16)

In their recommendations for 2003, the WHO and the International Society of Hypertension (ISH) defined three sets of risk factors required for monitoring in management of hypertension. *(Table 1.)* (28)

Based on this, a stratification of overall cardiovascular risk factors was provided. Three major risk categories - low, medium and high risk - were calibrated to effectively indicate absolute likelihood of developing a cardiovascular disease in the next 10 years as follows: (1) low risk – less then 15%; (2) medium risk – 15-20%; and (3) high risk – over 20%. *(Table 2.)*

3. Hypertension as a cardiovascular risk factor

Nearly 1 billion of people worldwide are suffering from hypertension. Population research studies showed that 15-37% of adult global population is stricken by hypertension. The WHO statistics in 2002 showed that hypertension is the third leading cause of the global burden of disease. Untreated and non-controlled hypertension as highly prevalent risk factor for cardiovascular disease results in cerebrovascular accidents, myocardial infarction, heart failure and dementia, kidney failure and blindness. (2,3,4).

Cardiovascular disease risk factors	Target organ damage (TOD)	Associated clinical condition (ACC)
1. SBP/DBP values (level 1-3) 2. Man > aged 55 years 3. Women > aged 65 years 4. Smoking 5. Total cholesterol > 6.1 mmol/l or LDL - cholesterol > 4.0 mmol/l 6. HDL - cholesterol Males < 1.0 mmol/l Females < 1.2 mmol/l 7. History of cardiovascular disease in the first degree relatives before the age of 50 8. Obesity, physical inactivity	1. Left ventricular hypertrophy 2. Microalbuminuria (20-300 mg/daily) 3. Radiological or ultrasound evidenced extensive atherosclerotic plaque (aorta, carotids, coronary, iliac or femoral arteries) 4. Grade 3 or 4 hypertensive retinopathy	1. Diabetes mellitus 2. Cerebrovascular conditions: • Stroke • Cerebral hemorrhage • Transitory ishemic attack (TIA) • Heart disease • Myocardial infarction • Angina pectoris • Coronary revascularization • Congestive coronary insufficiency 3. Kidney diseases • Plasma creatinine concentrations • Females > 1.4 mg/dl • Males > 1.5mg/dl (120, 133 µmol/l) • Albuminuria >300mg/dnevno 4. Peripheral arterial disease

Source: 2003 World Health Organization (WHO)/International Society of Hypertension (ISH) statement on management of hypertension

Table 1. Risk factors required for monitoring in hypertension management

Other risks and history of disease	Blood pressure (mmHg)		
	Grade 1 mild hypertension SBP 140-159 or DBP 90-99	Grade 2 medium hypertension SBP 160-179 or DBP 100-109	Grade 3 severe hypertension SBP ≥180 or DBP ≥110
No other risk factors	LOW	MEDIUM	HIGH
1-2 risk factors	MEDIUM	MEDIUM	HIGH
3 or more risk factors or damaged target organs or diabetes mellitus	HIGH	HIGH	HIGH

Source: 2003 World Health Organization (WHO)/International Society of Hypertension (ISH) statement on management of hypertension

Table 2. Stratification of risk in quantification of prognosis

Hypertension is estimated to cause 7.1 million of deaths worldwide or roughly 13% of total global morality. Significance of high blood pressure is becoming increasingly higher when it comes to disability caused by stroke and coronary ischemia, which expressed in DALY (Disability-Adjusted Life Year) that is 64.3 million DALYs of lost life or 4.5% of the total burden of disease. Each year globally there are 12 million fatal and approximately 20 million non-fatal myocardial infarctions, mostly in developing countries. Research showed that treated hypertension reduces risk of cerebrovascular accidents by 40% and risk of myocardial infarctions by 15%. (2,3,4)

Even with extensive knowledge about the pathophysiology and the epidemiology of hypertension, simple diagnostics, availability of efficient drugs, hypertension still has high prevalence and as a result introduction of an effective hypertension control represents considerable public health challenge. (18,19) Public health systems worldwide continue to cope with inadequate management of hypertension and there is a need to ensure constant improvement of management by health professionals in order to make sure that at least two thirds of treated patients suffering from hypertension reach adequate control of blood pressure.

In doing so it is necessary to perform control of major risk factors, such as smoking, obesity, increased total serum cholesterol and diabetes mellitus. (18,19) All this creates necessary prerequisites for setting up different methods of controlling hypertension that basically prevent continuation of costly cycle of clinical management of hypertension and the related complications.

Definitions of hypertension, in particular in public health sense, are essentially pragmatic. They can be used and they were also defined to characterize a group of individuals who potentially may benefit from specific treatment regimes - non-pharmacological and pharmacological. Definition of hypertension which is more then 30 years old and which says that *"Hypertension should be defined as the level of blood pressure which requires investigation and treatment to improve the condition"* indicates that any numerical definition and categorization should be flexible and based on evidenced risk and availability of effective and well-tolerated drugs. (20-24) Also clinically used definitions are rather arbitrary because of the nature of blood pressure distribution in the population. (25-27) Researchers have long discussed about threshold values of high blood pressure in different populations, in particular those threshold values that warrant therapeutic interventions. There is also variability in deciding the threshold values for evaluation of cardiovascular disease risk factor in individuals.

Problem-based approach to hypertension is twofold: (i) it is described as a separate clinical entity/condition and is classified as a prevalent cardiovascular disease. Also hypertension is a very important factor in development of morbidity and mortality that are caused by cardiovascular disease; or (ii) it is described as intermediary (biological) factor in development of cardiovascular disease and conditions of circulatory system. In both cases hypertension is recognized as "an entry point" for the management of cardiovascular disease.

The World Health Organization/International Society of Hypertension issued in 1999 and 2003 guides for the management (diagnostics and treatment) of hypertension. The European Society of Hypertension (ESH) and the European Society of Cardiology (ESC) did not develop their own guides but simply endorsed the WHO/ISH guides. As the number of population research studies and clinical trials in Europe increased and their results brought to light the new evidence, the European Society of Hypertension and the European Society of Cardiology developed for the first time in 2003 their own guides for the management of hypertension as a response to a suggestion by the WHO/ISH that regional experts should develop recommendations for the management of the disease based on regional conditions, depending on the degree of their health care and health care availability and their economic resources. (25) In 2007 these guides were updated based on the new clinical evidence. (28) As a result, a classification of blood pressure levels was made on the basis of the adopted definitions.(Table 3.)

Category*	Systolic pressure	Diastolic pressure
Optimal blood pressure	<120	<80
Normal blood pressure	120-129	80-84
High normal blood pressure	130-139	85-89
Grade 1 hypertension - mild	140-159	90-99
Grade 2 hypertension - medium	160-179	100-109
Grade 3 hypertension - severe	≥180	≥110
Isolated systolic hypertension	≥140	<90

Isolated systolic hypertension should be graded (1,2,3) according to systolic blood pressure values in the ranges indicated, provided that diastolic values are < 90mmHg. Grades 1, 2 and 3 correspond to classification in mild, moderate and severe hypertension, respectively. These terms have been now omitted to avoid confusion with quantification of total cardiovascular risk.

Source: 2007 Guidelines for the Management of Arterial Hypertension. The Task Force for the Management of Arterial Hypertension of the European Society of Hypertension (ESH) and of the European Society of Cardiology (ESC)

Table 3. Definitions and classification of blood pressure levels (mmHg)

4. Situational analysis in the Federation of Bosnia and Herzegovina

The Federation of Bosnia and Herzegovina is a part of Bosnia and Herzegovina. In April 1992, Bosnia and Herzegovina was internationally recognised as a new independent country and became a member of the United Nations. War broke out in 1992 and ended with the signing of the Dayton Peace agreement in December 1995. The Peace Agreement established Bosnia and Herzegovina as a country of two entities and one district - the Federation of Bosnia and Herzegovina, Republika Srpska and District Brcko. The war 1992-1995 caused drastically demographic and epidemiological changes in Bosnia and Herzegovina. (29,30)

The Federation of Bosnia and Herzegovina is currently going through a period of considerable political and economical transition which altogether has evident implications on the population's health status. Changed lifestyles are result of transitional socioeconomic changes. Over the past two decades health reports have constantly showed high mortality and morbidity rates for noncommunicable diseases, in particular cardiovascular disease.

Hospital discharge rate statistics for these diseases is not analyzed at the Federation of Bosnia and Herzegovina level. (32)

As the Federation of Bosnia and Herzegovina is currently going through a strong transitional and reform period of its socioeconomic development, its health system should be responsive to health and social needs of its population, especially at times when such needs turbulently change. Health system of the Federation of Bosnia and Herzegovina should be flexible and prompt to provide adequate and timely response to demographical and social changes, changes in epidemiological patterns of diseases, expectations of health care users for quality and their role in decision-making, inequity in health care system, and scientific an technological progress. (32,33)

According to the official statistics of the Federation BiH Statistics Office, population of the Federation of Bosnia and Herzegovina in 2009 reached 2,327,318 with average population density at 89 people per square kilometer. Population of the Federation of Bosnia and Herzegovina falls under the category of stationary/regressive population with 14% of people over 65+ years of age. In the overall structure of the population, female population accounts for 51%. (34) According to the World Health Organization (WHO) estimates, life expectancy at birth for males is 73 and for female 78.

The Federation of Bosnia and Herzegovina hypertension morbidity rate reported for 2009 was almost 12% increase compared to the time before 1992 when practically started the period of strong political and socio-economic transition. The hypertension morbidity rates are not reliable, primary as a result of inconsistency of the health statistics system. Statistics available on morbidity rates originate from the primary health care and as such they are simply tip of an iceberg. In fact the statistics is based on the patient-requested health care, not on actual health needs of population. Assessment of actual health needs of the population requires additional sensitive research, such as cross-sectional research population studies. (31) This was the original idea in designing this particular research and assessment of the health needs. (30)

In recent years, there have been several isolated population research studies in tthe Federation of Bosnia and Herzegovina which used different samples. Findings of one such study based on the CINDI methodology showed that unhealthy life habits have slightly increased in the population as a result of exposure to bad life habits such as smoking, unhealthy diet, physical inactivity, etc). (35) Wider public health implications of growingly unhealthy lifestyles are reflected in increased morbidity rates for chronic conditions and early disability, in particular those caused by cardiovascular disease. Statistics on awareness, treatment and control of hypertension in adult population of the Federation of Bosnia and Herzegovina are completely unreliable.

5. The case study

In order to effectively evaluate the prevalence of cardiovascular risk factors (overweight and obesity, smoking, history of hypercholesterolemia and diabetes mellitus) and also blood pressure values, a cross-sectional population study was carried out in the Federation of Bosnia and Herzegovina on a sample of adult population (aged 25-64 years), which was representative for the Federation of Bosnia and Herzegovina. (30)

The households were selected using the random sample method, following the survey conducted in the field. From each household one individual aged 25 to 64 years was selected. Stratified sampling allowed inclusion of both urban and rural areas within the selected municipalities.

Original size of the sample was 3,020 households/respondents, which is effectively the internationally recommended sample size for evaluation of noncommunicable diseases risk factors in adult population. The survey was carried out in the autumn of 2002. Compared to the original sample (3,020 people), response rate was very high (91.5 %). Female respondents made 59 % of the total sample.

Methodology of the survey fully complied with the international recommendations for survey protocol. (36-39) The survey involved interviews with and physicals measurements of individual respondents in their homes. The physicals measurements actually included blood pressure measurements.

Hypertension awareness in the respondents was evaluated through a question listed on the survey questionnaire about whether the respondents being informed on high blood pressure by health professionals.

Drug treatment of hypertension was evaluated by another question listed on the survey questionnaire. The term "treated" included the respondents who at that point were using antihypertensive drugs.

Control of hypertension was evaluated by the question on awareness of their hypertension, use of antihypertensive drugs and measured value of blood pressure.

The survey used a criterion for evaluation of hypertension prevalence which is normally used in population research studies. This criterion was based on the blood pressure threshold values and values of actual treatment by antihypertensive drugs. The respondents were hypertensive if they were using antihypertensive drugs and/or if their systolic blood pressure (SBP) was ≥ 140 mmHg and/or diastolic blood pressure (DBP) was ≥ 90 mmHg.

In addition to the above definitions, the research study also used the WHO/ISH definitions which categorize hypertension into three grades: mild, medium and severe. Following these definitions, **mild hypertension** included respondents who reported SBP of 140-159 mmHg and/or DBP of 90-99 mmHg; **medim hypertension** included respondents who reported SBP of 160-179 mmHg and/or DBP of 100-109 mmHg; and **severe hypertension** included respondents who reported SBP of > 180 mmHg and/or DBP of > 110mmHg. *(see Table 3)*

Limitation of the survey is reflected in the categorization of hypertensive respondents based on one off blood pressure measurement, which in fact may lead to overrated hypertension levels, especially in patients who reported threshold values of SBP of 140mmHg and/or DBP of 90mmHg.

Although cross-sectional research studies are not ideal tools for evaluation, they are necessary to obtain information about individuals who have no contact with health professionals in health care institution, individuals who are not aware of their hypertension, level of treatment and control of hypertension in different countries. Description of blood pressure patterns in the population and the underlying trends classified by age, sex, education and other socioeconomic variables, actually allows development of strategies for reduction of morbidity and mortality caused by high blood pressure.

5.1 Blood pressure

Mean value of SBP was under 140 mmHg, while the DBP mean value was above 80 mmHg in both male and female respondents. Reported values were higher in female respondents.

Age and gender structure showed that the lowest percentage of the respondents was from the youngest age group 25-34 years, males in particular. The highest number of respondents was from the age group 35-44 years, which proportionally included the highest number of females and males. *(See Figure 1.)*

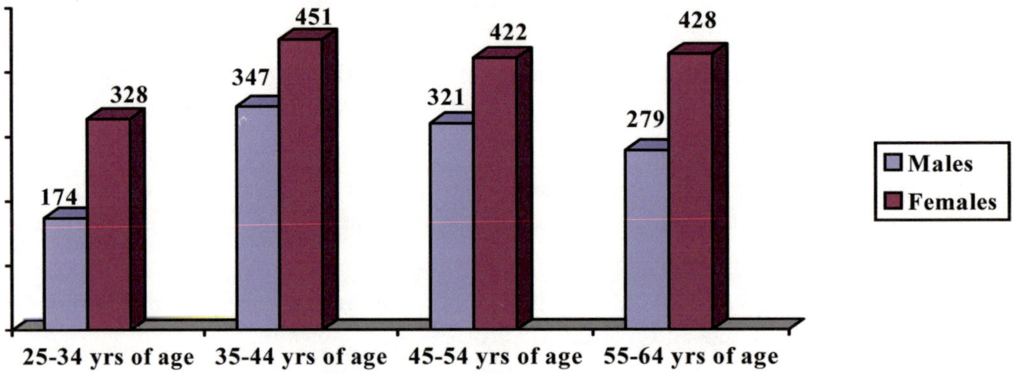

Fig. 1. Number of respondents by age and gender

$\chi^2(3)=12.5, p<.006$

Mean value of SBP in male respondents was 132 mmHg and in female respondents it was 135 mmHg. The difference was statistically significant ($p < 0.001$) *(See Table 4.).* Mean value of DBP was 84 mmHg in both genders. As with the SBP, mean value of DBP also increased with the age of the respondents.

5.2 Prevalence of hypertension

Following the definition of hypertension whereby the respondents were hypertensive if they were using antihypertensive drugs and/or if their SBP was ≥ 140 mmHg and/or DBP was ≥ 90 mmHg. Total of 41% respondents were hypertensive *(Table 5.)*

Prevalence of hypertension was 36% in male and 45% in female respondents. Proportion of the respondents with hypertension statistically increased to a significant degree in both female and male respondents ($p < 0.0001$), but slightly higher in female respondents in elderly age group (aged 45 to 64 years). *(See Table 6.).*

In addition to the above definitions, as already mentioned, the research study also used the WHO/ISH definitions which categorize hypertension into three grades: mild, medium and severe. Following these definitions, **mild hypertension** included respondents who reported

SBP of 140-159 mmHg and/or DBP of 90-99 mmHg; m**edim hypertension** included respondents who reported SBP of 160-179 mmHg and/or DBP of 100-109 mmHg; and **severe hypertension** included respondents who reported SBP of > 180 mmHg and/or DBP of > 110mmHg. *(See Table 3.)*

Age (years)	Males			Females		
	Mean value	(SD)	N	Mean value	(SD)	N
Systolic blood pressure						
25-34	124	(10.8)	172	119	(12.8)	325
35-44	128	(13.2)	346	126	(17.8)	450
45-54	134	(16.5)	320	141	(24.5)	419
55-64	142	(23.7)	279	150	(25.1)	426
Total	***132***	***(18.1)***	***1117***	***135***	***(24.2)***	***1620***
Diastolic blood pressure						
25-34	79	(8.2)	172	77	(8.6)	325
35-44	83	(8.0)	346	81	(10.1)	450
45-54	85	(9.1)	320	87	(12.3)	419
55-64	87	(10.9)	279	90	(12.9)	426
Total	***84***	***(9.4)***	***1117***	***84***	***(12.3)***	***1620***

Table 4. Systolic and diastolic blood pressure (mean value and SD), by age and gender

Age (Years)	Normotensive		Hypertensive	
	N	%	N	%
	Grade 1 hypertension			
25-34	422	88	58	12
35-44	572	73	213	27
45-54	372	50	365	50
55-64	220	31	482	69
Total	***1586***	***59***	***1118***	***41***

Table 5. Prevalence of hypertension by age

Prevalence of mild hypertension was equally distributed in both female and male respondents. Proportion of respondents suffering from mild hypertension statistically increased significantly with the age of both female and male respondents ($p < 0.0001$). Prevalence of moderate and severe hypertension was higher in female respondents. *(See Table 7.).*

Prevalence of hypertension on the threshold value of 140 and/or 90 mmHg among the adult population of the Federation of Bosnia and Herzegovina was higher than in some countries in this part of Europe, including Albania and Hungary. Cross-sectional research studies carried out in Albania and Hungary in recent years showed much lower prevalence of hypertension which in Albania was reported at 32% and in Hungary at 37%. (40,41)

Furthermore, compared to findings of research studies carried out in developed European counties (e.g. UK, Germany) in the past 10 years, where prevalence of hypertension was 38% and 32% respectively (and it was much lower in female respondents), prevalence of hypertension in the Federation of Bosnia and Herzegovina is quite high. (42,43) This altogether should be a challenge for public health of the Federation of Bosnia and Herzegovina in order to effectively identify potential additional risk factors.

Age (Years)	Normotensive		Hypertensive	
	N	%	N	%
Males				
25-34	145	88	20	12
35-44	254	75	86	25
45-54	190	60	129	40
55-64	120	43	158	57
Total	***709***	***64***	***393***	***36***
Females				
25-34	277	88	38	12
35-44	318	71	127	29
45-54	182	43	236	57
55-64	100	24	324	76
Total	***877***	***55***	***725***	***45***

* The respondent were classified as hypertensive if they were using antihypertensive drugs and/or if their systolic blood pressure was > 140 mmHg and/or diastolic blood pressure was > 90 mmHg
Males $\chi^2(3)=113.3$, $p<.0001$; Females $\chi^2(3)=377.6$, $p<.0001$

Table 6. Prevalence of hypertension by age and gender

Age (Years)	Normotensive		Grade 1 Mild hypertension		*Grade 2* Moderate hypertension		Grade 3 Severe hypertension	
	N	%	N	%	N	%	N	%
Males*								
25-34	151	88	18	10	2	1	1	1
35-44	261	75	73	21	9	3	3	1
45-54	196	61	91	28	27	9	6	2
55-64	131	47	88	32	37	13	23	8
Total	***739***	***66***	***270***	***24***	***75***	***7***	***33***	***3***
Females**								
25-34	290	89	32	10	3	1	0	0
35-44	330	73	92	20	19	5	9	2
45-54	193	46	126	30	59	14	41	10
55-64	123	29	134	31	109	26	60	14
Total	***936***	***58***	***384***	***24***	***190***	***12***	***110***	***6***

*$\chi^2(9)=128.6$, $p < .0001$
** $\chi^2(6)=394.2$, $p < .0001$

Table 7. Prevalence of hypertension by age and gender (clinical classification of hypertension)

5.3 Awareness of hypertension, treatment and control of hypertension

Almost 54% of hypertensive respondents were not aware of their hypertension. Very high 79% of the hypertensive respondents who are aware of their hypertension were pharmacologically treated, which indicates relatively good availability of antihypertensive drugs. Of the total number of respondents who were pharmacologically treated, the condition was adequately controlled in only 13%. Generally female respondents were more aware of their hypertension and they were more regularly treated and controlled then male respondents.

In the hypertensive respondents there was a statistically significant difference between the genders with respect to the degree of awareness, treatment and control of hypertension. There were 63% of hypertensive male respondents who were not aware of their hypertension as opposed to 50% of females in this particular category of respondents. Hypertension treated but not controlled respondents included 24% male and 34% female respondents. Percentage of the hypertensive respondents who were both treated and controlled was relatively low - 5% in male and 6% in female respondents. *(See Figure 2.)*

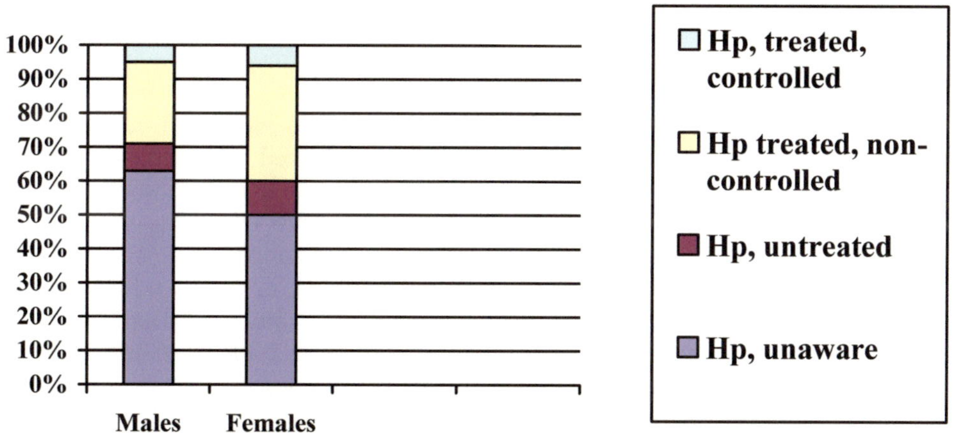

Fig. 2. Awareness, treatment and control in hypertensive respondents, by gender

In genders there was a statistically significant difference among the age groups with regards the degree of awareness of hypertension, treatment and control of hypertension. The degree of awareness of hypertension in both genders significantly increases with the age of the respondents. There were more hypertensive, treated, and non-controlled respondents in older age groups (45 to 64 years) and the portion significantly increased with the age of the respondents. Percentage of hypertensive, treated, and controlled respondents was low at males 5% and females 6%). *(Table 8.)*

The low rate of detection and control of hypertension in hypertensive respondents can be attributed to the lack of standardized integrated programs for reduction of hypertension or at least developed screening programs at the Primary health care (PHC) level. The degree of detection, treatment and control of hypertension increased with the age of the respondents as prevalence of hypertension increased.

	Hypertensive, Unaware		Hypertensive, untreated		Hypertensive, treated, non-controlled		Hypertensive, treated, controlled	
	N	%	N	%	N	%	N	%
Males								
25-34	19	95	0	0	1	5	0	0
35-44	75	87	6	7	1	1	4	5
45-54	81	63	15	12	28	22	5	4
55-64	74	47	11	7	63	40	10	6
Total	***249***	***63***	***32***	***8***	***93***	***24***	***19***	***5***
Females								
25-34	29	77	6	16	0	0	3	8
35-44	80	63	16	13	23	18	8	6
45-54	126	53	27	11	72	30	11	5
55-64	123	38	26	8	153	47	22	7
Total	***358***	***50***	***75***	***10***	***248***	***34***	***44***	***6***

Table 8. Awareness, treatment and control in hypertensive respondents by age and gender

6. Control of hypertension

Experiences of good practice exercised in various countries have showed that significant progress in health can be made through a well organized and focused approach to prevention, treatment and control of the disease, which should be a part of any health system. This is possible to achieve in social environments which support intervention programs in community. In order to make this happen, major changes need to be made in the areas of health policies, organization of health, training/academic education of health professional who also need to be properly equipped. Ultimately, such approaches do not require considerable resources compared to highly complex clinical interventions. (2,3,4)

Following the general managerial approach, the World Health Organization introduced in mid 1980s a number of integrated programs for prevention and control of disease that were defined as "*programs that combine resources and approaches to prevention and control of selected diseases and related conditions and programs that will allow managerial unification of activities that will lead to prevention and control of diseases and promotion of health in overall community.*" (4)

Integrated management of disease and risk factors is particularly recommended in countries with limited financial resources for health care. Mechanisms of such integrated approach can be used to evaluate actual health needs, develop manuals to be used at all levels of management, supervision, adequate treatment and mobilization of community in support of the population's health.

One of well-founded approaches and an example of good practice is Integrated Management of Childhood Illness (IMCI) which is very efficient and applicable in developing countries as more than 80 developing countries has adopted the IMCI as their national policy aimed at improving children's health. This approach allows provision of children's health care in an efficient and effective way. (2)

Since non-communicable diseases, in particular cardiovascular disease, are leading cause of global morbidity and mortality, defining an integrated management of cardiovascular disease, including risk factor management, represents a major challenge for the national health systems worldwide. The modeling of an integrated management of non-communicable diseases means improved supervision and monitoring, development and implementation of intervention prevention programs for different target population groups, implementation of intervention programs in the community and advocacy in public policies with considerable support for health care services. The model of integrated management should promote rational allocation of resources, evidence-based treatment, cost-effectiveness and self-management strategies aimed at achieving improved health outcomes through full involvement of the entire community. (44,45)

The integrated approach to control of hypertension is innovative in shifting the paradigm from "treatment of hypertension" to "management of hypertension" as an integrative program in control of risk factors such as high cholesterol, obesity and diabetes mellitus. This movement to an innovative approach is supported by evidence of cost-effectiveness of managerial approaches to the integrative control of hypertension in the population. Therefore the developing of an integrated hypertension management model at the level of the community should be supported in the country as the original, flexible approach and comprehensive package that combines different sustainable activities that will produce a synergic effect in fight against selected risk factors. (46-48)

Population approaches in dealing with the health needs of the population are the bigger challenge with the long-term results. Epidemiological theories confirmed by research studies have indicated that intensive treatment of individuals who are under a threat of high risk of developing a disease have actually yielded limited progress in reducing general risk in the population as opposed to the population approaches. (49-51)

This effectively corroborate the fundamental axiom of preventive medicine which says that a large number of people exposed to small risk can result in much bigger number of cases that the small number of people exposed to high risk.(2)

However, effective and efficient control of blood pressure in the population requires two approaches: *population approach and individual approach to high risk individuals.* Both approaches are necessary and complementary for effective control and management of hypertension in the community. It is important to specifically note that balanced combination of population preventive strategy and preventive strategy in dealing with the high risk individuals is vital for effective control of epidemic and growing burden of non-communicable in the community in general, in particular hypertension and cardiovascular disease. *(See Figure 3)* (2,4)

7. Strategies for reducing high blood pressure

Despite many efforts to diagnose and effectively treat hypertension, this condition is still the leading cause of cardiovascular morbidity and mortality. This is why it is very important to improve unsatisfactorily treatment and control of hypertension globally. According to the research studies published by the WHO, major barriers for adequate management of hypertension include lack of standardized clinical guides at the national level, inadequate training of health professionals in management of hypertension and poor availability of hypertension drugs at the Primary health care level. Development of management of hypertension in public health context represents the best way to introduce the management of cardiovascular risks. (52,53)

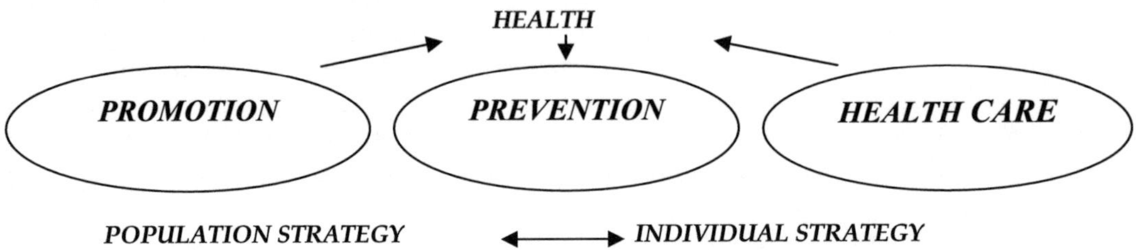

Fig. 3. Population vs. individual approach in improved health of the population

For the most part, successful implementation of guides and recommendations requires a multidisciplinary approach, from mass dissemination of recommendations, provision of public health education programs direction in the field, all the way to clinical treatment of ill patients. To achieve all this it is necessary to ensure involvement of lager number of stakeholders, from strategic to operational levels of management. Formal approval of guides essentially depends on national associations of hypertension and professional associations, in order to promote the proposed changes in behavior and improve prognosis for patients. (54-59)

Leading non-communicable diseases, including hypertension, are associated with common preventable risk factors – obesity, smoking and increased levels of fats in the blood. Better understanding of these risk factors and their determinants means better opportunities for prevention and control of the associated non-communicable diseases. Early detection and understanding of extent of this health issue, early warning and early response altogether allow timely prevention of future epidemic and "explosion" of risk factors. (60,61)

High rate of undetected hypertension and unsatisfactorily control of hypertension indicate that hypertension today is insufficiently and inadequately treated. This results in far reaching consequences in development of heart-, brains- and kidney-related conditions and eventually fatal outcomes. At this point the health system of the Federation of Bosnia and Herzegovina is treating adverse health outcome and the sequels. Number of complicated cardiac surgeries is on the rise and this in fact puts additional strain on already limited health sector budget allocations.

Lessons from many countries which developed the comprehensive policies showed that there is a significant reduction in mortality caused by cardiovascular disease. In Finland, for example, the comprehensive strategy that effectively combined prevention, promotion in the community and the approach to the treatment resulted in decrease of mortality rate by staggering 60%.

Two preventive strategies are described in the scientific literature: population and individual strategy.

Population strategy in reducing high blood pressure in countries throughout the world is very cost-effective – it is especially suitable for countries with limited resources such as Bosnia and Herzegovina. Population strategy allows potential control of incidence of disease in the population. With respect to hypertension, this approach includes reduction of mean value of blood pressure in the population by shifting the entire distribution towards the left lower values (*distributional transition* - a shift from the current values towards the desired value and planned scenario) and reduction of prevalence of high blood pressure and hypertension in adult population in elderly age as well. *(See Figure 4.)* Population approach strongly supports promotion and improvement of cardiovascular health of the population. INTERSALT study showed that population measures which can reduce mean value of systolic blood pressure by 2-3 mmHg can also reduce prevalence of hypertension in the population by one fifth at the age of 20 to 59 years. This means that organized, focused and controlled measures put in place in the population/community can successfully lead to distributional transition. (62)

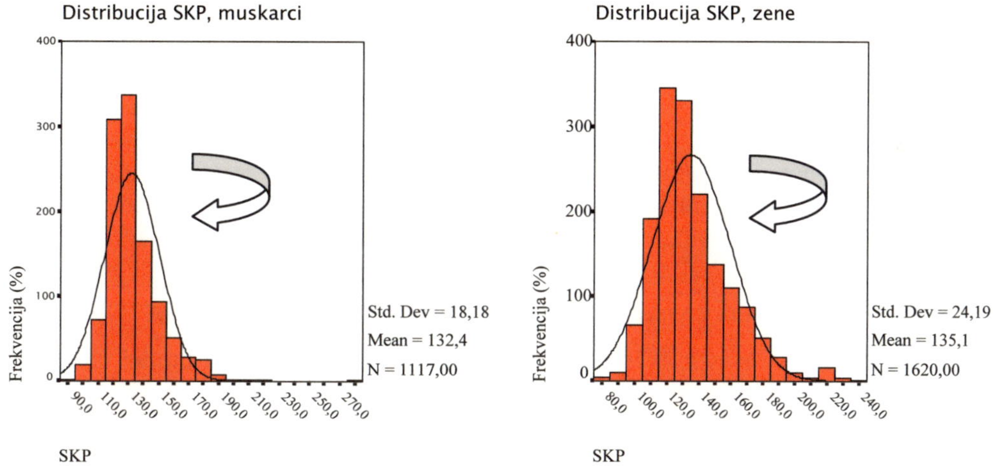

Fig. 4. Distribution of SBP in adult respondents and directions of distributional transition by gender

Population approach supports identification and modification of risk factors associated with different behaviors such as, for example, dietary habits, smoking and physical inactivity. Multiple interventions with regards the risk factors are possible by setting up health policies in the country through the multisectorial approaches in the community. Managerial approach to the population/community requires active involvement of large number of stakeholders from all three levels of management (strategic, tactical and operational) in health sector which is the primary public sector for the starting of such initiative.

It is described in the scientific literature that interventions aimed at changing the unhealthy lifestyles are very successful in reducing the absolute risk of development of hypertension in the population. (52,63,64) Preventive strategies implemented in young population, or rather in early stages of life, allow long-term potential for prevention of conditions which lead to development of hypertension and high blood pressure, as well as for reduction of overall morbidity and complications associated with conditions caused by high blood pressure. (53)

On the other hand, *individual approach* in prevention of disease does not provide a big picture of causes of diseases in the environment and projections of potential trends of the disease. However, it requires continuous and considerable screening of new highly risk individuals. Individual approach to high risk individuals with respect to hypertension includes detection, treatment and effective control of high blood pressure. Such approach requires effective treatment and both modification of lifestyle and pharmacological treatment.

It is necessary to create prerequisites necessary to study the approach to high-risk individuals which in fact primarily includes detection, early diagnosis and start of a treatment of hypertension. Changes to attitudes of health professionals in terms of the integrated hypertension management can be achieved through formal education of health professionals.

Based on the international recommendations, tables of cardiovascular risk stratification are recommended for management of hypertension at the level of an individual. Cardiovascular risk assessment systems have been for the most part developed on the findings of the Framingham Risk Score study. (65,66) Recent SCORE project developed the risk assessment tables to estimate the probability of developing fatal cardiovascular disease within the next 10 years, in particular for high-risk countries in the north of Europe and low-risk countries in the south of Europe.(67)) These categories can be used as indicators for assessment of relative risk in the population. It is recommended that the countries adapt the risk stratification tables and to introduce them in daily practice. The SCORE tables are based on risk assessment relative to values of cholesterol and blood pressure and age and gender.

8. Model of integrated hypertension management in community

Based on the survey results, it has become necessary to introduce a model of integrated management of hypertension in the Federation of Bosnia and Herzegovina at this point because of the relatively high prevalence of hypertension and leading cardiovascular risk factors.

In the countries with limited budgetary allocations for health, such as the Federation of Bosnia and Herzegovina, population prevention strategies are the most cost-effective solution. (2, 68) These strategies control incidence of risk factors in the population, their goal is to change health behavior and reduce exposure to risk factors and also to reduce risk in the entire population. Potential benefits are high but there are challenges as well because the community largely benefits from preventive measures while it seems that such measures produce limited benefits for an individual. This, on the other hand, may cause a negative motivation in the population and this is described as "preventive paradox." Therefore it is necessary to use the both approaches complementary. The key challenge is to find a suitable balance between the population approach and the approach to high-risk individuals. (69)

Managerial approach to the community (to the population) requires active involvement of large number of stakeholders from all three levels of management (strategic, tactical and operational) in health sector which is the primary public sector for the starting of such initiative.

Role of strategic management in the health sector (a country's government) in reduction of risk is significant. The government should act as an advisor in the initiative to reduce the risk factors – selected, highly prevalent in the population and widely distributed risks. One of potential instruments include the passing of legislation, which is more cost-effective as it is assumed that the legal regulations will more readily lead to changes in agreements rather than professional recommendations alone. Both approaches require consultations with a large number of active stakeholders and the multisectorial approach. *(See Table 9.,)* Unfortunately transition countries, such as the Federation of Bosnia and Herzegovina, have a poor regulatory structure and they are more dependable on the non-controlled market. Against such backdrop, it is necessary to select sustainable and implementable measures, including, for example, higher taxes on tobacco products, legislation on reduced salt content in industrially produced food products, use of mandatory content labeling of products, support for production of healthy food or subsidization of price of food produced by local producers.

Levels of management	Possible interventions	Responsible organizations	Theoretical coverage of population
Strategic management	1. Legal regulations on reduced content of salt in local industrially produced food products and mandatory food product content labeling	Government of the country	100%
Tactical management	1. Health education through mass media 2. Campaigns 3. Introduction of risk screenings 4. Development of diagnostics and therapeutic protocols 5. Training for health professionals 6. Development of reference programs such as the School of Hypertension in Community	Public health institutes, medical associations, professional associations, non-governmental organizations	60-80%
Operational management	1. Pharmacological treatment and patient education on lifestyles including dietary counseling for individuals with SBP over 160 mmHg or 140 mmHg. 2. Pharmacological treatment and patient education on lifestyles including dietary counseling for individuals with cholesterol serum concentration of over 5.7 mmol/l. 3. Nicotine replacement therapy with medical consultations by physician. 4. Triple therapy treatment for reduction of high blood pressure for individuals with absolute risk of cardiovascular events of 5% (15, 20, 25%) over the next 10 years. 5. Development of hypertension consultation facilities.	PHC Hospitals	26-41%

Table 9. Cost-effective interventions in reducing prevalence of hypertension

Role of tactical management in health sector, such as public health institutes, medical associations, professional physician associations, is reflected in designing, introducing and implementing intervention programs in the community through a series of mapped activities including preparation of culturally-sensitive promotional and preventive education messages, services aimed at supporting the changed lifestyles, introduction of risk screenings, development of diagnostic and therapeutic protocols, training for of health professionals and development of reference programs.

Role of operational management in the health sector, such as primary, secondary and tertiary health care levels (hospitals, clinics and health resorts) and non-governmental sector is reflected in the active implementation of recommendations, design and dissemination of written materials and active participation in the health training/education.

These interventions could be used as strategies in creation of population approach in management of hypertension.

Findings of this research study showed that prevalence of detection and prevalence of control of hypertension were relatively low, which further supports the importance of introducing the integrated management of hypertension.

Based on evaluation of prevalence of hypertension and distribution of major cardiovascular factors in the population research study, the managerial approach was assumed, through all developmental stages of the process (input, process and output) for for hypertension. *(See Figure 5.)*

Input included input variables (income) and resources (actual input).

Input variables (income) included:

1. High prevalence of hypertension in the population (41%),
2. High prevalence of selected major cardiovascular risk factors (27% in both genders)
3. High prevalence of smoking in young males aged 25 to 44 years (56%)
4. High prevalence of obesity in middle-aged women aged 35 to 54 years (35%).

Actual input included required resources:

1. Staff
2. Premises
3. Equipment
4. Time
5. Money

Process included supervision, stakeholders and activities.

1. **Supervision** included formal bodies such as steering committees of projects implemented in the community or intervention programs which targeted subgroups within the population.
2. **Implementers** included predominantly the health sector experts from different implementation sites (Family Medicine Ambulantas, work places, schools).
3. **Activities** were linked together through project cycles, with clearly defined goals, performance indicators and monitoring that was carried out. *(See Table10.)*

Output included output variables and outcome.

Output variables were:
1. Process evaluation of the project (resources, process, monitoring)
Outcome and impact was:
1. Degree of achieved value – achievement of the desired quantified goal.

GOAL - WHAT?	PROCESS - HOW?	LOCATION - WHERE?	TIME - WHEN?
1. Reduced prevalence of hypertension by 10% in adult population	Legal regulations on reduced content of salt in local industrially produced food products and mandatory food product content labeling	THE COMMUNITY **Coverage** 100% of the population	CONTINUOUSLY
2. Reduced mean value of blood pressure in the population (distributional transition) aimed at promoting and improving cardiovascular health of the population	Develop the reference program *the School of Hypertension in the Community*	THE COMMUNITY **Coverage** 100% of the population 1. Health professionals – Family Medicine teams (PHC) 2. Support groups – healthy population 3. Population under the risk 4. Representatives of mass media	ONE-YEAR CONTROLLED PROGRAM IN LOCAL DEMONSTRA-TIONAL AREAS
3. Reduced smoking by 10%, especially in young males	- Campaigns on possible use of nicotine replacement therapies with medical counseling by physician. - Health education through the mass media – TV shows on how to quit smoking	Big shopping centers, places which people of this age normally visit (entertainment and sports venues), sports non-governmental organizations, TV stations **Coverage** 55% of male population	ONE-YEAR CONTROLLED PROGRAM IN LOCAL DEMONSTRA-TIONAL AREAS
4. Reduced obesity by 10%, especially in middle-aged women	- Health education through the mass media – TV shows on importance of physical activity - On-the-job education - Promotion of recipes for low-calorie meals	TV stations big shopping centers, women's non-governmental organizations **Coverage** 40% of female population	ONE-YEAR CONTROLLED PROGRAM IN LOCAL DEMONSTRA-TIONAL AREAS

Table 10. Activities proposed in managerial process of intervention programs in the community – population approach

These interventions could be used as strategies in creation of population approach in management of hypertension. Findings of this research study showed that prevalence of detection and prevalence of control of hypertension were relatively low, which further supports the importance of introducing the integrated management of hypertension. The individual approach is better suited for high prevalence of hypertension. Compounded by the high prevalence of major cardiovascular factors, detection, adequate treatment and control are placed at (70)

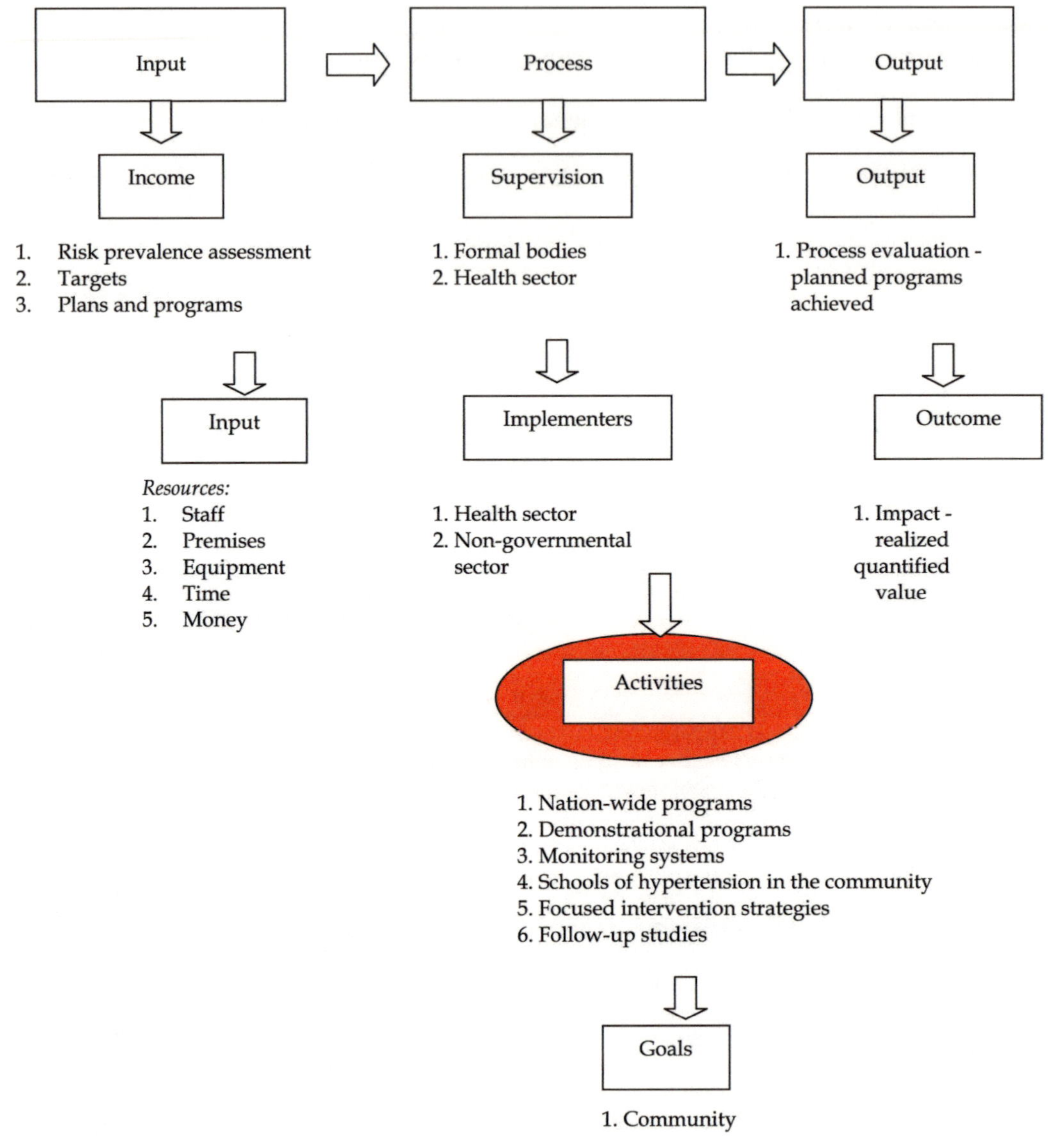

Fig. 5. Integrated management of blood pressure in the community (Intervention programs in the community)

9. Recommendations

1. Ensure support to healthy policies in the country by introducing a number of multisectorial approaches in the community that will allow multiple interventions in reducing the risk factors. The community is a significant partner and the vital point in achieving the goals that have been set.
2. It is necessary to develop a model of integrated management of hypertension and major cardiovascular risk factors as a comprehensive model introduced in the community that should be primarily directed towards modification of a detrimental lifestyle.

3. Health care should be restructured in order to effectively provide integrated health care through changed attitudes of health professionals, availability of technologies used for diagnostics and treatment of hypertension and improved quality of the referral system that will reduce inequities in the health.
4. With regards to the findings of the research study, purpose of the integrated hypertension program should be reduction of high blood pressure in adult population, with the following specific objectives -
   - Raise awareness of hypertension in hypertensive individuals through efficient *detection* of hypertensive individuals by health professionals through improved monitoring, in particular at the level of Primary health care;
   - Introduce standardized and suitable diagnostic and therapeutic protocols to be used by health professionals - efficient *monitoring and treatment of hypertension;*
   - Improve *control of hypertension* in hypertensive individuals;
   - Allow effective collection of data on epidemiology of hypertension.
5. Strong support to development of population approach in the managerial process of implementation of intervention programs of blood pressure control that will promote reduction of mean value of blood pressure in the population (distributional transition) in order to improve and advance cardiovascular health of the population.

In the light of the above recommendations, these activities should be focused on clear identification of health needs. Carefully planned, well designed and well implemented programs of disease control, either population or individual, represent a strong sole instruments to effectively deal with the problem of morbidity through the use of preventive measures. (71,72)

Prevention of disease is crucial to human development. Through such approach, it will be possible to reach different groups of the population, which will in turn facilitate equity in health. (31,33.)

10. References

[1] Health 21–Health for all in the 21.Century.WHO Regional Office for Europe.Copenhagen 1999.
[2] The World Health Report 2002:Reducing Risks, Promoting Healthy life. WHO 2002.
[3] The World Health Report 2003:Shaping the future.WHO 2003.
[4] Integrated management of cardiovascular risk: report of a WHO meeting Geneva, 9-12 July 2002. WHO 2002.
[5] Coca A. Actual blood pressure control: are we doing things right? J. Hypertension. 1998;16: S45-S51
[6] Kannel W.B. Elevated systolic blood pressure as a cardiovascular risk factor. American Journal of Cardiology. 2000;85:251-255.
[7] MacMahon B,Pugh T.F. Epidemiology:Principles and methods.Boston, 1970.
[8] Lilienfeld A.M, Lilienfeld D.E.Foundations of epidemiology.Oxford University Press 1980.
[9] Raljević E, Dilić M, Čerkez F. Prevencija kardiovaskularnih bolesti.Sarajevo 2003.
[10] Sholer C et all. Synthesis of findings and issues from community prevention trials.Annals of Epidemiology. 1997, S7:S54-S68.
[11] Winkleby MA, Jatulis DE, Frank E, Fortmann SP. Socioeconomic status and Health: How Education, Income, and Occupation Contribute to Risk Factors for Cardiovascular Disease.American Journal of Public Health. 1992;82(6):816-820.

[12] PREMIER Collaborative Research Group. Effects of comprehensive lifestyle modification on blood pressure control:Main results of the PREMIER Clinical Trial. JAMA.2003;289(16):2083-2093.
[13] Puska P, Tuomilehto J, Nissinen A, Vartiainen E. The North Karelia Project:20 year results and experiences. National Public Health Institute Finland KTL. Helsinki 1995.
[14] Puska P. Successful prevention of noncommunicable disease:25 year experiences with North Karelia Project in Finland. Public Health Medicine. 2002;4(1):5-7
[15] Puska P, Vartiainen E, Tuomilehto J. et all. Changes in premature deaths in Finland: successfull long-term prevention of cardiovascular diseases. Bulletin of the WHO. 1998;76(4):419-425.
[16] Nissinen A, Ximena B, Puska P. Community-based noncommunicable disease interventions:lessons from developed countries for developing ones. Bulletin of the World Health Organization. 2001, 79: 963-970.
[17] 2003 World Health Organization (WHO)/International Society of Hypertension (ISH) statement on management of hypertension. J. Hypertension.2003;21:1983-1992.
[18] He J, Muntner P, Chen J, Roccella EJ, Streiffer RH, Whelton PK Factors associated with hypertension control in the general population of the United States. Archives of Internal Medicine 2002;162:1051-1058.
[19] Coca A. Actual blood pressure control: are we doing things right? J. Hypertension. 1998;16:S45-S51
[20] Guibert R, Franco E.D. Choosing a definition of hypertension:impact on epidemiological estimates. J Hypertension. 1996;14(11):1275-1280
[21] Birkett N.J. The effect of alternative criteria for hypertension on estimates of prevalence and control. J. Hypertension.1997;15:237-244
[22] Le Pailleur C, Helft G, Landais P. Et all. The effects of talking, reading and silence on the «white coat» phenomenon in hypertensive patients.American Journal of Hypertension. 1998;11:203-207.
[23] Wilber JA, Barrow JG. Hypertension–a community problem. Am Journal of Medicine. 1972;52(5):653-663
[24] Bulpitt C.J. Epidemiology of hypertension. Elsevier 2000.
[25] 2003 European Society of Hypertension-European Society of Cardiology guidelines for the management of arterial hypertension - Guidelines Committee.J. Hypertension. 2003;21:1011-1053.
[26] 2003 World Health Organization (WHO)/International Society of Hypertension (ISH) statement on management of hypertension. J. Hypertension.2003;21:1983-1992.
[27] Chobanian A.V, Bakris G.L, Black H.R et all. The Seventh Report of the Joint National Committee on prevention, detection, evaluation and treatment oh high blood pressure–The JNC 7 Report. JAMA 2003; 289
[28] 2007 Guidelines for the Management of Arterial Hypertension. The Task Force for the Management of Arterial Hypertension of the European Society of Hypertension (ESH) and of the European Society of Cardiology (ESC). J. Hypertension 2007, 25:1105–1187
[29] Smajkic A et al. Social health consequences of the war in Bosnia and Herzegovina, Public Health Institute of BIH,Sarajevo 1995.
[30] Pilav A, Nissinen A, Haukkala A, Nikšić D, Laatikainen T. Cardiovascular Risk Factors in the Federation of Bosnia and Herzegovina. European Journal of Public Health 2006. 17:75-79
[31] Report on health status and organization of health care in the FBiH, Federal Public Health Institute, Sarajevo 2009.
[32] Strategic plan for Primary Health Care in the FBIH, Federal Ministry of Health, 2006.

[33] Strategic plan for health care development in the FBIH 2008-2018, Federal Ministry of Health
[34] Statistical Yearbook 2010. Federal Office for Statistics, Sarajevo 2010.
[35] Omanić A, Omanić J. Rezultati istraživačkog programa CINDI u Sarajevskom kantonu. Medicinski fakultet. Sarajevo 2002.
[36] WHO MONICA Project. Survey protocol. http://www.ktl.fi/publications/monica/index.html
[37] Prattala R, Helasoja V, Laaksonen M, Laatikainen T, Nikander P and Puska P. CINDI Health Monitor. Proposal for practical guidelines.WHO Regional Office for Europe. Publications of the National Public Health Institute,B14/2001.
[38] CINDI Protocol and Guidelines.WHO Regional Office for Europe Copenhagen.1996.
[39] Tolonen H, Kuulasmaa K, Laatikainen T et al. European Health Risk Monitoring Project. Recommendation for indicators, international collaboration, protocol and manual for operations for chronic disease risk factor surveys. http://www.ktl.fi/ehrm/
[40] Shapo L, Pomerleau J, McKee M. Epidemiology of hypertension and associated cardiovascular risk factors in a country in transition: a population based survey in Tirana City, Albania.J Epidemiol Community Health 2003; 57:734-739
[41] Jenei Z, Pall D, Katana E et al. The epidemiology of hypertension and its associated risk factors in the city of Debrecen, Hungary.Public Health 2002; 116:138-144.
[42] Primatesta P. Brookes M., Poulter NR. Improved hypertension management and control:results from the health survey for England 1998. Hypertension. 2001;38:827-832.
[43] Gasse C, Hense H-W, Stieber J. Et all. Assessing hypertension management in the community:trends of prevelence, detection tretment, and control of hypertension in the MONICA Project, Augsburg 1984-1995. J of Human Hypertension. 2001;15:27-36.
[44] Brownson R.C, Baker E.A, Leet T.L, Gillespie K.N. Evidence-based public health. Oxford University Press 2003.
[45] Merzel C, D'Affilitti J. Reconsidering community based health promotion:promise, performance and potential. Am J Public Health. 2003;93:557-574
[46] The Protocol for the WHO Study on the Effectiveness of Community-Based Programmes for the NCD Prevention and Control (COMPASS).WHO 2003.
[47] Bradley E.H, Tashonna W.R, Baker D, Schlesinger M. et all. Translating research into practice:Speeding the adoption of innovative health care programs. The Commonwealth Fund. July 2004.
[48] Israel B.A, Schulz A.J, Parker E.A, Becker A.B. Review of community-based research:Assesing partnership approaches to improve public health. Ann. Rev. Public Health. 1998;19:173-202.
[49] MacMahon B,Pugh T.F. Epidemiology:Principles and methods.Boston, 1970.
[50] Lilienfeld A.M, Lilienfeld D.E.Foundations of epidemiology.Oxford University Press 1980.
[51] Raljević E, Dilić M, Čerkez F. Prevencija kardiovaskularnih bolesti.Sarajevo 2003.
[52] Whelton P.K,Jiang H,Lawrence A.J. et all. Primary prevention of hypertension:Clinical and public health advisory from the National high blood pressure education program. JAMA. 2002;288(15):1882-1888.
[53] Kannel W.B, Garrison R.J, Dannenberg A.L et all. Secular blood pressure trends in normotensive persons:The Framingham study.Am Heart Journal.1993;125:1154-1158.
[54] Fields L.E,Burt V.L, Cutler J.A, Hughes J. Et all. The burden of adult hypertension in the United States 1999 to 2000. A Rising Tide. Hypertension.2004;44:389-404.
[55] Kastarinen MJ, Saloma VV, Vartiainen EA et al. Trend in blood pressure levels and control of hypertension in Finland from 1982-1997. J Hypertension 1998;16:1379-1387.

[56] Prevention and Treatment - Both work, says WHO Study on heart disease, Press Release WHO/10, February 2000.
[57] Milchak J.L, Carter B.L, James P.A, Ardery G. Measuring adherence to practice guidelines for the management of hypertension:An evaluation of the literature. Hypertension. 2004;44:602-608.
[58] Elder J.P, Ayala G.X, Harris S: Theories and Intervention approaches to health behaviour change in primary care.American Journal of Preventive medicine 1999;17(4):275-284
[59] Montgomery A.A, Fahey T, Peters T.J. et all. Evaluation of computer based clinical decision support sytem and risk chart for management of hypertension in primary care:randomised controlled trial.BMJ.2000;320:686-690.
[60] Kuulasmaa K, Tunstall-Pedoe H, Dobson A et all. For the WHO MONICA Project Estimation of contribution of changes in classic risk factors to trends in coronary-event rate across the WHO MONICA Project population. The Lancet 2000; 3555:675-687.
[61] Fuster V, Gotto A.M. Risk reduction.Circulation.2000;102:IV-94-IV-102.
[62] Carvalho JJM, Baruzzi RG, Howard P. Et all. Blood pressure in four remote populations in the INTERSALT study. Hypertension 1989;14:238-246.
[63] PREMIER Collaborative Research Group. Effects of comprehensive lifestyle modification on blood pressure control:Main results of the PREMIER Clinical Trial. JAMA. 2003;289(16):2083-2093.
[64] Geleijnse J.M,Kok F.J,Grobbee D.E. Impact of dietary and lifestyle factors on the prevalence of hypertension in Western population.European Journal of Public Health 2004;14:235-239.
[65] Kannel W.B. Risk stratification in hypertension:new insights from the Framingham study.Hypertension. 2000;13:3S-10S.
[66] Persson M, Carlberg B, Weinehall L, Nilsson L. Et all. Risk stratification by guidelines compared with risk assessment by risk equations applied to a MONICA sample. Journal of Hypertension. 2003;21:1089-1095.
[67] Conroy R.M, Pyorala K, Fitzgerald A.P, Sans S, Menotti A, De Backer G, De Bacquer D, Ducimetiere P, Jousilahti P, Keil U, Njřlstad I, Oganov R.G, Thomsen T, Tunstall-Pedoe H, Tverdal A, Wedel H, Whincup P, Wilhelmsen L, Graham I.M. on behalf of the SCORE project group. Estimation of ten-year risk of fatal cardiovasculardisease in Europe: the SCORE project. European Heart Journal 2003;24:987–1003
[68] Žarković G., Hrabač B., Nakaš B. Zdravstvena politika i upravljanje nacionalnim sistemima zaštite zdravlja:sa posebnim osvrtom na probleme bivših socijalističkih zemalja.ANU BIH. Sarajevo 1999.
[69] Egan B.M. hypertension in the 21st Century: The tide is rising; Our Daze Must End. Hypertension. 2004;44:389.
[70] Pilav A. Algorithm for the Control of Hypertension at Community Level. European Federation for Medical Informatics - Special Topic Conference 2007. Brioni, Croatia, May 30 – June 1, 2007
[71] Pilav A. Zdravstveni indikatori i značaj njihove primjene u svakodnevnom radu. Med. Arhiv. 1999;53 (4,supl. 3): 51-53
[72] Rychetnik L, Frommer M, Hawe P. Et all. Criteria for evaluating evidence on public health interventions.Journal of Epidemilogy and Community Health 56:119-127.2002.

20

Theoretical Identification of Behavioral Risk Factors Among Multiple Risk Factors Causing Morning Onset of Cardiac Events due to Circadian Variations

Fumiko Furukawa[1] and Tatsuya Morimoto[2]
[1]*School of Nursing, University of Shizuoka*
[2]*School of Pharmaceutical Sciences, University of Shizuoka*
Japan

1. Introduction

Circadian variations of cardiac events exist, although times of onset differ slightly between studies (Atkinson et al., 2010; Muller et al., 1989; Quyyumi, 1990; Scheer et al., 2010; Willich et al., 1987). However, several studies have confirmed the occurrence of more events in the morning than in the evening (Atkinson et al., 2010; Mulcahy et al., 1988; Scheer et al., 2010). Two peaks of onset of cardiac events were found: a high frequency of cardiac events in the hours after rising in the morning and in the evening hours (Atkinson et al., 2010; Hjalmarson et al., 1989; Mulcahy et al., 1988; Muller, 1987).

Because cardiac events occurred more frequently in the morning than at any other times of the day, the occurrences of these events are discussed relative to the time after awakening (Kiowski & Osswald, 1993). A specific single factor causing circadian variation in the morning has not been identified. It has been suggested that interactions between multiple factors during transition from the sleep state to the waking stage may occur simultaneously or as a self-sustaining reaction (Atkinson et al., 2010; Scheer et al., 2010).

Evidence regarding physiological risk factors for morning onset of cardiac events has been used when selecting the most appropriate time for taking antihypertensive or anti-arrhythmic medications (Athyros et al., 1998; Mulcahy, 1999; Redon, 2004). For example, Redon (2004) indicated that the angiotensin II blocker telmisartan with a long half-life given once daily is likely to confer benefit in terms of 24-hour blood pressure control and reduce early morning surge in blood pressure. Despite applications of this evidence to medical treatment, few studies examine use of behavioral risk factors related to morning onset of cardiac events. For example, final decisions based on evidence regarding the safest time to exercise during the day are still pending (Atkinson et al., 2006; Atkinson & Davenne, 2007; Murray et al.,1993; Shiotani et al., 2009; White, 2003).

Even though Ebrahim et al. (2006, 2011) indicated that intervention using educational method may be effective in reducing mortality in cardiac high risk population, few discussions have taken place regarding how to apply the current evidence regarding morning onset of cardiac events to patient education. In particular, knowledge about preventive strategies for self-care that minimize the chance of recurrent morning onset of cardiac events is lacking. Amazingly, most patient educational materials about cardiac disease do not contain information about risks of morning behaviors.

Although behavioral risk factors for cardiac events will not significantly influence daily life if they occur once in a while at an early age, human behaviors tend to be unconscious and habitual throughout life. By identifying behavioral risk factors among multiple risk factors that can trigger morning onset of cardiac events, patients with cardiac disease may be able to avoid life-threatening conditions and reconsider their daily lives, including the cycle of activity, rest, and sleep that is associated with quality of life (Baas, 2004; Condon & McCarthy, 2006; Kristofferzon et al., 2007; Noriss et al., 2004). By controlling behavioral risks among the multiple risk factors for cardiac events in the morning, it might be possible to reduce the frequency of early morning cardiac events.

Reviewing evidence regarding behavioral risk factors of morning onset of cardiac events may be helpful for health professionals including doctors and nurses in the cardiovascular community to educate the patients. Furthermore, interventions supported by research that ameliorate life-threatening conditions may improve the quality of patient education. Thus, the primary aim of this chapter is to identify behavioral risk factors among possible causes of morning onset of cardiac events. To develop interventions leading to evidence-based practice, the secondary aim is to suggest strategies for controlling behavioral risk factors that trigger morning onset of cardiac events.

2. Methods

Material reviewed in this chapter was based on journals reporting risk factors related to cardiac events. First, focus of the review was put on the physiological perspective in nature, and then behavioral risk factors were reviewed to suggest strategies for controlling such risk factors. Because physiological conditions are usually deteriorated by behavioral risk factors under the occurrence of cardiac events, it is importance to recognize how each physiological risk factor is progressed and interacted with each other (Deedwania, 1996). Recognition regarding physiological risk factors is also important to develop effective strategies for controlling behavioral risk factors (Baxendale, 1992).

The electronic databases of PubMed (1950 to 2011), CINAHL (1998 to 2011), and the COCHRANE Library (1998 to 2011) were searched for topics related to morning cardiac events and their mechanism. Key words were as follows: circadian variation, sleep, ischemic episodes, cardiac events, cardiac disease, autonomic nervous system activation, physical stress (abrupt upright posture), mental stress, endothelial response of the coronary blood vessels, morning surge of blood pressure, and blood components (Carnethon et al., 2002; Cooke-Ariel, 1998; Furukawa et al., 1998; Khoury et al., 1992; Scheer et al., 2010; Thrall et al., 2007; White, 2003). By searching the database for these key words, evidence regarding behavioral risks factors triggering morning cardiac events was identified, and preventive patient education strategies to decrease morning onset of cardiac events are proposed.

All journals used for this review were limited in only English language, and findings from the animal study were included to understand mechanism of the morning onset of cardiac events in patients with cardiac disease. Also the findings reported in the 1998 review

(Furukawa et al., 1998) were used in part in this review. Permission for utilization of the findings was obtained from the editor.

3. Results

Possible risk factors for cardiac events were as follows: 1) coronary artery blood flow dynamics during sleep; 2) physiology of sympathetic nervous system activation in the morning; 3) pathophysiology of sympathetic nervous system activation in the morning, including coronary blood flow, α- and β-adrenergic receptor responses of coronary artery endothelial cells to sympathetic nerves, platelet aggregation and atherosclerosis with sympathetic nervous activation, neurotransmitters and hormonal elements, and other risk factors for cardiac events, such as morning surge in blood pressure and seasonal variations; and 4) behavioral risk factors immediately after awakening, including abrupt changes of body position.

3.1 Coronary artery blood flow dynamics during sleep

Because of the sleeping state in relation to patterns of REM and non-REM sleep (Aserinsky & Kleitman, 1953; Jouvet, 1967; Steriade, 1992), the morning onset of cardiac events should be discussed from this point. One sleeping cycle is made up of one REM and one non-REM sleep period, and four to six cycles are repeated during the night in adults. Non-REM sleep has four sub-stages, from I to IV, during one cycle, and the depth of sleep increases progressively toward stage IV and then decreases in REM sleep. People wake up mostly at the end of the last rapid eye movement sleep (Willis, 1981).

During the night, arterial blood pressure falls progressively by 5% to 23% from the wakening state to stage IV of non-REM sleep (Martin, 1984). Giles (2005) indicated blood pressure in most people is from 10% to 20% lower than the mean daytime value (Giles, 2005). Cardiac output is minimized during the last rapid eye movement sleep period before arousal and is 25% lower than that during wakening (Martin, 1984). Changes in blood flow of the coronary artery vessels from the beginning of sleep to the time of awakening make insufficient blood flow in cardiac muscles at the time of restart of physical activity immediately upon awakening.

In healthy subjects, increased blood flow by sustained physical activity might lead to vasodilatation, which is induced by endothelial derived relaxing factor released from endothelial cells (Furchgott, 1983). This is a compensation mechanism to increase the blood supply to cardiac muscle. However, such mechanism may not work in patients with cardiac disease. The sudden rises in heart rate at each transition from non-REM sleep (deeper sleep) to REM sleep (lighter sleep), or increase in blood pressure at awakening may precipitate cardiac events (Viola et al., 2002).

3.2 Physiology of sympathetic nervous system activation in the morning

Coronary blood flow is determined by five factors (West, 1990): metabolic control (oxygen demand), coronary perfusion pressure, systolic compression, autonomic nervous system, and circulating catecholamine and other vasoactive substances. Determinants for coronary blood flow are conveyed by auto-regulatory mechanisms. Sympathetic nerve fibers stimulate α-adrenergic receptors of the endothelial cells to respond to vasoconstriction so as to increase coronary vascular resistance (Laxson et al., 1992; Baran et al., 1992; Quyyumi et al., 1992). Stimulation of β-adrenergic receptors of the endothelial cells is a response to coronary vasodilatation (Baran et al., 1992; Quyyumi et al., 1992).

Epinephrine, norepinephrine, and acetylcholine also act through adrenergic receptors of smooth muscle in the coronary arteries (Furchgott, 1983; Kuo et al., 1993). In the transition period from resting to activity in healthy person in the morning, coronary arteries of the human heart can receive signals normally from the sympathetic nervous system due to the increased physical and mental stress associated with awakening, and the compensatory mechanisms of the coronary artery function are well activated to meet oxygen demands.

3.3 Pathophysiology of sympathetic nervous system activation in the morning

In this section, 1) coronary blood flow, 2) α- and β-adrenergic receptor responses of coronary artery endothelial cells to the sympathetic nervous system, 3) platelet aggregation and atherosclerosis with sympathetic nervous activation, 4) neurotransmitters and hormonal elements under sympathetic nervous activation, and 5) other risk factors are reviewed.

3.3.1 Coronary blood flow

Ischemic episodes occur if the increase in coronary blood flow is inadequate for the myocardial oxygen demand. The frequency of ischemic episodes is maximized in the first 2 hours after awakening (Quyyumi, 1990; Rocco, 1990). Coronary spasms due to vasoconstriction are a trigger for ischemic episodes (Sugiishi & Takatsu, 1993). Coronary artery constriction is more severe in the early morning than in the late afternoon, and coronary blood flow at rest in the morning is lower than in the afternoon under comparable hemodynamic conditions (Fujita & Franklin, 1987).

Vascular resistance increases due to the decreased blood flow in patients with hypertrophy or elevated left ventricular diastolic pressure (Duncker et al., 1993). When coronary vascular resistance is increased in the morning, the ischemic threshold is lower than in the afternoon (Benhorin et al., 1993; Quyyumi et al., 1992). Also, the cardiac output during the last REM sleep period before arousal is lowest, and it is one fourth of that while wakening (Martin, 1984). These studies indicate that abrupt and vigorous physical stress becomes a risk factor for cardiac events.

3.3.2 α- and β-adrenergic receptor response of coronary artery endothelial cells to the sympathetic nervous system

The vascular endothelium modifies the contractile characteristics of vascular smooth muscle (Greenberg et al., 1990). When the vasodilator response to acetylcholine in endothelial dysfunction is eliminated, the coronary perfusion rate increases (Furchgott et al., 1980). Endothelial injury initiated by atherosclerotic change leads to plaque formation in a variety of conditions (Zemel & Sowers, 1990; Baxendale, 1992).

Similarly, injury to the endothelial wall triggers monocyte and platelet aggregation, which leads to release of growth factors into the smooth muscle of coronary arteries (Lucchesi,

1990). In particular, the injured endothelial vessel wall produces a paradoxical response that alters the normal response against α- and β-receptors on the vessel walls (Ludmer et al., 1986). The neural sympathetic tone, which increases in the morning, may cause an increased stimulation of α-adrenergic receptors, leading to coronary and peripheral vasoconstriction.

The presence of enough β-adrenergic receptors is necessary to adapt to the increased oxygen demand (Hammond et al., 1992; Figueras & Lindon, 1995). However, the number of β-adrenergic receptors decreases if there is volume overload-induced myocardial hypertrophy, or if the endothelial cells of the coronary artery are impaired (Figueras & Lidon, 1995; Hammond et al., 1992). Patients with unstable angina during bed rest and with significant coronary disease demonstrate a lower ischemic threshold early in the morning (Figueras & Lindon, 1995). Usually, plasma levels of norepinephrine are increased and myocardial levels of norepinephrine are decreased in patients with fewer β-adrenergic receptors (West, 1990; Hammond et al., 1992). The increased plasma norepinephrine over-stimulates sympathetic nervous activity and acts mostly on α-adrenergic receptors, causing vessel constriction (Hammond et al., 1992; Kuo et al., 1993; West, 1990).

3.3.3 Platelet aggregation and atherosclerosis with sympathetic nervous activation

Accelerated platelets aggragation is one of significant risk factors for the morning onset of ischemic episodes (Andrews et al., 1996; Quyyumi, 1990; Braunwald, 1995). The plasma levels of fibrin peptide (thrombin generator) in patients with variant angina are significantly higher from midnight to early morning than other times (Masuda et al., 1994). The plasma norepinephrine concentration (Brezinski et al., 1988), renin activity, and angiotensin II concentration (Oparil et al., 1970; Schachter, 2004) are all increased with change of platelet levels.

Activated platelets release potent vasoactive factors due to adherence of atherosclerotic plaque and cause vasoconstriction or vasospasms (Kaul et al., 1993; Vanhoutte & Huston, 1985). A plaque rupture associated with well-developed atherosclerotic conditions in the coronary artery is often occurred in the morning as sympathetic activity is upregulated, and this induced increase in blood pressure (Shimada et al., 2001; Stone, 1990). Fibrinogen is also involved in this process (Palmieri et al., 2003), and leads to increased blood viscosity (Jay et al., 1990; Lowe et al., 1980).

Plasma fibrinogen has further been found to stimulate red cell aggregation in familial hypercholesterolemia (Jay et al., 1990). The increased fibrinogen and red blood cells lead to increased blood viscosity (Yarnell et al., 1991). In addition, body fluid during sleep usually shifts from the vascular space to the interstitial space (Jacob et al., 1998). These conditions may lead to vasoconstriction and cause vessel occlusion in the presence of atherosclerosis and physical stress in the morning.

3.3.4 Neurotransmitters and hormonal elements

Neurotransmitters and hormonal elements such as epinephrine, norepinephrine, neuropeptide Y, and acetylcholine also participate in cardiac events through aggregation (Eisenhofer et al., 1992; Pernow et al., 1988; Svendsen et al., 1990; Yang & Levy, 1993) and interrelations with endothelial dysfunction (Ludmer et al., 1986), sympathetic nervous system activation (Drager et al., 2009), degrees of coronary blood flow (Fujita & Franklin, 1987; Kuo et al., 1993; Young & Vatner, 1986), level of co-existing atherosclerosis (Ludmer et al., 1986), sleep cycle during the morning transitional phase (Culebras, 1992; Steriade, 1992; Viola et al., 2002), and sleep duration (Cappuccio et al., 2011).

In particular, plasma epinephrine and norepinephrine levels were shown to increase rapidly while plasma volume induced by an abrupt upright posture fell by 13% over 14 minutes (Jacob et al., 1998). Epinephrine approached baseline values by 20 minutes of standing, but norepinephrine spillover increased by 80% and clearance decreased by 30% with 30 minutes of standing (Jacob et al., 1998). Inhibition of the morning surge in catecholamine levels may reduce the risk of thrombotic vascular events in atherosclerosis (Andwers et al., 1999).

3.3.5 Other risks factors

The morning increase in blood pressure, called the morning surge, is one of the risk factors for cardiac events (Giles, 2005; Ohkubo et al., 2008; White, 2001). In addition, morning onset of cardiac events might occur more easily in winter if the body is suddenly exposed to a cold environment (Peters et al., 1996). Mental stress also may cause stress-induced cardiac arrhythmic vulnerability associated with sudden cardiac death (Critchley et al., 2005).

3.4 Behavioral risk factors immediately after awakening

Physical activity, such as standing up immediately after awakening, affects the blood components. In healthy men, a significant change in platelet aggregation occurs as a result of a compensatory homeostatic mechanism against the immediate change to the upright position (Muller et al., 1989; Krantz et al., 1996). Adaption to the change of position after awakening causes persistent platelet aggregation for the next 90 minutes; this platelet aggregation is greater than walking up and down stairs. (Muller et al., 1989). If activities such as walking up and down stairs are performed immediately after waking, platelet aggregation becomes greater than just staying in the upright position (Muller et al., 1989). Because the abrupt upright position after awakening brings a significant change in platelet aggregation with persistent manner, patients with cardiac disease may experience an adverse effect of exercise in the morning (Hilberg et al., 2000).

Also, the upright posture from spine position made plasma volume fell by 13% over approximately 14 minutes in healthy subjects, after which time it remained relatively stable (Jacob et al., 1998). This occurs as a result of compensatory homeostatic mechanisms responding to the initial decrease in central blood and stroke volume from the heart induced by the physical stress (Ahmadizad et al., 2006; Thrall et al., 2007). The sudden rises in heart rate in this case may occur to compensate cardiac output based on the intense of activity. These changes in platelet aggragation and plasma volume occurred in healthy subjects may become severe triggers of cardiac events for patients with cardiac disease.

4. Discussion and conclusion

Cardiac events often occur in the morning after awakening. Many studies report similar findings in terms of the circadian variation of the cardiac events. The significant behavioral risk factor was an abrupt upright position at awakening and seriously acted on physiological risk factors at the occurrence of the cardiac events. The most plausible underline cause of cardiac events in the morning in patients with progressed atherosclerosis was activation of the sympathetic nervous system due to activity immediately upon rising (Kiowski & Osswald, 1993; Stone, 1990; Umemura et al., 1987). Studies on physical stress for cardiac disease under variety of settings were available (Camici et al., 1992; Herd, 1991), but only a few studies of the relation between physical stress and morning onset of the cardiac events were found. The activation of the sympathetic nervous system by physical activity after rising (Umemura et al., 1987) should be considered in relation to levels of atherosclerosis and sleeping stages. The nature of sleep (Culebras, 1992; Steriade, 1992) plays an important role in the morning onset of cardiac events.

A shift change of domination in the autonomic nervous system occurs upon awakening, so that the sympathetic nervous system is activated to prepare for physical and mental activities in the morning. The morning surge of blood pressure can be explained by this shift change, because the sympathetic nervous system is activated by exogenous factors (Leary et al., 2002; van Eekelen et al., 2004a). It should be noted that domination of the sympathetic nervous system in the morning may play a major role on the occurrence of cardiac events (Atkinson et al., 2010; van Eekelen et al., 2004a, 2004b).

In particular, patients who have atherosclerosis may experience a paradoxical response in their vessels under sympathetic nervous system activation with abrupt physical activities undertaken after awakening in the morning (Ludmer et al., 1986). Atherosclerosis triggers cardiac events by creating a paradoxical response in the injured endothelial cells of coronary vessels, providing the greatest vulnerability to sympathetic nervous activity (Ludmer et al., 1986). Thus, normal daytime activity may become a powerful stimulus if it is undertaken in the morning by patients with coronary artery disease (Freed et al., 1989; Herd, 1991; Meller et al., 1979).

It can be assumed that we might experience cardiac events at the time of awakening in the morning because our lives repeat to follow a daily active-sleep cycle, and nobody can develop atherosclerosis with aging. The last REM sleep at the time of awakening is needed to create a smooth transition from parasympathetic to sympathetic nervous activation. As one study indicated, REM sleep works to increase pulse rate (Martin, 1984). The last REM sleep may bring a wake-up ready condition by increasing pulse rate through gradually stimulating the sympathetic nervous system (Martin, 1984) and decreasing parasympathetic nervous system activation (van Eekelen et al., 2004a). Using evidence on the nature of sleep is beneficial if strategies for controlling the morning onset of cardiac events are developed.

Waking-up at REM sleep, not at non-REM sleep may be important for decreasing cardiac events in the morning. REM sleep provide a waking-up ready condition to cardiovascular system. To facilitate waking-up at rapid eye movement sleep, it is better to avoid utilizing an alarm clock, and use non-artificial stimuli such as sunlight providing a natural wake-up call. People should sleep with the shades and curtains open so that they are woken up with natural sunlight that will lead us to wake up at REM sleep.

Similarly, it is important for patients with cardiac disease to not wake up in the morning during non-REM sleep. Because coronary blood flow is the lowest at the last non-REM sleep (Martin, 1984), cardiac output in patients with cardiac disease might not respond adequately to a sudden increase of coronary blood flow at the time of wakening (Kuo et al., 1993), so that supply and demand become unbalanced (Li, 2003). If patients with cardiac disease show non-movement of eyelids, smooth movement of the chest, and quiet breathing indicating non-REM sleep (Aserinski & Kleitman, 1953; Aserinski & Kleitman, 2003), it is better for them to be left until waking-up by themselves.

In addition to sensitivity to REM sleep and non-REM sleep, levels of catecholamine and coronary tone should be considered because they are lowest just before awakening (Linsell et al., 1985). During the transitional phase from sleep state to physical activity state in patients with atherosclerosis, insufficient oxygen supply to the heart occurs. The high levels of catecholamine at awakening may produce a severe paradoxical response to the coronary vessel wall in patients with progressing atherosclerosis, leading to vasospasm (Ludmer et al., 1986). Such vasospasms might trigger a cardiac event. Atherosclerosis of artery walls develops over a long period and progresses with a high-fat diet and a sedentary lifestyle. The cardiovascular system should be maintained in a healthy condition by an adequate caloric intake and an active lifestyle (Ebrahim et al., 2011). From the viewpoint of human evolution, modern life with excess caloric intake and sedentary lifestyles may contribute to the increased number of cardiac events that occur in the morning.

Although atherosclerotic changes are significantly associated with aging, platelet aggregation may not be. Platelet aggregation has shown to be triggered in healthy young people who assume an abrupt upright position in the morning (Muller et al., 1989; Tofler et al., 1987) and works with fibrinogen levels to significantly contribute to morning onset of cardiac events (Braunwald, 1995). Abruptly assuming an upright position immediately after awakening is now a known risk factor for cardiac events, and may create a life-threatening condition in patients with the major cardiac risk factors. However, such behavior seems to be recognized as a small factor that can be modified, and the effects of this change have not been studied.

Abrupt changes in blood pressure and heart rate due to adoption of an upright position after awaking in the morning may trigger platelet aggregation, enhancing the degree of occlusion of the coronary artery with aging (Storm et al., 1989). Once platelet aggregation occurs, it lasts for hours (Muller et al., 1989). Activated platelets release potent vasoactive factors due to adherence of atherosclerotic plaque, and cause vasoconstriction or vasospasms (Kaul et al., 1993; Vanhoutte & Huston, 1985). This phenomenon may create a morning peak in cardiac events. Patients with cardiac disease should take their time getting up in the morning, engaging only in slow activities until platelet aggregation subsides. Furthermore, they should maintain ideal fibrinogen levels by taking part in regular exercise (Furukawa et al., 2008).

Cold temperatures with seasonal variations at the transitional phase in the morning are also a risk factor triggering cardiac events (Peters et al., 1996). These temperatures may increase blood pressure by constricting peripheral vessels. Increased blood pressure might create rupture of the vessel's wall and release clots, leading to ischemic events (Shimada et al., 2001). Here again, rupture of the vessel wall leads to an increase in platelets (Shimada et al., 2001). Abruptly assuming an upright posture, which causes platelet aggregation, will precipitate ischemic events during a few hours after awakening in the morning. Therefore, before patients rise from bed, they should lay quietly in bed for a few minutes.

In general, four strategies are recommended to reduced cardiac events in the early morning, especially for people with any cardiac disease: waking up at the end of rapid eye movement sleep, laying in bed for a few minutes after awakening, slowly raising the body from bed, and staying relaxed at least 30 minutes after awakening. Staying relaxed in 30 minutes is suggested because the once increased norepinephrine spillover by standing mostly decreased after 30 minutes (Jacob et al., 1998). Relaxation therapy is also recommended in the morning to control sympathetic nervous activation in patients with cardiac disease (Benson et al., 1974; Guzzetta, 1989; Hoffman et al., 1982; Melville, 1987).

From a preventive perspective for self-care, health professionals might intervene in awakening behavior to control one of the risk factors that triggers cardiac events in the morning. Based on findings of this review, an experimental study should be conducted to identify the effects of interventions associated with the four wakening behaviors identified.

In conclusion, evidence indicates that activation of the sympathetic nervous system due to physical stress in the morning is a significant factor causing morning cardiac events in relation to the pattern of REM and non-REM sleep stages in patients with atherosclerosis. In addition to controlling the major cardiac risk factors causing cardiac events, four strategies for controlling the abrupt upright position at wakening should be included in patient education to reduce cardiac events for patients with cardiac disease. These strategies include waking up at the end of REM sleep, laying in bed for a few minutes after awakening, slowly raising the body from bed, and staying relaxed at least 30 minutes after awakening. Health professionals play vital roles on identifying novel behavioral risk factors that trigger morning cardiac events. Because it is important to maintain continuity of the activity, rest, sleep cycle of daily life in patients with cardiac disease, strategies for patient education should focus on preventive behaviors that control triggers of cardiac events.

5. Clinical implications for managing behavioral risk factors for morning cardiac events

Health professionals should develop educational strategies to reduce the frequency of cardiac events by modifying the patient behaviors such as abruptly assuming an upright position upon awakening in the morning. When patients wake up, they should stay in bed for few minutes and slowly sit up, then stand and walk in relaxed manner. In addition, running up and down stairs, smoking, mental stress, and other behaviors immediately after awakening should be avoided.

6. References

Ahmadizad, S., EI-Sayed, M.S., & Maclaren, D.P. (2006). Responses of Platelet Activation and Function to a Single Bout of Resistance Exercise and Recovery. *Clinical Hemorheology and Microcirculation,* Vo.35, No.1-2, pp159-168, ISSN 1386-0291

Andrews, N.P., Goldstein, D.S., & Quyyumi, A.A. (1999). Effect of Systemic Alpha-2 Adrenagic Blockade on the Morning Increase in Platelet Aggragation in Normal Subjects. *American Journal of Cardiology,* Vol.84, No.3, pp. 316-320, ISSN 0002-9149

Andrews, N.P.,Gralnick, H.R., & Merryman, P., et al. (1996). Mechanisms Underlying the Morning Increase in Platelet Aggregation: a Flow Cytometry Study. *American Journal of Cardiology,* Vol.28, No.7, pp.1789-1795,ISSN 0002-9149

Aserinsky, E., & Kieitman, N.(1953). Regularly Occurring Periods of Eye Motility and Concomitant Phenomena during Sleep. *Science,* Vol.118, No.3062, pp. 273-274, ISSN 0036-8075

Aserinsky, E. & Kleitman, N. (2003). Regularly Occurring Periods of Eye Motility and Concomitant Phenomena during Sleep. 1953. *Journal of Neuropsychiatry Clinical Neuroscience,* Vol.15, No.4, pp. 454-455, ISSN 0895-0172

Athyros, V.G., Didangelos, T. P., & Karamitsos, D. T., et al. (1998).Long-term Effect of Converting Enzyme Inhibition on Circadian Sympathetic and Parasympathetic Modulation in Patients with Diabetic Autonomic Neuropathy. *Acta Cardiologica,* Vol.53, No.4, pp.201-109, ISSN 0001-5385

Atkinson, G. & Davenne, D. (2007). Relationship between Sleep, Physical Activity and Human Health. *Physiology & Behavior,* Vol.90, No.2-3, pp. 229-235, ISSN 0031-9384

Atkinson, G., Jones, H. & Ainslie, P.N. (2010). Circadian Variation in the Circulatory Responses to Exercise: Relevance to the Morning Peaks in Strokes and Cardiac Events. *European Journal of Applied Physiology,* Vol.108, No.1, pp. 15-29, ISSN 1439-6319.

Atkinson, G., Drust, B., & George, K. (2006). Chronobiological Considerations for Exercise and Heart Disease. *Sports Medicine,* Vol.36, No.6, pp. 487-500, ISSN 0112-1642

Baran, K.W., Bache, R.J., & Dai, X.Z., et al. (1992).Effect of α- adrenergic Blocked with Prazosin on Large Coronary Diameter during Exercise. *Circulation,* Vol.85, No. 3, pp. 1139-1145, ISSN 0009-7322

Baas, L.S. (2004). Self-care Resources and Activity as Predictors of Quality of Life in Persons after Myocardial Infarction. *Dimensions of Critical Care Nursing,* Vol.23, No.3, pp. 131-138, ISSN 0730-4625

Baxendale, L.M. (1992). Pathophysiology of Coronary Artery Disease. *Nursing Clinic of North America,*Vol.27, No.1, pp143-152, ISSN 0029-6465

Benhorin, J., Banai, S., & Moriel, M., et al. (1993). Circadian Variations in Ischemic Threshold and Their Relation to the Occurrence of Ischemic Episodes. *Circulation,* Vol.87, No.3, pp. 808-814, ISSN 0009-7322

Benson, H., Rosner, B.A., & Marzetta, B.R., et al (1974). Decreased Blood Pressure in Pharmacologically Treated Hypertensive Patients Who Regularly Elicited the Relaxation Response. *Lancet,* Vol.1, No.7852, pp. 289-291, ISSN 0140-6736

Braunwald, E. (1995). Morning Resistance to Thrombolytic Therapy. *Circulation,* Vol.91, No.5, pp. 1604-1606, ISSN 0009-7322

Brezinski, D.A., Tofler, G.H., & Muller, J.E., et al.(1988). Morning Increase in Platelet Aggragability. Association with Assumption of the Upright Posture. *Circulation,* Vol.78, No. 1, pp. 35-40, ISSN 0009-7322

Camici, P.G., Gistri,R., & Lorenzoni, R., et al. (1992). Coronary Reserve and Exercise ECG in Patients with Chest Pain and Normal Coronary Angiograms. *Circulation,* Vol.86, No.1, pp179-186, ISSN 0009-7322

Cappuccio, F.P., Cooper, D., & D'Elia, L., et al. (2011). Sleep Duration Predicts Cardiovascular Outcomes: a Systematic Review and Meta-analysis of Prospective Studies. *European Heart Journal,* Vol.32, No.12, pp.1484-1492, ISSN 0195-668X

Carnethon, M.R., Liao, D., & Evans, G.W., et al. (2002). Does the Cardiac Autonomic Response to Postural Change Predict Incident Coronary Heart Disease and

Mortality? The Atherosclerosis Risk in Communities Study. *American Journal of Epidemiology,* Vol.155, No.1, pp. 48-56, ISSN 0002-9262

Condon, C. & McCarthy, G. (2006). Lifestyle Changes Following Acute Myocardial Infarction: Patients Perspectives. *European Journal of Cardiovascular Nursing,* Vol.5, No.1, pp. 37-44, ISSN 1479-5151

Cooke-Ariel, H. (1998). Circadian Variation in Cardiovascular Function and their Relation to the Occurrence and Timing of Cardiac Events. *American Journal of Health-System Pharmacy,* Vol. 55, Suppl.3, pp.S5-S11, ISSN 1079-2082

Critchley, H.D., Taggart, P., & Sutton, P.M., et al. (2005). Mental Stress and Sudden Cardiac Death: Asymmetric Midbrain Activity as a Linking Mechanism. *Brain,* Vol.128, (Pt 1), pp. 75-85, ISSN 0006-8950

Culebras, A. (1992). The Neurology of Sleep: Introduction. *Neurology,* Vol. 42, (7 Supple 6), pp. 6-8, ISSN 0028-3878

Deedwania, P.C. (1996). Hemodynamic Changes as Triggers of Cardiovascular Events. *Cardiology Clinics,* Vol.14, No.2, pp. 229-238, ISSN 0733-8651

Drager, L.F., Ueno, L.M., & Lessa, P.S., et al. (2009). Sleep-related Changes in Hemodynamic and Autonomic Regulation in Human Hypertension. *Journal of Hypertension,* Vol.27, No.8, pp. 1655-1663, ISSN 0263-6352

Duncker, D.J., Zhang, J., & Bache, R, J. (1993). Coronary Pressure-flow Relation in Left Ventricular Hypertrophy. Importance of Changes in Back Pressure versus Changes in Minimum Resistance. *Circulation Research,* Vol.72, No. 3, pp579-587, ISSN 0009-7330

Ebrahim, S., Beswick, A., & Burke, M. et al. (2006). Multiple Risk Factor Interventions for Primary Prevention of Coronary Heart Disease. *Cochrane Database System Reviews (Online),* (4), CD001561. ISSN 1469-493X

Ebrahim, S., Taylor, F.,& Ward, K., et al. (2011). Multiple Risk Factor Interventions for Primary Prevention of Coronary Heart Disease. *Cochrane Database System Reviews (Online),* (1), CD001561. ISSN 1469-493X

Eisenhofer, G., Esler, M.D., & Meredith, I.T., et al. (1992). Sympathetic Nervous Function in Human Heart as Assessed by Cardiac Spillovers of Dihydroxyphenylglycol and Norepinephrine. *Circulation,* Vol.85, No.5, pp. 1775-1785, ISSN 0009-7322

Figueras, J., & Lidon, R.M. (1995). Early Morning Reduction in Ischemic Threshold in Patients with Unstable Angina and Significant Coronary Disease. *Circulation,* Vol. 92, No.7, pp. 1737-1742, ISSN 0009-7322

Freed, C.D., Thomas, S.A., & Lynch, J.J., et al. (1989). Blood Pressure, Heart Rate, and Heart Rhythm Changes in Patients with Heart Disease during Talking. *Heart & Lung,* Vol.18, No.1, pp. 17-22, ISSN 0147-9563

Fujita, M. & Franklin, D. (1987). Diurnal Changes in Coronary Blood Flow in Conscious Dogs. *Circulation,* Vol.76, No.2, pp. 488-491, ISSN 0009-7322

Furchgott, R.F., & Zawadzki,J.V. (1980).The Obligatory Role of Endothelial Cells in the Relaxation of Arterial Smooth Muscle by Acethlcholine. *Nature,* Vol.288 , No.5789, pp.373-376, ISSN 0028-0836

Furchgott, R.F. (1983). Role of Endothelium in Responses of Vascular Smooth Muscle. *Circulation Research,* Vol.53, No.5, pp. 557-573, ISSN 0009-7330

Furukawa, F., Kazuma, K., & Kojima, M., et al. (2008). Effects of an Off-site Walking Program of Fibrinogen and Exercise Energy Expenditure in Women. *Asian Nursing Research,* Vol.2, No.1, pp. 35-45, ISSN 1976-1317

Furukawa, F., Nagano, M., & Ueda, E., et al. (1998). Mechanisms of Ischemic Morning Episodes of Coronary Artery Disease Following Awakening: a Review. *Tenri Medical Bulletin,* Vol.1, No.1, pp. 126-138, ISSN 1433-1817

Giles, T. (2005). Relevance of Blood Pressure Variation in the Circadian Onset of Cardiovascular Events. *Journal of Hypertension Supplement,* Vol.23, Suppl 1, pp. S35-S39, ISSN 0952-1178

Greenberg, S.S., Diecke, F.P., & Peevy, K., et al.(1990). Release of Norepinephrine from Adrenagic Nerve Endings of Blood Vessels is Modulated by Endothelium-derived Relaxing Factor. *American Journal of Hypertension,*Vol.3, No.3, pp. 211-218, ISSN 0895-7061

Guzzetta, C.E. (1989). Effects of Relaxation and Music Therapy on Patients in a Coronary Care Unit with Presumptive Acute Myocardial Infarction. *Heart & Lung,* Vol.18, No.6, pp. 609-619, ISSN 0147-9563

Hammond, H.K., Roth, D.A., & Insel, P.A., et al. (1992). Myocardial Beta-adrenergic Receptor Expression and Signal Transduction after Chronic Volume-overload Hypertrophy and Circulatory Congestion.*Circulation,*Vol.85, No.1, pp. 269-280, ISSN 0009-7322.

Herd, J.A. (1991). Cardiovascular Response to Stress. *Physiological Reviews,* Vol.71, No.1, pp. 305-330, ISSN 0031-9333

Hilberg, T., Nowacki, P.E., & Muller-Berghaus, G., et al. (2000). Changes in Blood Coagulation and Fibrinolysis Associated with Maximal Exercise and Physical Conditioning in Women Taking Low Dose Oral Contraceptives. *Journal of Science and Medicine in Sport,* Vol.3, No.4, pp.383-390, ISSN 1440-2440

Hjalmarson, A., Gilpin, E.A., & Nicod, P., et al.(1989). Differing Circadian Patterns of Symptom Onset in Subgroups of Patients with Acute Myocardial Infarction. *Circulation,* Vol.80, No.2, pp. 267-275, ISSN 0009-7322

Hoffman, J.W., Benson, H., & Arns,P.A., et al. (1982). Reduced Sympathetic Nervous System Responsivity Associated with the Relaxation Response. *Science,* Vol.215, No.4529, pp. 190-192, ISSN 0036-8075

Jacob, G., Ertl, A.C., & Shannon, J.R., et al. (1998). Effect of Standing on Neurohumoral Responses and Plasma Volume in Healthy Subjects. *Journal of Applied Physiology,* Vol.84, No.3, pp. 914-921, ISSN 8750-7587

Jouvet, M. (1967).Neurophysiology of the States of Sleep. *Physiological Reviews,* Vol.47, No.2, pp.117-177, ISSN 0031-9333

Jay, R.H., Rampling, M.W., & Betteridge, D.J. (1990). Abnormalities of Blood Rheology in Familial Hypercholesterolaema: Effects of Treatment. *Atherosclerosis,* Vol.85, No,2-3, pp. 249-256, ISSN 0021-9150

Kaul, S., Waack, B.J., & Padgett, R.C., et al. (1993).Altered Vascular Responses to Platelets from Hypercholesterolemic humans, .*Circulation Research,* Vol.72, No.4, pp. 737-743, ISSN 0009-7330.

Khoury, A.F., Sunderajan, P., & Kaplan, N.M. (1992). The Early Morning Rise in Blood Pressure is Related Mainly to Ambulation. *American Journal of Hypertension,* Vol. 5, No.(6 Pt 1), pp. 339-344, ISSN 0895-7061

Kiowski, W., & Osswald, S. (1993).Circadian Variation of Ischemic Cardiac Events. *Journal of Cardiovascular Pharmacology,* Vol.21, Suppl 2, ppS45-S48, ISSN 0160-2446

Krantz, D.S., Kop,W.J., & Gabbay, F.H., et al.(1996). Circadian Variation of Ambulatory Myocardial lschermia: Triggering by Daily Activities and Evidence for an Endogenous Circadian Component. *Circulation,* Vol.93, No.7, pp. 1364-1371, ISSN 0009-7322

Kristofferzon, M.L., Lofmark, R., & Carlsson, M. (2007). Striving for Balance in DailyLlife: Experiences of Swedish Women and Men Shortly after a Myocardial Infarction, *Journal of Clinical Nursing,*Vol.16, No.2, pp. 391-401, ISSN 0962-1067.

Kuo, L.,Arko, F., & Chilian, W.M., et al. (1993). Coronary Vascular Responses to Flow and Pressure, *Circulation Research,* Vol.72, No.3, pp. 607-615, ISSN 0009-7330

Laxson, D.D., Dai, X.Z., & Homan, D.C., et al. (1992). Coronary Vasodilator Reserve in Ischemic Myocardium of the Exercising Dog.*Circulation,*Vol.85, No.1, pp. 313-322, ISSN 0009-7322

Leary, A.C., Struthers, A.D., & Donnan, P.T., et al. (2002). The Morning Surge in Blood Pressure and Heart Rate is Dependent on Levels of Physical Activity after Waking. *Journal of Hypertension,* Vol.20, No.5, pp. 865-870, ISSN 0263-6352

Linsell, CR., Lightman, S.L., & Mullen, P.E., et al.(1985). Circulation Rhythms of Epinephrine and Norepinephrine in Man. *Journal of Clinical Endocrinology & Metabolism.* Vol. 60, No.6, pp.1210-1215, ISSN 0021-972X

Lowe, G.D., Drummond, M.M., & Lorimer, A,R., et al. (1980). Relation between Extent of Coronary Artery Disease and Blood Viscosity. *British Medical Journal,* Vol.280, No.6215, pp. 673-674, ISSN 0959-8138

Li, J.J. (2003). Circadian Variation in Myocardial Ischemia: the Possible Mechanisms Involving in this Phenomenon. *Medical Hypotheses,* Vol.61, No.2, pp. 240-243, ISSN 0306-9877

Lucchesi, B. (1990). Myocardial Ischemia, Reperfusion, and Free Radical Injury. *American Journal of Cardiology,* Vol.65, No.19, pp.141-231, ISSN 0002-9149

Ludmer, P.L., Selwyn, A.P., & Shook, T.L., et al.(1986). Paradoxical Vasoconstriction Induced by Acetylcholine in Atherosclerotic Coronary Arteries. *The New England Journal of Medicine,* Vol. 315, No.17, pp. 1046-1051, ISSN 0028-4793

Martin, R.J. (1984). Cardiorespiratory Disorders during Sleep. 2nd. Future Pub Co., ISBN 978-0-87993-208-4, New York, USA

Masuda, T., Ogawa, H., & Miyao, Y. (1994). Circadian Variation in Fibrinolytic Activity in Patients with Variant Angina. *British Heart Journal,* Vol.71, No.2, pp.156-161, ISSN 0007-0769

Meller, J., Goldsmith, S. J., & Rudin, A. (1979). Spectrum of Exercise Thallium-201 Myocardial Perfusion Imaging in Pateints with Chest Pain and Normal Coronary Angiograms. *American Journal of Cardiology,* Vol.43, No.4, pp. 717-723, ISSN 0002-9149

Melvile, S.B. (1987). Relaxation Techniques in Acute Myocardial Infarction: the Theoretic Rationale. *Focus on Critical Care,* Vol.14, No.1, pp. 9-11, ISSN 0736-3605

Mulcahy, D.(1999). "Circadian" Variation in Cardiovascular Events and Implications for Therapy? *Journal of Cardiovascular Phamacology,* Vol.34, Suppl 2, pp. S3-S8, Disscussion, S29-S31, ISSN 0160-2446

Mulcahy, D., Keegan, J., & Cunningham, D., et al. (1998). Circadian Variation of Total Ischemic Burden and Its Alteration with Anti-anginal Agents. *Lancet,* Vol.2, No.8614, pp. 755-759, ISSN 0140-6736

Muller, J.E., Ludmer, P.L., & Willich, S.N., et al. (1987). Circadian Variation in the Frequency of Sudden Cardiac Death. *Circulation*, Vol.75, No. 1, pp. 131-138, ISSN 0009-7322

Muller, J.E., Tofler, G.H., & Stone, P.H. (1989). Circadian Variation and Triggers of Onset of Acute Cardiovascular Disease. *Circulation,* Vol. 79, No.4, pp. 733-743, ISSN 0009-7322

Murray, P.M., Herrington, D.M., & Pettus, C.W., et al. (1993).Should Patients with Heart Disease Exercise in the Morning or Afternoon. *Archives of Internal Medicine,* Vol.153, No.7, pp. 833-836, ISSN 0003-9926

Norris, C.M., Ghali, W.A., & Galbraith, P.D., et al. (2004). Women with Coronary Artery Disease Report Worse Health-related Quality of Life Outcomes Compared to Men. Health and Quality of Life Outcomes, Vo.2, No. 21, pp.1-11 (page number not for citation pruposes), Published online 2005 May 5 doi:10. ISSN 1186/1477-7525-2-21.

Ohkubo, T., Metoki, H., & Imai, Y. (2008). Prognostic Significance of Morning Surge in Blood Pressure: Which Definition, Which Outcome? *Blood Pressure Monitoring,* Vol.13, No,3, pp.161-162, ISSN 1359-5237

Oparil, S., Vassaux, C., & Sanders, C.A., et al. (1970).Role of Renin in Acute Postural Hemostasis.*Circulation,*Vol.41, No.1, pp. 89-95, ISSN 0009-7322.

Palmieri, V., Celentano, A., & Roman, M.J., et al. (2003). Relation of Fibrinogen to Cardiovascular Events is Independent of Preclinical Cardiovascular Disease: the Strong Heart Study. *American Heart Journal,* Vol.145, No.3, pp. 467-474, ISSN 0002-8703

Pernow, J., Lundberg, J.M., & Kaijser, L. (1988). Alph-adrenoceptor Influence on Plasma Level of Neuropeptide Y-like Immunoreactivity and Catecholamines during Rest and Sympathoadrenal Activation in Humans. *Journal of Cardiovascular Phamacology,*Vol.12, No.5, pp. 593-599, ISSN 0160-2446

Peters R.W., Brooks, M.M., & Zoble, R.G., et al. (1996). Chronobiology of Acute Myocardial Infarction: Cardiac Arrhythmia Suppression Trial (CAST) Experience. *The American Journal of Cardiology, Vol.*78, No.11, pp.1198-1201, ISSN 0002-9149

Quyyumi, A.A. (1990).Circadian Rhythms in Cardiovascular Disease. *American Heart Journal.*Vol.120, No.3, pp.726-733, ISSN 0002-8703

Quyyumi, A.A., Panza, J.A., & Diodati,J.G., et al. (1992). Circadian Variation in Ischemic Threshold: A Mechanimic Underlying the Circadian Variation in Ischemic Events. *Circulation,* Vol.86, No.1, pp. 22-28, ISSN 0009-7322

Redon, J. (2004). The Normal Circadian Pattern of Blood Pressure: Implications for Treatment. *International Journal of Clinical Practice,*Vol.58, Supplement 145, pp. 3-8 ISSN 1368-504X

Rocco, M.B. (1990). Timing and Triggers of Transient Myocardial Ischemia. *American Journal of Cardiology.*Vol.66, No.16, pp. 18G-21G, ISSN 0002-9149

Schachter, M. (2004).Diurnal Rhythms, the Rennin-angiotensin System and Antihypertensive Therapy. *British Journal of Cardiology,* Vol.11, No. 4, pp. 287-290, ISSN 0969-6113

Scheer, F.A., Hu, K., & Evoniuk, H., et al. (2010). Impact of the Human Circadian System, Exercise, and Their Interaction on Cardiovascular Function. *Proceeding of National*

Academy of Science of the United States of America, Vol. 107, No.47, pp20541-20546, ISSN 0027-8424

Shimada, K., Kario, K., & Umeda, Y., et al. (2001). Early Morning Surge in Blood Pressure. *Blood Pressure Monitoring,* Vol.6, No.6, pp. 349-353, ISSN 1359-5237

Shiotani, H., Umegaki, Y., & Tanaka, M.., et al. (2009).Effects of Aerobic Exercise on the Circadian Rhythm of Heart Rate and Blood Pressure. *Chronobiology International,* Vol.26, No.8, pp. 1636-1646, ISSN 0742-0528

Steriade, M. (1992). Basic Mechanisms of Sleep Generation. *Neurology,* Vol.42, 7Supple 6, pp. 9-17, ISSN 0028-3878

Stone, P.H. (1990). Triggers of Transient Myocardial Ischemia: Circadian Variation and Relation to Plaque Rupture and Coronary Thrombosis in Stable Coronary Artery Disease. *American Journal of Cardiology.*Vol.66, No.16, pp. 32G-36G, ISSN 0002-9149

Storm, D.S., Metzger, B.L., & Therrien, B. (1989). Effects of Age on Autonomic Cardiovascular Responsiveness in Healthy Men and Women. *Nursing Research,* Vol.38, No.6, pp. 326-300, ISSN 0029-6562

Sugiishi, M., & Takatsu, F. (1993). Cigarette Smoking is a Major Risk Factor for Coronary Spasms. *Circulation,* Vol. 87, No.1, pp. 76-79, ISSN 0009-7322

Svendsen, J.H., Sheikh, S.P., & Jorgensen, J., et al. (1990). Effect of Neuropeptide Y on Regulation of Blood Flow Rate in Canine Myocardium. *American Journal of Physiology,* Vol.259, No.6, pt 2, pp.H1709-H1717, ISSN 0363-6135

Thrall, G., Lane, D., & Carroll, D., et al. (2007). A Systematic Review of the Prothrimbotic Effects of an Acute Change in Posture: a Possible Mechanism Underlying the Morning Excess in Cardiovascular Events? *Chest,* Vol.132, No.4, pp. 1337-1347, ISSN 0012-3692

Tofler, G.H., Brezinski, D., & Schafter, A.I., et al. (1987). Concurrent Morning Increase in Platelet Aggregability and the Risk of Myocardial Infarction and Sudden Cardiac Death. *New England Journal of Medicine,* Vol.316, No.24, pp. 1514-1518, ISSN 0028-4793

Umemura, S., Tochikubo, O., & Noda, K. (1987). Changes in Blood Pressure and Plasma Norepinephrine during Sleep in Essential Hypertension. *Japanese Circulation Journal.* Vol. 51, No.11, pp1250-1256, ISSN 0047-1828

van Eekelen, A.P., Houtveen, J.H. & Kerkhof, G.A. (2004a). Circadian Variation in Cardiac Autonomic Activity: Rreactivity Measurements to Different Type of Stressors. *Chronobiology International,* Vol.21, No.1, pp107-129, ISSN 0742-0528

van Eekelen, A.P., Houtveen, J.H., & Kerkhof, G.A.(2004b).Circadian Variation in Base Rate Measures of Cardiac Autonomic Activity. European Journal of Applied Physiology, Vol.93, No.1-2. pp.39-46, ISSN 1439-6319

Vanhoutte, A.M., & Huston, D.S. (1985).Platelets, Endothelium and Vasospasm. *Circulation,* Vol.72, No.4, pp. 728-743, ISSN 0009-7322

Viola, A.U., Simon, C., & Ehrhart, J., et al. (2002). Sleep Processes Exert a Predominant Influence on the 24-h Profile of Heart Rate Variability. *Journal of Biological Rhythms,* Vol.17, No.6, pp. 539-547, ISSN 0748-7304

West, J.B. (1990). *Best and Taylor's Physiological Basis of Medical Practice.* 12thed, Williams & Wilkins, ISBN 0-683-08947-1, Baltimore, USA

White, W.B. (2001). Cardiovascular Risk and Therapeutic Intervention for the Early Morning Surge in Blood Pressure and Heart Rate. *Blood Pressure Monitoring,* Vol.6, No.2, pp.63-72, ISSN 1359-5237

White, W.B. (2003). Relevance of Blood Pressure Variation in the Circadian Onset of Cardiovascular Events. *Journal of Hypertension, Supplement,* Vol. 21(S6), pp. S9-S15, ISSN 0952-1178

Willich, S.N., Levy, D., & Rocco, M.B., et al. (1987). Circadian Variation in the Incidence of Sudden Cardiac Death in the Framingham Heart Study Population. *American Journal of Cardiology,* Vol.60, No.10, pp.801-806, ISSN 0002-9149

Willis, W.D. & Grossman, R.G. (1981).*Medical Neurobiology.* 3rd CV Mosby Co, ISBN 978-0-8016-5582-1, St. Luis, USA

Yang, T., & Levy, M.N. (1993). Effects of Intense Antecedent Sympathetic Stimulation on Sympathetic Neurotransmission in the Heart. *Circulation Research,*Vol.72, No.1, pp. 137-144, ISSN 0009-7330

Yarnell, J.W., Baker, I.A., & Sweetnam, P.M., et al. (1991). Firbirnogen, Viscosity, and White Blood Cell Count are Major Risk Factors for Ischemic Heart Disease. The Caerphilly and Speedwell Collaborative Heart Disease Studies. *Circulation,* Vol.83, No.3, pp.836-844, ISSN 0009-7322

Young, M.A., &Vatner, S.F. (1986). Regulation of Large Coronary Arteries. *Circulation Research,* Vol.59, No.6, pp. 579-596, ISSN 0009-7330

Zemel, P.C. , & Sowers, J.R. (1990). Relation between Lipids and Atherosclerosis: Epidemiologic Evidence and Clinical Implications. *American Journal of Cardiology,* Vol.66, No. 21, pp.71-121, ISSN 0002-9149

21

Health Related Quality of Life in Coronary Patients

María Dueñas, Alejandro Salazar, Begoña Ojeda and Inmaculada Failde
Preventive Medicine and Public Health Department, University of Cádiz, Spain

1. Introduction

The increase observed in the survival of patients with ischemic cardiopathy, together with the effect of the disease on the social, professional, and family life of those suffering from it, have led researchers to consider that the traditional ways of measuring morbidity and mortality are not adequate for assessing the potential benefits of health care interventions. For this reason, there is common agreement on the need to use an indicator of subjective assessment of health, and of health related quality of life (HRQL), as a complementary criterion for monitoring the results of medical interventions in these patients.

The term "quality of life" (QoL) or health related quality of life (HRQL) came into use during the 1970s as a multidimensional concept reflecting the overall subjective condition of the physical and mental welfare of the individual, which is a consequence not only of the disease but also of the family and social conditions forming the patient's environment.

The assessment of these patients' HRQL has been tackled by several authors using both disease-specific and generic instruments such as the Nottingham Health Profile, the Sickness Impact Profile, the SF-36 or the SF-12 health questionnaire. Both types of instrument have advantages and disadvantages, and they may provide additional information since they quantify the patient's overall health.

Using different multidimensional measures, poorer HRQL has been observed in patients with Acute Myocardial Infarction (AMI) and angina pectoris than in other populations, and these differences have been related to low social class, female sex, the presence of mental disorders and the severity of the clinical condition.

Measuring changes in the HRQL of coronary patients is also important as a way of assessing interventions and predicting needs for social care, because it has been shown that the focus of attention in the immediate period following a cardiac attack is generally the physical functioning, but following discharge from hospital and in the longer term, general health, vitality, social and emotional functions could be at least as important.

In this chapter, we aim to provide an overview of the concept of HRQL and the usefulness of this measure from the perspective of a coronary patient. Likewise, we intend to review the main instruments used to assess HRQL and we analyse the factors that have been seen to affect the quality of life of these patients.

2. Quality of Life and heart disease

2.1 The concept of Quality of Life and Health-Related Quality of Life

Quality of Life has generated interest for many years, and as early as 384-322 BC Aristotle noted "the good life" or "doing well" to be the same as "being happy". However, the advent of this concept as it is known today, and concern for its systematic and scientific assessment, is relatively recent. In the field of health sciences, one of the most important advances in recent decades has been to recognise that patients' perspective of their illness is just as legitimate and valid as that of healthcare professionals. This has led to the need to define the concept of Health Related Quality of Life (HRQL) and to its assessment as a way of subjectively measuring its effect on a disease. In addition, its treatment is considered with growing frequency as an indicator of the advances and innovations in healthcare services (Casas Anguita et al., 2001).

The most widely accepted definition of Quality of Life at the present time was proposed in 1994 by the World Health Organization (WHO); it is considered as an individual's perception of their position in life in the context of the culture and value systems in which they live and in relation to their goals, expectations, standards and concerns (Group, World Health Organization Quality of Life (WHOQOL), 1993). The term Health-Related Quality of Life (HRQL) emerged later to distinguish between QoL in its more general sense and the requirements of clinical medicine and clinical trials, and thus remove ambiguity. Shumaker et al. defined it as people´s subjective evaluations of the influences of their current health status, health care, and health promoting activities on their ability to achieve and maintain a level of overall functioning that allows them to pursue valued life goals and that is reflected in their general well-being. Although there is disagreement about which dimensions should be included in HRQL assessments, these authors have specified that the domains of functioning that are critical to HRQL include: social, physical and cognitive functioning; mobility and self-care; and emotional well-being (Shumaker & Berzon, 1995).

HRQL acts as a point of reference for measuring the effect of a disease on the individual, and is described and characterized by the patients themselves as the result of their appraisal of their health care (Urzúa M, 2010). One unifying and non-controversial theme throughout all the approaches is that this concept can only be assessed by subjective measures. It is precisely their subjective and multidisciplinary nature that has led to them being more widely used to complement the traditional physiological and biological measures of health status. However, their assessment requires instruments with suitable psychometric properties, something which must be taken into consideration before their implementation.

2.2 Assessing Quality of Life in coronary patients

One area of health care that has taken particular interest in the concept and measurement of Health-Related Quality of Life involves patients with coronary heart disease. This disease, besides being the main cause of death worldwide, has significant physical, emotional and social consequences for sufferers, so assessing their quality of life is not only necessary for assessing the success of a treatment or operation, but also for highlighting certain problems which are not assessed by traditional methods and that may be of use for modifying or improving the treatment given, or for providing alternatives that improve patients' clinical course (Fayers & Machin, 2007). Considering that the management of coronary artery disease mainly involves leading a healthy life style, instruments for measuring HRQL are one of the best ways of providing an assessment of the experience of the patients themselves with regard to their health problems in areas such a physical, emotional or social functioning, role accomplishment, pain and fatigue (Asadi-Lari et al., 2003).

Despite the accepted interest in the assessment of HRQL in coronary patients, one of the main problems posed in clinical practice is the choice of the right instrument. When choosing a tool to assess HRQL, researchers or clinicians must first consider whether the chosen instrument has really been developed and validated in a population with similar characteristics, and if it covers all the aspects that it is important to assess in coronary patients.

To be used with confidence, the tools must have a series of characteristics such as: validity, or the degree to which it measures what it aims to measure; reliability, or the degree to which a measure provides similar values for people with the same quality of life; and sensitivity to change, or the degree to which a measure manages to detect significant changes appropriate to clinical changes (Cepeda-Valery et al., 2011). Furthermore, these tools must be complete; that is, they must include all the aspects that may be affected by the disease and they should be easy to score and interpret. This last aspect is of utmost importance in clinical settings as being quick and easy to use are necessary qualities under these circumstances (McDowell & Newell, 1996).

The most widely-used tools for measuring the HRQL of coronary patients can be grouped in two types: generic and specific (Table 1). Both kinds have pros and cons, and deciding which to use depends on the type of intervention to be assessed and the aims to be reached. In general, generic tools are able to detect the effects on the health of a broad range of patients and diseases and so comparisons can be established between the effect of heart disease and that of other chronic diseases such as diabetes or COPD on HRQL. However, generic measures are less sensitive at detecting the effect that the specific symptoms of heart disease have on a patient's life.

		Dimensions	Items
Generic	SF-36	8	36
	SF-12		12
	EroQol (EQ-5D)	5	16
Specific	Seattle Angina Questionnaire (SAQ)	5	19
	The Angina Pectoris Quality of Life Questionnaire (APQLQ)	4	22
	Myocardial Infarction Dimensional Assessment Scale (MIDAS)	7	35
	The MacNew Heart Disease Health-related Quality of Life instrument (MacNew)	3	27
	Cardiovascular Limitations and Symptoms Profile (CLASP)	9	37

Table 1. Health Related Quality of Life Instruments for Coronary Disease

The IQOLA project (International Quality of Life Assessment) (Alonso et al., 2004; Gandek et al., 1998), which studied the general population in eight countries, is one of the few projects to examine the impact of a series of chronic diseases, including coronary disease, on HRQL. In this project, which used the SF-36 health questionnaire to assess HRQL, it is interesting to note how quality of life is affected in different ways depending on the chronic disease analysed. At the present time, the Medical Outcomes Study 36-item Short-Form Health Survey (SF-36) used in this project is the most valid instrument for measuring the quality of life of patients with coronary disease and its use has been proven in the clinical forms of both angina and myocardial infarction (Failde & Ramos, 2000). Likewise, it is an appropriate tool for use in patients who undergo heart surgery and as an evaluative measure in intervention programmes (Brown et al., 1999; Dougherty et al., 1998; Hawkes & Mortensen, 2006; Yu et al., 2003).

There are two versions of the SF-36 health questionnaire. Version 1, developed by Ware et al in the USA in 1992 (Ware et al., 1993) and version 2, revised and published by Ware himself (Ware, 2000). The latter, an improved version of the original, is made up of 36 items grouped into 8 dimensions: Physical Functioning (10 items), Social Functioning (2 items), Role-Physical (4 items) , Role-Emotional (3 items), Mental Health (5 items), Vitality (4 items), Bodily Pain (2 items), and General Health (6 items). For each of the 8 dimensions, the items are coded, aggregated and transformed to a scale ranging from 0 (the worst state of health for that dimension) to 100 (the best state of health). The instrument was not designed to produce of global index. However, it is possible to calculate two summary scores by combining the scores of each dimension: the physical and mental summary measures (PCS and MCS).

One of the short forms of this questionnaire, the SF-12, has also been shown to possess suitable psychometric properties for use in this field of medicine, and has been shown to have the advantage of being quicker to carry out while achieving the same results as the SF-36 (Failde et al., 2009). However, some studies carried out on patients after an acute myocardial infarction have found that the results of the SF-12 may not detect significant differences between the domains of QL affected by the disease, although this has been improved in version 2 of the questionnaire, in which it is possible to assess the same 8 dimensions included in the SF-36, and the summary dimensions (physical and mental). In patients with a recent myocardial infarction, the SF-36 has also been shown to be more sensitive at detecting improvements in HRQL after active intervention (Thompson & Yu, 2003).

Another of the most widely-used instruments for assessing HRQL is the EuroQol (EQ-5D). Like the SF-36, this questionnaire can be applied to a wide range of diseases. It provides a simple descriptive profile and a single index value for health status. The EQ-5D has three parts. The first enables the respondent to define their health status in accordance with the EQ-5D multi-attribute scale and is composed of 5 dimensions (mobility, self-care, usual activities, pain/discomfort, and anxiety/depression). Each of these has 3 levels of severity, where a higher score corresponds with a worse health status. The second part is a visual analogical scale ranging from 0 (worst health status imaginable) to 100 (best health status imaginable). The third part gathers other anonymous data to provide a demographic characterization of the group studied (Williams, 1990). This questionnaire has been validated among populations with heart disease and has been shown to possess good psychometric characteristics when compared with other previously-validated generic tools used with these populations (Ellis et al., 2005; Nowels et al., 2005).

In a recently published review it was revealed that the Stratification of EQ-5D index scores by disease severity decreased from a mean of 0.78 (SD 0.18) to 0.51 (SD 0.21) for mild to severe disease in heart failure patients and from 0.80 (SD 0.05) to 0.45 (SD 0.22) for mild to severe disease in angina patients (Dyer et al., 2010).

Unlike the generic tools mentioned previously, specific instruments which have been developed for one particular disease assess the effect that the disease, in this case coronary artery disease, has on the different dimensions of HRQL. This improves their sensitivity at detecting the clinical changes in the symptoms that most frequently affect individuals. They are also less likely to have a floor or ceiling effect, with high percentages of patients with minimum or maximum scores in the survey not being observed. On the other hand, a drawback with regard to generic tools is that they do not allow for comparisons between groups of patients with different diseases (Thompson & Yu, 2003).

In the field of cardiology, several scales have been developed that are specifically designed to assess the HRQL of patients with angina, myocardial infarction or heart failure. Among the specific tools for assessing the HRQL of patients with angina, one of the most widely used is the Seattle Angina Questionnaire (SAQ) (Spertus et al., 1995). This questionnaire comprises 19 items that quantify 5 relevant clinical domains for coronary disease: physical limitations of the patient due to angina; angina frequency (assessing the frequency of symptoms and the use of medication); angina stability (measuring recent changes in symptoms); treatment satisfaction (assessing general satisfaction, and satisfaction with the treatment and the doctor's explanations); and disease perception (measures the effect of angina on quality of life). All the items use 5 or 6 point descriptive scales. The global score is calculated by adding the score of the items within each dimension and transforming them to a scale of 0 to 100, where the highest scores show better functioning (less physical limitations, less angina, and better quality of life). Regarding its psychometric properties, it appears to have good validity characteristics (Dougherty et al., 1998) and each domain and dimension of the SAQ has been independently validated, proving to be both reliable and sensitive to clinical changes. Furthermore, several studies show that the questionnaire correlates well with variables that influence the disease such as age and gender (Cepeda-Valery et al., 2011).

The Angina Pectoris Quality of Life Questionnaire (APQLQ) (Marquis et al., 1995a) developed in France is another specific instrument for use with coronary patients. It comprises 22 items grouped into 4 domains: physical activity, somatic symptoms, emotional distress, and life satisfaction. The correlations with the SF-36 dimensions were consistent with what was expected. Its reliability, concurrent and clinical validity allowed its use in clinical trials. The distribution of the scores of the APQLQ according to the clinical severity of Angina Pectoris (AP) was as hypothesized: the more severe the AP, the more impaired the Quality of Life (Marquis et al., 1995b).

As with patients with Angina Pectoris, it is important to assess the HRQL of patients who have suffered a myocardial infarction as it provides a holistic examination of the results of treatment and does not only focus on the physical component. A few years ago, a group from the UK developed and validated a specific instrument for this kind of patients (Thompson & Roebuck, 2001) which is commonly used nowadays. Known as the Myocardial Infarction Dimensional Assessment Scale (MIDAS), this tool comprises a 35-item self-administered questionnaire covering seven dimensions related to health status (physical activity, insecurity, emotional reaction, dependency, diet, concerns over medications and side effects). The MIDAS showed excellent content validity, good criterion validity with good internal consistency, and sensitivity to change. Compared with other already validated questionnaires such as the SF-36, this tool showed a good correlation in most of the variables.

The MacNew Heart Disease Health-related Quality of Life instrument (MacNew) is a self-administered scale, a modified version of the original Quality of life after Myocardial Infarction Questionnaire (QLMI) (Oldridge et al., 1991). It is designed to assess the effect of coronary heart disease and its treatment (initially myocardial infarction, then extended to include angina pectoris) on everyday activities, and physical, emotional and social functioning. It comprises 27 items grouped into 3 dimensions: physical limitations, emotional functioning and social functioning. This new version of the instrument has good psychometric properties of validity, reliability and sensitivity to change, and is of proven use with patients after myocardial infarction. (Höfer et al., 2004).

Finally, it should be noted that it is sometimes difficult to establish an accurate diagnosis of coronary disease. It could begin with angina and proceed to a myocardial infarctus or heart failure. In these cases the Cardiovascular Limitations and Symptoms Profile (CLASP) can be extremely useful for assessing HRQL. The main advantage of this instrument is that it makes it possible to assess HRQL through different clinical situations, and is especially useful to check whether symptoms worsen or new ones develop. The CLASP, with 37 items grouped into 9 different dimensions (4 related to symptomatology and 5 with physical limations), can identify where there are difficulties for a patient, their importance, and the best treatment in each case. This instrument has been shown to be a reliable, valid and sensitive measure of health-related quality of life in patients with chronic stable angina (Lewin et al., 2002). However, further research is required before it can be recommended for routine use in clinical practice.

2.3 Factors related to Health Related Quality of Life in coronary patients

As mentioned above, quality of life measures have gained increasing attention as outcome variables in studies of cardiovascular disease in addition to the objective measures of cardiovascular status (Kaplan, 1988). Also, one main goal of coronary artery by-pass grafting (CABG) after a coronary event is to relieve angina and thereby to improve physical activity. This has consequences for work, leisure, mood, social, sexual activities, and also over quality of life (Duits et al., 1997).

Several studies carried out in coronary patients after CABG have shown some improvements in physical, social and sexual functioning (Stanton et al., 1984) as well as working status (Folks et al., 1986) 6 months after the intervention; and decreased anxiety, depression, fatigue, and sleep problems have been also reported at this time in this patients (Jenkins et al., 1983). On the other hand, some authors have found improvements in performance of everyday activities, mental state, and family life one year post-surgery (Mayou & Bryant, 1987) with general health status becoming very similar with those from a normal population (Caine et al., 1991).

Cross-sectional studies carried out in patients with angina and myocardial infarctus have shown that the SF-36 health questionnaire is a valid and reliable instrument for detecting differences between groups of coronary patients defined by age, gender, socio-economic status, and clinical condition (Hemingway et al., 1997a, 1997b), and that it is a useful tool in patients with stable angina (Charlier et al., 1997; Permanyer-Miralda et al., 1991). Likewise, it has been demonstrated using this tool that coronary patients have worse HRQL than general population (Figure 1) (Soto Torres et al., 2004); also being female, being older, not being married, having a history of the disease and having a mental illness are factors affecting the QoL of these patients. Moreover, patients with unstable angina have been found to have a worse QoL than those who suffered an AMI (Soto et al., 2005).

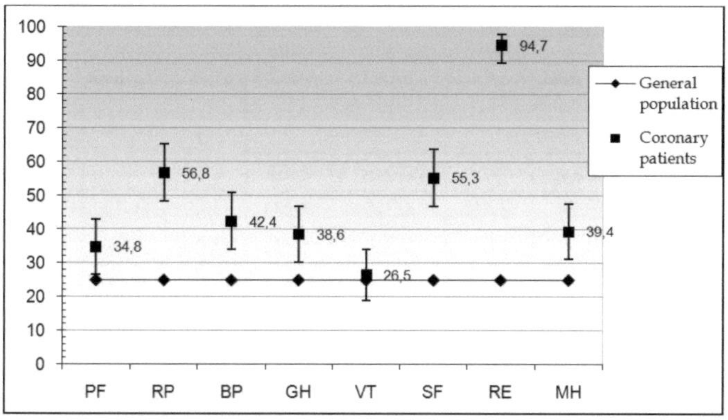

Fig. 1. Percentage of coronary patients below the 25th percentile of the general population, with the corresponding 95% confidence intervals. PF: Physical Functioning. RP: Role Physical . BP: Bodily Pain. GH: General Health. VT: Vitality. SF: Social Functioning. RE: Role Emotional. MH: Mental Health.

Despite this, and the fact that HRQL is a useful indicator of results in coronary patients who undergo revascularization, there are not many follow-up studies that analyse the evolution of HRQL and assess the effect of clinical and socio-demographic variables on the different clinical forms of the disease (angina vs myocardial infarction), even though it would be advisable to identify predictive factors to improve the development of interventions for subjects at risk (Bryant & Mayou, 1989).

Failde et al., in a study carried out in patients affected by both unstable angina and myocardial infarction (Failde & Soto, 2006), observed a significant decrease at 3 months of follow-up in the physical functioning, general health, and vitality dimensions, and the physical component summary (PCS) of the SF-36 health questionnaire. Also, the same authors have recently shown that HRQL is significantly impaired in coronary patients just after hospital discharge, with improvements being produced at 6 months, especially in the dimensions of the SF-36 related to bodily pain, general health, vitality, and the physical component summary (PCS) (Table 2) (data not yet published). In the same way, Höfer et al. (Höfer et al., 2006) also observed a significant positive change over time for the physical component summary dimension (PCS) of the SF-36, but not for the mental component summary dimension (MCS). However, other authors (Elliott et al., 2003; Mancuso et al., 2000; Wells et al., 1989) have shown that the SF-36 MCS is a good indicator of depression in general and diseased populations and Tavella et al. (Tavella et al., 2010) have even established a threshold score on the SF-36 MCS that would categorise a population with cardiac disease into depressed and non-depressed patients.

In the analysis of the factors affecting the change of HRQL in coronary patients Failde et al. observed that revascularization, age, and the interaction between a previous history of Coronary Heart Disease (CHD) and the presence of one or more risk factors affected negatively the physical component summary of the SF-36 at 3 months of follow-up (Failde & Soto, 2006). Also, studying the factors related to HRQL at 6 months, the same authors observed that depression, assessed by the 28-item General Health Questionnaire, a previous history of Coronary Heart Disease (CHD), or the associated comorbidity had a negative effect on quality of life, with a worse clinical course in these patients when compared with those without these conditions.

	BASELINE N=175		3 MONTHS N=80		6 MONTHS N=47		p	p^1	p^2	Partial eta-squared
	Mean	SD	Mean	SD	Mean	SD				
PF	61.9	28.9	66.9	27.9	63.4	30.0	0.67	0.41	1.00	0.004
RP	53.2	48.5	70.7	41.8	72.8	42.6	0.04	0.14	0.13	0.085
BP	56.6	29.1	60.5	27.4	67.5	25.6	0.01	0.89	0.02	0.148
GH	57.9	19.9	65.7	19.5	65.4	18.6	0.01	0.00	0.01	0.155
VT	59.7	30.7	69.7	27.4	68.3	26.7	0.04	0.09	0.13	0.084
SF	74.5	34.4	83.7	28.3	83.5	30.2	0.09	0.24	0.28	0.060
RE	76.6	39.8	80.1	39.1	84.4	36.0	0.27	1.00	0.82	0.026
MH	64.9	18.4	67.8	21.5	67.7	17.9	0.19	0.48	0.58	0.036
PCS	40.6	12.1	44.4	9.7	44.5	11.4	0.01	0.03	0.04	0.122
MCS	47.9	10.9	49.8	11.9	50.2	9.7	0.15	0.75	0.46	0.043

Table 2. Mean (SD) of SF-36 dimensions at baseline and during follow-up. PF: physical functioning; RP: role physical; BP: body pain; GH: general health. VT: vitality; SF: social functioning; RE: role emotional; MH: mental health; PCS: physical component summary; MCS: mental component summary. ANOVA test with the Bonferroni test for post hoc comparisons. p: comparison at three times; p^1: comparison between baseline and 3 months; p^2: comparison between baseline and 6 months. No significant differences were observed between 3 months and 6 months. Partial eta-squared: as an effect size estimator that describes the proportion of variability that exists in each dimension of the SF-36 during the follow-up. (0.01: Small; 0.06: Medium; 0.14: Large)

This results are in agreement with Ormel et al. (Ormel et al., 2007) and Höfer et al. (Höfer et al., 2005) who found that depression and anxiety are the most significant factors influencing HRQL in patients with heart disease, and with McBurney et al. (McBurney et al., 2002), who observed that the presence of other illnesses had a negative effect on the PCS-12 seven months after an AMI, and that having more comorbidity tends to lower HRQL in all dimensions.

Dickens et al. (Dickens et al., 2011) in a prospective cohort study conducted to investigate the impact of depression on subsequent HRQL in subjects with CHD, identified a number of cognitive targets for psychological interventions in these patients, namely a perceived tendency to avoid physical activity, increased somatic awareness, perceived symptom burden, and emotional impact of heart disease. In the Dickens´ study, when the results are controlled for demographic and medical variables, depression was associated with a subsequent worse score in the physical component summary of the SF-36, but when anxiety, awareness of somatic symptoms, and negative illness perceptions were added to the regression model, depression no longer continued to be a significant independent factor. Maladaptive cardiac related health behaviour, like a high-fat diet, no regular exercise, being stressed or smoking, among others, were not related to the SF-36 physical component summary, so could not mediate the relationship between depression and the physical component summary (Baron & Kenny, 1986).

The associations between HRQL and patients' age, gender and whether or not they have undergone revascularization have been constantly studied, but the results are still inconclusive. Older age has been found to be associated with better postoperative mental health in these patients (Rumsfeld et al., 2004). However, Miller and Grindel (Miller & Grindel, 2001) reported that both preoperative health status and physiological, psychological and social recovery of older and younger patients were similar after CABG.

It has also been observed (Duenas et al., 2011) that being female negatively affects HRQL, and most studies suggest that women do not cope as well physically and psychosocially as men. However, it remains unclear why gender-related differences in HRQL exist among coronary patients (Van Jaarsveld et al., 2002).

Several authors have shown that women with coronary disease report significantly poorer physical functioning and mental health than men (Dixon et al., 2000; Ghali et al., 2002; Norris et al., 2004; Shumaker et al., 1997; Wiklund et al., 1993) and that this effect is mediated in some cases by its interaction with other variables such as a history of the illness or the mental health status. Norris et al. (Norris et al., 2007) also showed that, after adjusting for clinical and psychosocial covariables, the physical HRQL differences between men and women did not disappear. In addition, others authors have shown that smoking, regular alcohol consumption, and overweight are the most common risk factors for worse HRQL in men, while psychological distress, role pressure, and less strenuous exercise are more characteristic of women (Verbrugge, 1989).

Prior data suggest that women with cardiac disease are more likely than men to be confronted with continuing demands in the home environment, and may be more likely to neglect health care needs (Emery et al., 2004). Thus, Emery et al. hypothesized that quality of life would be more strongly associated with social support among women than among men.

Recently, a study analysing gender differences in the outcome of HRQL in coronary patients (Duenas et al., 2011), found that baseline scores in the SF-36 were lower among women. Also, the men had a better clinical course at 6 months in most of the physical dimensions, and social functioning. Meanwhile, the women only improved in the physical component summary, role physical and social functioning. This is partly in accordance with the results obtained by Emery and co-workers, (Emery et al., 2004) which show that men and women have increased scores in physical health over time, but women have significantly lower scores in physical dimensions across all assessments. Likewise, Duenas et al reported that the variables most strongly associated with an unfavourable evolution of HRQL in men were deterioration in mental health and angina frequency. Likewise, mental health was also a determining factor in the evolution of women's quality of life, although this was also affected by other variables, such as a clinical history of the disease, angina frequency and undergoing revascularization during the follow-up (Duenas et al., 2011). In this respect, it is worth highlighting that revascularization was carried out earlier in the men, which may have conditioned the worse clinical course observed in the women, who suffered higher frequencies of angina and rehospitalisation during follow-up. Hemingway et al. (Hemingway et al., 2006) and Aguado-Romero and co-workers (Aguado-Romeo et al., 2006) detail the tendency to operate less on women with coronary disease than on men, although the latter try to justify these differences by referring to limitations in their data.

Thus, other factors, such as the perception that women have a lower pre-test probability of infarction, may influence the clinician´s discharge decision (Willingham & Kilpatrick, 2005) and the different attitude to treatment among women may be another determining factor.

On the other hand, several studies have found that the evolution of HRQL differs between men and women after coronary surgery. Phillips et al. (Phillips Bute et al., 2003) concluded that women do not obtain the same benefit from CABG surgery as men, and that the difference cannot be attributed to preoperative divergence. One possible explanation for this is that women´s compromised HRQL is less related to cardiac health than men´s, with other environmental and/or personality variables related to quality of life affecting women more than men (Phillips Bute et al., 2003).

Finally, another important factor related to the HRQL of patients with coronary disease is familial support (Rantanen et al., 2008). Patients who receive only limited support from significant others have been reported to suffer more anxiety and depressive symptoms than patients who receive more (Okkonen & Vanhanen, 2006) and patients have reported a better HRQL than their peers when they have received much social support (Bosworth et al., 2000; Woloshin et al., 1997; Yates, 1995).

Research results explaining the relationship between HRQL for CABG patients and social support have been contradictory, however, and social support received from family members and other significant others has shown no significant association with patients' functional capacity (Barry et al., 2006; Hamalainen et al., 2000). However, ready access to concrete support, does seem to correlate with positive changes in mental health (Barry et al., 2006).

3. Conclusion

HRQL is an essential primary outcome measure in coronary patients. Several instruments, both generic and specific, have proven to be of use for its assessment, showing differences between different groups of patients affected by the disease. In addition, several variables related to patients' clinical evolution and history of the disease have been shown to be related to HRQL, with worse results among women, subjects with previous history of CHD, and those with another comorbidity.

Mental health has been shown to significantly affect the evolution of HRQL in these patients. However, the systematic assessment of this variable is not common. Therefore, more emphasis needs to be placed on the systematic assessment of mental status specially in women, and the development of patient-oriented programs which reduce mental disturbances, and on providing increased social support for this at-risk population in particular.

4. References

Aguado-Romeo, M.J., Marquez-Calderon, S., Buzon-Barrera, M.L. & por los investigadores del grupo VPM-IRYSS-Andalucia. (2006). Differences between women's and men's access to interventional cardiovascular procedures at public hospitals in Andalusia (Spain). *Revista espanola de cardiologia*, Vol.59, No.8, (August 2006), pp. 785-793, ISSN 0300-8932; 0300-8932

Alonso, J., Ferrer, M., Gandek, B., Ware Jr., J.E., Aaronson, N.K., Mosconi, P., Rasmussen, N.K., Bullinger, M., Fukuhara, S., Kaasa, S. & Leplège, A. (2004). Health-related quality of life associated with chronic conditions in eight countries: Results from the International Quality of Life Assessment (IQOLA) Project. *Quality of Life Research*, Vol.13, No.2, (March 2004), pp. 283-298

Asadi-Lari, M., Packham, C. & Gray, D. (2003). Is quality of life measurement likely to be a proxy for health needs assessment in patients with coronary artery disease? *Health and Quality of Life Outcomes*, Vol.1, No.50, (October 2003), pp. 1-8

Baron, R.M. & Kenny, D.A. (1986). The moderator-mediator variable distinction in social psychological research: conceptual, strategic, and statistical considerations. *Journal of personality and social psychology*, Vol.51, No.6, (December 1986), pp. 1173-1182, ISSN 0022-3514; 0022-3514

Barry, L.C., Kasl, S.V., Lichtman, J., Vaccarino, V. & Krumholz, H.M. (2006). Social support and change in health-related quality of life 6 months after coronary artery bypass grafting. *Journal of psychosomatic research*, Vol.60, No.2, (February 2006), pp. 185-193, ISSN 0022-3999; 0022-3999

Bosworth, H.B., Siegler, I.C., Olsen, M.K., Brummett, B.H., Barefoot, J.C., Williams, R.B., Clapp-Channing, N.E. & Mark, D.B. (2000). Social support and quality of life in patients with coronary artery disease. *Quality of life research : an international journal of quality of life aspects of treatment, care and rehabilitation*, Vol.9, No.7, (November 2000), pp. 829-839, ISSN 0962-9343; 0962-9343

Brown, N., Melville, M., Gray, D., Young, T., Munro, J., Skene, A.M. & Hampton, J.R. (1999). Quality of life four years after acute myocardial infarction: Short form 36 scores compared with a normal population. *Heart*, Vol.81, (November 1999), pp. 352-358

Bryant, B. & Mayou, R. (1989). Prediction of outcome after coronary artery surgery. *Journal of psychosomatic research*, Vol.33, No.4, (January 1989), pp. 419-427, ISSN 0022-3999; 0022-3999

Caine, N., Harrison, S.C., Sharples, L.D. & Wallwork, J. (1991). Prospective study of quality of life before and after coronary artery bypass grafting. *BMJ (Clinical research ed.)*, Vol.302, No.6775, (March 1991), pp. 511-516, ISSN 0959-8138; 0959-535X

Casas Anguita, J., Ramon Repullo Labrador, J. & Pereira Candel, J. (2001). Measurements of quality of life related with health. Basic concepts and cultural adaptation. *Medicina clinica*, Vol.116, No.20, (June 2001), pp. 789-796, ISSN 0025-7753; 0025-7753

Cepeda-Valery, B., Cheong, A.P., Lee, A. & Yan, B.P. (2011). Measuring health related quality of life in coronary heart disease: The importance of feeling well. *International journal of cardiology*, Vol.149, No.1, (May 2011), pp. 4-9

Charlier, L., Dutrannois, J. & Kaufman, L. (1997). The SF-36 questionnaire: a convenient way to assess quality of life in angina pectoris patients. *Acta Cardiologica*, Vol.52, No.3, pp. 247-260, ISSN 0001-5385; 0001-5385

Dickens, C., Cherrington, A., McGowan, L. & Taylor, C.B. (2011). Do Cognitive and Behavioral Factors Mediate the Impact of Depression on Medical Outcomes in

People with Coronary Heart Disease? *Journal of cardiopulmonary rehabilitation and prevention*, Vol.31, No.2, (March 2011), pp. 105-110, ISSN 1932-751X; 1932-7501

Dixon, T., Lim, L.L., Powell, H. & Fisher, J.D. (2000). Psychosocial experiences of cardiac patients in early recovery: a community-based study. *Journal of advanced nursing*, Vol.31, No.6, (June 2000), pp. 1368-1375, ISSN 0309-2402; 0309-2402

Dougherty, C.M., Dewhurst, T., Nichol, W.P. & Spertus, J. (1998). Comparison of three quality of life instruments in stable angina pectoris: Seattle Angina Questionnaire, Short Form Health Survey (SF-36), and Quality of Life Index-Cardiac Version III. *Journal of clinical epidemiology*, Vol.51, No.7, (July 1998), pp. 569-575, ISSN 0895-4356; 0895-4356

Duenas, M., Ramirez, C., Arana, R. & Failde, I. (2011). Gender differences and determinants of health related quality of life in coronary patients: a follow-up study. *BMC cardiovascular disorders*, Vol.11, (May 2011), pp. 24, ISSN 1471-2261; 1471-2261

Duits, A.A., Boeke, S., Taams, M.A., Passchier, J. & Erdman, R.A. (1997). Prediction of quality of life after coronary artery bypass graft surgery: a review and evaluation of multiple, recent studies. *Psychosomatic medicine*, Vol.59, No.3, (June 1997), pp. 257-268, ISSN 0033-3174; 0033-3174

Dyer, M.T.D., Goldsmith, K.A., Sharples, L.S. & Buxton, M.J. (2010). A review of health utilities using the EQ-5D in studies of cardiovascular disease. *Health and Quality of Life Outcomes*, Vol.8, No.13, (January 2010), pp. 1-12

Elliott, T.E., Renier, C.M. & Palcher, J.A. (2003). Chronic pain, depression, and quality of life: correlations and predictive value of the SF-36. *Pain medicine*, Vol.4, No.4, (December 2003), pp. 331-339, ISSN 1526-2375; 1526-2375

Ellis, J.J., Eagle, K.A., Kline-Rogers, E.M. & Erickson, S.R. (2005). Validation of the EQ-5D in patients with a history of acute coronary syndrome. *Current medical research and opinion*, Vol.21, No.8, (August 2005), pp. 1209-1216

Emery, C.F., Frid, D.J., Engebretson, T.O., Alonzo, A.A., Fish, A., Ferketich, A.K., Reynolds, N.R., Dujardin, J.P., Homan, J.E. & Stern, S.L. (2004). Gender differences in quality of life among cardiac patients. *Psychosomatic medicine*, Vol.66, No.2, (April 2004), pp. 190-197, ISSN 1534-7796; 0033-3174

Failde, I., Medina, P., Ramírez, C. & Arana, R. (2009). Assessing health-related quality of life among coronary patients: SF-36 vs SF-12. *Public health*, Vol.123, No.9, (September 2009), pp. 615-617

Failde, I. & Ramos, I. (2000). Validity and reliability of the SF-36 Health Survey Questionnaire in patients with coronary artery disease. *Journal of clinical epidemiology*, Vol.53, No.4, (April 2000), pp. 359-365

Failde, I.I. & Soto, M.M. (2006). Changes in Health Related Quality of Life 3 months after an acute coronary syndrome. *BMC public health*, Vol.6, (Jan 27), pp. 18, ISSN 1471-2458; 1471-2458

Fayers, P.M. & Machin, D. (2007). *Quality of life: The assessment, analysis and interpretationof patient-reported outcomes* (2), Wiley, ISBN 13 978-0-470-02450-8, Chichester, England

Folks, D.G., Blake, D.J., Fleece, L., Sokol, R.S. & Freeman, A.M.,3rd. (1986). Quality of life six months after coronary artery bypass surgery: a preliminary report. *Southern medical journal*, Vol.79, No.4, (April 1986), pp. 397-399, ISSN 0038-4348; 0038-4348

Gandek, B., Ware, J.E., Aaronson, N.K., Apolone, G., Bjorner, J.B., Brazier, J.E., Bullinger, M., Kaasa, S., Leplege, A., Prieto, L. & Sullivan, M. (1998). Cross-validation of item selection and scoring for the SF-12 Health Survey in nine countries: Results from the IQOLA Project. *Journal of clinical epidemiology*, Vol.51, No.11, (November 1998), pp. 1171-1178

Ghali, W.A., Faris, P.D., Galbraith, P.D., Norris, C.M., Curtis, M.J., Saunders, L.D., Dzavik, V., Mitchell, L.B., Knudtson, M.L. & Alberta Provincial Project for Outcome Assessment in Coronary Heart Disease (APPROACH) Investigators. (2002). Sex differences in access to coronary revascularization after cardiac catheterization: importance of detailed clinical data. *Annals of Internal Medicine*, Vol.136, No.10, (May 2002), pp. 723-732, ISSN 1539-3704; 0003-4819

Group, World Health Organization Quality of Life (WHOQOL). (1993). Study protocol for the World Health Organization project to develop a Quality of Life. *Quality of Life Research*, Vol.2, No.2, (April 1993), pp. 153-159, ISSN 0962-9343 (Print) 0962-9343 (Linking)

Hamalainen, H., Smith, R., Puukka, P., Lind, J., Kallio, V., Kuttila, K. & Ronnemaa, T. (2000). Social support and physical and psychological recovery one year after myocardial infarction or coronary artery bypass surgery. *Scandinavian Journal of Public Health*, Vol.28, No.1, (March 2000), pp. 62-70, ISSN 1403-4948; 1403-4948

Hawkes, A.L. & Mortensen, O.S. (2006). Up to one third of individual cardiac patients have a decline in quality of life post-intervention. *Scandinavian Cardiovascular Journal*, Vol.40, No.4, (August 2006), pp. 214-218

Hemingway, H., McCallum, A., Shipley, M., Manderbacka, K., Martikainen, P. & Keskimaki, I. (2006). Incidence and prognostic implications of stable angina pectoris among women and men. *JAMA : the journal of the American Medical Association*, Vol.295, No.12, (March 2006), pp. 1404-1411, ISSN 1538-3598; 0098-7484

Hemingway, H., Nicholson, A., Stafford, M., Roberts, R. & Marmot, M. (1997a). The impact of socioeconomic status on health functioning as assessed by the SF-36 questionnaire: the Whitehall II Study. *American Journal of Public Health*, Vol.87, No.9, (September 1997), pp. 1484-1490, ISSN 0090-0036 (Print) 0090-0036 (Linking)

Hemingway, H., Stafford, M., Stansfeld, S., Shipley, M. & Marmot, M. (1997b). Is the SF-36 a valid measure of change in population health? Results from the Whitehall II Study. *BMJ (Clinical research ed.)*, Vol.315, No.7118, (November 1997), pp. 1273-1279, ISSN 0959-8138; 0959-535X

Höfer, S., Doering, S., Rumpold, G., Oldridge, N. & Benzer, W. (2006). Determinants of health-related quality of life in patients with coronary artery disease. *European Journal of Cardiovascular Prevention & Rehabilitation*, Vol.13, No.3, (June 2006), pp. 398-406, ISSN 1741-8267

Höfer, S., Benzer, W., Alber, H., Ruttmann, E., Kopp, M., Schüssler, G. & Doering, S. (2005). Determinants of health-related quality of life in coronary artery disease patients: A prospective study generating a structural equation model. *Psychosomatics*, Vol.46, No.3, (June 2005), pp. 212-223

Höfer, S., Lim, L., Guyatt, G. & Oldridge, N. (2004). The MacNew Heart Disease Health-related Quality of Life instrument: A summary. *Health and Quality of Life Outcomes*, Vol.2, No.3, (January 2004), pp. 1-8

Jenkins, C.D., Stanton, B.A., Savageau, J.A., Denlinger, P. & Klein, M.D. (1983). Coronary artery bypass surgery. Physical, psychological, social, and economic outcomes six months later. *JAMA : the journal of the American Medical Association*, Vol.250, No.6, (August 1983), pp. 782-788, ISSN 0098-7484; 0098-7484

Kaplan, R.M. (1988). Health-related quality of life in cardiovascular disease. *Journal of consulting and clinical psychology*, Vol.56, No.3, (June 1988), pp. 382-392, ISSN 0022-006X; 0022-006X

Lewin, R.J.P., Thompson, D.R., Martin, C.R., Stuckey, N., Devlen, J., Michaelson, S. & Maguire, P. (2002). Validation of the cardiovascular limitations and symptoms profile (CLASP) in chronic stable angina. *Journal of cardiopulmonary rehabilitation*, Vol.22, No.3, (June 2002), pp. 184-191

Mancuso, C.A., Peterson, M.G. & Charlson, M.E. (2000). Effects of depressive symptoms on health-related quality of life in asthma patients. *Journal of general internal medicine*, Vol.15, No.5, (May 2000), pp. 301-310, ISSN 0884-8734; 0884-8734

Marquis, P., Fayol, C. & Joire, J.E. (1995a). Clinical validation of a quality of life questionnaire in angina pectoris patients. *European heart journal*, Vol.16, No.11, (November 1995), pp. 1554-1560, ISSN 0195-668X; 0195-668X

Marquis, P., Fayol, C., Joire, J.E. & Leplege, A. (1995b). Psychometric properties of a specific quality of life questionnaire in angina pectoris patients. *Quality of life research : an international journal of quality of life aspects of treatment, care and rehabilitation*, Vol.4, No.6, (December 1995), pp. 540-546, ISSN 0962-9343; 0962-9343

Mayou, R. & Bryant, B. (1987). Quality of life after coronary artery surgery. *The Quarterly journal of medicine*, Vol.62, No.239, (March 1987), pp. 239-248, ISSN 0033-5622; 0033-5622

McBurney, C.R., Eagle, K.A., Kline-Rogers, E.M., Cooper, J.V., Mani, O.C.M., Smith, D.E. & Erickson, S.R. (2002). Health-related quality of life in patients 7 months after a myocardial infarction: Factors affecting the short form-12. *Pharmacotherapy*, Vol.22, No.12, (December 2002), pp. 1616-1622

McDowell, I. & Newell, C. (1996). *Measuring Health: A Guide to Rating Scales and Questionnaires* (2), Oxford University Press, ISBN 0-19-510371-8, New York, USA

Miller, K.H. & Grindel, C.G. (2001). Recovery from coronary artery bypass surgery: age-related outcomes. *Outcomes management for nursing practice*, Vol.5, No.3, (September 2001), pp. 127-133, ISSN 1093-1783; 1093-1783

Norris, C.M., Hegadoren, K. & Pilote, L. (2007). Depression symptoms have a greater impact on the 1-year health-related quality of life outcomes of women post-myocardial infarction compared to men. *European Journal of Cardiovascular Nursing*, Vol.6, No.2, (June 2007), pp. 92-98, ISSN 1474-5151 (Print) 1474-5151 (Linking)

Norris, C.M., Ghali, W.A., Galbraith, P.D., Graham, M.M., Jensen, L.A., Knudtson, M.L. & APPROACH Investigators. (2004). Women with coronary artery disease report worse health-related quality of life outcomes compared to men. *Health and quality of life outcomes*, Vol.2, (May 2004), pp. 21, ISSN 1477-7525; 1477-7525

Nowels, D., McGloin, J., Westfall, J.M. & Holcomb, S. (2005). Validation of the EQ-5D quality of life instrument in patients after myocardial infarction. *Quality of Life Research*, Vol.14, No.1, (February 2005), pp. 95-105

Okkonen, E. & Vanhanen, H. (2006). Family support, living alone, and subjective health of a patient in connection with a coronary artery bypass surgery. *Heart & lung : the journal of critical care*, Vol.35, No.4, (August 2006), pp. 234-244, ISSN 0147-9563; 0147-9563

Oldridge, N., Guyatt, G., Jones, N., Crowe, J., Singer, J., Feeny, D., McKelvie, R., Runions, J., Streiner, D. & Torrance, G. (1991). Effects on quality of life with comprehensive rehabilitation after acute myocardial infarction. *The American Journal of Cardiology*, Vol.67, No.13, (May 1991), pp. 1084-1089, ISSN 0002-9149; 0002-9149

Ormel, J., Von Korff, M., Burger, H., Scott, K., Demyttenaere, K., Huang, Y.Q., Posada-Villa, J., Pierre Lepine, J., Angermeyer, M.C., Levinson, D., de Girolamo, G., Kawakami, N., Karam, E., Medina-Mora, M.E., Gureje, O., Williams, D., Haro, J.M., Bromet,

E.J., Alonso, J. & Kessler, R. (2007). Mental disorders among persons with heart disease - results from World Mental Health surveys. *General hospital psychiatry*, Vol.29, No.4, (August 2007), pp. 325-334, ISSN 0163-8343 (Print) 0163-8343 (Linking)

Permanyer-Miralda, G., Alonso, J., Anto, J.M., Alijarde-Guimera, M. & Soler-Soler, J. (1991). Comparison of perceived health status and conventional functional evaluation in stable patients with coronary artery disease. *Journal of clinical epidemiology*, Vol.44, No.8, pp. 779-786, ISSN 0895-4356; 0895-4356

Phillips Bute, B., Mathew, J., Blumenthal, J.A., Welsh-Bohmer, K., White, W.D., Mark, D., Landolfo, K. & Newman, M.F. (2003). Female gender is associated with impaired quality of life 1 year after coronary artery bypass surgery. *Psychosomatic medicine*, Vol.65, No.6, (December 2003), pp. 944-951, ISSN 1534-7796; 0033-3174

Rantanen, A., Kaunonen, M., Sintonen, H., Koivisto, A.M., Astedt-Kurki, P. & Tarkka, M.T. (2008). Factors associated with health-related quality of life in patients and significant others one month after coronary artery bypass grafting. *Journal of Clinical Nursing*, Vol.17, No.13, (July 2008), pp. 1742-1753, ISSN 1365-2702; 0962-1067

Rumsfeld, J.S., Ho, P.M., Magid, D.J., McCarthy, M.,Jr, Shroyer, A.L., MaWhinney, S., Grover, F.L. & Hammermeister, K.E. (2004). Predictors of health-related quality of life after coronary artery bypass surgery. *The Annals of Thoracic Surgery*, Vol.77, No.5, (May 2004), pp. 1508-1513, ISSN 0003-4975; 0003-4975

Shumaker, S.A. & Berzon, R.A. (1995). *The International assessement of health related quality of life: Theory, Translation, Measurement and Analysis* (1), Rapid Communications of Oxford Ltd., ISBN 1-85650-004-7, New York, USA

Shumaker, S.A., Brooks, M.M., Schron, E.B., Hale, C., Kellen, J.C., Inkster, M., Wimbush, F.B., Wiklund, I. & Morris, M. (1997). Gender differences in health-related quality of life among postmyocardial infarction patients: brief report. CAST Investigators. Cardiac Arrhythmia Suppression Trials. *Women's health (Hillsdale, N.J.)*, Vol.3, No.1, (Spring 1997), pp. 53-60, ISSN 1077-2928; 1077-2928

Soto Torres, M., Marquez Calderon, S., Ramos Diaz, I., Barba Chacon, A., Lopez Fernandez, F. & Failde Martinez, I. (2004). Health-related quality of life in coronary heart disease compared to norms in Spanish population. *Quality of life research : an international journal of quality of life aspects of treatment, care and rehabilitation*, Vol.13, No.8, (October 2004), pp. 1401-1407, ISSN 0962-9343; 0962-9343

Soto, M., Failde, I., Marquez, S., Benitez, E., Ramos, I., Barba, A. & Lopez, F. (2005). Physical and mental component summaries score of the SF-36 in coronary patients. *Quality of life research : an international journal of quality of life aspects of treatment, care and rehabilitation*, Vol.14, No.3, (April 2005), pp. 759-768, ISSN 0962-9343; 0962-9343

Spertus, J.A., Winder, J.A., Dewhurst, T.A., Deyo, R.A., Prodzinski, J., McDonell, M. & Fihn, S.D. (1995). Development and evaluation of the Seattle Angina Questionnaire: A new functional status measure for coronary artery disease. *Journal of the American College of Cardiology*, Vol.25, No.2, (February 1995), pp. 333-341

Stanton, B.A., Jenkins, C.D., Savageau, J.A. & Thurer, R.L. (1984). Functional benefits following coronary artery bypass graft surgery. *The Annals of Thoracic Surgery*, Vol.37, No.4, (April 1984), pp. 286-290, ISSN 0003-4975; 0003-4975

Tavella, R., Air, T., Tucker, G., Adams, R., Beltrame, J.F. & Schrader, G. (2010). Using the Short Form-36 mental summary score as an indicator of depressive symptoms in patients with coronary heart disease. *Quality of life research : an international journal of quality of life aspects of treatment, care and rehabilitation*, Vol.19, No.8, (October 2010), pp. 1105-1113, ISSN 1573-2649; 0962-9343

Thompson, D.R. & Yu, C.-M. (2003). Quality of life in patients with coronary heart disease-I: Assessment tools. *Health and Quality of Life Outcomes*, Vol.1, No.42, (September 2003), pp. 1-5

Thompson, D.R. & Roebuck, A. (2001). The measurement of health-related quality of life in patients with coronary heart disease. *The Journal of cardiovascular nursing*, Vol.16, No.1, (October 2001), pp. 28-33

Urzúa M, A. (2010). Health related quality of life: Conceptual elements. *Revista Médica de Chile*, Vol.138, No.3, (March 2010), pp. 358-365

Van Jaarsveld, C., Sanderman, R., Ranchor, A., Ormel, J., van Veldhuisen, D. & Kempen, G. (2002). Gender-specific changes in quality of life following cardiovascular disease: a prospective study. *Journal of clinical epidemiology*, Vol.55, No.11, (November 2002), pp. 1105-1112, ISSN 0895-4356

Verbrugge, L.M. (1989). The twain meet: empirical explanations of sex differences in health and mortality. *Journal of health and social behavior*, Vol.30, No.3, (September 1989), pp. 282-304, ISSN 0022-1465; 0022-1465

Ware, J.E. (2000). SF-36 Health Survey update. *Spine*, Vol.25, No.24, (December 2000), pp. 3130-3139

Ware, J.E., Snow, K.K., Kosinski, M. & Gandek, B. (1993). *SF-36 Health Survey: Manual and Interpretation Guide* (1), ISBN 1891810006 (user's manual) 1891810065, Boston, USA

Wells, K.B., Stewart, A., Hays, R.D., Burnam, M.A., Rogers, W., Daniels, M., Berry, S., Greenfield, S. & Ware, J. (1989). The functioning and well-being of depressed patients. Results from the Medical Outcomes Study. *JAMA : the journal of the American Medical Association*, Vol.262, No.7, (August 1989), pp. 914-919, ISSN 0098-7484; 0098-7484

Wiklund, I., Herlitz, J., Johansson, S., Bengtson, A., Karlson, B.W. & Persson, N.G. (1993). Subjective symptoms and well-being differ in women and men after myocardial infarction. *European heart journal*, Vol.14, No.10, (October 1993), pp. 1315-1319, ISSN 0195-668X; 0195-668X

Williams, A. (1990). EuroQol - A new facility for the measurement of health-related quality of life. *Health Policy*, Vol.16, No.3, (December 1990), pp. 199-208

Willingham, S.A. & Kilpatrick, E.S. (2005). Evidence of gender bias when applying the new diagnostic criteria for myocardial infarction. *Heart (British Cardiac Society)*, Vol.91, No.2, (February 2005), pp. 237-238, ISSN 1468-201X; 1355-6037

Woloshin, S., Schwartz, L.M., Tosteson, A.N., Chang, C.H., Wright, B., Plohman, J. & Fisher, E.S. (1997). Perceived adequacy of tangible social support and health outcomes in patients with coronary artery disease. *Journal of general internal medicine*, Vol.12, No.10, (October 1997), pp. 613-618, ISSN 0884-8734; 0884-8734

Yates, B.C. (1995). The relationships among social support and short- and long-term recovery outcomes in men with coronary heart disease. *Research in nursing & health*, Vol.18, No.3, (June 1995), pp. 193-203, ISSN 0160-6891; 0160-6891

Yu, C.M., Li, L.S.W., Ho, H.H. & Lau, C.P. (2003). Long-term changes in exercise capacity, quality of life, body anthropometry, and lipid profiles after a cardiac rehabilitation program in obese patients with coronary heart disease. *The American Journal of Cardiology*, Vol.91, No.3, (February 2003), pp. 321-325

22

Anger, Hostility and Other Forms of Negative Affect: Relation to Cardiovascular Disease

Marco A.A. Torquato Jr., Bruno P.F. de Souza,
Dan V. Iosifescu and Renerio Fraguas
University of São Paulo, Institute of Psychiatry, Brazil

1. Introduction

The link between psychological factors and cardiovascular disease goes far beyond well-established psychiatric diagnoses such as major depressive disorder, generalized anxiety disorder or panic disorder. The literature describes several mental and behavioral concepts which are not captured in the current nomenclature as independent mental disorders but show some degree of association with cardiovascular disease. We will discuss them in this chapter under the larger category of "negative affect". The most common constructs we subsume in this category are Anger, Hostility, Aggressiveness, Negative Emotion, Negative Affectivity, Vital Exhaustion (VE), Type D Personality, and Type A Behavior Pattern (TABP). We chose the "negative affect" category as a mean to discuss together these different mood states having in common their potential negative impact on the cardiovascular system.

Some of these constructs have different definitions and are measured by diverse instruments. This variety of approaches reflects the complexity of the field and explains, at least in part, some disparity in results relating them to cardiovascular disease.

In this chapter, we review these constructs included in "negative affect" and the instruments that have been developed to assess them. Additionally, we will review the studies investigating their relationship with cardiac conditions, emphasizing the pathophysiological mechanisms that could mediate the relationship between negative affect and cardiac pathology . Finally, we will discuss potential treatments of negative affect and their eventual impact on cardiac conditions.

2. The mix of concepts: Hostility, anger, aggression and other negative affect

Over the past decades, a large number of studies have investigated the association between negative affect and coronary heart disease (CHD). Many were cross-sectional case-control studies, which have been criticized for the recall bias of the CHD diagnosis and for the memory distortion (Chida and Steptoe 2009). More recently, several prospective longitudinal studies with more rigorous methodology have also been developed. Notwithstanding, results from this studies are not homogeneous, with both positive and negative results. Although more rigorous in their methodology, the prospective studies use diverse and partially overlapping concepts to define negative affect associated with CHD (Table 1). Since each study analyzes only a single psychological construct at a time and since these concepts are only partially overlapping, it is not surprising to note the conflicting results in the literature. In addition, the single-factor approach ignores the clustering of psychosocial risk factors for physical disease, which may act synergistically (Suls and Bunde 2005). Another view, from a twin-designed study, is that some of this negative affect concepts may have a single common genetic factor and a nonshared environmental factor, i.e., enviroments uncorrelated between twins, such as accidents.(Raynor, Pogue-Geile et al. 2002).

Type A Behavior Pattern	Type D Personality	Vital exhaustion	Hostility	Anger	Aggression	Negative Affectivity	Negative emotions
An action-emotion complex induced by environmental factors, involving psychomotor mannerisms, vigorous voice, hard-driving, time envolvement-pressured job, competitiveness, impatience and easy triggering anger and hostility (Friedman and Rosenman 1959)	Negative affectivity, social inhibition and feeling of distress (Denollet 1998).	An unusual tiredness, increased irritability and feelings of demoralization (Appels, Hoppener et al. 1987).	A tendency to view the world in a negative, cynical fashion; a primarily cognitive construct involving negative attitude toward others, consisting of enmity, denigration, and ill will (Smith, Glazer et al. 2004).	An affective experience, ranging in intensity from mild annoyance to fury and outrage. Two subtypes "anger-out", a combination of anger and aggression and "anger-in", a tendency to feel anger and suppress it (Schulman and Stromberg 2007).	A physical or verbal behavior including attacking destructive or hurtful actions, may be considered a personality trait.	Abroadband personality dimension caracterized by a general disposition to chronically experience anxiety, sadness, guilt, anger, irritability, and other negative emotions.	Depression, anger, anxiety and hostility are emotions that range from normal to pathological in a continuum (Kubzansky and Kawachi 2000; Kubzansky, Davidson et al. 2005; Kubzansky 2007).

Table 1. Concepts.

Some authors have proposed that anger, hostility and aggression should be considered a syndrome and other include anger and hostility in the concept of aggression. For others, hostility is characterized by interrelated elements of cynical beliefs and attributions, angry emotional states, and aggressive or antagonistic behaviors. Martin et al. advocate for the standardization of these concepts emphasizing that anger corresponds to *affect*, aggression to *behavior*, and hostility (or cynicism) to *cognition*. Together the three constructs form a three-factor "ABC" model of trait anger (Martin, Watson et al. 2000).

Aside from hostility, anger and aggression, VE and distressed personality are more complex concepts. Although they overlap partially, these constructs include specific patterns and aspects not captured by general scales for hostility, anger and aggression. Last but not least, the concept of negative affectivity posits that these symptoms represent markers of a trait characterized by hypersensitivity to negative stimuli (Watson and Clark 1984) and the concept of negative emotions postulate the existence of a continuum across these affective states.

3. Depression: The mix beyond the negative affects

Beyond negative affect, depression and, secondarily, anxiety have the strongest evidence for associations with CHD, even after controlling for traditional CHD risk factors, such as serum cholesterol, blood pressure, and smoking. Intriguingly, as it has been pointed out by Suls and Bunde, there is an appreciable construct and measurement overlap across anger, anxiety, and depression, which creates ambiguity both for theory testing and for interpretation of available evidence (Suls and Bunde 2005). Ravaja et al., have proposed that depression would be a moderator of the relationship between cardiovascular risk factors and anger (Ravaja, Kauppinen et al. 2000). They reported a negative association between hostility and cardiovascular risk factors in patients with high depressive tendencies. Patients with severe depression and lack of anger or hostility would represent the most severe form of exhaustion where the individual had "given-up"(Ravaja, Kauppinen et al. 2000).

Irritability has been considered a diagnostic feature of MDD in children and adolescents (American Psychiatric Association 1994). Actually, a hostile depressive subtype has been proposed in 1966 (Overall, Hollister et al. 1966). However, unfortunately, most standard rating scales of depressive symptom severity do not specifically measure irritability (Hamilton 1960; Montgomery and Asberg 1979). A particular form of irritable depression marked by recurrent anger attacks, spontaneous episodes characterized by feelings of rage and symptoms of physiologic arousal similar to panic attacks and accompanied by chronic irritability, has been reported to occur in 20-60% of patients with unipolar depression and nearly two-thirds of patients with bipolar depression (Perlis, Smoller et al. 2004) (Baker, Dorzab et al. 1971; Overall, Goldstein et al. 1971; Snaith and Taylor 1985) (Gould, Ball et al. 1996; Fava, Uebelacker et al. 1997; Morand, Thomas et al. 1998; Mischoulon, Dougherty et al. 2002; Posternak and Zimmerman 2002; Dougherty, Rauch et al. 2004). Data have suggested that depression with anger may be associated with distinct abnormalities of subcortical white matter structure (Iosifescu, Renshaw et al. 2007) and brain metabolism (Dougherty, Rauch et al. 2004), and possibly with increased serotonergic dysfunction (Fava, Vuolo et al. 2000). It is possible that anger may be a marker of a depressive variant with increased cardiovascular risk (Fava, Abraham et al. 1996; Painuly, Sharan et al. 2005; Fraguas, Iosifescu et al. 2007). Anger attacks in MDD patients were independently associated with smoking (for periods >11 years) and with total serum levels of cholesterol ≥ 200mg/dL, after adjusting for age, gender, BMI, and baseline severity of depression (Fraguas, Iosifescu et al. 2007).

Major depression is a mental disorder and has reliable operational diagnostic criteria. However, the limit between major depressive disorder and subsyndromal depressive symptoms and the relevance of irritability/anger/hostility in depressed patients involve multiple non answered questions. For example, little is known about the distinction between irritable depression and depression with comorbid personality disorders or other psychiatric diagnoses associated with high rates of irritability. The interaction between temperament, personality is a complex phenomenon (Clark, Watson et al. 1994). The nature of depressive symptoms may be influenced by personality traits; in this model, irritability may be one manifestation of sensitivity to negative stimuli (Watson and Clark 1984), or interpersonal sensitivity(Bagby, Kennedy et al. 1997). Also, increased anxiety levels may define a specific subtype of MDD (Fava, Alpert et al. 2004) and irritability is often manifested in the presence of increased anxiety (as an inadequate response of individuals overwhelmed by stress and anxiety); in a factor analysis, this continuum of symptoms in depression appears to be best captured by a common anxiety/irritability factor (Gullion and Rush 1998).

4. Instruments

The variety of instruments (Table 2) used to evaluate negative affect makes standardization or even comparison between studies difficult (Davidson 2008). We describe the instruments when addressing each "negative affect" construct separately (Item 6). However, some general limitations should be discussed. For example, some instruments are composed of multidimensional items mixing several concepts and including definitional caveats. For example, the Potential for Hostility subcomponent of the Structured Inverview for the TABP

Type A Behavior Pattern	Type D Personality	Vital exhaustion	Hostility	Anger	Agresssion
Among the self-report instruments there is the Jenkins Activity Scale (JAS) (Jenkins, Rosenman et al. 1967) and the Framingham Type A scale (FTAS) (Levenkron, Cohen et al. 1983). Among the instruments used by an interviewer there is the Rosenman and Friedman structured interview (MacDougall, Dembroski et al. 1979).	The Type D Scale-14 (DS14) evaluate the two components of Type D, the negative affectivity and social inhibition (Denollet 2005).	The 21-item Maastricht Questionnaire evaluates VE including factors such as depressive symptoms, sleep problems and lack of concentration (Appels, Hoppener et al. 1987).	The Cook and Medley Hostility scale (CMHS, or Ho scale) includes 50 items, true or false, evaluates cynicism and distrust (Smith, Glazer et al. 2004); the Buss-Durkee Hostility Inventory (Buss and Durkee 1957) assesses expressive hostility or antagonism (physical and verbal aggression) and neurotic or experiential hostility; the Interpersonal Hostility Assessment Technique (IHAT) is a structured interview that classifies the hostile behavior in four styles (Brummett, Maynard et al. 2000).	The Anger Expression scales (Spielberger et al., 1985), and Framingham Anger Reaction or Expression Scales (Haynes, Feinleib et al. 1980; Eaker, Pinsky et al. 1992); the Spielberger State-Trait Anger Expression Inventory is a self-report Inventory and assess anger expression ("anger-in" and "anger out"); the Anger Attacks Questionnaire evaluates the presence of anger attacks, spells of anger that are inappropriate to the situation and have physical features resembling panic attacks(Fava, Rosenbaum et al. 1991).	The Aggressio n Questionn aire (AQ), developed by Buss and Perry (1992) contains subscales to measure anger, hostility and verbal and physical aggression (Buss and Perry 1992).

Table 2. Instruments

has elements of hostile cynicism and anger affect , although it primarily assesses antagonistic expression (Dembroski, MacDougall et al. 1989). In addition, the same questionnaires identified as measures of anger and hostility by some authors are described as measures of aggression by others (Felsten and Hill 1999).

Raynor et al., using twin analyses, found that covariation among the Beck Depression Inventory, the Interpersonal Support Evaluation List and the Cook-Medley Hostility Scale could be explained by a single common genetic factor and a common nonshared environmental factor. They challenged the conventional approach of examining these psychosocial variables as independent risk factors for cardiovascular disease and argued for the importance of investigating specific causes for their covariation(Raynor, Pogue-Geile et al. 2002).

Devidson et. al. (Davidson 2008) performed a comparative analysis between the association of different instruments for measuring anger and hostility and CHD. The Minnesota Multiphasic Personality Inventory (MMPI) and the Cook-Medley Hostility Scale (CMHS) were positively associated with CHD in populations with and without psychiatric pathology. The Spielberger Trait Anger Scale (TAS) tended to show higher association with CHD compared with the overall effect in disease studies, while the Spielberger anger expression scale showed no association with CHD.

5. Neurophysiological bases for the relationship between negative affect and the cardiovascular system

Many authors attribute the possible influence of psychological traits on CHD to the impact of these affect states on promoting cardiovascular high-risk behaviors such as smoking, poor eating habits, low physical activity, poor sleep quality and low adherence to drug treatment (Scherwitz, Perkins et al. 1992). However, physiological pathways have been studied, suggesting that these affective constructs may be associated with autonomic, inflammatory and neuroendocrine changes that increase the risk for CHD (Table 3). Aspects of the proposed mechanisms of impact on the cardiovascular system are also discussed in the each of the negative affect categories in section 6.

The *reactivity hypothesis* offers a comprehensive model to understand the mechanisms connecting negative affect and increased cardiovascular morbidity. This hypothesis states that exaggerated physical or psychological responses can identify individuals at increased risk of cardiovascular disease. Based on this model, psychological traits and states would lead to increased risk through cardiovascular and neuroendocrine responses to environmental stressors. Lovallo and Gerin (2003)(Lovallo and Gerin 2003), divided the physiological mechanisms responsible for cardiovascular reactivity in three levels: 1) exaggerated cognitive-emotional responses; 2) increased brain stem and hypothalamus responsiveness; 3) Abnormalities in peripheral tissue modifications. In this paper, we discuss the first level, since it concerns the influence of personality traits on physiological responses of the organism.

Neurophysiologically, Lovallo and Gerin (2003)(Lovallo and Gerin 2003), outline two brain circuits through which the frontal lobe modulates and controls emotions. The first one includes the premotor region of the frontal cortex, connected to the anterior cingulate cortex, responsible for the selection of motor responses due to a motivated behavior. The second involves the orbital prefrontal cortex, which regulates the activity of the brain stem and hypothalamus secondary to the conscious evaluation of external events. It is worth mentioning the important connection of the orbital prefrontal cortex to the ventromedial prefrontal cortex, which has extensive dopaminergic and serotonergic areas, and is activated by signals ascending from the amygdala, the bed nuclei of the stria terminalis and septal regions. Thus, this second circuit would provide "emotional color" to the experiences.

After the cognitive and emotional evaluation, such areas send signals to the hypothalamus and brain stem, originating a wide range of physiological, endocrine, visceral and motor changes. Thus, specific cognitive and affective dispositions would lead to specific (and possibly persistent) changes in these systems (Lovallo and Gerin 2003).

This model is supported by several studies (Everson, McKey et al. 1995; Drevets 1999; Schaefer, Abercrombie et al. 2000; Pizzagalli, Pascual-Marqui et al. 2001) which indicate the importance of the quality of the stressor event (and not just its intensity) in the increased reactivity in susceptible individuals.

5.1 Proposed mechanisms: Chronic versus acute risk

The impact of negative affect on the cardiovascular system may be chronic or acute. For instance, hostility may be a personality trait with considerable stability across years and can be considered a character trait. In this situation the negative affect may chronically contribute to the morbidity of the cardiovascular system such as an association with increased levels of cholesterol (Table 3) (Dujovne and Houston 1991). On the other hand, anger attacks occurring episodically may acutely damage the cardiovascular system, such as an anger attack causing a heart attack (Mittleman, Maclure et al. 1995).

Regarding emotional states precipitating acute cardiac events, the evidence is very robust. Epidemiological studies have shown a significant increase of sudden cardiac death in populations submitted to disasters such as wars or earthquakes. In records of patients with implantable cardioverter-defibrillator (ICD), it was noticed that individual intense emotions such as anger or anxiety could trigger arrhythmias in susceptible patients. Lampert R et al, 2002, (Lampert, Joska et al. 2002) conducted a controlled prospective study, where ICD patients were requested to record in a diary the intensity of their emotions in the 15 minutes before shocks and, also, during the two hours to 15 minutes before the shock. As a control, the study assessed the diaries of the same patients during the same periods, one week after the shocks registration. Patients identified anger significantly more in the 15 minutes before the shock than during the control period. The association between the shocks and acute anger showed to be higher than the association with other measured emotions such as joy, sadness, worry and anxiety. The same group had previously reported that induced arrhythmias in patients undergoing mental stress (eg, performing arithmetic calculation or remembering stressful events) were faster in onset and more difficult to be extinguished than in those without such exposure.

Regarding psychological precipitants for acute myocardial infarction (MI), Culic V., et al, 2005 (Culic, Eterovic et al. 2005), performed a meta-analysis which found that emotional stress could immediately precedes MI in 7% of all cases of MI.

The relevance of considering both patterns is that affective traits may increase the frequency of acute subtle cardiovascular episodes.

Type A Behavior Pattern	Type D Personality	Vital exhaustion	Hostility	Anger
-Short-term responses to stress in physiological variables that are controlled by sympathetic nervous system(Oishi, Kamimura et al. 1999); - Increased cardiovascular risk factors as atherogenic lipid profile(Niaura, Stoney et al. 1992), -Increased thickness of the carotid intima-media (Keltikangas-Jarvinen, Hintsa et al. 2007).	-Overstated cardiovascular activity in daily life, mediated by an enhanced sympathetic drive and decreased vagal control of the heart including endothelial function, platelet function, altered lipid profile, altered activity of the hypothalamus-pituitary-adrenal cortex (HPA) axis and enhanced inflammatory activity of the immune system; -Increased negative behavioral factors; enhanced cortisol reactivity to stress and heightened blood pressure reactivity (Habra, Linden et al. 2003).	-Decreased ACTH and cortisol activation of inflammation; decreased slow wave sleep; reactivated cytomegalovirus fosters growth of atherosclerosis; -Increased production of cytokines and decreased negative feedback from the HPA-axis upon the sympathic adrenomedular system.	-Increased blood pressure, heart rate, and levels of norepinephrine, cortisol and testosterone after stress (Suarez, Kuhn et al. 1998); -Decreased adaptation of blood pressure and heart rate to different stressors (mainly those related to interpersonal activities).(Everson, McKey et al. 1995).	-Increased levels of catecholamines and decreased vagal stimulation; increased risk of cardiac arrhythmias (Verrier, Calvert et al. 1975; Stopper, Joska et al. 2007; Ziegelstein 2007; Yu-Wai-Man, Griffiths et al. 2010); -Increased hypertension (Ohira 2010).

Table 3. Proposed Mechanisms

6. The negative affects

6.1 Type A Behavior Pattern (TABP)

The TABP was described by Meyer Friedman and Ray Rosenman, two American cardiologists in the decade of 1950. The TABP is an action-emotion complex induced by environmental factors, involving psychomotor mannerisms, vigorous voice, hard-driving, time envolvement-pressured job, competitiveness, impatience and easy triggering anger and hostility (Friedman and Rosenman 1959) (Table 1). During the decades of 1960 and 1970 various studies demonstrated a significant association between high levels of TABP measures and the development of cardiovascular disease (Jenkins, Rosenman et al. 1974; Rosenman, Brand et al. 1976). However, subsequent studies found did not confirm the relevance of the TABP as a predictor of CHD (Ragland and Brand 1988; Ragland and Brand 1988; Schulman and Stromberg 2007). Therefore, many researchers changed the focus of their research to assess whether some aspects of the TABP, particularly anger and hostility, would be more closely linked with the development of heart disease.

Both self-report and investigator-administered instruments have been developed to recognize TABP. Among the self-report instruments are the Jenkins Activity Scale (JAS) (Jenkins, Rosenman et al. 1967) and the Framingham the Type A scale (FTAS) (Levenkron, Cohen et al. 1983). A reliable investigator-administered instrument is the Rosenman and Friedman structured interview (MacDougall, Dembroski et al. 1979). Use of this structured interview may result in different association with CHD than the self report evaluation (Dembroski, MacDougall et al. 1985; Schulman and Stromberg 2007), raising questions on the reliability of the self-report instruments.

6.2 Hostility

Various studies combine under the single label of hostility a variety of manifestations of anger and aggression. Nevertheless, those represent distinct cognitive, emotional and behavioral characteristics. Essentially, hostility generally reflects a person's tendency to view the world in a negative, cynical fashion. Smith et al (Smith, Glazer et al. 2004) define hostility as a primarily cognitive construct involving "negative attitude toward others, consisting of enmity, denigration, and ill will". The author describes its components: the cynicism (i.e., a belief that others are motivated primarily by selfish concerns); the mistrust (an expectation that people will tend to be hurtful); and denigration (i.e., a devaluation of other people's motivation and goals). Other authors define hostility as "antagonistic interpersonal attitude" including cognitions (cynicism and hostile attributions), affect (hostile emotions) and behaviors (aggressive responses) (Barefoot JC LI. The assessment of anger and hostility. In: Siegman AW, Smith TW, eds Anger, Hostility, and the Heart Hillsdale, NJ: Lawrence Erlbaum 1994:43- 66.

It is clear that these definitions, as well as the personality traits they originate from, are highly correlated and overlapping. Smith and Glazer (Smith, Glazer et al. 2004) point out the correlation among these phenomena, emphasizing that anger, hostility and aggression are not just different names for the same construct. Consequently, one could not presume that they have similar associations with cardiovascular pathology. Suarez et al (Suarez, Kuhn et al. 1998) conducted a randomized study in which men, stratified by high or low scores on the Ho scale, underwent an anagram-solving task while experiencing alternatively harassing and not harassing comments from the researcher. It was observed that, compared to men with low levels of hostility, those with higher scores on Ho scale showed greater increase in blood pressure, heart rate, and levels of norepinephrine, cortisol and testosterone. Interestingly, such increase occurred only during (and shortly after) the aversive comments. In a similar study Everson et al (Everson, McKey et al. 1995) evaluated men with high and low levels of hostility. They found that men with low levels of hostility experienced rapid adaption of heart rate and blood pressure elevations to task repetition, while men with high hostility experienced even larger increases in their rates of heart rate and blood pressure after repetitions of aversive tasks. From these two studies it can be concluded that personality traits influence physiological responses to different stressors, particularly those related to interpersonal activities. Smith and Glazer (Smith, Glazer et al. 2004) point out other social stressors also related to high reactivity among hostile individuals, such as recalling and discussing past anger-inducing events, discussions, watching anger-inducing movies and self-disclosure of personal problems. Some authors have emphasized the relevance of higher cynical hostility (Chaput, Adams et al. 2002). Various studies and meta-analyses have supported the role of hostility in increasing the risk of CHD and even cardiac death (Booth-Kewley and Friedman 1987; Friedman and Booth-Kewley 1987; Miller, Smith et al. 1996).

A variety of instruments have been used to evaluate hostility and the differences among them indicate the distinction among the subjacent concepts.

The Cook and Medley Hostility scale (CMHS, or Ho scale) consists of 50 items taken from the Minnesota Multiphasic Personality Inventory to be answered true or false. CMHS can be interpreted as a measure of cynicism and distrust (Smith, Glazer et al. 2004). This is a comprehensive scale that has been correlated with other features outside of the concept of hostility, such as neuroticism, depression and anxiety (Barefoot, Dodge et al. 1989; Steinberg and Jorgensen 1996). Although frequently used, its internal reliability is low and some authors advise to analyze its subscales separately(Barefoot, Dodge et al. 1989).

The Buss-Durkee Hostility Inventory (Buss and Durkee 1957) assesses mainly two interconnected dimensions: the expressive hostility or antagonism (physical and verbal aggression) and the neurotic or experiential hostility, which involves subjective experiences like resentment, suspicion, mistrust and irritation.

The Interpersonal Hostility Assessment Technique (IHAT) developed by Barefoot and colleagues (Brummett, Maynard et al. 2000), is a structured interview that classifies hostile behaviors in four types, based on the style (rather than content) of the responses to interviewer: direct challenges to the interviewer, indirectly or more subtle challenges, hostile withholding of information or evasion of the question, and irritation (Brummett, Maynard et al. 2000).

Although consistently associated with increased cardiovascular morbidity, the effect size of hostility has been considered low and its clinical relevance has been questioned by some authors (Myrtek 2001).

6.3 Anger

The concept of anger usually refers to an unpleasant emotion ranging in intensity from irritation or annoyance to fury or rage. Feelings of anger are elicited in situation of being treated unjustly and is accompanied by subjective arousal. As a personality trait it can be defined as the characteristic to experience frequent and pronounced episodes of this emotion.

Another relevant aspect of anger is its expression. In this context, two subtypes have been defined: "anger-out", a personality trait derived from a combination of anger and aggression (i.e, the expression of aggressive behavior when angry) and “anger- in”, a tendency to feel anger and suppress it (Schulman and Stromberg 2007) . Anger is viewed by other authors (Norlander and Eckhardt 2005) as a multidimensional construct, involving physiological, behavioral, cognitive and phenomenological components. Scales have been developed to evaluate various aspects of anger. The Anger-Out scale of the Spielberger et al. (1985) Anger-Expression Questionnaire evaluates tendencies to express aggression outwardly using a self-report questionnaire format, whereas the Anger-In scale purportedly measures tendencies to suppress or withhold anger.

Evaluated as a trait, anger significantly predicted occurrence of another MI (Denollet and Brutsaert 1998). More recently, Ohira (Ohira 2010), 2010, in the Circulatory Risk in

Communities Study (CIRCS), evaluated the association of depressive symptoms, tension and anger expression with the incidence of cardiovascular disease in Japanese population. It was a pioneering study, since all previous relevant data are mostly limited to Western populations. As an instrument for measuring tension and anger expression, Ohira and colleagues used the Spielberger anger expression scale and the Framingham Tension Scale to evaluate 6292 men and women. In a cross-sectional examination, "anger-out" was inversely associated with hypertension in men. In longitudinal observation, anger-in score was positively associated with hypertension in men, even after further adjustment for BMI, alcohol intake and systolic blood pressure levels at baseline.

Besides working chronically as a personality trait, episodes of anger may acutely cause negative impact on the cardiovascular system. Anger attacks have been associated with sudden cardiac death, MI and ventricular arrhythmias.

Among the pathophysiological mechanisms linking anger attacks and acute cardiovascular changes, two are most studied: modifications in autonomic regulation and electrophysiological changes. The autonomic dysregulation caused by anger and other emotions is well described. Experimental studies show that intense emotional factors increase the level of catecholamines and decrease vagal stimulation. Other findings suggest that cardiac sympathetic activation (and the decrease of vagal stimulation) is arrhythmogenic (Lampert 2010). Of note, Verrier et al (Verrier, Calvert et al. 1975) reported the stimulation of the posterior hypothalamus (which increases sympathetic cardiac stimulation) produced a 40% reduction of the threshold for induction of ventricular fibrillation in dogs. Regarding arrhythmogenic electrophysiological changes induced by stress, interesting results were obtained by analyzing the T-wave alternation. This measure is considered a marker of the heterogeneity of repolarization and therefore to have a major role in arrhythmogenesis. T-wave alternation was enhanced during mental stress (Kovach, Nearing et al. 2001). In a previous study, increased T-wave alternation among patients experiencing emotional stressors correlated to a higher incidence of shocks of implantable cardioverter-defibrillator (ICD) which were in turn induced by acute ventricular arrhythmias (Stopper, Joska et al. 2007). Moreover, it is noteworthy that recent evidence obtained from neuroimaging studies using positron emission tomography suggest that the laterality of brain activity during stress is related to an increased susceptibility to ventricular arrhythmias (Ziegelstein 2007).

Psychological interventions may be used to improve the management of anger, and anger attacks may also decrease significantly with antidepressant treatment, particularly in those with depression (Fava, Rosenbaum et al. 1991; Fava, Alpert et al. 1996).

6.4 Type D

Type D personality, also known as *distressed* personality, is a construct that has also been associated with cardiovascular disorders. The core symptoms of this construct are *negative affectivity* and *social inhibition* (Denollet 1998). The *negative affectivity* refers to a tendency to experience distress over time and in various situations (Watson and Pennebaker 1989), while *social inhibition* refers to the tendency of consciously inhibit the expression of these negative emotions in social situations. A high score on both traits denotes those with a Type D personality (Pedersen and Denollet 2003). Therefore, the base of this construct is not just experiencing negative emotions, but the combination of negative emotion and suppressed emotional expression. Consequently, those with this personality experience distress which is not easily shared with others. Type D personality may be identified with the DS14, an instrument developed specifically to obtain standard assessment of negative affectivity and social inhibition (Denollet 2005).

Several studies established Type D personality as an independent predictor of cardiac mortality in patients with CHD (Denollet, Sys et al. 1995; Denollet, Vaes et al. 2000). It has also been reported that Type D personality increases the risk of sudden cardiac arrest (Appels, Golombeck et al. 2000) and is an independent predictor of mortality in patients with decreased left ventricular ejection fraction after MI (Denollet and Brutsaert 1998).

Direct mechanisms proposed for the impact of Type D personality in the cardiovascular system include cardiovascular autonomic nervous system activity, endothelial function, platelet function and altered lipid profile. Type D personality has been associated with greater cortisol reactivity to stress, heightened blood pressure reactivity (Habra, Linden et al. 2003) and increased circulating levels of the pro-inflammatory cytokine tumor necrosis factor (TNF-α) and TNF-α soluble receptors 1 and 2 (Denollet, Conraads et al. 2003).

6.5 Vital exhaustion

The most common definition of VE characterizes this condition by an unusual fatigue, increased irritability and feelings of demoralization. The assessment of VE can be made with the 21-item Maastricht Questionnaire (Appels, Hoppener et al. 1987) and, although there is an overlap between VE and depressive symptoms, there is evidence these are distinct conditions (Kopp, Falger et al. 1998).

Various studies have associated VE with CHD and chronic heart failure (Appels, Kop et al. 1995; Pedersen and Middel 2001; Smith, Gidron et al. 2009). VE has been associated with a twofold to threefold increased risk of mortality and morbidity in patients with CHD (Kop, Appels et al. 1994; Appels, Kop et al. 1995). It has also been associated with sudden cardiac arrest and adverse cardiac events in patients that underwent successful angioplasty(Kop, Appels et al. 1994; Appels, Golombeck et al. 2000). A recent study showed that four distinct VE trajectories may be found in cardiac patients: low VE, decreasing VE, increasing VE and severe VE; the last two (increasing VE and severe VE) trajectories were predictors of poor cardiovascular prognosis (Smith, Kupper et al. 2010).

Several possible biological pathways may link VE with cardiovascular disease. VE has been associated with increased lipid metabolism (van Doornen and van Blokland 1989), reduced fibrinolytic capacity (Kop, Hamulyak et al. 1998; van Diest, Hamulyak et al. 2002), parasympathetic withdrawal (Watanabe, Sugiyama et al. 2002), reduced heart rate recovery after exercise (von Kanel, Barth et al. 2009), increased levels of cytokines (van der Ven, van Diest et al. 2003; Janszky, Lekander et al. 2005), decreased slow wave sleep, reactivated cytomegalovirus fosters growth of atherosclerosis, decreased negative feedback from the HPA-axis onto the sympathetic-adrenomedular system (Appels 2004) and hypocortisolemia (Keltikangas-Jarvinen, Raikkonen et al. 1996; Nicolson and van Diest 2000).

Treatment of VE aims to reduce stressors causing exhaustion and to support recovery by promoting rest and by making rest more efficient. Group discussions may be used to identify stressors in the family and work domain, and to help patients to cope with these stressors. The process includes an evaluation of the optimum length of resting time, teaching relaxation exercises designed to make rest more efficient, stimulation of physical exercise and homework assignments(Appels 2004).

6.6 Aggression

Aggression refers to a physical or verbal behavior, typically defined as attacking, destructive, or hurtful actions. Aggressive behavior may be precipitated by anger, but it may be motivated by many other factors as well. Aggression may be considered a personality trait in those who tend to frequently exhibit such behavior. The Aggression Questionnaire (AQ), developed by Buss and Perry (1992) (Buss and Perry 1992), contains subscales to measure anger, hostility and verbal and physical aggression.

6.7 Negative affectivity and negative emotion

Watson & Clark (1984) have proposed the existence of a broadband personality dimension referred to as negative affectivity(Watson and Clark 1984). This construct includes all negative emotions and is characterized by a general disposition to chronically experience anxiety, sadness, guilt, anger, irritability, and other negative emotions.

These individuals tend to be internally focused and attuned to somatic sensations. This tendency leads them to experience body sensations as symptoms of physical illness.

Some data have offered a support for increased risk of CHD in individuals with increased levels of negative affectivity (Frasure-Smith and Lesperance 2003).

Besides negative affectivity, some studies have referred to depression, anger, anxiety and hostility as negative emotions. According to Kubzansky et al. anger, anxiety and depression are the three negative emotions with the largest evidence linking them etiologically to the development of CHD (Kubzansky and Kawachi 2000; Kubzansky, Davidson et al. 2005; Kubzansky 2007). According to these authors emotions occur in a continuum ranging from normal to pathological and there is evidence of a dose response between negative emotions and CHD risk (Kubzansky and Kawachi 2000; Everson-Rose and Lewis 2005; Rozanski, Blumenthal et al. 2005). Possibly all these negative emotions work as a general stressor of the cardiovascular system (Todaro, Shen et al. 2003). In the INTERHEART, a case-control study, the authors performed an analysis using a score integrating psychosocial factors including depression, locus of control, perceived stress and life events. They found that psychosocial factors had a greater relative risk of MI than well-established risk factors such as hypertension, abdominal obesity and diabetes (Yusuf, Hawken et al. 2004).

7. Treatment

Various strategies have been developed to treat negative affect (Table 4). Most of them focused in reducing TABP, including education about CHD and TABP; Relaxation Training (Relaxation excercises of the "deep-muscle" or "acobsonian"); Cognitive Therapy including restructuring techniques such as the identification and modification of TABP cognitions (e.g.,

"I have to get there faster" is changed to "I'm going fast enough"). Specific techniques are the *Imaging* strategy that includes imagining rousing situations such as a traffic jam or confrontation with a boss and the training to apply specific coping skills such as relaxation training or cognitive restructuring; the *Behavior Modification* that includes rehearsing of Type B coping skills through role playing or behavioral prescriptions that are given to be carried out between sessions; the *Emotional Support* that includes the encouragement to ventilate the painful affects and experiences in an empathic atmosphere. There is also the *Psychodynamic Interpretation* that includes the use of psychodynamic interpretations of the unconscious motives and conflicts underlying TABP (Nunes, Frank et al. 1987). A meta-analysis of 18 controlled studies of psychological treatment of TABP revealed an effect size of 0.61±0.21 indicating a reduction approximately by half a standard deviation (Nunes, Frank et al. 1987).

Type A Behavior Pattern	Type D Personality	Vital exhaustion	Hostility	Anger	Aggression
-Education about CHD and TABP; -Relaxation Training: Relaxation excercises; -Cognitive Therapy including cognitive restructuring techniques and also psychodynamic interpretation (Nunes, Frank et al. 1987)	-Patients may benefit from psychological treatment to deal with threatening issues and lighten the symptoms.	-Reduction of the stressors that cause exhaustion, -Support recovery by promoting rest and by making rest more efficient; -Group discussions may be used to identify stressors in the family and work domain, and to help patient in coping with these stressors; -Stimulation of physical exercise (Appels 2004).	-Cognitive-behavior interventions may reduce measures of hostility (Sloan, Shapiro et al. 2010); -SSRIs may reduce hostile affect (Kamarck, Haskett et al. 2009).	-Cognitive-behavioral and skills-based approaches may reduce anger (Blake and Hamrin 2007). -Anger attacks may decrease with SSRIs particularly in depressed patients (Fava, Rosenbaum et al. 1991; Fava, Alpert et al. 1996)	-SSRIs may reduce, physical and verbal aggression in women (Kamarck, Haskett et al. 2009).

Table 4. Treatments

There is no well-established treatment for type D personality, but these patients may benefit from psychological treatment to deal with threatening issues and lighten the symptoms. Interventions for VE focus on reducing the stressors associated with the exhaustion and support recovery by promoting rest and by making rest more efficient. Group discussions may be used to identify stressors in the family and work domain, to help patients to cope with these stressors and to stimulate physical exercise (Appels 2004). Kamark et al (Kamarck, Haskett et al. 2009) studied people with high hostility scores and with no Axis I diagnosis medicated with citalopram or placebo. The citalopram group showed significant reductions in state anger, and hostile affect, while physical and verbal aggression was reduced among women.

Cognitive-behavior interventions have shown to be effective in reducing measures of hostility and improving cardiac autonomic modulation (Sloan, Shapiro et al. 2010). In addition, Cognitive-behavioral and skills-based approaches may be effective in reducing anger and aggression in youth (Blake and Hamrin 2007). Anger attacks (Fava, Rosenbaum et al. 1991; Fava, Alpert et al. 1996) decreased significantly with fluoxetine treatment in depressed patients.

8. Discussion

Several studies have linked negative affect with cardiovascular morbidity. However, due to discrepancies among results, there is still some controversy regarding the existence, nature and magnitude of their relationship. In this context, Schulman and Stromberg, 2007, (Schulman and Stromberg 2007) conducted a review of the meta-analyses and systematic reviews on this subject. As inclusion criteria, the authors used the Database of Abstracts of Reviews of Effects (DARE) criteria and they chose to include only those reviews and meta-analyses which had measured the magnitude of the effect of anger, hostility and TABP on the cardiovascular outcomes. The final analysis included five systematic reviews (Hemingway and Marmot 1999; Rozanski, Blumenthal et al. 1999; Kuper, Marmot et al. 2002; Suls and Bunde 2005). As a common result, they showed positive results between TABP, hostility, anger and CHD in healthy populations. For individuals with heart disease the review showed conflicting results. The authors concluded that TABP, hostility, anger and anger expression may not constitute a risk factor for worse prognosis in all patient samples, and their effects would be more significant in a previously healthy population. In such patients negative affect could harm the cardiovascular system directly or indirectly by increasing cardiovascular risk factors such as hypertension and atherosclerosis (Matthews, Owens et al. 1998; Pollitt, Daniel et al. 2005).

In a more recent review and meta-analysis, Chida and Steptoe (2009) (Chida and Steptoe 2009) selected only prospective cohort studies, exploring the causal association of measures of anger and hostility and heart disease. A total of 21 cohorts with healthy patients at baseline with 71 606 individuals, and 18 cohorts of patients with existing CHD with 8120 individuals were included. These studies were published between 1983 and 2006 and performed in a wide range of countries (Europe, America and Australia). This meta-analysis found that 28% of studies with healthy individuals and 26.3% of studies with CHD patients showed significant harmful effects. The overall combined hazard ratio (HR) was 1.19 (95% CI 1.05 to 1.35) for the healthy population and 1.23 (95% CI 1.08 to 1.42) for the disease population, indicating a positive association. In subgroup analysis, it was found that cohorts with longer follow-up periods showed higher HR than the overall effect both in studies with healthy and with CHD individuals. Also, in studies with CHD patients, the HR was sustained even after controlling for baseline disease status and treatment (1.20 95% CI 1.0 to 1.44). Focusing on mortality analyses, a positive association was also found between anger and hostility and cardiovascular mortality. Thus, this review emphasizes the increased risk of negative affect for those with established CHD, in contrast to the results of Schulman and Stromberg.

The development of a validated gold standard for the assessment of negative affect is necessary to allow the comparison between studies. Moreover, the concepts of anger and hostility do not include a clear cutoff for its morbidity and consequently data about their prevalence, course, comorbidity and treatment response are lacking. Besides this difference in instruments, there is also a disagreement concerning the results of clinical studies focused on the relationship between psychological traits and cardiovascular disease.

Undeniably, a consistent body of evidence links negative affect with heart disease. In addition, the efficacy of psychotherapeutic interventions in cardiac patients was recently demonstrated (Linden, Phillips et al. 2007). While the clinical use of screening instruments for anger and hostility is not yet a reality, in the future the multi-disciplinary approach involving psychological techniques, possibly specifically focused on these traits, might become an important strategy in the management of patients with CHD. Moreover, recent advances in our understanding of pathophysiology involving physical and emotional changes will potentially allow specific case definitions and possible targeted drug therapies for certain forms of negative affect.

9. References

American Psychiatric Association (1994). Diagnostic and Statistical Manual of Mental Disorders. Washington, DC, American Psychiatric Association.

Appels, A. (2004). "Exhaustion and coronary heart disease: the history of a scientific quest." Patient Educ Couns 55(2): 223-229.

Appels, A., B. Golombeck, et al. (2000). "Behavioral risk factors of sudden cardiac arrest." J Psychosom Res 48(4-5): 463-469.

Appels, A., P. Hoppener, et al. (1987). "A questionnaire to assess premonitory symptoms of myocardial infarction." Int J Cardiol 17(1): 15-24.

Appels, A., W. Kop, et al. (1995). "Vital exhaustion, extent of atherosclerosis, and the clinical course after successful percutaneous transluminal coronary angioplasty." Eur Heart J 16(12): 1880-1885.

Bagby, R. M., S. H. Kennedy, et al. (1997). "Personality and symptom profiles of the angry hostile depressed patient." J Affect Disord 45(3): 155-160.

Baker, M., J. Dorzab, et al. (1971). "Depressive disease: classification and clinical characteristics." Compr Psychiatry 12(4): 354-365.

Barefoot, J. C., K. A. Dodge, et al. (1989). "The Cook-Medley hostility scale: item content and ability to predict survival." Psychosom Med 51(1): 46-57.

Blake, C. S. and V. Hamrin (2007). "Current approaches to the assessment and management of anger and aggression in youth: a review." Journal of child and adolescent psychiatric nursing : official publication of the Association of Child and Adolescent Psychiatric Nurses, Inc 20(4): 209-221.

Booth-Kewley, S. and H. S. Friedman (1987). "Psychological predictors of heart disease: a quantitative review." Psychol Bull 101(3): 343-362.

Brummett, B. H., K. E. Maynard, et al. (2000). "Reliability of interview-assessed hostility ratings across mode of assessment and time." J Pers Assess 75(2): 225-236.

Buss, A. H. and A. Durkee (1957). "An inventory for assessing different kinds of hostility." J Consult Psychol 21(4): 343-349.

Buss, A. H. and M. Perry (1992). "The aggression questionnaire." J Pers Soc Psychol 63(3): 452-459.

Chaput, L. A., S. H. Adams, et al. (2002). "Hostility predicts recurrent events among postmenopausal women with coronary heart disease." Am J Epidemiol 156(12): 1092-1099.

Chida, Y. and A. Steptoe (2009). "The association of anger and hostility with future coronary heart disease: a meta-analytic review of prospective evidence." J Am Coll Cardiol 53(11): 936-946.

Clark, L. A., D. Watson, et al. (1994). "Temperament, personality, and the mood and anxiety disorders." J Abnorm Psychol 103(1): 103-116.

Culic, V., D. Eterovic, et al. (2005). "Meta-analysis of possible external triggers of acute myocardial infarction." Int J Cardiol 99(1): 1-8.

Davidson, K. W. (2008). "Emotional predictors and behavioral triggers of acute coronary syndrome." Cleve Clin J Med 75 Suppl 2: S15-19.

Dembroski, T. M., J. M. MacDougall, et al. (1989). "Components of hostility as predictors of sudden death and myocardial infarction in the Multiple Risk Factor Intervention Trial." Psychosom Med 51(5): 514-522.

Dembroski, T. M., J. M. MacDougall, et al. (1985). "Components of Type A, hostility, and anger-in: relationship to angiographic findings." Psychosom Med 47(3): 219-233.

Denollet, J. (1998). "Personality and coronary heart disease: the type-D scale-16 (DS16)." Ann Behav Med 20(3): 209 215.

Denollet, J. (2005). "DS14: standard assessment of negative affectivity, social inhibition, and Type D personality." Psychosom Med 67(1): 89-97.

Denollet, J. and D. L. Brutsaert (1998). "Personality, disease severity, and the risk of long-term cardiac events in patients with a decreased ejection fraction after myocardial infarction." Circulation 97(2): 167-173.

Denollet, J., V. M. Conraads, et al. (2003). "Cytokines and immune activation in systolic heart failure: the role of Type D personality." Brain Behav Immun 17(4): 304-309.

Denollet, J., S. U. Sys, et al. (1995). "Personality and mortality after myocardial infarction." Psychosom Med 57(6): 582-591.

Denollet, J., J. Vaes, et al. (2000). "Inadequate response to treatment in coronary heart disease : adverse effects of type D personality and younger age on 5-year prognosis and quality of life." Circulation 102(6): 630-635.

Dougherty, D. D., S. L. Rauch, et al. (2004). "Ventromedial prefrontal cortex and amygdala dysfunction during an anger induction positron emission tomography study in patients with major depressive disorder with anger attacks." Archives of General Psychiatry 61(8): 795-804.

Drevets, W. C. (1999). "Prefrontal cortical-amygdalar metabolism in major depression." Annals of the New York Academy of Sciences 877: 614-637.

Dujovne, V. F. and B. K. Houston (1991). "Hostility-related variables and plasma lipid levels." Journal of behavioral medicine 14(6): 555-565.

Eaker, E. D., J. Pinsky, et al. (1992). "Myocardial infarction and coronary death among women: psychosocial predictors from a 20-year follow-up of women in the Framingham Study." Am J Epidemiol 135(8): 854-864.

Everson, S. A., B. S. McKey, et al. (1995). "Effect of trait hostility on cardiovascular responses to harassment in young men." International journal of behavioral medicine 2(2): 172-191.

Everson-Rose, S. A. and T. T. Lewis (2005). "Psychosocial factors and cardiovascular diseases." Annu Rev Public Health 26: 469-500.

Fava, M., M. Abraham, et al. (1996). "Cardiovascular risk factors in depression. The role of anxiety and anger." Psychosomatics 37(1): 31-37.

Fava, M., J. Alpert, et al. (1996). "Fluoxetine treatment of anger attacks: a replication study." Ann Clin Psychiatry 8(1): 7-10.

Fava, M., J. E. Alpert, et al. (2004). "Clinical correlates and symptom patterns of anxious depression among patients with major depressive disorder in STAR*D." Psychol Med 34(7): 1299-1308.

Fava, M., J. F. Rosenbaum, et al. (1991). "Anger attacks in depressed outpatients and their response to fluoxetine." Psychopharmacology bulletin 27(3): 275-279.

Fava, M., L. A. Uebelacker, et al. (1997). "Major depressive subtypes and treatment response." Biol Psychiatry 42(7): 568-576.

Fava, M., R. D. Vuolo, et al. (2000). "Fenfluramine challenge in unipolar depression with and without anger attacks." Psychiatry Research 94(1): 9-18.

Felsten, G. and V. Hill (1999). "Aggression Questionnaire hostility scale predicts anger in response to mistreatment." Behaviour research and therapy 37(1): 87-97.

Fraguas, R., D. V. Iosifescu, et al. (2007). "Major depressive disorder with anger attacks and cardiovascular risk factors." Int J Psychiatry Med 37(1): 99-111.

Frasure-Smith, N. and F. Lesperance (2003). "Depression and other psychological risks following myocardial infarction." Arch Gen Psychiatry 60(6): 627-636.

Friedman, H. S. and S. Booth-Kewley (1987). "The "disease-prone personality". A meta-analytic view of the construct." Am Psychol 42(6): 539-555.

Friedman, M. and R. H. Rosenman (1959). "Association of specific overt behavior pattern with blood and cardiovascular findings; blood cholesterol level, blood clotting time, incidence of arcus senilis, and clinical coronary artery disease." J Am Med Assoc 169(12): 1286-1296.

Gould, R. A., S. Ball, et al. (1996). "Prevalence and correlates of anger attacks: a two site study." J Affect Disord 39(1): 31-38.

Gullion, C. M. and A. J. Rush (1998). "Toward a generalizable model of symptoms in major depressive disorder." Biol Psychiatry 44(10): 959-972.

Habra, M. E., W. Linden, et al. (2003). "Type D personality is related to cardiovascular and neuroendocrine reactivity to acute stress." J Psychosom Res 55(3): 235-245.

Hamilton, M. (1960). "A rating scale for depression." J Neurol Neurosurg Psychiatry 23: 56-62.

Haynes, S. G., M. Feinleib, et al. (1980). "The relationship of psychosocial factors to coronary heart disease in the Framingham Study. III. Eight-year incidence of coronary heart disease." Am J Epidemiol 111(1): 37-58.

Hemingway, H. and M. Marmot (1999). "Evidence based cardiology: psychosocial factors in the aetiology and prognosis of coronary heart disease. Systematic review of prospective cohort studies." BMJ 318(7196): 1460-1467.

Iosifescu, D. V., P. F. Renshaw, et al. (2007). "Major depressive disorder with anger attacks and subcortical MRI white matter hyperintensities." J Nerv Ment Dis 195(2): 175-178.

Janszky, I., M. Lekander, et al. (2005). "Self-rated health and vital exhaustion, but not depression, is related to inflammation in women with coronary heart disease." Brain Behav Immun 19(6): 555-563.

Jenkins, C. D., R. H. Rosenman, et al. (1967). "Development of an objective psychological test for the determination of the coronary-prone behavior pattern in employed men." J Chronic Dis 20(6): 371-379.

Jenkins, C. D., R. H. Rosenman, et al. (1974). "Prediction of clinical coronary heart disease by a test for the coronary-prone behavior pattern." N Engl J Med 290(23): 1271-1275.

Kamarck, T. W., R. F. Haskett, et al. (2009). "Citalopram intervention for hostility: results of a randomized clinical trial." Journal of consulting and clinical psychology 77(1): 174-188.

Keltikangas-Jarvinen, L., T. Hintsa, et al. (2007). "Type A eagerness-energy across developmental periods predicts adulthood carotid intima-media thickness: the Cardiovascular Risk in Young Finns Study." Arteriosclerosis, thrombosis, and vascular biology 27(7): 1638-1644.

Keltikangas-Jarvinen, L., K. Raikkonen, et al. (1996). "Vital exhaustion, anger expression, and pituitary and adrenocortical hormones. Implications for the insulin resistance syndrome." Arterioscler Thromb Vasc Biol 16(2): 275-280.

Kop, W. J., A. P. Appels, et al. (1994). "Vital exhaustion predicts new cardiac events after successful coronary angioplasty." Psychosom Med 56(4): 281-287.

Kop, W. J., K. Hamulyak, et al. (1998). "Relationship of blood coagulation and fibrinolysis to vital exhaustion." Psychosom Med 60(3): 352-358.

Kopp, M. S., P. R. Falger, et al. (1998). "Depressive symptomatology and vital exhaustion are differentially related to behavioral risk factors for coronary artery disease." Psychosom Med 60(6): 752-758.

Kovach, J. A., B. D. Nearing, et al. (2001). "Angerlike behavioral state potentiates myocardial ischemia-induced T-wave alternans in canines." Journal of the American College of Cardiology 37(6): 1719-1725.

Kubzansky, L. D. (2007). "Sick at heart: the pathophysiology of negative emotions." Cleve Clin J Med 74 Suppl 1: S67-72.

Kubzansky, L. D., K. W. Davidson, et al. (2005). "The clinical impact of negative psychological states: expanding the spectrum of risk for coronary artery disease." Psychosom Med 67 Suppl 1: S10-14.

Kubzansky, L. D. and I. Kawachi (2000). "Going to the heart of the matter: do negative emotions cause coronary heart disease?" J Psychosom Res 48(4-5): 323-337.

Kuper, H., M. Marmot, et al. (2002). "Systematic review of prospective cohort studies of psychosocial factors in the etiology and prognosis of coronary heart disease." Semin Vasc Med 2(3): 267-314.

Lampert, R. (2010). "Anger and ventricular arrhythmias." Curr Opin Cardiol 25(1): 46-52.

Lampert, R., T. Joska, et al. (2002). "Emotional and physical precipitants of ventricular arrhythmia." Circulation 106(14): 1800-1805.

Levenkron, J. C., J. D. Cohen, et al. (1983). "Modifying the Type A coronary-prone behavior pattern." J Consult Clin Psychol 51(2): 192-204.

Linden, W., M. J. Phillips, et al. (2007). "Psychological treatment of cardiac patients: a meta-analysis." Eur Heart J 28(24): 2972-2984.

Lovallo, W. R. and W. Gerin (2003). "Psychophysiological reactivity: mechanisms and pathways to cardiovascular disease." Psychosom Med 65(1): 36-45.

MacDougall, J. M., T. M. Dembroski, et al. (1979). "The structured interview and questionnaire methods of assessing coronary-prone behavior in male and female college students." J Behav Med 2(1): 71-83.

Martin, R., D. Watson, et al. (2000). "A three-factor model of trait anger: dimensions of affect, behavior, and cognition." J Pers 68(5): 869-897.

Matthews, K. A., J. F. Owens, et al. (1998). "Are hostility and anxiety associated with carotid atherosclerosis in healthy postmenopausal women?" Psychosom Med 60(5): 633-638.

Miller, T. Q., T. W. Smith, et al. (1996). "A meta-analytic review of research on hostility and physical health." Psychol Bull 119(2): 322-348.

Mischoulon, D., D. D. Dougherty, et al. (2002). "An open pilot study of nefazodone in depression with anger attacks: relationship between clinical response and receptor binding." Psychiatry Res 116(3): 151-161.

Mittleman, M. A., M. Maclure, et al. (1995). "Triggering of acute myocardial infarction onset by episodes of anger. Determinants of Myocardial Infarction Onset Study Investigators." Circulation 92(7): 1720-1725.

Montgomery, S. A. and M. Asberg (1979). "A new depression scale designed to be sensitive to change." Br J Psychiatry 134: 382-389.

Morand, P., G. Thomas, et al. (1998). "Fava's Anger Attacks Questionnaire: evaluation of the French version in depressed patients." Eur Psychiatry 13(1): 41-45.

Myrtek, M. (2001). "Meta-analyses of prospective studies on coronary heart disease, type A personality, and hostility." Int J Cardiol 79(2-3): 245-251.

Niaura, R., C. M. Stoney, et al. (1992). "Lipids in psychological research: the last decade." Biological psychology 34(1): 1-43.

Nicolson, N. A. and R. van Diest (2000). "Salivary cortisol patterns in vital exhaustion." J Psychosom Res 49(5): 335-342.

Norlander, B. and C. Eckhardt (2005). "Anger, hostility, and male perpetrators of intimate partner violence: a meta-analytic review." Clin Psychol Rev 25(2): 119-152.

Nunes, E. V., K. A. Frank, et al. (1987). "Psychologic treatment for the type A behavior pattern and for coronary heart disease: a meta-analysis of the literature." Psychosom Med 49(2): 159-173.

Ohira, T. (2010). "Psychological distress and cardiovascular disease: the Circulatory Risk in Communities Study (CIRCS)." J Epidemiol 20(3): 185-191.

Oishi, K., M. Kamimura, et al. (1999). "Individual differences in physiological responses and type A behavior pattern." Applied human science : journal of physiological anthropology 18(3): 101-108.

Overall, J. E., B. J. Goldstein, et al. (1971). "Symptomatic volunteers in psychiatric research." J Psychiatr Res 9(1): 31-43.

Overall, J. E., L. E. Hollister, et al. (1966). "Nosology of depression and differential response to drugs." JAMA 195(11): 946-948.

Painuly, N., P. Sharan, et al. (2005). "Relationship of anger and anger attacks with depression: a brief review." Eur Arch Psychiatry Clin Neurosci 255(4): 215-222.

Pedersen, S. S. and J. Denollet (2003). "Type D personality, cardiac events, and impaired quality of life: a review." Eur J Cardiovasc Prev Rehabil 10(4): 241-248.

Pedersen, S. S. and B. Middel (2001). "Increased vital exhaustion among type-D patients with ischemic heart disease." J Psychosom Res 51(2): 443-449.

Perlis, R. H., J. W. Smoller, et al. (2004). "The prevalence and clinical correlates of anger attacks during depressive episodes in bipolar disorder." J Affect Disord 79(1-3): 291-295.

Pizzagalli, D., R. D. Pascual-Marqui, et al. (2001). "Anterior cingulate activity as a predictor of degree of treatment response in major depression: evidence from brain electrical tomography analysis." The American journal of psychiatry 158(3): 405-415.

Pollitt, R. A., M. Daniel, et al. (2005). "Mediation and modification of the association between hopelessness, hostility, and progression of carotid atherosclerosis." J Behav Med 28(1): 53-64.

Posternak, M. A. and M. Zimmerman (2002). "Anger and aggression in psychiatric outpatients." J Clin Psychiatry 63(8): 665-672.

Ragland, D. R. and R. J. Brand (1988). "Coronary heart disease mortality in the Western Collaborative Group Study. Follow-up experience of 22 years." Am J Epidemiol 127(3): 462-475.

Ragland, D. R. and R. J. Brand (1988). "Type A behavior and mortality from coronary heart disease." N Engl J Med 318(2): 65-69.

Ravaja, N., T. Kauppinen, et al. (2000). "Relationships between hostility and physiological coronary heart disease risk factors in young adults: the moderating influence of depressive tendencies." Psychological Medicine 30(2): 381-393.

Raynor, D. A., M. F. Pogue-Geile, et al. (2002). "Covariation of psychosocial characteristics associated with cardiovascular disease: genetic and environmental influences." Psychosom Med 64(2): 191-203; discussion 204-195.

Rosenman, R. H., R. J. Brand, et al. (1976). "Multivariate prediction of coronary heart disease during 8.5 year follow-up in the Western Collaborative Group Study." Am J Cardiol 37(6): 903-910.

Rozanski, A., J. A. Blumenthal, et al. (2005). "The epidemiology, pathophysiology, and management of psychosocial risk factors in cardiac practice: the emerging field of behavioral cardiology." J Am Coll Cardiol 45(5): 637-651.

Rozanski, A., J. A. Blumenthal, et al. (1999). "Impact of psychological factors on the pathogenesis of cardiovascular disease and implications for therapy." Circulation 99(16): 2192-2217.

Schaefer, S. M., H. C. Abercrombie, et al. (2000). "Six-month test-retest reliability of MRI-defined PET measures of regional cerebral glucose metabolic rate in selected subcortical structures." Human brain mapping 10(1): 1-9.

Scherwitz, L. W., L. L. Perkins, et al. (1992). "Hostility and health behaviors in young adults: the CARDIA Study. Coronary Artery Risk Development in Young Adults Study." Am J Epidemiol 136(2): 136-145.

Schulman, J. K. and S. Stromberg (2007). "On the value of doing nothing: anger and cardiovascular disease in clinical practice." Cardiol Rev 15(3): 123-132.

Sloan, R. P., P. A. Shapiro, et al. (2010). "Cardiac autonomic control and treatment of hostility: a randomized controlled trial." Psychosomatic medicine 72(1): 1-8.

Smith, O. R., Y. Gidron, et al. (2009). "Vital exhaustion in chronic heart failure: symptom profiles and clinical outcome." J Psychosom Res 66(3): 195-201.

Smith, O. R., N. Kupper, et al. (2010). "Vital exhaustion and cardiovascular prognosis in myocardial infarction and heart failure: predictive power of different trajectories." Psychol Med: 1-8.

Smith, T. W., K. Glazer, et al. (2004). "Hostility, anger, aggressiveness, and coronary heart disease: an interpersonal perspective on personality, emotion, and health." J Pers 72(6): 1217-1270.

Snaith, R. P. and C. M. Taylor (1985). "Irritability: definition, assessment and associated factors." Br J Psychiatry 147: 127-136.

Steinberg, L. and R. S. Jorgensen (1996). "Assessing the MMPI-based Cook-Medley Hostility Scale: the implications of dimensionality." J Pers Soc Psychol 70(6): 1281-1287.

Stopper, M., T. Joska, et al. (2007). "Electrophysiologic characteristics of anger-triggered arrhythmias." Heart rhythm : the official journal of the Heart Rhythm Society 4(3): 268-273.

Stopper, M., T. Joska, et al. (2007). "Electrophysiologic characteristics of anger-triggered arrhythmias." Heart Rhythm 4(3): 268-273.

Suarez, E. C., C. M. Kuhn, et al. (1998). "Neuroendocrine, cardiovascular, and emotional responses of hostile men: the role of interpersonal challenge." Psychosom Med 60(1): 78-88.

Suls, J. and J. Bunde (2005). "Anger, anxiety, and depression as risk factors for cardiovascular disease: the problems and implications of overlapping affective dispositions." Psychol Bull 131(2): 260-300.

Todaro, J. F., B. J. Shen, et al. (2003). "Effect of negative emotions on frequency of coronary heart disease (The Normative Aging Study)." Am J Cardiol 92(8): 901-906.

van der Ven, A., R. van Diest, et al. (2003). "Herpes viruses, cytokines, and altered hemostasis in vital exhaustion." Psychosom Med 65(2): 194-200.

van Diest, R., K. Hamulyak, et al. (2002). "Diurnal variations in coagulation and fibrinolysis in vital exhaustion." Psychosom Med 64(5): 787-792.

van Doornen, L. J. and R. W. van Blokland (1989). "The relation of type A behavior and vital exhaustion with physiological reactions to real life stress." J Psychosom Res 33(6): 715-725.

Verrier, R. L., A. Calvert, et al. (1975). "Effect of posterior hypothalamic stimulation on ventricular fibrillation threshold." The American journal of physiology 228(3): 923-927.

von Kanel, R., J. Barth, et al. (2009). "Heart rate recovery after exercise in chronic heart failure: Role of vital exhaustion and type D personality." J Cardiol 53(2): 248-256.

Watanabe, T., Y. Sugiyama, et al. (2002). "Effects of vital exhaustion on cardiac autononomic nervous functions assessed by heart rate variability at rest in middle-aged male workers." Int J Behav Med 9(1): 68-75.

Watson, D. and L. A. Clark (1984). "Negative affectivity: the disposition to experience aversive emotional states." Psychol Bull 96(3): 465-490.

Watson, D. and J. W. Pennebaker (1989). "Health complaints, stress, and distress: exploring the central role of negative affectivity." Psychol Rev 96(2): 234-254.

Yu-Wai-Man, P., P. G. Griffiths, et al. (2010). "Multi-system neurological disease is common in patients with OPA1 mutations." Brain : a journal of neurology 133(Pt 3): 771-786.

Yusuf, S., S. Hawken, et al. (2004). "Effect of potentially modifiable risk factors associated with myocardial infarction in 52 countries (the INTERHEART study): case-control study." Lancet 364(9438): 937-952.

Ziegelstein, R. C. (2007). "Acute emotional stress and cardiac arrhythmias." JAMA 298(3): 324-329.

23

"Recognizing Hunger" – A Training to Abate Insulin Resistance, Associated Subclinical Inflammation and Cardiovascular Risks

Mario Ciampolini
Università di Firenze,
Italy

1. Introduction

1.1 Background

People cannot share subjective sensations with others as they do with sounds and figures. Subjective sensations guide the intake. In this chapter, subjective sensations of hunger that induce intake, become objective (verifiable by others, reproducible and comparable) by the association with measurements of blood glucose concentration (BG). This is possible after about two weeks of training with BG measurements. Subjective sensations become thus a meal by meal information tool on energy balance. Respecting the arousal of the validated sensation before any intake was useful to treat infants with chronic non-specific diarrhea (Ciampolini et al. 1990). In a health policy for cardiovascular risk prevention, for a suppression of subclinical inflammation and for a decrease or maintenance of a stable body weight, treating functional intestinal disorders means treating a reversible condition like insulin resistance to prevent irreversible events. Functional intestinal disorders are also capable to give valid motivation to patients for training (see further "Training to...").

Subjective signals that promote intake are reported by many researchers (Harshaw, 2008). In past investigations, we suggested subjects to find a subjective target (initial hunger, IH) before intake on the first day, and measuring blood glucose concentration as a marker of this target on the first and subsequent days (Ciampolini & Bianchi, 2006a).

In our experience, less than 10% of healthy people report never perceiving any kind of hunger. No perception may depend on insulin resistance or non-insulin dependent diabetes (NIDD). With the word hunger, all over the world, healthy subjects report gastric pangs or sensations of gastric emptiness. In other circumstances, the subject's definition is inadequate. Subjects trained to "hunger recognition" were able to assess current value of blood glucose with a fairly low estimation error from measurement (Figure 1) both when they either recognized or denied hunger (Figure 2, Ciampolini & Bianchi, 2006a). Subjects who denied hunger, reported mental and/or physical sensations of weakness. They reported these sensations from 10% to 45% of instances of eating induction. In these instances, animals actually show a decrease of resting metabolic rate (RMR). In this report, with the term "initial hunger" (IH) we indicate gastric, physical and mental sensations that are associated with a low error of estimation of BG measurement after training (Ciampolini & Bianchi, 2006a).

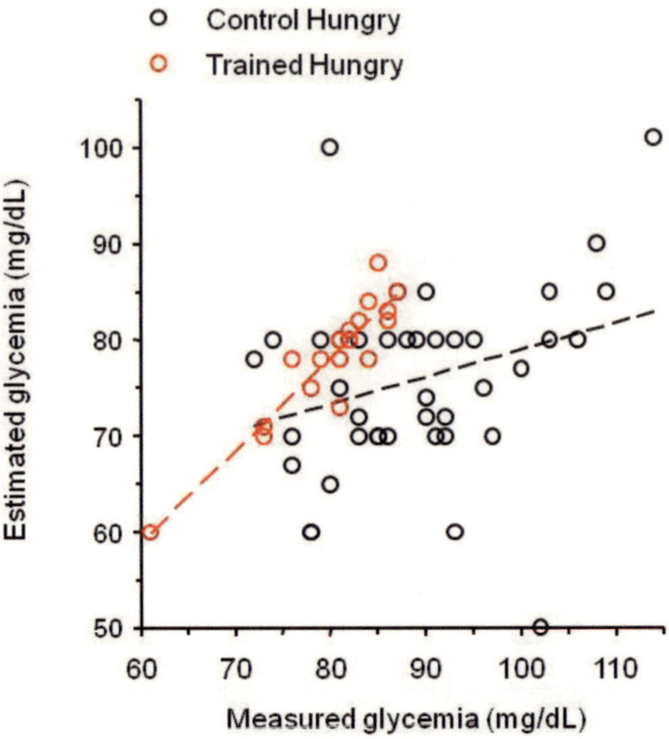

Fig. 1. Estimated *vs.* measured blood glucose of subjects reporting to be hungry at the final laboratory investigative session.
Hollow red circles, trained hungry subjects (n = 18); hollow black circles, control (untrained) hungry subjects (n = 42). Linear correlation was significant for the trained data (dashed red line; r = 0.92; p = 0.0001) but not for the control data (dashed black line; r = 0.29, p = 0.06). (By kind permission of the Authors: Ciampolini & Bianchi, 2006a).

We named intake adaptation to IH arousal before meals three times a day as initial hunger meal pattern (IHMP) (Ciampolini et al. 2010°; 2010b; Ciampolini & Sifone, 2011). This is a meal pattern based on "recognizing hunger". We use these two simple words in this report to be more evocative than by using the term IHMP. We chose the assessment of the validated sensation and of BG measurement before meals for six reasons: first, because before meals people sometimes recognise definite hunger sensations, and are able to validate them through BG measurement (Ciampolini & Bianchi, 2006a). Second, a BG measurement (as well as validated hunger sensations, initial hunger, IH) is an evaluation of either sufficiency or excess of energy intake at previous meal, and is useful in planning meal sizes (Ciampolini et al. 2010; 2010b; Ciampolini & Sifone, 2011). Third, 7 day-food-diary reporting consecutive 21 BG measurements and meal compositions may prove to be a highly effective educational instrument to evaluate intake meal by meal as suggested in point two. Fourth, a mean of pre-meal BG sequence informs on lowest mean energy availability for the body. "Mean BG" is a metabolic characterization of an individual, energy meal pattern (fifth), which is standard in metabolic time and allows comparisons and classifications better than daily energy intake (Ciampolini & Sifone, 2011). Sixth, mean BG measures the blood function of providing energy to body tissues (Ciampolini & Sifone, 2011).

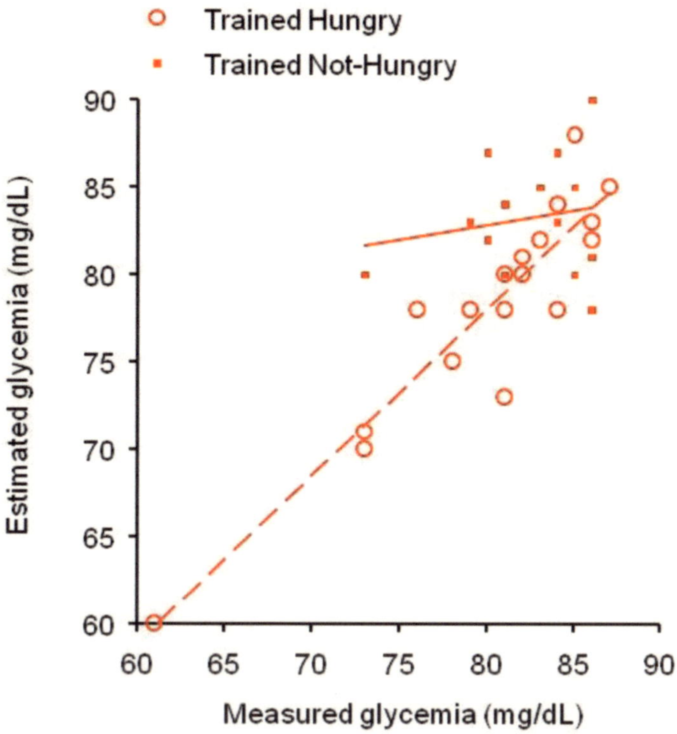

Fig. 2. Estimated *vs* measured blood glucose (BG) of trained subjects with BG below 87 mg/dL at the final session.
The highest BG measured in trained hungry subjects was 87 mg/dL. Below this value of measured BG, 18 subjects reported to be hungry (hollow red circles) and 14 subjects were not hungry (filled red squares). The errors in estimation (estimated BG value less measured one) showed no significant difference between the two groups. (By kind permission of the Authors: Ciampolini & Bianchi, 2006a).

Meal adaptation to "recognizing hunger" decreased mean BG, metabolic risks, insulin resistance and overweight in the trained group compared to control subjects (Ciampolini et al. 2010b). The global response in mean BG and the global improvement overlooks differences in single meal patterns, insulin sensitivity and health at recruitment and in response to training. If mean BG is maintained as a personal habit, the differences may explain huge risk differences that can be personally felt and corrected by "recognizing hunger".

1.2 Investigation aims

After suspension of food intake and initial identification of the first sensation of hunger, can a subject show a stable recognition of the same hunger sensation by coincidence between BG estimation and measurement? Can a subject maintain a meal rhythm based on recognition of the same subjective sensation (IH)? Can few subjects maintain the rhythm before any training? Can the trained rhythm decrease metabolic risk factors? Can prevent malnutrition and slightly depressed BG? Can decrease body weight in overweight people and in subjects with insulin resistance? The demonstration of these effects show that the achieved rhythm (mean BG) is homeostatic rather than being an artifact, i.e. maintains a BG that is constant and both sufficient for activity and body weight maintenance, and effective in risk prevention. Informed people may approximate this *reference* model in eating as much as they can.

1.3 Subjects

A total of 181 subjects were recruited by the Paediatric Gastroenterology Unit of Florence University, a third level referring center, between 1995 and 2000 (Ciampolini et al. 2010). Subjects were gastroenterology patients between 18 and 60 years of age with functional bowel disorders, a self recovering disease. Subjects showed no morphological, physical or biochemical signs of organic disease. Subjects with impaired glucose tolerance (fasting plasma-glucose > 115 mg/dL (6.4 mmol/l)), as well as subjects suffering from non-insulin dependent diabetes mellitus (NIDDM), celiac, inflammatory bowel, liver, heart, brain and kidney diseases were excluded from recruitment. At end of investigation, 149 completed the protocol. 120 served for the metabolic study. All 149 were used for the body weight study. Informed consent was obtained from all participants. The local Hospital Ethics Committee approved the study in compliance with the Helsinki Declaration.

2. Metabolic study on 120 subjects

2.1 Design

All 120 subjects who completed the protocol were fully assessed at recruitment (before training), clinically only after the first 7 weeks of training, and completely at the end of the investigation (total investigation 5 months). In 31 control subjects, we investigated whether food intake is habitual, ie, maintaining the same meal pattern by "mean BG". Moreover, habits in BG maintenance may be personal, ie, sharply defined from most others. In all 120 subjects, we calculated mean confidence interval at recruitment (0.95%) for this purpose, and we stratified all 120 subjects in groups that contained subjects without significant differences in mean BG. Some subjects who had low mean BG at recruitment might fail any response to "recognizing hunger", because their meal pattern lowers mean BG to the point of imminent subjective insufficiency (see description of training) (Ciampolini et al. 2010a; 2010b; Ciampolini & Sifone, 2011). We decided to find the most significant cutoff point on the basis of individual response in mean BG (decrease), either significant or not. After finding the cutoff, we separately investigated (at recruitment and during "recognizing hunger" 5 months from recruitment, compared with controls) the association of subjects with low mean BG (LBG) and high mean BG (HBG) with insulin area under curve (AUC), and indices of insulin sensitivity and beta cell function (primary endpoints). Analyses were also performed on BG AUC, measurements of BG and insulin concentrations during oral glucose tolerance test (GTT), mean BG, and glycated hemoglobin (HbA1c) values (secondary endpoints). Data are presented post hoc division. Data without division have also been published and are not reported here (Ciampolini et al. 2010b).

2.2 Assessment of metabolic and health conditions

Additional analyses were performed on energy balance, cardiovascular status, well-being, and nutrition. i) Energy balance during the 5-month investigation interval was assessed through measurement of arm and leg skin-fold thickness changes, by measurements of body weight and body mass index (BMI) and by assessment of reported energy and vegetable intake (Ciampolini et al. 1987; Ciampolini et al. 1990; Ciampolini & Bianchi, 2006a; Ciampolini et al. 2010; 2010b; Ciampolini & Sifone, 2011) ii) Cardiovascular status was assessed by systolic and diastolic blood pressures, plasma LDL cholesterol/HDL cholesterol ratio, triglycerides, and HDL cholesterol. iii) Structured interviews ascertained the number of days in which each of five functional symptoms (diarrhea, vomiting, headache, epigastric or abdominal pain) occurred during the previous three months (Ciampolini et al. 1987; Ciampolini et al. 1990). The hours of daily physical activity and time spent in bed reported in the seven-day diary were also assessed. iv) Nutrition was assessed by monitoring blood hemoglobin (Hb), mean cellular volume (MCV), transferrin saturation, plasma ferritin, zinc, folates, and vitamin B12 (Ciampolini et al. 1990).

2.3 Training to "recognizing hunger"

The trained group exercised regularly under tutorial assistance for seven weeks, and maintained the new strategies of food consumption and energy expenditure for further three months without any assistance. On the first day, subjects suspended food intake until arousal of a sensation of hunger, generally epigastric hunger (Ciampolini & Bianchi, 2006a). Meal consumption delayed two hours in average, 0 - 48 hours in range. At first arousal subjects memorized the sensation, measured BG by a portable instrument (See, please later) and consumed a meal. The energy content was calibrated to a further hunger arousal before the planned, subsequent mealtime. After 3 - 14 days of this training, subjects became aware of current BG state before meals by sensations (Ciampolini et al. 2010; 2010b; Ciampolini & Sifone, 2011). After showing association with constant BG, we named the three sensations of epigastric hunger, physical or mental weakness as "Initial Hunger" (IH). IH was maintained pre-meal, adjusting meal sizes, composition or timing of food intake. After a few days of trials and errors, and sometimes irregular mealtimes, subjects were able to arrange their intake so that IH appeared before the usual three mealtimes per day with an average error of half-an-hour in 80% of instances in adults and 90% in children ("recognizing hunger" or initial hunger meal pattern, IHMP) (Ciampolini et al. 1987; Ciampolini et al. 1990; Ciampolini & Bianchi, 2006a; Ciampolini et al. 2010; 2010b; Ciampolini & Sifone, 2011; Ciampolini et al. 2001; Ciampolini, 2006b). Thus, subjects chose BG the first day on hunger sensations, in subsequent days learned the food amount per meal, and confirmed the chosen sensation as reference for intake by showing the same BG attainment before each meal. Both control (N = 31) and trained (N = 89) subjects had the same information on food energy contents, on recommended vegetable intake and physical activity amount per day.

2.4 BG measurements

Subjects measured by themselves capillary blood by glucometer (a portable device for whole blood glucose measurement: Glucocard Memory; Menarini Diagnostics; Florence, Italy) within the 15 minutes before each meal. Accuracy of measurements by the glucometer was validated against periodic measurements by hospital autoanalyzer. Subjects avoided BG measurements taken less than 1 hour after consuming even few grams of food, after changes in ambient temperature, after physical activity such as walking or cycling, or being feverish, or under psychic stress because BG in these circumstances is higher than 1 hour after cessation of the transient metabolic condition (Ciampolini & Bianchi, 2006a). Seven-day home diaries reported BG measurements before the three main meal times, energy and vegetable intake, hours in bed and hours spent during physical and outdoor activities (weekly mean and SD) and presence or absence of pre-prandial sensation of epigastric hunger (Ciampolini et al. 1987; Ciampolini et al. 1990; Ciampolini et al. 2001; Ciampolini & Bianchi, 2006a; Ciampolini, 2006b; Ciampolini & Sifone, 2011). Subjects compiled the diaries before training, after seven weeks and at the end of investigation. Our previous studies include more details on validation of BG estimation compared to BG measurements; comparison of energy intake and total energy expenditure as assessed by doubly labelled water in infants (Ciampolini, 2006b); glycated hemoglobin (HbA1c); methods for anthropometric measurements, structured interviews, and relevant clinical blood tests.

2.5 Preliminary findings and subgrouping

2.5.1 Stratification of 120 subjects by significant differences in mean pre-prandial BG

At recruitment, mean BG was distributed from 64.5 to 109.9 mg/dL in all 120 subjects, but the mean confidence interval (95%) of diary measurements around mean BG was ± 3.84 mg/dL. In Figure 3, all 120 subjects were stratified in ten groups by increasing mean BG at recruitment. Each of ten stratifications included subjects who showed no difference in mean for BG ($P > 0.05$), but excluded subjects who had significant differences (Armitage & Berry, 1994).

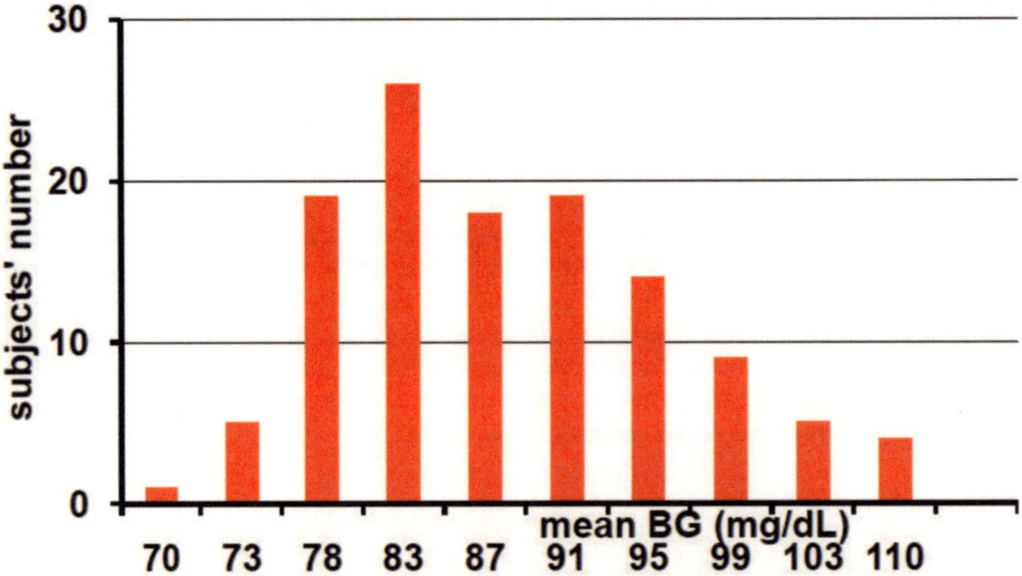

Fig. 3. Increasing sequence of mean blood glucose (mean BG) of all 120 trained and control subjects divided in 10 strata (columns) by significance of differences in mean BG at recruitment.

Strata consist of subjects with no significant difference in mean BG inside the stratum. Moreover each stratum excludes subsequent subjects whose mean BG is significantly higher than that of the first subject in the stratum. Column height shows the first component. Mean blood glucose reported in sequentially increasing order at recruitment, not in linear correlation with segment length on the x-axis scale. (By kind permission of the Authors: Ciampolini & Sifone, 2011).

2.5.2 Stability of mean BG in 31 control subjects

31 control subjects maintained a stable mean BG after 5 months (from 85.2 ± 8.1 mg/dL to 85.3 ± 7.6 mg/dL). The absolute pre/post change (increase or decrease) was 6.0 ± 4.6 mg/dL with a confidence interval (95%) from 3.1 mg/dL to 8.9 mg/dL.

2.5.3 LBG and HBG subgroups by response to "recognizing hunger"

Figure 4 shows the increasing mean BG sequence in 89 trained subjects and their response to "recognizing hunger" training. Significant decrease of mean BG by the end of the investigation occurred mainly in subjects with high mean BG at recruitment, whereas mean BG remained relatively constant in subjects with low BG at recruitment. A cutoff value (demarcation point) of mean BG that most significantly divided these two subgroups was identified, being 81.8 mg/dL (Figure 4: mean BG changes: post-minus pre-values as a function of the BG means at recruitment). 34 subjects below this "cutoff" (demarcation point) formed the low BG (LBG) subgroup. 55 subjects over this cutoff formed the high mean BG subgroup (HBG). Similarly, the BG value of 81.8 mg/dL was used to divide control subjects into LBG and HBG control subgroups (Tables 1 and 2).

2.6 Results from subgroups and discussion

2.6.1 Clinical events

About one third of subjects already maintained a mean LBG by free personal choice at recruitment. Others, motivated by bowel disorders, considered compliance as difficult before training and easy after training. Yet, the easy maintenance and the rapid recovery allowed sustained compliance. The functional disorder was significantly associated with high mean BG (and insulin resistance etc.) in HBG subjects, and possibly with high standard deviation of BG in LBG subjects (Table 2). In infants we suggested that positive balance of energy stimulates a diarrheic feedback (Ciampolini et al. 1990; Ciampolini et al. 1996). In the trained HBG group (Table 3), the decreases in days with abdominal pain or stomach-ache, were significant and significantly larger than in the control HBG group. In a national assistance design of risk prevention, recurrences of bowel disorder are sufficiently diffuse and sufficiently disturbing to motivate balance correction (training "recognizing hunger") and to improve insulin sensitivity in large part of population.

2.6.2 Stressful states

A large number of evidence shows an association between the emotional state of central nervous system and high levels of serotonin, cortisol, cortisol releasing factor and glucose in blood and/or mucosa (De Giorgio & Camilleri, 2004; Gershon, 1999; Spiller, 2008; Bischoff et al. 2009; van den Wijngaard et al. 2010; Wang et al. 2003; Lal et al. 2001; Ohman & Simrén, 2010; Spiller, 2008). These factors activate mast cells (Sand et al. 2009) and disrupt motility, secretion and absorption in mucosa (Dinan et al. 2006; Rana, 2009).

Persistence of these biological, infective stimuli and/or psychophysical stresses modify activity of monocytes, macrophages and mast cells, and together alter the neuro-endocrine system, and increase intestinal permeability. Bacterial biofilms may develop inside the alimentary canal and produce endotoxins that invade blood and all tissues (Ciampolini et al.

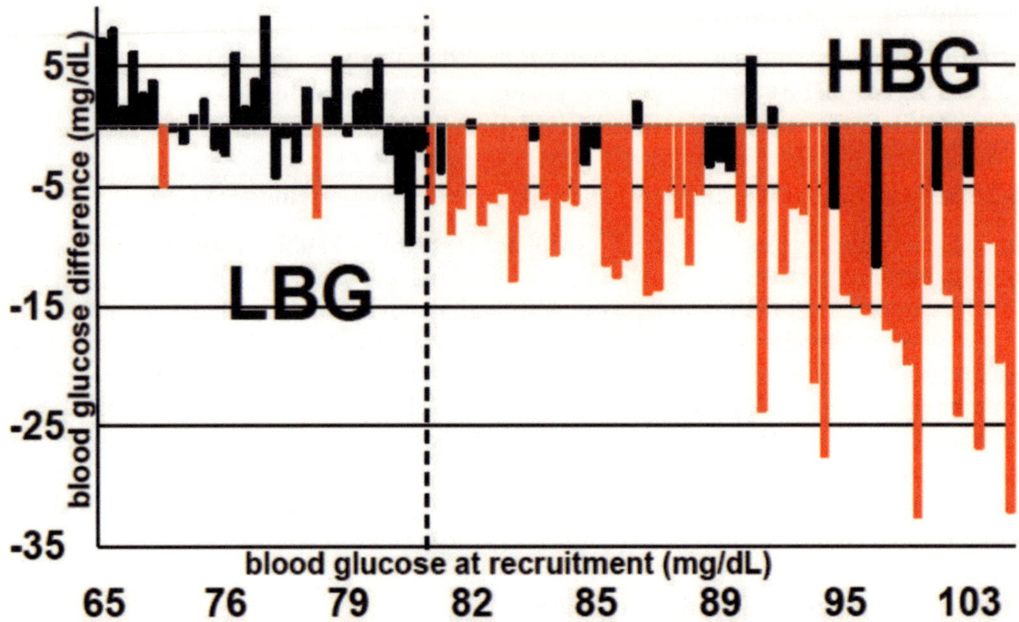

Fig. 4. Difference after training versus value in mean blood glucose for each trained subject at recruitment.

Column height shows 5-month post less pre mean blood glucose difference from 7d-diary in each trained subject. Significant decreases in red and not significant changes in black. Mean blood glucose reported in sequentially increasing order at recruitment, not in linear correlation with segment length on the x-axis scale. The dashed division indicates the most significant division between subjects who showed no mean blood glucose decrease after training (LBG group, n = 34 subjects) and those who showed significant decrease of mean blood glucose (HBG group, n = 55 subjects; $\chi 2$ analysis: P = 0.00001). This threshold blood glucose (demarcation point) is 81.8 mg/dl (4.5 mmol.l) at recruitment. (By kind permission of the Authors Ciampolini & Sifone, 2011).

1996). Locally, an inflammatory process develops in mucosa and may persist for months and years. (Tornblom et al. 2002; Ohman, L. & Simrén, 2010; Spiller, 2008). Locally, the process is minimal, because of intestinal tolerance (Brandtzaeg et al. 1989). Inside the intestine, a minority (10% - 20%) of bacterial species are immunogenic although being incapable of promoting a general illness such as Salmonella species do (van der Waaij et al. 1996). Immunogenic bacteria induce a huge biological activity of human immune system and a deep functional alteration (Reaven, 2006; Festa et al. 2000). Body tissues develop a pro-inflammatory state (subclinical inflammation, a synonym) that is sterile, ineffective and dangerous for body tissues in the intestine, vascular bed and elsewhere (Reaven, 2006; Festa et al. 2000). The invasion of body tissues by bacterial products and endotoxins sustains subclinical inflammation and causes the slow progression of many chronic diseases.

The start of the subclinical inflammatory process is controversial. Stress is associated with a condition of high BG and insulin resistance. This condition is causally associated with a "pro-inflammatory state" or "subclinical inflammation". General acceptance of this causal association took unfortunately 80 years (Kylin, 1923; Randle et al. 1963; Festa et al. 2000; Reaven, 2006). Stressed people may eat as usually, and even more, disregarding any hunger or signs of low BG (Robbins & Fray, 1980; Flaa et al. 2008). This meal pattern can maintain intestinal disorders for years (Zwaigenbaum et al.1999), and may contribute to current epidemic of insulin resistance, obesity (Flaa et al. 2008), subclinical inflammation and vascular diseases (Reaven, 2006; Festa et al. 2000; Kahna et al. 2005; Cefalu, 2005; Moller & Flier, 1991; Mather & Verma, 2005; Weiss et al. 2004). On the contrary, "recognizing hunger" prescribes transient suspension of intake during stress and in the subsequent hours until BG lowering (Table 7). Implementation of "recognizing hunger" definitively stopped intestinal disorders in adults (Table 3) and relapses in children (Ciampolini et al. 1987; Ciampolini et al. 1990; Ciampolini et al. 1991; Ciampolini et al. 1994; Ciampolini et al. 1996; Ciampolini et al. 2000; Ciampolini & Sifone, 2011).

2.6.3 Subjective and objective assessments

The training was subjective. Subjects learned to recognize IH in the first day and adapted intake to the arousal of this target sensation three times a day. The BG association checked the consistency of the recognition ("recognizing hunger").

	Low BG group				High BG group			
	Control		Trained		Control		Trained	
	Recruit-ment	After 5 mo.	Recruit-ment	After 5 mo.	Recruit-ment	After 5 mo.	Recruit-ment	After 5 mo.
Number of subjects and Gender	8 F + 4 M		21 F +13 M		6 F + 13 M		25 F + 30 M	
Schooling (years)[1]	12.0±3.2		12.9±2.7		9.8±4.4		11.4±3.7	
Age (years)[1]	28.3±8.2		32.2±8.5		30.5±9.2		32.8±11.4	
BMI	21.8±3.4	21.9±3.1	22.6±3.3	22.0±2.7**,b	22.4±5.1	23.0±4.1	23.2±4.0	22.1±3.4**,a***,b
Weight (Kg)	57.5±8.4	57.7±8.9	62.4±11.1	60.8±9.9*,b	60.9±12.2	62.9±8.4	65.2±13.4	62.7±12.1**,a***,b
Arm skin-fold thickness (mm)	15.6±9.8	15.7±9.5	15.4±8.4	13.3±6.4*,b	14.9±10.2	13.9±7.2	16.4±7.9	12.8±6.0*,a**,b
Leg skin-fold thickness (mm)	21.7±13.5	21.7±13.4	20.1±10.8	17.3±8.0**,b	20.0±11.8	18.6±9.4	22.5±11.4	17.5±8.8*,a,**,b

Values are expressed as means ± SD. [1], values at the beginning of the study. *Asterisks* indicate a significant difference (Student's *t*-test: *, $P < 0.05$; **, $P < 0.01$; ***, $P < 0.001$) on pre/post difference *vs.* respective control group (*a*), or *vs.* value of the same group at recruitment (*b*).

Table 1. Group composition and effects of training on anthropometry in low and high BG subjects.

.	Low BG group				High BG group			
	Control		Trained		Control		Trained	
	Recruitment	After 5 mo.	Recruitment	After 5 mo.	Recruitment	After 5 mo.	Recruitment	After 5 mo.
Mean pre-meal BG (mg/dL)	76.9 ± 3.4	79.1±3.5	76.6±3.7	77.2±4.2	90.4±5.3	89.2±6.9	91.6±7.7***,c	81.0±7.7 ***,a ***,b
BG diary SD (mg/dL) [1]	7.6±2.3	8.7±1.7**b	6.8±3.0	5.4±2.3 *,a **,b	9.0±3.3	9.3±3.9	9.4±4.8**,c	6.6±2.6**,a ***,b
Glycated Hb (%)	4.38±0.29	4.53±0.35	4.50±0.30	4.43±0.31	4.65±0.38	4.83±0.39	4.81±0.44***,c	4.56±0.47 ***,a ***,b
Insulin AUC[2] (mU L-1 3h-1)	192±106	243±133	180±98	183±83*,a	222±81	215±98	244±138*,c	164±92**,a ***,b
Insulin peak (mU L-1)	66±30	83±41	62±44	58±30	75±33	68±36	79±46**,c	54±29*,a ***,b
Insulin sens. (index)[3]	14.6±7.2	11.8±5.8	15.9±8.3	15.7±9.0	6,0±2.2	6,8 ± 3,9	5.9±3.3***,c	9.8±5.6**,a ***,b
Insulingenic index [4]	0.9 ±0.6	0.8±0.6	0.9±0.9	1.0±0.7	1.1±1.2	0.7±0.7	1.0±0.7	1.4±1.1*a *,b
BG AUC (mg/dL)	547±117	542±126	548±73	537±81	627±101	598±107	639±98***,c	567±91***,b
BG peak (mg/dL)	124±25	124±30	119±22	122±24	136±22	128±27	145±27***,c	128±27***,b
Energy intake (kcal/d)	1803±567	1565±677	1568±612	1303±590***,b	1887±599	1703±557	1872±655*,c	1251±470 ***,a ***,b
Meals per day[5]	3.7±0.7	3.8±0.6	3.8±0.6	3.5±0.5**,b	4.0±0.7	3.9±0.7	3.9±0.7	3.7±0.7***,b
Vegetable intake (g/d)	272±265	292±223	388±257	492±217*,b	127±128	166±218	287±223*,c	392±251**,b
Fruit intake (g/d)	183±177	188±205	233±152	334±315	183±133	147±113	214±150	290±219*,a *,b

[1] diary SD refers to the mean of the mean BG standard deviations of 21 measurements reported by each of 7d diary.
[2] AUC = area under GTT curve.
[3] Whole body insulin sensitivity index (Matsuda & DeFronzo, 1999).
[4] Insulinogenic index of beta cell function (Wiesli et al. 2004).
[5] Meal was an event of higher intake than 20 kcal.

Values are expressed as mean ± SD. Peak values include different observations from those at 30′ during GTT. *Asterisks* indicate a significant difference (Student's *t*-test: *, $P < 0.05$; **, $P < 0.01$; ***, $P < 0.001$) on pre/post difference *vs.* respective control group (*a*), or *vs.* the value of the same group at recruitment (*b*), or *vs.* the value of LBG trained group at recruitment (*c*).

Table 2. Effects of training on metabolic and intake parameters in low and high BG subjects

We assume that a week sequence of BG measurements before meals shows the least energy availability to body cells in that week, and the mean value at this metabolic moment represents the standardized parameter that we needed in the evaluation of habitual energy balance (meal pattern) in relation to its main function, provision of energy to body. Mean BG was maintained as a habit in control subjects, i.e. for a longer period than a week, and was personal, at different level from one person to another. Before initial abstinence from food (before training), HBG subjects habitually forestalled the arousal of the physiological regulation mechanism and maintained positive energy balance. On the basis of the high standard deviation of BG (Table 2 and 7), the meal pattern of untrained LBG subjects was irregular from a meal to another in comparison with during "recognizing hunger", despite of null balance, of low mean BG and weight stability in a long period (see, please, later). We cannot conclude that LBG coincided with "recognizing hunger" (See, please, later).

2.6.4 Unremitting adjustment to energy expenditure

The food diary with pre-prandial BG measurements served moreover as an educational instrument. We trained (and checked) "recognizing hunger" in adjusting intake to sensations meal by meal by the reported diary. Changes in skinfold thickness, i.e. five-month energy balance, showed reliability of the reported "recognizing hunger" (Tables 1 and 7). Within this view, dieting represents a rough attempt to achieve an ideal (?) weight without understanding and implementing the necessary meal by meal adjustments to expenditure.

2.6.5 Sufficient intake by "recognizing hunger"

As regards normal-weight subjects, trained HBG but not LBG subjects showed a cumulative balance that was negative in the 5 months, and the longitudinal difference was significant in comparison with control subjects (Table 7). The significant decrease of glycated hemoglobin (Table 2) and of body weight, BMI and arm and leg skin-fold thickness in HBG group and the stability of LBG group (Table 7), confirmed the persistence of reliability throughout 5 months of this investigation, and also the meal adjustments by "recognizing hunger" to expenditure. The maintenance of previous physical activities in all trained subjects and the improvement in nutrition parameters in HBG subgroup (Table 3) demonstrate that meals taken by trained subjects were sufficient to meet energy needs. This confirms earlier controlled, randomised studies in children with chronic non-specific diarrhea, in which daily activity was preserved and body weight increased normally after seven months, 4 years and 12 years of complying with a pediatric adaptation of the present training (Ciampolini et al. 1990).

We adapted "recognizing hunger" to infants, and the initial request of children substituted initial hunger (Initial Request Meal Pattern, IRMP) (Ciampolini et al. 1990). In 73 infants (Ciampolini, 2006b), the cutoff at 81.2 mg/dL divided subjects with low mean BG from those with high mean BG at recruitment by the highest significance. By this division, 18 infants showed low mean BG and 55 infants showed high mean BG at recruitment. This cutoff in infants is quite similar to the cutoff (81.8 mg/dL) that we found in adults in the present chapter and to the cutoff found in prevention of non-insulin dependent diabetes in Israeli recruits (Tirosh et al. 2005).

In the same preliminary work (Ciampolini, 2006b), we reported a significant 15% - 16% decrease in RMR by respiratory calorimetry and in total daily expenditure (TDE) by doubly labeled water in 24 infants from before training to during IRMP (Ciampolini, 2006b). IRMP decreases mean BG, RMR and TDE in infants. We interpreted the three decreases during IRMP (Vs. meal pattern at recruitment) as an elimination of forestalling IH, i.e. leaving behind meal by meal positive balance and acquiring null balance in blood. Taking together the investigations on children and adults, "recognizing hunger" decreased mean BG, RMR and TDE, meal by meal positive balance in blood, insulin resistance, intestinal disorders, and vascular risks (subclinical inflammation). Table 4 has not been published, except for 6 groups. There are findings on mean BG from 9 different groups.

		Control		Trained	
		Recruitment	After 5 mo.	Recruitment	After 5 mo.
Well being trial	Vomiting (days with vom./90 days)	0.1±0.3	0.1±0.2	0.2±0.9	0.1±0.5
	Headache (days with pain/90 days)	12.3±27.8	8.8±20.9	6.2±13.4	1.9±4.9**,b
	Diarrhoea (days with diarrhoea/90 days)	2.0±0.6	0.6±1.4	5.6±15.7	0.6±2.8 **,b
	Abdominal pain (days with pain/90 days)	5.8±20.5	5.9±20.6	7.6±13.6	1.0±2.0 ***,a ***,b
	Stomach ache (days with pain/90 days)	7.3±11.0	2.2±4.6	7.5±11.4	0.5±1.9 ***,a ***,b
	Outdoor and gym hours (hours/d)	4.3±3.4	3.8±3.4	3.5±2.9	4.2±2.9 *,a
	Bedtime (hours/d)	8.4±0.7	8.3±0.9	7.91.0	7.7±1.1
Cardio vascular trial	Systolic blood pressure (mm Hg)	114.7±15.0	112.3±12.2	114.1±16.4	106.3±15.2 **,b
	Diastolic blood pressure (mm Hg)	64.7±12.1	69.2±11.0	70.4±12.6	65.5±11.5 **,a *,b
	Triglycerides (mg/dL)	87.7±65	68.0±36	73.8±30.7	71.3±33.2
	HDL cholesterol (mg/dL)	52.9±14.3	44.9±14.9	45.4±14.6	52.0±13.9 **,a **,b
	LDL cholest./HDL cholest. ratio	2.1±0.9	2.7±1.5	2.9±1.5	2.3±1.2 **,a **,b
Nutrition trial	Hemoglobin (g/dL)	13.3±0.6	13.5±0.9	13.3±1.5	13.4±1.4
	MCV (micr3)	86.9±5.5	85.6±3.7	87.4±6.5	87.2±6.4
	Transferrin Sat. (%)	45.9±17.8	43.8±15.0	37.1±16.9	40.3±17.0
	Ferritin (ng/ml)	42.7±41.8	42.4±17.3	63.1±58.5	68.4±56.6
	Zn (micrgr/dL)	86.0±29.2	80.1±14.5	77.8±24.4	81.9±20.7
	Folates ng/ml	7.9±4.4	8.3±4.3	9.6±4.6	11.3±4.9
	B12 (pg/ml)	567±465	438±149	544±262	590±264

*, suppressed for Bonferroni correction. **, ***, a and b symbols as in Table 2.

Table 3. Effects of training on well-being, cardiovascular, and nutrition parameters in HBG groups.

2.6.6 Diabetes prevention

It is interesting that insulin production decreases with increasing non-insulin dependent diabetes (NIDD) duration and HbA1c height (Wiesli et al. 2004). In this investigation, the HBG control subgroup decreased insulinogenic index of beta cell function whereas the HBG trained subgroup increased it (Table 2). The difference between control and trained subgroups was significant, this implies higher insulin production, preservation of beta cell function and the possibility of an innovative therapy designed to preserve or even improve functional beta-cell mass by "recognizing hunger" (Wiesli et al. 2004). In a longitudinal investigation of 13,163 subjects a fasting plasma glucose of ≥ 87 mg/dL (4.8 mmol/l) was found to be associated with an increased risk of non insulin-dependent diabetes (NIDD) in men compared to those whose fasting plasma glucose was < 81 mg/dL (4.5 mmol/l) (Tirosh et al. (2005). Assessment and classification of meal habits allows correction toward metabolic risk decrease as in Framingham studies (Singer et al. 1992).

Training [1]	Before	After
34 adults (BMI from 17 to 40)[2]	76.6 ± 3.7 2	77.2 ± 4.2
12 adults, ctrl[2]	76.9 ± 3.4	No training
18 diarrheic infants	77.1 ± 3.8	75.2 ± 6.9
9 normalweight adults, ctrl	77.3 ± 3.9	No training
26 normalweight adults, [2]	76.5 ± 3.9	76.7 ± 4.1
8 overweight adults, ctrl	77.4 ± 3.6	No training
12 overweight adults	77,1 ± 3,1	77,2 ±4,8
41 HBG adults [23]	91.7 ± 7.8	78.5 ± 6.8
41 HBG infants [4]	92,3 ± 7,7	74,7 ± 5,1

[1] Trained subjects show mean BG both before and after training. No training refers to subjects kept as control (ctrl).
[2] Mean ± SD of mean diary of 21 pre-prandial BG in a week in mg/dL, (present report, subchapter 2).
[3] 41 of 55 adults of mixed body mass index (BMI) and mean BG > 81.8 mg/dL at recruitment who significantly decreased mean BG after training "recognizing hunger" (present report, subchapter 2).
[4] 41 of 55 HBG infants of 73 recruited for diarrhea, who showed arm skin-fold thickness on 15th percentile of normal reference. They significantly decreased mean BG from > 81.1 mg/dL, the level at recruitment. Further 18 of 73 diarrheic infants appear in the third line.

Table 4. Occurrence of low mean blood glucose (LBG) either by free, spontaneous choice (Before) or after training (After) "recognizing hunger" in 9 different groups

2.6.7 Diabetes treatment

In this report, "recognizing hunger" either prevented or cured insulin resistance and NIDD in young, clinically healthy, adults with "normal" BG. A condition of insulin sensitivity suppresses subclinical inflammation (pro-inflammatory state) and the associated functional disorders and evolving vascular diseases (Reaven, 2006; Festa et al. 2000; Kahna et al. 2005; Cefalu, 2005; Moller & Flier, 1991; Mather & Verma, 2005; Weiss et al. 2004). "Recognizing hunger" might be helpful also to some people with NIDD. Unfortunately, "recognizing hunger" contrasts the currently prevailing idea of constancy in time of daily energy intake. NIDD patients may have no hunger sensation at all. Absent arousal of hunger yet facilitates low energy intake. As an extreme example, two meals per day of 50 grams of fish and salad, 100 kcal per meal produced rapid and large weight loss and recovery of hunger sensations after adequate weight loss. Some of these lowered weight people may show low estimation error of BG after training "recognizing hunger" (Ciampolini & Bianchi, 2006a). The low error validates "recognizing hunger", and prevents regaining body weight (Table 7),(Ciampolini et al. 2010; 2010b; Ciampolini & Sifone, 2011). Thus, adaptation of "recognizing hunger" to treating aged people with fully developed NIDD requires further investigation, and suggests that current treatment practices shall survive for part of patients.

2.6.8 Prevention of vascular diseases

In tables 2 and 3, the untrained meal pattern of HBG subjects was positively associated with energy intake, mean BG, insulin resistance, glycated hemoglobin, diastolic blood pressure, high LDL to HDL cholesterol ratio, and low HDL cholesterol. Briefly, these associations form the 'metabolic syndrome, which is strongly associated with development of bacteria in small intestine (Ciampolini et al. 1996), high absorption of microbial antigens (Brandtzaeg et al. 1989; Kinugasa et al. 2000; Perez et al. 2007), subclinical inflammation and vascular diseases (Reaven, 2006; Festa et al. 2000; Kahna et al. 2005; Cefalu, 2005; Moller & Flier, 1991; Mather & Verma, 2005; Weiss et al. 2004). Subclinical inflammation develops in blood and on endothelia, and may become clinically relevant in every tissue for local presence of additional inflammatory factors. Bronchitis becomes respiratory distress, and ankle trauma becomes local arthritis. "Recognizing hunger" was associated with lowering the habitual BG and disappearing of metabolic syndrome and risks of vascular disease. "Recognizing hunger" decreased body weight in normal weight adults who were insulin resistant, and in overweight adults (BMI > 25)."Recognizing hunger" decreased insulin resistance index, HbA1c, and increased the insulinogenic index of beta cell function in 55 HBG of 89 trained subjects as compared to control subjects. In future investigations on the risks due to high blood pressure, "recognizing hunger" and achievement of insulin sensitivity may prove far better than drug control of blood pressure and thrombotic tendency.

2.6.9 "Recognizing hunger" fading and overlapping over HBG

Mean BG had little absolute change (13.2% ± 10.1% of the range at recruitment in mean BG in the 120 investigated subjects: 64.5 mg/dL to 109.9 mg/dL) in control subjects over 5 months. The division of all 120 subjects in ten strata at recruitment was a classification of associated meal pattern. Subjects chose "recognizing hunger" at the lowest level of BG availability during the day. No surprise if "recognizing hunger" largely coincides with LBG meal patterns. The point of mean inversion was at 81.8 mg/dL. However, 27 out of 89 subjects further persisted at HBG level at final investigation although 15 out of 27 were within LBG limits after seven weeks training. Six of the 27 subjects were engaged in heavy handwork during cool winters. The six subjects had a mean BG of 86.4 ± 4.0 mg/dL that showed no difference from 87.1 ± 5.3 mg/dL in 21 out of all 27 other subjects. They reported pre-prandial IH and were insulin sensitive (Table 5). IH developed in these heavy outdoor workers at higher levels than 81.8 mg/dL for high expenditure (Table 5). The division between compliance and no compliance with "recognizing hunger" is statistically strong at

81.8 mg/dL, but single subjects who actually comply with "recognizing hunger" may show higher mean BG than 81.8 mg/dL, an overlapping over HBG.

	6 HBG [1]	21 HBG [2]
Mean Blood glucose (mg/dL)	86.4 ± 4.0	87.1 ± 5.3
Final insulin AUC (mU $L^{-1}3h^{-1}$)	124 ± 26	207± 99 **
Final blood glucose AUC (mg $dL^{-1}3h^{-1}$)	536 ± 56	601 ± 82 *
Insulin Sensitivity Index	11.4 ± 2.9	6.68 ± 4.0 ***
Beta cell Function Index	1.29 ± 0.66	1.43 ± 1.22

*, **, *** symbols as in Table 2.

[1] Six HBG subjects reported to make heavy handwork all day in outdoor environment during cold winter and to practice "recognizing hunger". No significant differences in the five parameters from recruitment. At recruitment mean BG = 86.9±5.3 mg/dL.

[2] 21 HBG subjects included 15 that were LBG after seven weeks training (clinical assessment) and six who had higher mean BG than 100 mg/dL at recruitment.

Table 5. Effects of heavy outdoor work[1] in 27 trained subjects who remained with high BG at investigation end.

3. Body weight study on 149 subjects

3.1 Effects of "recognizing hunger"

The study on 120 adults included 30 overweight (OW) subjects. This number was not sufficient to draw separate conclusions on responses of LBG and HBG OW subjects to "recognizing hunger". We had however treated and investigated also OW subjects who had not performed blood examinations. We thus could add 29 OW subjects to the 120 subjects that we reported up to now (Table 6). We trained these OW subjects and collected 7-d-food intake diaries like in previous investigation. We randomized 90 NW subjects separately from 59 who were OW to the control and the trained groups. We assigned both control and trained, NW and OW subjects to LBG and HBG subgroups on the basis of diary mean BG. The cutoff was 81.8 mg/dL (Figure 4) (Ciampolini et al. 2010a; Ciampolini & Sifone, 2011).

"Recognizing hunger" (IHMP) led to loss of weight in subjects who are either OW or who are of NW with HBG (Table 7). In NW LBG subjects, weight was maintained (Ciampolini et al. 2010a). The division between normal-weight and overweight people is based on a significant increase of vascular diseases over the limit of 25 for BMI. About 20% of people below 25 BMI is at increased risk for vascular diseases (Colditz, 2004; Weiss et al. 2004). The present report is in agreement with this statement: forty of 55 HBG subjects were NW and insulin-resistant (Table 2 and 7). Maintenance of high BG and of the associated insulin resistance provokes the increased risk, although subjects may have a small fat increase, insufficient to overcome the limit of 25 BMI, and insufficient to be classified as overweight (Table 7). Insulin resistance is a sort of fattening that remains below 25 BMI in lean subjects, and is thus un-apparent even by an esthetical evaluation. People with thin bones and thin muscles are at high risk of intentional fat accumulation (and associated insulin resistance). They may increase subcutaneous fat to improve their figure, and become insulin-resistant by remaining NW or even thin!

NORMAL-WEIGHT								
	Low BG group				High BG group			
	Control		Trained		Control		Trained	
	Baseline	After 5 mo.	Baseline	After 5 mo.	Baseline	After 5 mo.	Baseline	After 5 mo.
Number of subjects and gender	5 F + 4 M		16 F +10 M		3 F + 12 M		19 F + 21 M	
Schooling[1]	11.8±3.5		13.3±2.9		10.3±4.7		11.2±3.8	
Age[1]	27.9±8.2		31.0±8.9		29.3±2.5		29.7±8.9	
Subjects showing BG decrease[2]	0/9 (0.0%)		3/26 (11.5%)		6/15 (40.0%)		33/40 (82.5%)**,a	
BG group mean pre-meal[3]	77.3±3.9	79.8±3.7	76.5±3.9	76.7±4.1	90.7±5.2	89.7±6.6	91.4±7.7	80.1±6.6 ***,a***,b
Subjects < 81.8 mg/dL[4]	9	7	26	22	0	1	0	25***,a
Vegetable intake[5]	228±217	238±226	403±273	504±235	133±151	142±158	247±240	368±246 *,a**,b
Fruit intake[5]	150±122	146±75	246±162	376±346	161±91	143±123	201±157	291±218 *,a*,b
OVER-WEIGHT								
	Low BG group				High BG group			
	Control		Trained		Control		Trained	
	Baseline	After 5 mo.	Baseline	After 5 mo.	Baseline	After 5 mo.	Baseline	After 5 mo.
Number of subjects and gender	6 F + 2 M		9 F +3 M		7 F + 6 M		14 F + 12 M	
Schooling[1]	11.8±3.0		12.3±2.6		10.6±4.0		11.9±3.3	
Age[1]	32.8 ±12.7		35.0±6.7		34.3±15,4		37.5±15.3	
Subjects showing BG decrease[2]	1/8 (12.5%)		2/12 (16.7%)		2/13 (15.4%)		22/26 (84.6%)***,a	
BG group mean pre-meal[3]	77.4±3.6	81,8±6.9	77,1±3,1	77,2±4,8	90,9±7,1	93,9±4,8	91,3±6,5	79,6±7.5 ***,a***,b
Subjects < 81.8 mg/dL[4]	8	5	12	10*,a	0	0	0	19***,a
Vegetable intake[5]	194±95	373±232	333±169	514±197	278±225	460±284 *,b	247±160	420±224 ***,b
Fruit intake[5]	138±121	182±219	214±138	223±124	226±168	167±121	225±116	286±191

Values are expressed as means ± SD. [1], years at the beginning of the study. [2],Number of subjects who significantly decreased mean pre-meal diary BG . [3],Mean pre-meal of diary blood glucose, mg/dL, LBG = lower than 81.8 mg/dL. HBG = higher than 81.8 mg/dL [4], Number of subjects who fell into the LBG at end of the study. [5], grams/d. *Asterisks* indicate significant differences (Student's *t*-test or Yates test: *, P < 0.05; **, P < 0.01; ***, P < 0.001) *vs.* respective control group values based on "post – pre" measurements (*a*), or *vs.* baseline values of the same group (*b*).

Table 6. Normal- and over-weight groups divided by low and high mean pre-meal diary blood glucose (BG). Composition and compliance at baseline and at investigation end.

3.2 Possible mechanisms and explanations

We suggested above (background) that IH may begin an important afferent arm of a physiological regulation mechanism that provides meal-by-meal feedback on energy need thus optimizing energy intake (Ciampolini et al. 1996). Subjects who are overweight and those who are normal-weight but have pre-meal HBG forestalled this homeostatic mechanism. Restoring the homeostatic mechanism would explain our finding that "recognizing hunger" (IHMP) leads to loss of weight in OW and NW HBG subjects but not in NW LBG subjects (Ciampolini et al. 2010a).

3.3 Training period and 7-day diaries

Implementation of "recognizing hunger" was associated with significant decrease of mean weekly BG as compared to control subjects. Glycated haemoglobin reflects the average BG over a 4 month period (Singer et al. 1992) and the lowered glycated haemoglobin (table 2) and significant weight loss observed in this study are unlikely to have occurred in the final week. These data suggest that awareness of IH indeed preceded final diary BG measurements, and was not significantly affected by it.

	Low BG group				High BG group			
	Control		Trained		Control		Trained	
	Baseline	After 5 mo.	Baseline	After 5 mo.	Baseline	After 5 mo.	Baseline	After 5 mo.
NORMAL-WEIGHT								
Energy intake[1]	1794±587	1660±732	1518±586	1357±628	2034±528	1886±417	1852±697	1270±457 **,a***,b
Diary BG SD[2]	8,0±2,4	9,1±1,7	6,3±3,0	5,2±1,8 **,a*,b	8,6±2,2	8,5±2,4	9,1±3,9	6,6±2,5 **,a***,b
BMI[3]	20.3±1,7	21.0±2.8	21.1±1.8	20.7±1.6	20.2±2.3	21.4±2.1	21.8±2.4	20.7±1.9 ***,a***,b
Weight[4]	55.2±7.7	57.0±9.6	57.9±7.8	57.0±7.6	57.5±6.9	60.9±6.4	61.4±10.4	58.9±9.6 ***,a***,b
Arm skinfold thickness[5]	12.9±5.3	14.7±7.7	12.6±6.6	11.3±5.0	11.3±4.3	11.7±4.2	14.1±7.0	11.6±5.7 **,a***,b
Leg skinfold thickness[5]	17.9±8.7	18.6±11.0	17.6±9.3	15.9±7.7	16.0±6.6	15.6±6.5	20.4±10.3	16.2±8.4 **,a***,b
OVER-WEIGHT								
Energy intake[1]	1611±471	1257±629	1618±616	950±448**,b	1799±701	1343±489 *,b	1820±570	1123±503 ***,b
Diary BG SD[2]	9.1±4.5	8.2±2.6	7.9±2.9	4,8±2.0 **,b	8.7±4.2	9.4±4.5	10.4±5.4	7.1±4.0 **,a**,b
BMI[3]	29.1±7.9	28.9±7.6	27.9±2.0	26.5±1.9 *,a***,b	29.2±3.9	27.8±4.2 *,b	29.0±4.1	26.5±4.0 ,a*,***b
Weight[4]	74.5±18.3	74.1±17.9	77.0±9.5	73.0±9.1 *,a***,b	77.1±16.2	73.7±15.9 *,b	78.5±10.6	71.8±10.7 *,a***,b
Arm skinfold thickness[5]	25.3±10.8	23.3±8.7 **,b	25.9±7.0	21.8±6.4 *,b	25.5±9.9	19.6±6.8	25.7±10.2	19.09±8.2 ***,b
Leg skinfold thickness[5]	33.7±13.7	30.3±12.6 **,b	32.5±12.1	26.6±10.3 ***,b	34.9±13.1	29.4±9.8** ,b	31.9±13.1	24.4±10.3 ***,b

[1] Kcal/d. [2], mg/dL; diary SD refers to BG SD of 21 measurements reported by each of 7d diary. [3] body weight kg/square height meters. [4] Kg [5] mm. *Asterisks* indicate significant differences as in Table 1.

Table 7. Effects of training (IHMP) on diary reports and anthropometry in normal- and over-weight groups divided by low and high mean pre-meal BG.

3.4 Clinical and research implications: Advantages over conventional dieting

3.4.1 Restraint approach

Control subjects were encouraged to lose weight and can be considered to represent a conventional restraint approach to dieting. Although control OW HBG subjects significantly lost weight in the first two months, they significantly increased their energy intake and BG during the last three months of the study and lost no further weight. This is consistent with a "restrained" eating pattern. Control OW LBG subjects showed a mean pre-meal BG just at 81.8 mg/dL at the end of the study indicating that without training, their meals remained partly conditioned, thus explaining firstly, their overweight status, and secondly, their failure to lose weight. Thus the findings in the two control OW subgroups (LBG and HBG) are consistent with the fact that restraint-type dieting tends to give short term results that are not sustained.

Weight cycling is a well-described phenomenon (Colditz, 2004). In the first phase of the cycle intake is conditioned or non-homeostatic. This leads to positive energy balance and weight increase. In the second phase OW subjects restrain their eating to lose weight. Most likely, the OW LBG subgroup was in this second phase at baseline. In the post-absorptive state, OW subjects have been shown to mobilise three times greater amounts of energy from reserve tissues to blood compared to NW subjects (Corcoran et al. 2007). By attending to preprandial arousal of IH, trained OW LBG subjects had to adjust meal energy intake downwards sufficiently to take into account the increased availability of energy owing to postabsorptive energy release, hence their lower energy intake (about 300 kcal per day) compared to trained LBG NW subjects (Table 7). During established application of "recognizing hunger", OW subjects reported that, provided meals were not delayed, their hunger was of no greater intensity nor more prolonged than NW subjects. Moreover, despite significantly higher body weight and lower energy intake than NW LBG subjects, trained OW LBG subjects showed the same mean preprandial BG as trained NW subjects (Table 6 and 7). These findings have at least three important clinical and research implications:

Trained OW subjects do not need to endure more prolonged or more intense hunger than trained NW subjects in order to lose weight.

The IHMP ("recognizing hunger") allows loss of weight without compromising energy availability for day-to-day energy need. The input of fatty acids from fat tissues to blood is limited in the overweight. Diets with lower mean content than 900 kcal a day may yield insufficient energy for body functions. That preprandial BG in the OW LBG group was the same as the NW LBG group indicates that in the OW LBG group a sufficiently high BG concentration was maintained for immediate energy needs. SD of diary BG in trained OW groups significantly decreased and regressed to that of NW groups further suggesting that under the IHMP ("recognizing hunger") OW groups adapted energy intake to metabolic need. In the absence of energy deprivation, less cycling of intake among trained OW groups would be expected.

An important subgroup exists (NW HBG) who appear NW by BMI criteria but who may nevertheless be at risk of weight related complications since they lose weight and decrease BG to a concentration comparable to the LBG group when trained to "recognizing hunger" (Tables 5 and 6).

3.4.2 Food composition approach (increased vegetables)

After 5 months, no significant difference was found in vegetable intake between control and trained subjects. At the end of the study controls did not attain significantly lower BG or body weight than the trained group although they had been encouraged to lose weight. This implies that high vegetable intake alone is insufficient in preventing conditioned meals and lowering high BG (Tables 6 and 7).

3.4.3 Advantages of immediate feedback

Subjects following the IHMP ("recognizing hunger") receive meal-by-meal subjective feedback from physiological signals (Ciampolini et al. 1996). These signals map closely to BG and allow subjects to eat in an unconditioned manner without self-imposed restraint or the necessity to seek any particular goal weight. The resulting improved energy balance leads to loss of weight. "Normal weight" is an artificial construct based on population statistics and may not apply to a given individual. Recommendations of goal weight may be unhelpful for some subjects to whom the goal may seem arbitrary and daunting especially if it is to be achieved by dietary restraint. The IHMP ("recognizing hunger") obviates the need for pursuit of a statistical norm and allows each individual to find his or her physiological norm.

This approach could thus prove useful in the clinical setting since it removes major obstacles to weight loss - the need for restraint, the need for dietary change, and the need to attain an arbitrary weight goal.

3.5 General interpretation

Even before any training, a consistent minority maintains a meal pattern that is similar to "recognizing hunger", and is similarly associated with improved insulin sensitivity (Table 2) and normal weight (Table 7) (Ciampolini et al. 2010; 2010b; Ciampolini & Sifone, 2011). Others may easily and reliably learn "recognizing hunger" (IHMP) to improve insulin sensitivity and lose weight, and can easily maintain this meal pattern below the age of 60 years. The IHMP ("recognizing hunger") could therefore be an important tool in the clinical management of overweight and obese patients and could have implications for health policy in the prevention of a wide range of metabolic and vascular disorders.

4. Conclusions

People share sounds and figures with other people but not subjective sensations. Subjective sensations guide the intake, but nobody knows sensations reported from others. Present investigation validated initial hunger (IH) by BG, and created a rhythm of meals at the arousal of IH, which decreased vascular risks. A three-times- daily meal pattern ("recognizing hunger" or IHMP) was associated with low mean blood glucose (LBG) and sustained regression of overweight and of the fat excess that is associated with insulin resistance, metabolic syndrome, subclinical inflammation and vascular diseases. Post hoc division of NW and OW subjects into subgroups with mean pre-meal BG either lower or higher than 81.8 mg/dL suggests body weight maintenance in NW subgroup with low mean BG and decrease in those who were either OW or HBG NW. The method was more effective than restraint-type dieting in a 5 month trial. IH, validated by BG, may represent the recovery of a vital afferent arm of the body's homeostatic energy regulation system allowing sustained self-regulation of energy intake.

Present findings suggest that the current epidemic of insulin resistance and overweight may have its origin in the non-cognizance of hunger - the physiological signals of energy insufficiency to body cells. Lack of a subjective limit in intake (a similar limit to arousal of initial hunger) explains current epidemic of insulin resistance and overweight, This may owe to forestalling such signals in early life and subsequent reinforcement of this behavior pattern. Training "recognizing hunger" rationalized the arousal of the subjective, validated limit in order to acquire and maintain energy homeostasis in blood, and decrease vascular risks. The achieved rhythm (mean BG) is homeostatic rather than being an artifact, i.e. maintains a BG that is constant and both sufficient for activity and body weight maintenance, and effective in the prevention and treatment of diabetes and obesity and a range of associated disorders and thus lessen the high economic burden of health services in industrialized societies.

5. Acknowledgments

The author wish to thank Laura Chiesi and Stefania Bini MD for dietary analyses, Riccardo Bianchi, David Lovell-Smith, Andrea Giommi (Statistics professor) and Stella Zagaria for technical support and insights, Stephen Buetow, Tim Kenealy, Chris Harshaw, Simon Thornton, Kent Berridge, James Gibbs, Charlotte Erlanson-Albertsson and Michael Hermanussen for helpful insights on earlier drafts of this paper. This research was supported by the Italian Ministry of University, Research, Science and Technology grants for the years 1998–2002 and ONLUS Nutrizione e Prevenzione, Firenze for years 2003–2008. The authors declare that they have no competing interests.

6. List of abbreviations

IHMP: Initial hunger meal pattern = "Recognizing Hunger"
AUC: area under curve at GTT
BMI: body mass index (body weight in kg/square height in m)
BG: blood glucose concentration (glycemia)
GTT: oral glucose tolerance test
HBG: high mean BG (> 81.8 mg/dL)
LBG: low mean BG (< 81.8 mg/dL)
NIDD: non-insulin dependent diabetes
Mean BG: mean of 21 pre-prandial blood glucose measurements reported by 7 day diary
Diary-BG standard deviation: Mean pre-meal blood glucose standard deviation reported by 7 day diary
BG estimation: During training: writing the expected BG value in the minute before measuring the blood sample by glucometer. After training and validation: evaluating one's own current BG value without measurement.

7. References

Armitage, P. & Berry, G. (1994). Statistical Methods in Medical Research, Blackwell, Oxford, UK, 3rd edition.

Brandtzaeg, P. et al. (1989). Immunobiology and immunopathology of human gut mucosa: humoral immunity and intreaepithelial lymphocytes. Gastroenterology, 97, 1562-1584.

Bischoff, S.C. et al. (2009). Role of serotonin in intestinal inflammation: knockout of serotonin reuptake transporter exacerbates 2,4,6-trinitrobenzene sulfonic acid colitis in mice. Am. J. Physiol. Gastrointest. Liver Physiol., 296, G685-G695.

Cefalu, W.T., (2005). Glycemic Control and Cardiovascular Disease – Should We Reassess Clinical Goals?. N. Engl. J. Med., 353, 2707-2709.

Ciampolini, M. et al. (1987). Internal stimuli controlled lower calorie intake: effects after eight months in toddler's diarrhoea. Ital. J. Gastroenterology, 19, 201–204.

Ciampolini, M. et al. (1990). Normal Energy intake range in children with chronic nonspecific diarrhea: association of relapses with the higher level. J. Pediatric Gastroenterology and Nutrition, 11, 342–350.

Ciampolini, M. et al. (1991). Decrease in serum IgE associated with limited restriction in energy intake to treat toddler's diarrhea. Physiology and Behavior, 49, 155–160.

Ciampolini, M. et al. (1994). Same growth and different energy intake over four years in children suffering from chronic non-specific diarrhea. International J. Obesity, 18, 17–23.

Ciampolini, M. et al. (1996). Microflora persistence on duodeno-jejunal flat or normal mucosa in time after a meal in children. Physiology and Behavior, 60, 1551-1556.

Ciampolini, M. et al. (2000). Attention to metabolic hunger and its effects on Helicobacter pylori infection. Physiology and Behavior, 70, 287–296.

Ciampolini, M. et al. (2001). Attention to metabolic hunger for a steadier (SD decrease to 60%), slightly lower glycemia (10%), and overweight decrease (Abstract). Appetite, 37, 123-172.

Ciampolini, M. & Bianchi, R. (2006a). Training to estimate blood glucose and to form associations with initial hunger. Nutrition and Metabolism, 3, 42

Ciampolini, M., (2006b). Infants do request food at the hunger blood glucose level, but adults don't any more (Abstract). Appetite, 46, 345.

Ciampolini, M. et al. (2010a). Sustained self-regulation of energy intake. Loss of weight in overweight subjects. Maintenance of weight in normal-weight subjects. Nutrition and Metabolism, 7, 4

Ciampolini, M. et al. (2010b). Sustained Self-Regulation of Energy Intake: Initial Hunger Improves Insulin Sensitivity. J. Nutrition and Metabolism, Article ID 286952.

Ciampolini, M. & Sifone, M. (2011). Differences in maintenance of mean blood glucose (BG) and their association with response to "Recognizing Hunger". International J. Gen. Med., 4, 403-412

Colditz, G.A. (2004) Weight Cycling and the Risk of Developing Type 2 Diabetes among Adult Women in the United States. Obesity Res., 12, 267-274.

Corcoran, M.P. et al., (2007). Skeletal muscle lipid deposition and insulin resistance: effect of dietary fatty acids and exercise. Am. J. Clin. Nutr., 85, 662-677.

De Giorgio, R. & Camilleri, M. (2004). Human enteric neuropathies: morphology and molecular pathology. Neurogastroenterol. Motil., 16, 515-531.

Dinan,T.G. et al. (2006). Hypothalamic-pituitary-gut axis dysregulation in irritable bowel syndrome: plasma cytokines as a potential biomarker? Gastroenterology, 130, 304-311.

Festa, A. et al. (2000). Chronic subclinical inflammation as part of the insulin resistance syndrome: the Insulin Resistance Atherosclerosis Study (IRAS). Circulation, 102, 42–47.

Flaa, A. et al. (2008). Does sympathoadrenal activity predict changes in body fat? An 18-y follow-up study. Am. J. Clin. Nutr., 87, 1596-1601.

Gershon, M.D., (1999). Review article: roles played by 5-hydroxytryptamine in the physiology of the bowel. Aliment. Pharmacol. Ther., 13(Suppl 2), 15-30.

Harshaw, C. (2008). Alimentary epigenetics: A developmental psychobiological systems view of the perception of hunger, thirst and satiety. Developmental Review, 28, 541-569.

Kahna, R. et al. (2005). The metabolic syndrome (Correspondence). Lancet, 366, 1921-1922.
Kinugasa, T. et al. (2000). Claudins regulate the intestinal barrier in response to immune mediators. Gastroenterology, 118, 1001-1011.
Kylin, E. (1923). Studien ueber Hypertonie-Hyperglykamie-Hyperurikamie syndrome., Zentralblatt fur innere Medizin, 44.
Lal, S. et al. (2001). Vagal afferent responses to fatty acids of different chain length in the rat., Am. J. Physiol. Gastrointest. Liver Physiol. 281, G907-G915.
Mather, K. & Verma, S. (2005). Function determines structure in the vasculature: lessons from insulin resistance. Am. J. Physiol. Regul. Integr. Comp. Physiol., 289, R305-R306.
Matsuda, M. & DeFronzo, R.A. (1999). Insulin sensitivity indices obtained from oral glucose tolerance testing: comparison with the euglycemic insulin clamp. Diabetes Care, 22, 1462–1470,
Moller, D.E. & Flier, G.S. (1991). Insulin resistance—mechanisms, syndromes, and implications. N. Engl. J. Med., 325, 938–948.
Ohman, L. & Simrén, M. (2010). Pathogenesis of IBS: role of inflammation, immunity and neuroimmune interactions. Nat. Rev. Gastroenterol. Hepatol., 7,163-173.
Perez PF et al. (2007). Bacterial Imprinting of the Neonatal Immune System: Lessons From Maternal Cells? Pediatrics, 119, e724-e732.
Rana, S.V., (2009). Role of serotonin in gastrointestinal motility and irritable bowel syndrome. Clin. Chim. Acta., 403, 47-55.
Randle, P.J. et al. (1963). The glucose-fatty acid cycle: its role in insulin sensitivity and the metabolic disturbances of diabetes mellitus. Lancet, 93, 785-789.
Robbins, T.W. & Fray, P.J. (1980). Stress induced eating: fact, fiction or misunderstanding? Appetite, 1, 103-133.
Reaven, G.M. (2006). The metabolic syndrome: is this diagnosis necessary? Am. J. Clin. Nutr., 83, 1237–1247.
Sand, E. et al. (2009). Mast cells reduce survival of myenteric neurons in culture. Neuropharmacology, 56, 522-30.
Singer, D.E. et al. (1992). Association of HbA(1c) with prevalent cardiovascular disease in the original cohort of the Framingham Heart Study. Diabetes, 41, 202–208.
Spiller, R. (2008). Serotonin and GI clinical disorders. Neuropharmacology, 55, 1072-1080.
Tirosh, A. et al. (2005). Normal Fasting Plasma Glucose Levels and Type 2 Diabetes in Young Men. N. Engl. J. Med., 353, 1454-1462.
Tornblom, H. et al. (2002). Full-thickness biopsy of jejunum reveals inflammation and enteric neuropathy in irritable bowel syndrome. Gastroenterology, 123, 1972-1979.
van den Wijngaard, R.M. et al. (2010). Peripheral relays in stress-induced activation of visceral afferents in the gut. Auton. Neurosci.,153, 99-105.
van der Waaij, L. A. et al. (1996). In vivo IgA coating of anaerobic bacteria in human faeces. Gut, 38, 348-354
Wang, H. et al. (2003). Nicotinic acetylcholine receptor alpha7 subunit is an essential regulator of inflammation. Nature, 421, 384-388.
Weiss, M.D. et al. (2004). Obesity and the Metabolic Syndrome in Children and Adolescents. N Engl J Med, 350, 2362-2374.
Wiesli, P. et al. (2004). Islet secretory capacity determines glucose homoeostasis in the face of insulin resistance. Swiss Medical Weekly, 134, 37-38, 559–564.
Zwaigenbaum, L. et al. (1999). Highly somatizing young adolescents and the risk of depression. Pediatrics, 103, 1203-1209.

24

Effects of Dietary Fiber Intake on Cardiovascular Risk Factors

Sara Arranz[1,2], Alex Medina-Remón[2,3],
Rosa M. Lamuela-Raventós[2,3] and Ramón Estruch[1,2,*]
[1]*Department of Internal Medicine, Hospital Clinic, Institut d'Investigacions Biomédiques August Pi i Sunyer (IDIBAPS), University of Barcelona, Barcelona,*
[2]*CIBEROBN Fisiopatología de la Obesidad y la Nutrición and RETIC RD06/0045 Alimentación Saludable en la Prevención Primaria de Enfermedades Crónicas: la Red Predimed, Instituto de Salud Carlos III,*
[3]*Nutrition and Food Science Department, CeRTA, INSA, Pharmacy School, University of Barcelona, Barcelona, Spain*

1. Introduction

A healthy dietary pattern is characterized by a high consumption of non-refined grains, legumes, nuts, fruits and vegetables; relatively high intake of total fat, mainly derived from olive oil; moderate to high intake of fish and poultry; dairy products (usually as yogurt or cheese) in small amounts; low consumption of red meat and meat products; and moderate alcohol intake, usually in the form of red wine with meals (Willett et al., 1995). Therefore, a high consumption of fiber-rich foods is one of the characteristic features of a healthy diet. Dietary fiber (DF) has received much attention in nutritional epidemiology. Observational studies have consistently shown that DF intake is associated with reduced cardiovascular risk, including ischemic heart disease (Rimm et al., 1996a; Todd et al., 1999; Liu et al., 2002; Mozaffarian et al., 2003a) and stroke (Ascherio et al., 1998; Oh et al., 2005; Salmeron et al., 1997)), and a lower risk of diabetes (Meyer et al., 2000; Liu, 2003b). Clinical trials have also suggested that DF supplementation has beneficial effects on risk factors, such as blood pressure, serum lipids, insulin sensitivity and diabetic metabolic control (Streppel et al., 2005b; Brown et al., 1999; Anderson et al., 2000; Chandalia et al., 2000a; Ludwig et al., 1999).

1.1 Dietary fiber: Definition and classification

The role of DF in nutrition and health is well established (Anderson et al., 1990; Englyst, Wiggins, & Cummings, 1982). Knowledge of the beneficial effects of high DF diets toward the prevention of cardiovascular diseases and several types of cancer, as well as the inclusion of DF supplements in slimming diets, has led to the development of a large and

---

* Corresponding Author

yielding market for DF-rich products. Commonly consumed products include traditional foods (meat, dairy products, breakfast cereals, biscuits, breads, etc.) enriched with different amounts of fiber from various sources, as well as dietary supplements including tablets, capsules, etc.

Traditionally, DF referred to plant cell wall components that are not digestible by human or other mammalian gastrointestinal tract enzymes, but that may be degraded by anaerobic bacteria in the colon (Trowell, 1972). The recognition that polysaccharides added to foods, notably hydrocolloids, could have similar effects to those originating from plant cell walls led to a redefinition of dietary fiber to include "polysaccharides and lignin that are not digested in the human small intestine" (Trowell et al., 1976).

Non-starch polysaccharides (NSP) are the main constituents of DF and include a host of different polymers, highly variable in terms of molecular size and structure, as well as in monomeric composition. The main classes of non-starch polysaccharides are cellulose, hemicelluloses, pectins, and other hydrocolloids. However, some authors (Saura-Calixto F, 1988) have reported that a significant part of the starch content in foods, namely, resistant starch (RS) escapes digestion and absorption in the human small intestine, along with other dietary substances not included in the DF definition such as protein, oligosaccharides and certain polyphenolic compounds (Cummings & Macfarlane, 1991; Bravo, 1998; Saura-Calixto F, 1988; Asp et al., 1996; Prosky, 1999).

In general, the definition and delimitation of DF has been much debated and related both to physiological considerations and to methods that can be used for DF analysis in foods (Asp, van Amelsvoort, & Hautvast, 1996; Englyst, H.N. and Hudson, G.J., 1996; Englyst & Englyst, 2005; Englyst, Liu, & Englyst, 2007; IoM (Institute of Medicine), 2005; FAO/WHO (Food and Agriculture Organization/World Health Organization), 1998; EFSA (European Food Safety Authority), 2007).

Therefore, DF constitutes a heterogeneous group of compounds. The components included in DF can be classified according to their chemical properties, such as their ability to dissolve in water (soluble vs. insoluble fibers), their ability to be fermented by the colonic microflora (fermentable vs. non-fermentable fibers), or their viscosity (viscous vs. non-viscous fibers) (Slavin et al., 2009) (see Figure 1).

Thus, cellulose is insoluble in water, whereas pectins and hydrocolloids, such as guar gum and mucilages, may form highly viscous water solutions. RS is insoluble and indigestible due to its physical form or enclosure in cellular structures, whereas resistant oligosaccharides are readily soluble in water but do not form viscous solutions. The terms "soluble" and "insoluble" DF have been used in the literature to differentiate between viscous, soluble types of fiber (e.g. pectins) and insoluble components such as cellulose. The distinction was mainly based on their different physiological effects. However, this differentiation is method-dependent, and solubility does not always predict physiological effects.

According to this controversy, the U.S. Food and Nutrition Board (FNB) defines "total DF" as the sum of "DF", consisting of non-digestible carbohydrates and lignin that are intrinsic and intact in plants, and "functional fiber", consisting of isolated, non-digestible carbohydrate components with demonstrated beneficial physiological effects in humans (IoM (Institute of Medicine), 2005). The rationale behind this differentiation is that there is epidemiological evidence for the beneficial effects of foods naturally high in DF, such as whole-grain cereals, some fruits and vegetables, and that DF can be regarded as a marker of such foods. The argument that the term "dietary fiber" should be restricted to non-starch polysaccharides of cell wall origin (Englyst, K.N. & Englyst, H.N., 2005; Englyst, K.N. Liu, & Englyst, H.N., 2007) has a similar rationale. Consequently, according to the FNB, documentation of the beneficial effects of added, functional fiber is required for inclusion in "total dietary fiber".

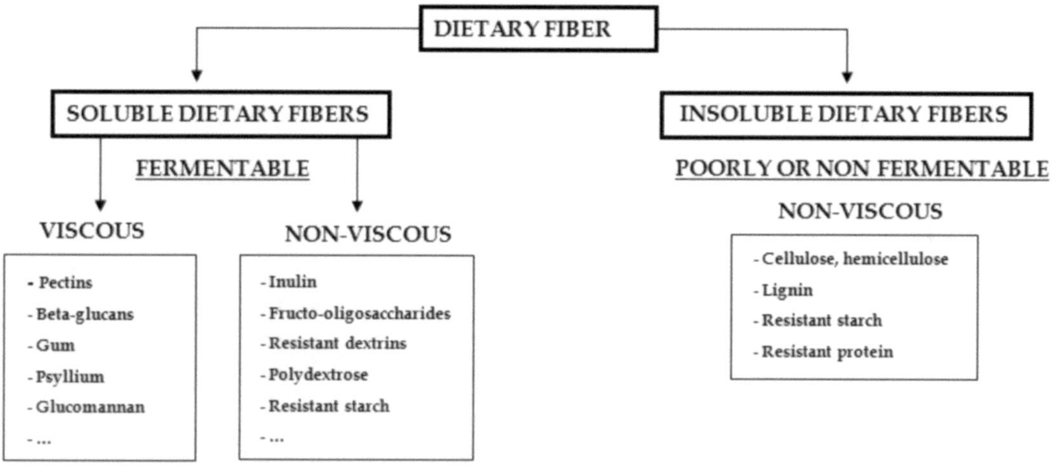

Fig. 1. Classification of dietary fiber according to chemical properties.

Based on this opinion, DF is defined as non-digestible carbohydrates plus lignin and it can be divided into different types:

- Non-starch polysaccharides (NSP) - cellulose, hemicelluloses, pectins, hydrocolloids (i.e. gums, mucilages, -glucans).
- Resistant oligosaccharides - fructo-oligosaccharides (FOS), galacto-oligosaccharides (GOS), other resistant oligosaccharides.
- Resistant starch - consisting of physically enclosed starch, some types of raw starch granules, retrograded amylose, chemically and/or physically modified starches.
- Lignin associated with the dietary fiber polysaccharides.

1.2 Methods for analysis of dietary fiber

Enzymatic-gravimetric or enzymatic-chemical methods for DF cover NSP, analytically resistant starch and lignin. However, as DF is a mixture of chemically heterogeneous carbohydrate components, several analytical methods are currently required to measure all fractions. Methods measuring only NSP (Englyst, H.N. & Hudson, G.J., 1996) give lower estimates than methods for total dietary fiber in foods containing resistant starch, and/or lignin. On the other hand, methods determining DF, including resistant starch, measure mainly retrograded amylose, resistant to the enzymes used in the assay. Finally, resistant oligosaccharides and inulin are not included in any of the current methods for total DF, and therefore need to be measured separately and subsequently added to the total fiber estimate (Cho et al., 1997; Champ et al., 2001, 2003)

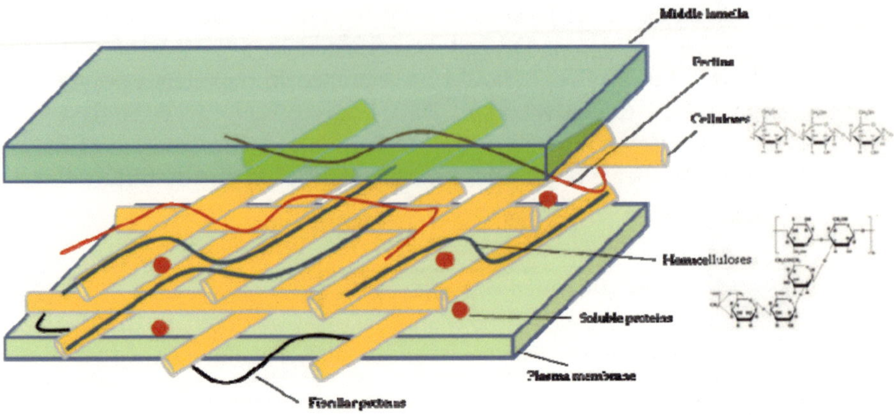

Fig. 2. The components that are part of the primary structure of the plant cell wall.

Total DF (TDF) can also be analysed by a combined enzymatic and gravimetric method, as the sum of insoluble DF (IDF) and soluble DF (SDF) which has been described in section 32.1.17 of the AOAC International Official Methods of Analysis (see Figure 3) based on previous work by Prosky et al. (Prosky et al., 1988). Another enzymatic-chemical method accepted for official action by the AOAC for the determination of TDF is one based on assays for components of TDF - neutral sugars, uronic acid residues and Klason lignin (section 45.4.11 AOAC). Starch is removed enzymatically and soluble polymers are precipitated with ethanol. Precipitated and insoluble polysaccharides are hydrolyzed using sulfuric acid and the released neutral sugars are quantitated as alditol acetates using gas-liquid chromatography. Uronic acids in the acid hydrolysate are determined by colorimetry. Klason lignin is determined gravimetrically.

However, other authors (Mañas & Saura-Calixto, 1995) have reported some methodological errors associated with precipitation and the enzymatic steps of the AOAC method. Subsequently, Saura-Calixto et al. (2000) proposed an alternative methodology to the AOAC definition of DF that measure the "indigestible fraction" (IF) of foods. The proposed method is an attempt to quantify, in a single analysis, the major non-digestible components in plant foods. This method is based on a concept of the IF that includes the main food constituents with nutritional relevance not available in the small intestine. In this method, samples are analyzed as eaten (fresh, boiled, or fried) and analytical conditions (pH, temperatures, incubation times) are close to physiological ones.

1.3 Dietary fiber content in foods

As we have mentioned before, DF occurring in foods and food products can be considered to consist mainly of cellulose, hemicelluloses, pectic substances, hydrocolloids (gums and mucilages), resistant starches, and resistant oligosaccharides.

SDF includes pectin, beta-glucans, inulin, fructans, oligosaccharides, some hemicelluloses, guar and gums. Food sources rich in SDF include legumes, vegetables, fruits, oat bran and pysllium seeds. IDF includes hemicellulose, cellulose, resistant starch and lignin. The main source of this kind of DF is whole grain. Vegetables and fruits contain both soluble and insoluble fiber, but depending on the vegetable and fruit type or maturity, the soluble to insoluble fiber ratio may vary.

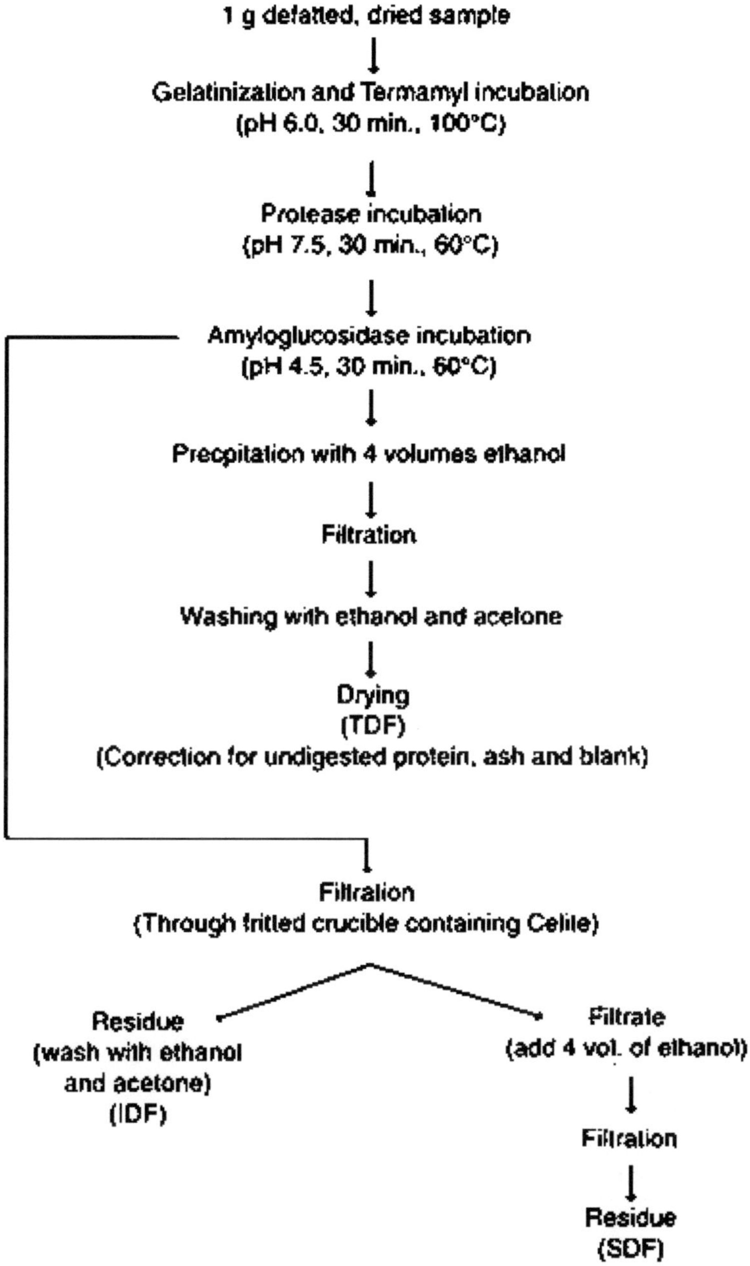

Fig. 3. Scheme of analysis of TDF by the AOAC method (section 32.1.17of AOAC, 1995).

Table 1 includes data of soluble and IDF content in some DF rich foods analyzed according to AOAC methodology. The most complete database on DF content is the USDA National Nutrient Database for Standard Reference, Release 23 (USDA). Other institutions such as FAO have also published a database on food composition, INFOODS Food Composition Database for Biodiversity (FAO).

Fiber Food Source	Insoluble DF *	Soluble DF *	Total DF
Vegetables, raw			
Broccoli, raw	0.44	3.06	3.50
Cabbage, green, raw	0.46	1.79	2.24
Carrots, raw	0.49	2.39	2.88
Cauliflower, raw	0.47	2.15	2.62
Cucumber, raw, with peel	0.20	0.94	1.14
Lettuce, iceberg, raw	0.10	0.88	0.98
Onion, mature, raw	0.71	1.22	1.93
Pepper, sweet, green, raw	0.53	0.99	1.52
Tomatoes, red, ripe, raw	0.15	1.19	1.34
Spinach, raw	0.77	2.43	3.20
Beans, green, fresh, microwaved	1.38	2.93	4.31
Carrots, fresh, microwaved	1.58	2.29	3.87
Peas, green, froz., microwaved	0.94	2.61	3.54
Potato, white, boiled, w/o skin	0.99	1.06	2.05
Fruits			
Apple (Red delicious), raw, ripe w/skin	0.67	1.54	2.21
Avocado (Calfornia, Haas), raw, ripe	2.03	3.51	5.53
Bananas, raw, ripe	0.58	1.21	1.79
Grapefruit, raw, white, ripe	0.58	0.32	0.89
Grapes, raw, ripe	0.24	0.36	0.6
Mango, raw, ripe	0.69	1.08	1.76
Nectarine, raw, ripe, w/skin	0.98	1.06	2.04
Oranges (Navel), raw, ripe	1.37	0.99	2.35
Orange juice, retail, from concentrate	0.28	0.03	0.31
Peaches, raw, ripe, w/skin	1.31	1.54	2.85
Pears, raw, ripe, w/skin	0.92	2.25	3.16
Pineapple, raw, ripe	0.04	1.42	1.46
Plum, raw, ripe, w/skin	1.12	1.76	2.87
Prunes, pitted	4.50	3.63	8.13
Watermelon, raw, ripe	0.13	0.27	0.40
Baked products			
Bread, wheat	1.26	2.13	3.38

Fiber Food Source	Insoluble DF *	Soluble DF *	Total DF
Bread, whole-wheat	1.26	4.76	6.01
Bread, rye	1.62	2.84	4.46
Bread, reduced-calorie, white	1.01	8.46	9.47
Cereal grains and pasta			
White rice, long grain, cooked	0.00	0.34	0.34
Spaghetti, cooked	0.54	1.33	2.06
Cornflakes	4.28	0.5	3.78
Brown rice, long grain, cooked	0.44	2.89	3.33
Corn, sweet, white, cooked, boiled, drained, without salt	0.62	3.32	3.94
Oat bran, cooked	0.42	1.23	1.65
Legumes			
Chick peas, canned, drained	0.41	5.79	6.19
Cowpeas, canned, drained	0.43	4.11	4.53
Lentils, dry, cooked, drained	0.44	5.42	5.86
Pinto beans, canned, drained	0.99	5.66	6.65
Red kidney beans, can, drained	1.36	5.77	7.13
Split peas, dry, cooked, drained	0.09	10.56	10.65

Table 1. List of food with their insoluble, soluble, and total fiber content (g/100 g edible food portion as eaten). * Data from Li et al., (Liu et al., 2002) and Marlett et al. (Marlett et al., 1992). Soluble and insoluble DF fractions were analyzed according to the AOAC Method 991.43.

1.4 Dietary fiber intake

Typical intakes of carbohydrates and DF are presented for children and adolescents in 19 countries and for adults in 22 countries in Europe included in the EFSA Panel on Dietetic Products, Nutrition, and Allergies (EFSA Journal 2010). The data refer to individual based food consumption surveys conducted from 1994 onwards. Most studies comprise national representative population samples. The data were derived from national reports and from a published overview (Elmadfa, 2009).

The National Academies Press also published in their web (www.nap.edu) the book titled "Dietary Reference Intakes for Energy, Carbohydrate, Fiber, Fat, Fatty Acids, Cholesterol, Protein, and Amino Acids (Macronutrients)" in which Chapter 7 entitled "Dietary, Functional, and Total Fiber" summarizes the DF intake in the American population shown in the USDA database.

Table 2 shows the DF intake in the United States and European population adapted from the two most referenced databases (USDA and EFSA).

Life stage group	Total dietary fiber intake (USDA) g/day [a]	Total dietary fiber intake (EFSA) g/day [b]
Infants		
0–6 month	ND	ND
7–12 month	ND	ND
Children		
1–3 year	19	12–15
4–8 year	25	11–20
Males		
9–13 year	31	13–27
14–18 year	38	15–33
19–34 year	38	16–26
35-64 year	30	17–27
Females		
9–13 year	26	13–25
14–18 year	26	14–27
19–34 year	25	15–24
35-64 year	21	15–26

[a] Dietary reference intake values reported by the USDA (see www.nap.edu)

[b] Dietary Reference intake values reported by the EFSA (EFSA Panel on Dietetic Products, Nutrition, and Allergies (NDA), 2010).

ND = Not determinable due to lack of data of adverse effects in this age group and concern with regard to the lack of ability to handle excess amounts.

Table 2. Dietary reference intakes of dietary fiber in United States and European population.

2. Main effects of dietary fiber

The physiological effects of DF result from its chemical and physical properties. Degradability, molecular weight, viscosity, particle size, cation exchange properties, organic acid absorption, and water-holding capacity are examples of such properties. Degradability enables the utilization of fiber in intestinal fermentation by colonic bacteria. Fermentation decreases the fecal pH and increases the bacterial biomass leading to an increase in faecal output and the production of gases and short-chain fatty acids (SCFAs). Viscous or soluble fibers form a gel by binding water and thereby decrease the gastric emptying rate and rate of absorption of glucose, triglycerides, and cholesterol. Large particle size and water holding capacity decrease transit time by increasing faecal bulk, which prevents constipation and dilutes carcinogenic compounds in the alimentary tract. Physicochemical properties are specific to different fibers and can change during cooking or digestion.

It is well known that DF plays important roles in the health of humans and in meeting the nutritional needs of animals. Much of the recent literature is focused on the ability of certain DF types to affect different physiological systems. Part of that research aims to understand how DF influences the characteristics and fermentation patterns of the intestinal microbiome in humans (Meyer & Stasse-Wolthuis, 2009; Roberfroid et al., 2010). Consequently, it is possible to understand the prebiotic function of fibers using new DNA sequencing procedures that permit complete characterization of the bacterial populations (microbiome). One of the products of fermentation, butyrate, is able to regulate gene transcription which affects cell proliferation, differentiation, and apoptosis of colon cells (Wilson et al., 2010; Crim et al., 2008). The overall goals of these studies are to determine why some individuals are more at risk to develop diseases and some animals are more efficiently using their food for production purposes, as well as to identify dietary modifications that improve animal production efficiency and human health.

3. Mechanisms of the beneficial effects of dietary fiber

Clinical recommendations for DF are routinely provided to improve gastrointestinal function, increasing laxation and reducing diverticular disease (Hall et al., 2010). In addition, an increase in the consumption of foods containing fiber is recommended to reduce obesity, type 2 diabetes mellitus (T2DM), cardiovascular disease and some cancers.

In this section we describe the mechanisms by which DF achieves its health effects focused on cardiovascular risk factors.

3.1 Body weight

DF can modulate body weight by various mechanisms, including promoting satiation, decreasing absorption of macronutrients, and altering the secretion of gut hormones.

Fiber rich foods usually have lower energy content, which contributes to a decrease into the energy density of the diet. Foods rich in fiber need to be chewed longer, leading to an increase in the time needed to eat the food and in the feeling of satiety. A number of studies (Slavin, 2005; Howarth et al., 2001a; Pereira & Ludwig, 2001) have shown that different DF affect subjective appetite, acute energy intake, long-term energy intake and body weight differently. The physicochemical properties of fibers may contribute to this variation. Fibers which make up viscous solutions and are more soluble and fermentable also delay the passage of food from the stomach to the duodenum and contribute to an increase in satiety and a decrease in energy intake. In the intestine, incorporation of fiber may complicate the interactions between digestive enzymes and their substrates, thereby slowing down the absorption of nutrients. It is also important to note that the effects of DF consumption on body weight may be related to different gut hormones which regulate satiety, energy intake and/or pancreatic functions (Aleixandre & Miguel, 2008).

3.2 Hypocholesterolemic action

The hypocholesterolemic action of fiber is partly mediated by a lower absorption of intestinal bile acid because of interruption of the enterohepatic bile acid circulation, thus increasing fecal bile acid loss, and its synthesis in liver (Morgan et al., 1993; Anderson et al., 1984). The physicochemical properties of soluble fiber result in important modifications in volume, bulk and viscosity in the intestinal lumen, which alter the metabolic pathways of hepatic cholesterol and lipoprotein metabolism, also resulting in the lowering of plasma LDL cholesterol. Other studies suggest that DF increases the enzymatic activity of cholesterol-7-αhydroxylase, the major regulatory enzyme in the hepatic conversion of cholesterol to bile acids (Roy et al., 2002) contributing to a higher depletion of hepatic cholesterol. Jones and co-workers (Jones et al., 1993) described a reduction in hepatic lipogenesis stimulated by insulin. It has also been suggested that the fermentation of DF by the intestinal microflora could modify the short chain fatty acid production thereby reducing acetate and increasing propionate synthesis. This, in turn, reduces the endogenous synthesis of cholesterol, fatty acids and very low density lipoproteins (Wolever et al., 1995; Wong et al., 2006).

Traditional dietary patterns, characterized by high fiber content, have been associated with lower rates of coronary disease. However, it should be taken into account that foods rich in fiber are also usually rich in a wide range of other bioactive substances which have a clear role in the prevention of cardiovascular disease (Craig, 1997; Hu & Willett, 2002; Buttriss & Benelam, 2010). Likewise, the beneficial effect of diets enriched in fiber on the lipid profile could also be explained by the fact that these diets are traditionally low in fat (especially saturated fat) and promote satiety and, therefore, help to protect against overweight and obesity (Mann, 2007).

3.3 Glucose tolerance and insulin sensitivity

Some studies have shown that soluble fiber plays an important role in controlling postprandial glycemic and insulin responses because of its effect on gastric emptying and macronutrient absorption from the gut (Slavin et al., 1999). Surprisingly, prospective studies have found that insoluble fiber, but not soluble fiber, is inversely related to the incidence of T2DM. In contrast, in postprandial studies, meals containing sufficient quantities of β-glucan, psyllium, or guar gum have decreased insulin and glucose responses in both healthy individuals and patients with T2DM. Diets enriched sufficiently in soluble fiber may also improve overall glycemic control in T2DM.

The association between the consumption of low dietary glycemic index (GI) foods and a lower risk of T2DM has been reported in several prospective studies (Salmeron et al., 1997), generally suggesting a preventive role of low GI diets. One of the largest was the 16-year follow-up of the Nurses' Health Study from 1980 including 3300 incident cases of type 2 diabetes, where the association between high glycemic load and the risk of developing T2DM was confirmed (Hu et al., 2001). A more recent meta-analysis of 37 prospective observational studies reported that diets with a high GI independently increased the risk of T2DM, providing protection similar to or higher than whole grains or fiber (Barclay et al., 2008). Similarly, a recent Cochrane database review concluded that low-GI diets can improve glycemic control in diabetic patients (Thomas & Elliott, 2009). However, not all investigators have reported similar findings: A well designed, controlled trial in well-controlled T2DM without oral antidiabetic therapy or insulin showed no effect on glycated hemoglobin, although a reduction in C-reactive protein and postprandial glucose was observed (Wolever et al., 2008).

To date, the physiopathologic mechanisms that explain the beneficial effects of fiber on glycemic control have still not been clearly delimited.

3.4 Blood pressure

Observational and experimental studies have reported that increased DF was associated with a lower risk of hypertension or lower self-reported blood pressure (BP), in both normotensive and hypertensive subjects (Ascherio et al., 1992; Beilin, 1994; He & Whelton, 1999). Subjects consuming a vegetarian diet are generally at lower risk of developing hypertension. However, it is unknown whether this can be ascribed to the high fiber content of the diet because vegetarians—apart from differences in lifestyle— also have higher intakes of potassium, magnesium, and polyunsaturated fatty acids and a lower intake of saturated fat.

The differences observed in BP response might be explained by fiber dose, type of fiber consumed, or better compliance with dietary supplements than with high-fiber diets (He & Whelton, 1999).

3.5 C-reactive protein

C-reactive protein (CRP) is a marker of acute inflammation recently recognized as an independent predictor of future cardiovascular disease and diabetes.

Several studies have reported that DF intake is inversely associated with serum concentrations of CRP (Butcher & Beckstrand, 2010; Oliveira et al., 2009). The mechanisms of change in CRP levels as a result of DF intake are still largely unknown; possibilities include DF slowing the absorption of glucose, fiber-rich meal modulation of cytokine responses blunting oxidative stress and inflammation, and the production of anti-inflammatory cytokines by gut flora exposed to fiber.

4. Epidemiological studies

Several limitations are common to all prospective studies examining the relationship between foods and nutrients and disease risk. The lack of consistency in the methods used for the measurement of different classes and subgroups of dietary fiber, especially the NSP, complicates comparisons between the results of studies and their extrapolation into nutritional recommendations. However, prospective epidemiological studies provide strong evidence for a protective role of wholegrain cereals, fruits and vegetables and dietary patterns characterized by relatively high intakes of such foods.

While a high consumption of DF derived from cereals is also associated with a reduced risk of cardiovascular disease, it is not clear whether this cardioprotection can entirely be attributed to the polysaccharides per se. Even the best prospective studies cannot conclusively eliminate the possibility of residual confounding, thus recommendations regarding the intake of carbohydrates in relation to cardiovascular disease also depend on the intervention studies described below.

4.1 Body weight

Large prospective studies have reported that consumption of DF is inversely associated with weight and weight gain. A high intake of DF may assist weight loss because of the incomplete digestion and absorption of energy from this type of carbohydrates and the bulky nature of high-fiber foods, with increased demands on chewing and subsequent distension and delayed emptying of the stomach, promoting satiety and thereby curtailing energy intake.

Reviews of randomized trials in adults have shown weight loss in a majority of studies with no differences between fiber types or between fiber occurring in foods or in supplements

(Pereira & Ludwig, 2001; Howarth et al., 2001a). Results from seven prospective cohort studies show an inverse relationship between weight gain and baseline intake or change in fiber intake among adults during follow-up periods of up to 12 years (Lairon, 2007; Koh-Banerjee et al., 2004).

The CARDIA (The Coronary Artery Risk Development in Young Adults) study, a multicenter population-based cohort study carried out over 10 years, examined 2909 young individuals to determine the relationship between total dietary fiber intake and plasma insulin concentrations, weight and other cardiovascular disease risk factors. After adjusting for BMI and multiple dietary and potential non-dietary confounders, the study reported an inverse association between total fiber intake, plasma insulin concentrations and body weight gain (Ludwig et al., 1999) suggesting that fiber may play an important role in the prevention of insulin resistance and obesity. Individuals consuming higher amounts of fiber had a lower weight gain compared to those consuming lower amounts, independently of the level of total fat consumed. Similarly, in the Nurses' Health Study cohort Liu (2003) showed that women in the highest quintile of DF intake had a 49% lower risk of major weight gain than women in the lowest quintile.

Kromhout et al. (2001) investigated the association between DF and indicators of body fat in a cross-cultural study of 16 cohorts of 12 763 middle-aged men in seven countries, between 1958 and 1964. The average DF intake was inversely related to population average subscapular skinfold thickness and body mass index.

Alfieri et al. (1995) assessed the total fiber intake by means of 3-day food records in 3 population groups (one normal, one moderately and one severely obese group). These authors showed that fiber intake was significantly higher in the normal weight group and was inversely associated with BMI after adjusting for several potential confounders. Recently, new research conducted as part of the PREDIMED study has also shown a significant inverse relationship between TDF consumption and body mass index or abdominal circumference (Estruch et al., 2009).

In an observational study looking at the effect of overall diet on body composition in obese and lean subjects it was demonstrated that lean men and women had significantly higher fiber intake versus obese males and females (27.0 g/d and 22.7 g/d vs. 22.0 g/d and 15.0 g/d respectively) (Miller et al., 1994). These results were supported in another study with a cohort of over 5000 subjects, which showed that higher fiber intake is associated with a lower body mass index (BMI) in both men and women (Appleby et al., 1998).

In a prospective cohort with 252 premenopausal, non-smoker women free from serious disease, Tucker & Thomas (2009) conducted a study to determine whether changes in fiber intake (total, soluble, and insoluble) influence the risk of gaining weight and body fat over time (20 months). Increasing DF significantly reduces the risk of women gaining weight and fat. For each 1 g increase in total fiber consumed, weight decreased by 0.25 kg (P = 0.0061) and fat decreased by 0.25 percentage point (P = 0.0052). Controlling for potential confounders did not affect the relationships, except for changes in energy intake, which weakened the associations by 24-32%. Soluble and insoluble fibers were borderline predictors of changes in weight and fat.

Studies on children eating mixed diets do not indicate adverse effects on growth due to high fiber intake. On the other hand, there are studies indicating that DF intake can contribute to lowering the risk of obesity in this population group (Edwards & Parrett, 2003).

In conclusion, increased intake of DF, both from naturally fiber-rich foods and added fiber or fiber supplements, has been shown to be related to improved weight maintenance in adults and sustained weight reduction in overweight subjects. Estimated intakes associated with this effect in adults are in the order of >25 g DF per day (from wholegrain cereals, fruit and vegetables).

4.2 Hypocholesterolemic action

DF has a potentially important effect on lipids and lipoproteins when consumed in plant foods or as supplements. Viscous subgroups of DF, including pectins, b-glucans, glucomannans, guar and psyllium, which are generally water soluble, all lower total and LDL cholesterol between 5 and 10 g/day, lowering LDL by about 5% (Truswell, 2002).

A cross-sectional epidemiological data, based on the EURODIAB Complications Study, which included over 2000 patients in 31 European centers, showed an inverse association between DF intake and HbA_{1c} and LDL cholesterol (in men only) and a positive association with HDL cholesterol in men and women (Toeller et al., 1999).

In an analysis of dietary factors and cardiovascular risk performed in a sample of 3,452 Swiss adults, it was observed that a healthy diet characterized by high consumption of DF was associated with lower rates of serum triglycerides and higher HDL-c (Berg et al., 2008). A 10-year study of a cohort of 2,909 healthy adults aged between 18 and 30 showed a strong negative association between fiber intake and blood pressure and levels of triglyceride, HDL cholesterol, LDL cholesterol, and fibrinogen even after adjusting for confounding factors (Ludwig et al., 1999). In a cohort of 316 Japanese-Brazilian subjects, a decrease of 12.5 mg/dl was observed in the serum total cholesterol levels ($P < 0.05$) for each increase of 10 g in the consumption of DF intake in a 7- year follow up (de Castro et al., 2006). Wu et al. (2003) studied a cohort of 573 adults aged between 40 and 60 and found and inverse relationship between the ratio of TC/HDL-c and the total intake of DF ($P = 0.01$); the ratio of TC/HDL-c has been proposed as a good indicator of cardiovascular risk.

Van Dam RM, et al. (2003) performed a cross-sectional study of 19,750 randomly selected men and women aged 20-65 y from 3 Dutch municipalities. Three dietary factors were identified: Cosmopolitan pattern (rich in fried vegetables, salad); traditional pattern (rich red meat) and refined pattern (rich sugar-beverages and white bread). A higher adherence to the Cosmopolitan pattern was significantly associated with lower blood pressure and higher HDL-c concentrations; the traditional dietary pattern was associated with higher blood pressure and higher concentrations of HDL cholesterol, total cholesterol, and glucose; and the refined dietary pattern was associated with higher total cholesterol concentrations.

Whole grain was also inversely associated with total cholesterol (P for trend = 0.02), LDL cholesterol (P for trend = 0.04), and 2-h glucose (P for trend = 0.0006) in a cross-sectional analysis of 1516 community-dwelling participants in the Baltimore Longitudinal Study of Aging. Associations between cereal fiber and anthropometrics and plasma lipids were similar (Newby et al., 2007).

In conclusion, viscous types of DF mainly from fruits, vegetables and whole grains may contribute to reducing total and LDL-cholesterol concentrations. The effects are limited to amounts usually consumed from foods.

4.3 Glycemic index and Type 2 diabetes mellitus

Glycemic control is of crucial importance in the management of T2DM. Few intervention studies have investigated the effects of fiber intake on measures of glucose tolerance or insulin sensitivity, but recent observations have shown the favourable effects of a diet with abundant fiber-rich foods, particularly whole grain, bran and germ intake, on the risk of T2DM (Murakami et al., 2005; Krishnan et al., 2007; Schulze et al., 2007; de Munter et al., 2007).

In the Nurses' Health Study, wholegrain consumption appeared to be protective for T2DM. When comparing the highest and lowest quintiles of intake, the age and energy adjusted relative risk was 0.62 (95% CI: 0.53, 0.71). Further adjustment for other risk factors did not appreciably alter this risk estimate (Liu et al., 2000; Salmeron, et al., 1997) virtually identical risk reduction was observed among men participating in the Health Professionals Study (Fung et al., 2002). A relative risk of 0.63 was reported in association with three or more servings/day of wholegrain. In the Iowa Women's Health Study, postmenopausal women in the upper quintile of wholegrain consumption (more than 33 servings per week) were 20% less likely to develop T2DM than those in the lowest quintile (fewer than 13 servings per week) (Meyer et al., 2000). Cereal fiber appears to be associated with a protective dose-response effect that is present after controlling for a range of potentially confounding factors. The role of whole grains and DF in diabetes has been reviewed in detail by Venn and Mann (Venn & Mann, 2004).

Two large cross-sectional studies, using validated food frequency questionnaires to assess nutrient intake and either the frequently sampled intravenous glucose tolerance test or homoeostasis model assessment for insulin resistance, found that intake of DF was inversely associated with the probability of having insulin resistance (Lau et al., 2005; Liese et al., 2005) and it was possible to demonstrate that fiber was associated with increased insulin sensitivity even after adjustment for body mass index.

During 8 years of follow-up (1995-2003) 1964 incident cases of T2DM were reported in a prospective cohort study including 41,186 participants of the Black Women's Health Study without a history of diabetes or CVD. Daily consumption of whole grain was associated with a lower risk of T2DM compared with consumption less than once a week. After mutual adjustment, the hazard ratio was 0.73 (0.63-0.85; P for trend = 0.0001) for whole grains (van Dam et al., 2006).

Krishnan S et al. (2007) examined the association of glycemic load, GI, and cereal fiber with risk of T2DM in 59000 black women with T2DM, CVD or cancer from the Black Women's Health Study. During 8 years of follow-up, there were 1,938 incident cases of diabetes. GI was positively associated with the risk of diabetes: the incidence rate ratios (IRR) for the highest quintile relative to the lowest was 1.23 (95% CI, 1.05-1.44). Cereal fiber intake was inversely associated with the risk of T2DM with an IRR of 0.82 (95% CI, 0.70-0.96) for the highest *vs.* the lowest quintiles of intake. Stronger associations were seen among women with a body mass index lower than 25: IRRs for the highest *vs.* the lowest quintile were 1.91

(95% CI, 1.16-3.16) for GI (P =0.12) and 0.41 (95% CI, 0.24-0.72) for cereal fiber intake (P= 0.05).

In conclusion, increasing intakes of foods rich in DF are associated with a reduced risk of developing T2DM. DF intakes associated with favorable effects are about 25 to 30 g per day, although the contribution of DF per se to this effect remains to be established.

4.4 Blood pressure

Increased DF has been associated with a lower risk of hypertension, and a meta-analysis of clinical studies of fiber supplementation also supports an inverse association between fiber and blood pressure.

In a cross-sectional study, Lairon D et al. (2007) determined the quintiles of fiber intake from dietary record, separately for 2532 men and 3429 women. The highest total DF and insoluble DF intakes were associated with a significantly ($P < 0.05$) lower risk of overweight and elevated waist-to-hip ratio, BP, plasma apolipoprotein (apo) B, apo B:apo A-I, cholesterol, triacylglycerols, and homocysteine. Fiber from cereals was associated with a lower body mass index, BP, and homocysteine concentration; fiber from vegetables with a lower BP and homocysteine concentration; and fiber from fruit with a lower waist-to-hip ratio and BP. Fiber from dried fruit or nuts and seeds was associated with a lower body mass index, waist-to-hip ratio, and fasting apo B and glucose concentrations.

Estruch et al. (2009) analyzed 772 cardiovascular high-risk subjects (age 69±5 years). On randomization they were assigned to a low-fat diet or two recommendations for increasing vegetable, fruit and legume intake. Body weight, waist circumference and mean systolic and diastolic BP significantly decreased across the quintiles of fiber intake (P<0.005).

In a meta-analysis of randomized placebo-controlled trials to estimate the effect of fiber supplementation on BP overall and in population subgroups, fiber supplementation (average dose, 11.5 g/d) changed systolic BP by –1.13 mm Hg (95% CI: –2.49 to 0.23) and diastolic BP by –1.26 mm Hg (–2.04 to –0.48). Reductions in BP tended to be greater in older (>40 years) and in hypertensive populations than in younger and in normotensive subjects (Streppel et al., 2005).

4.5 Cardiovascular disease

Many epidemiological studies have evaluated the effects of DF on the risk of coronary heart disease (CHD) (Rimm et al., 1996; Todd et al., 1999; Liu et al., 2002; Mozaffarian et al., 2003). Most likely, as assessed in prospective studies, DF intake with the usual diet is a marker of healthy food choices with an overall cardiovascular benefit, while changing the diet to increase DF at late stages, when clinical consequences of atherosclerosis have developed, may not be protective.

A meta-analysis, involving four of the largest studies published, suggested a 28% reduction in the risk of CHD on comparing individuals in the highest and lowest quintiles of intake of whole grains (relative risk 0.72, 95% confidence intervals: 0.48, 0.94) (Anderson, 2003).

After adjustment for cardiovascular risk factors, in the Iowa Women's Health Study the relative risks for cardiovascular disease were 1.0, 0.96, 0.71, 0.64 and 0.70 in ascending quintiles of whole grain intake, *P* <0.02 (Jacobs et al., 1998). The Nurses' Health Study (Liu et al., 2000) observed risk reductions of magnitude similar to those observed for CHD (relative risk 0.69, 95% CI: 0.50, 0.98 when comparing the highest relative to the lowest quintile of intake of whole grains).

The suggestion that reduced cardiovascular risk principally results from consumption of wholegrain rather than DF was supported by findings from the Iowa Women's Health Study. CHD rates were compared in women consuming similar amounts of cereal fiber from either predominantly refined grain sources or predominantly wholegrains. After adjustments, all-cause mortality was significantly lower, and CHD appreciably (though not statistically significantly) reduced among the latter group (Jacobs et al., 2000).

In the Nurses' Health Study and the Health Professionals' Study (Hu et al., 2000; Fung et al., 2001), factor analysis was used to examine the association between CHD and the two major dietary patterns identified: "western" characterized by higher intakes of red and processed meats, sweets and desserts, French fries and refined grains and 'prudent' characterized by higher intakes of fruit, vegetables, legumes, fish, poultry and wholegrains. After adjustment for cardiovascular risk factors, the prudent diet score was associated with relative risks of 1.0, 0.87, 0.79, 0.75 and 0.70 from the lowest to the highest quintiles. Conversely, the relative risks across increasing quintiles of the western pattern score were 1.0, 1.21, 1.35, 1.40 and 1.64. The patterns were also related to biochemical markers of CHD.

The effect of DF may be largely explained by fiber derived from wholewheat, rye or pumpernickel breads, in a multicenter study among 3588 men and women aged 65 years or older and free of known CVD at baseline (Mozaffarian et al., 2003). During a mean follow-up of 8.6 years, there were 811 incident CVD events. After adjustment for different confounder factors, cereal fiber consumption was inversely associated with incident CVD (*P* for trend=0.02), with 21% lower risk (HR: 0.79; 95% CI: 0.62-0.99) in the highest quintile of intake, compared with the lowest quintile. In similar analyses, neither fruit fiber intake (*P* for trend=0.98) nor vegetable fiber intake (*P* for trend=0.95) were associated with incident CVD.

Furthermore, in a combined analysis of 10 prospective cohort studies conducted in the USA and Europe Pereira et al. (2004) showed a 25% decrease in the risk of CHD for each 10 g increase in fiber intake, after adjusting for several dietary and cardiovascular confounding factors. A relative risk of 0.90 (95% CI: 0.77, 1.07 that is not statistically significant) was reported for total CHD events for each 10 g/day increase in cereal fiber. When considering CHD deaths, the relative risk, 0.75 (95% CI: 0.63, 0.91) was statistically significant, the association being independent of a number of dietary factors and other cardiovascular risk factors.

Recently, Streppel et al. (2008) also observed that CHD mortality and all-cause mortality were reduced by 17% and 9%, respectively for every additional 10 g of DF per day, with no clear associations for different types of DF.

4.6 Inflammatory markers

CRP is an inflammatory marker useful in the prediction of coronary events. Results from recent epidemiologic studies have consistently shown an inverse association between DF intake and plasma CRP levels. In a recent study, both increasing fiber intake by about 30 g/day from a diet rich in fiber or from a supplement reduced the levels of CRP.

Jenkins et al. (2003) reported reduced CRP levels in hyperlipidaemic patients consuming a high carbohydrate diet rich in viscous fiber-containing foods. However, the diets were also high in nuts (almonds), plant sterols and soy proteins, and it is therefore impossible to disentangle separate effects. A recent study (Kasim-Karakas et al., 2006) found that when carbohydrate replaced a substantial proportion of dietary fat under eucaloric conditions, the levels of several inflammatory markers increased along with an increase in triglycerides.

Data from the Massachusetts Hispanic Elders Study (Gao et al., 2004) obtained from 445 Hispanic and 154 non-Hispanic white elders showed that greater frequency of fruit and vegetable intake, which are reach in fiber, was associated with lower CRP and homocysteine concentrations. With each additional serving of fruit and vegetable intake, the risk of having high CRP (>10 mg/l) and homocysteine concentrations decreased by 21% and 17%, respectively.

The relation between DF and CRP was examined from 1999 to 2000 in 3,920 participants in the National Health and Nutrition Examination Survey (Ajani, Ford, & Mokdad, 2004). DF intake was inversely associated with serum CRP concentrations: The adjusted odds ratio for increased CRP levels (>3 mg/l) was 0.59 (P = 0.006) for the highest quintile of fiber intake compared with the lowest. The results were not affected after exclusion of persons with diabetes, cancer, CVD, or CRP levels >10 mg/l. The results of Ajani et al. confirmed the previous findings (King et al., 2003).

5. Clinical trials

Most of the data available on disease prevalence and events are from epidemiological studies. However, it is necessary to also resort to clinical trials to test effects of different types and sources of DF on cardiovascular risk factors taking into account a specific population.

5.1 Body weight

Although epidemiological data and mechanistic studies support the contention that fiber has beneficial effects on body weight regulation; there has been inconsistent data from randomized controlled clinical trials that have evaluated how body weight is affected by supplementing fiber in the diet (Rodriguez-Moran et al., 1998; Birketvedt et al., 2000; Pittler & Ernst, 2001).

In a systematic review, Howarth et al. (2001) analyzed several clinical trials conducted in small and heterogeneous population samples over relatively short periods of time (from 1 to 12 months). The findings were that the intake of 12 g fiber/day resulted in a decrease of 10% in energy intake and a body weight loss of 1.9 kg over 3.8 months, with this effect on body weight loss being greater in obese subjects.

Esposito et al. (2004) explored the possible mechanisms underlying a dietary intervention and randomized 180 patients (99 men, 81 women) with the metabolic syndrome to a Mediterranean-style diet (instructions about increasing daily consumption of whole grains, vegetables, fruits, nuts, and olive oil) versus a cardiac prudent diet with fat intake less than 30%. After 2 years, body weight decreased more in the intervention group than in the control group, even after controlling for weight loss, inflammatory markers, such as IL-6, IL-7, IL-18, and CRP.

In randomized placebo-controlled studies, 176 overweight or obese men and women were included to receive either active fiber substance or placebo during a five-week observation period. The fiber supplements consisted of the viscous fibers glucomannan (Chrombalance), glucomannan and guar gum (Appe-Trim) and glucomannan, guar gum and alginat (Glucosahl). All fiber supplements plus a balanced 1200 kcal diet induced a significant weight reduction more than placebo and diet alone, during the observation period (Birketvedt et al., 2005).

Salas-Salvador et al. (2008) evaluated the effect of a mixed fiber supplement on body-weight loss, in 200 overweight or obese patients in a parallel, double-blind, placebo-controlled clinical trial. Weight loss tended to be higher after both doses of fiber (-4.52 ± 0.56 and -4.60 ± 0.55 kg) than placebo (-0.79 ± 0.58 kg); the differences in changes between groups were not statistically significant. Postprandial satiety increased in both fiber groups compared to the placebo. Estruch et al. (2009) analyzed 772 cardiovascular high-risk subjects that were assigned to a low-fat diet or two recommendations for increasing the intake of vegetables, fruit and legumes. Body weight, waist circumference and BP significantly decreased across the quintiles of fiber intake (P=0.04).

In a dietary intervention involving 107 overweight and obese children it was shown that low GI diets are more effective in reducing weight than low-fat diets (Spieth et al., 2000). The BMI of subjects assigned to the low GI diet reduced significantly in comparison to those on the low-fat diet across all three tertiles (<28.3 kg/m^2, 28.3–34.9 kg/m^2 and >34.9 kg/m^2). The mean overall reduction was 1.53 kg/m^2 vs. 0.06 kg/m^2 ($P < 0.001$). Another study showed that low GI diets result in the greatest reduction in fat mass, especially in women (McMillan-Price et al., 2006).

5.2 Serum lipids

Several studies have shown that a high consumption of DF, particularly soluble fiber (pectin, guar gumm, β-glucans, glucomannan, and psyllium), significantly decreases serum levels of total and LDL cholesterol (Anderson, 2000; Brighenti, 2007). Other clinical trials support the hypocholesterolemic effects of soluble fiber derived both from supplements or fiber derived from foods in patients at high risk of cardiovascular disease.

In a double-blind placebo-controlled study, Rodríguez-Morán M et al., (1998) determined the plasma-lowering effects of *Plantago psyllium*, as an adjunct to dietary therapy, on lipid and glucose levels, in patients with T2DM. The study included 125 subjects undergoing a 6-week period of diet counseling followed by a 6-week treatment period in which *Plantago psyllium* or placebo was given in combination with a low fat diet. No significant changes were observed in the patient's in either group. Fasting plasma glucose, total cholesterol, LDL-c, and triglyceride levels, showed a significant reduction ($P < 0.05$), whereas HDL-c increased significantly ($P < 0.01$) following *Psyllium* treatment.

A meta-analysis carried out by Brown et al. (1999) indicates that the effects of different types of viscous fibers on TC concentrations are modest. These results were obtained from 67 experimental metabolic studies carried out on 2,990 subjects showing that for each gram of soluble fiber added to the diet, the TC and the LDL-c concentration decreased by 1.7 mg/dL and 2.2 mg/dL, respectively.

In a meta-analysis of 8 controlled trials, it was observed that the hypolipidemic effects of physillium in hypocholesterolemic individuals already consuming a low-fat diet achieved reductions with diet only. Results confirm that *Psyllium* significantly lowers an additional 4% of serum total and cholesterol and an additional 7% relative of LDL-c concentrations in comparison to a placebo group consuming a low fat diet (Anderson, 2000).

In a randomized, crossover study Maki KC et al. (2007) compared the effects of consuming high-fiber oat and wheat cereals on postprandial metabolic profiles in healthy men. Twenty-seven subjects received oat (providing 5.7 g/day beta-glucan) or wheat (control) cereal products, in random order, incorporated into their usual diets for two weeks. Peak triglyceride concentration was lower after oat vs. wheat cereal consumption. Mean area under the triglyceride curve also tended to be lower.

In a recent parallel, double-blind, placebo-controlled clinical trial, 200 overweight or obese patients were randomized to receive a mixed dose of soluble fiber (3 g *Plantago ovata husk* and 1 g glucomannan) or a placebo twice or three times daily in the context of an energy-restricted diet for a period of 16 weeks. Differences in plasma LDL-c changes between the groups were significant, with greater reductions in the two fiber supplemented groups in comparison to the placebo (Salas-Salvado et al., 2008).

Insoluble fiber, such as that from wheat or cellulose, has not been reported to have any significant effect on blood cholesterol (Jenkins et al., 2000; Sola et al., 2007), possibly because of the presence, along with DF, of several bioactive and antioxidant phytochemical substances in foodstuffs (Salas-Salvado et al., 2006) or because of the effect that fiber has on blood pressure, body weight and postprandial glycemia or insulin levels.

5.3 Glycemic index and type 2 diabetes mellitus

On glycemic control, several randomized controlled trials have been performed to determine the effect of DF on insulin sensitivity, blood glucose control and hypoglycemic episodes. However, all were short-term studies. A whole grain diet led to a postprandial improvement in insulin sensitivity when compared to a refined grain diet. Plasma glucose concentrations were significantly lower for the high fiber diet than for the low-fiber diet. In clinical studies using fiber supplements, it appears that only soluble fiber plays a significant role in reducing postprandial glycemia. However, prospective epidemiological studies have shown that insoluble fiber, but not soluble fiber, from natural food sources was inversely related to the risk of diabetes.

Giacco and co-workers (Giacco et al., 2000) carried out a 6-month randomized parallel study comparing a diet containing 50 g/d of soluble fiber with a diet containing only 15 g/d of fiber. Thirty-two patients (intervention group) and 31 patients (control group) were randomized to follow a high-fiber or low-fiber diet for a 24-week period. This study confirmed the potential for around 40 g/d DF (half of the soluble type from legumes, fruits and vegetables) to improve glycemic control. They found an improvement in the daily blood glucose profile and the HbA_{1c} levels, as well as a marked reduction in the number of hypoglycemic events.

Chandalia et al. (2000) also demonstrated that high-fiber diets contributed to better metabolic control in 13 T2DM diabetic patients. In a cross-over study, patients were randomized to a diet containing a moderate amount of fiber (8 g of soluble fiber and 16 g insoluble fiber) or to a diet containing a high amount of fiber (25 g of soluble fiber and 25 g insoluble fiber). Plasma glucose concentrations were significantly lower for the high fiber than for the low-fiber diet.

In a controlled 6-week study, overweight hyperinsulinaemic adults consumed diets providing 55% energy from carbohydrate and 30% from fat, Pereira et al. (Pereira et al., 2002) observed that insulin sensitivity measured by a euglycemic hyperinsulinaemic clamp was appreciably improved in the wholegrain compared with the refined grain diet. Fasting insulins and area under the 2-h insulin curve were lower, despite body weight not being significantly different in the two diets. In this intervention, carbohydrates were derived from predominantly wholegrain or refined grain cereals, with DF content of the wholegrain diet 28 g compared with 17 g on the refined grain diet. DF was predominantly from cereal sources. Total carbohydrate and fat and fat sources were virtually identical in the two diets. Rye bread has also been shown to improve insulin sensitivity in overweight and obese women too (Juntunen et al., 2003).

Likewise, Weicker and co-workers (Weickert et al., 2006) used the same method to measure insulin sensitivity in overweight and obese women and found that this increased after 3 days of a diet containing bread enriched with insoluble fiber compared to another diet containing white bread

In a recent 6-month parallel, randomized clinical trial composed of 210 patients with T2DM the patients were randomized to either a high cereal fiber diet (GI = 80.8) or a low GI diet (GI = 69.6). The low GI diet resulted in statistically significant reductions in fasting plasma glucose and HbA_{1c} (Jenkins et al., 2008). The results of this study confirm the notion that high fiber diets in a low GI setting are more effective in managing and preventing T2DM in comparison with high fiber diets that have medium or high GI.

A recent meta-analysis of randomized controlled trials looking at the effect of legumes on glycemic markers concluded that legumes as part of a high fiber diet significantly reduce fasting blood glucose and glycated proteins (Sievenpiper et al., 2009).

5.4 Inflammatory markers

In hyperlipidemic patients a reduction was founded in CRP levels (28% vs. baseline) following a whole diet approach, which was low in saturated fat and included viscous fibers, almonds, soy protein, and plant sterols being comparable to statin therapy (33% reduction of CRP levels) and independent of changes in body weight. The diet also induced a reduction in lipids that was comparable to lovastatin therapy (Jenkins et al., 2003). They reported reduced CRP levels in hyperlipidemic patients consuming a high carbohydrate diet rich in viscous fiber-containing foods. However, the diets were also high in nuts (almonds), plant sterols and soy proteins, and it was therefore impossible to disentangle separate effects.

Kasim-Karakas et al. (2006) found that when carbohydrates replaced a substantial proportion of dietary fat under eucaloric conditions in post-menopausal women, the levels of several inflammatory markers increased along with an increase in triglycerides. However, when the participants consumed the 15% fat diet *ad libitum* under free living conditions, they lost weight and triglyceride and the levels of inflammatory markers decreased. In another study, Estruch et al. (2009) analyzed 772 cardiovascular high-risk subjects concluding that plasma concentrations of CRP decreased in parallel with increasing DF (P=0.04).

A review of seven clinical trials of at least 2 weeks in duration, with an increased and measurable consumption of DF, reported significantly lower CRP concentrations of 25-54% with increased DF consumption with dosages ranging between 3.3-7.8 g/MJ. The seventh trial with *Psyllium* fiber supplementation failed to lower CRP levels significantly in overweight/obese individuals. Weight loss and altered fatty acid intakes were present in most of the studies (North et al., 2009). The mechanisms are inconclusive but may involve the effect of DF on weight loss, and/or changes in the secretion, turnover or metabolism of insulin, glucose, adiponectin, interleukin-6, free fatty acids and triglycerides.

6. Conclusions

Based on epidemiological and clinical studies that have attributed important health effects to fiber, several organizations such as the American Dietetic Association and the Institute of Medicine recommend an intake of 14 g of DF per 1,000 kcal, or 25 g/day for adult women and 38 g/day for adult men, to protect against the risk of CHD and T2DM and improved weight maintenance. However, in most Western countries, the current intakes of DF are below those recommended with, for instance, an average consumption of 19 and 16 g per day for men and women, respectively. In order to improve the DF intake of the population, national dietary guidelines usually recommend the consumption of high-fiber foods.

Since no biomarker of DF intake is available, food frequency questionnaire (FFQ) data is the only source of information on food consumption, including DF. FFQs are known to contain measurement errors, a reason why energy intake should be included as a covariate in the models to achieve the equivalent of an isoenergetic diet and thereby overcome this problem.

The evidence available shows that the intake of foods that are high in fiber has clear benefits regarding lipid profile and other cardiovascular risk factors. Although some studies of fiber supplements have shown positive effects on the lipid profile, the number of adults who adhere to the use of fiber supplements tends to be low. Likewise, these effects are modest when compared with a whole foods approach that encourages the consumption of fiber-rich foods.

Epidemiologic studies show that intact fruit, vegetables, whole grains, nuts and legumes, all of which are rich in potentially cardioprotective components, protect the body from cardiovascular diseases and mortality. There is debate in relation to cereals that are especially rich in insoluble fiber, but some studies have shown an inverse association between their intake and blood pressure. However, in clinical studies, only soluble viscous fiber has been demonstrated to have metabolic advantages. This paradox can be explained by the fact that food rich in fiber contains other phytochemical compounds that have been demonstrated to modulate inflammation, oxidation, insulin resistance and cholesterol metabolism.

Consequently, a Mediterranean-style diet rich in fiber-rich foods should be recommended to reduce the risk of cardiovascular disease.

7. Acknowledgments

The authors are grateful for the support granted by the Spanish Minister of Health (RETIC G03/140 and RD06/0045), the Spanish Minister of Science and Innovation (AGL2010-22319-C03-02), the FIS 070473, Centro Nacional de Investigaciones Cardiovasculares (CNIC06) and CIBEROBN that is an initiative of Instituto de Salud Carlos III, Spain. Sara Arranz received support from the Sara Borrell postdoctoral program with reference CD10/00151 supported by the Instituto de Salud Carlos III, Spain.

8. References

Ajani, U. A., Ford, E. S., & Mokdad, A. H. (2004). Dietary fiber and C-reactive protein: findings from national health and nutrition examination survey data. *The Journal of nutrition, 134*(5), 1181-1185.

Aleixandre, A., & Miguel, M. (2008). Dietary fiber in the prevention and treatment of metabolic syndrome: a review. *Critical reviews in food science and nutrition, 48*(10), 905-912.

Alfieri, M. A., Pomerleau, J., Grace, D. M., & Anderson, L. (1995). Fiber intake of normal weight, moderately obese and severely obese subjects. *Obesity research, 3*(6), 541-547.

Anderson, J. W. (2003). Whole grains protect against atherosclerotic cardiovascular disease. *The Proceedings of the Nutrition Society, 62*(1), 135-142.

Anderson, J. W. (2000). Dietary fiber prevents carbohydrate-induced hypertriglyceridemia. *Current atherosclerosis reports, 2*(6), 536-541.

Anderson, J. W. et al. (2000). Cholesterol-lowering effects of psyllium intake adjunctive to diet therapy in men and women with hypercholesterolemia: meta-analysis of 8 controlled trials. *The American Journal of Clinical Nutrition, 71*(2), 472-479.

Anderson, J. W., Deakins, D. A., Floore, T. L., Smith, B. M., & Whitis, S. E. (1990). Dietary fiber and coronary heart disease. *Critical reviews in food science and nutrition, 29*(2), 95-147.

Anderson, J. W., Story, L., Sieling, B., Chen, W. J., Petro, M. S., & Story, J. (1984). Hypocholesterolemic effects of oat-bran or bean intake for hypercholesterolemic men. *The American Journal of Clinical Nutrition, 40*(6), 1146-1155.

Appleby, P. N., Thorogood, M., Mann, J. I., & Key, T. J. (1998). Low body mass index in non-meat eaters: the possible roles of animal fat, dietary fibre and alcohol. *International journal of obesity and related metabolic disorders : journal of the International Association for the Study of Obesity, 22*(5), 454-460.

Ascherio, A. et al. (1992). A prospective study of nutritional factors and hypertension among US men. *Circulation, 86*(5), 1475-1484.

Ascherio, A. et al. (1998). Intake of potassium, magnesium, calcium, and fiber and risk of stroke among US men. *Circulation, 98*(12), 1198-1204.

Asp, N. G., van Amelsvoort, J. M., & Hautvast, J. G. (1996). Nutritional implications of resistant starch. *Nutrition research reviews, 9*(1), 1-31.

Barclay, A. W. et al. (2008). Glycemic index, glycemic load, and chronic disease risk--a meta-analysis of observational studies. *The American Journal of Clinical Nutrition, 87*(3), 627-637.

Beilin, L. J. (1994). Vegetarian and other complex diets, fats, fiber, and hypertension. *The American Journal of Clinical Nutrition, 59*(5 Suppl), 1130S-1135S.

Berg, C. M. et al. (2008). Food patterns and cardiovascular disease risk factors: the Swedish INTERGENE research program. *The American Journal of Clinical Nutrition, 88*(2), 289-297.

Birketvedt, G. S., Aaseth, J., Florholmen, J. R., & Ryttig, K. (2000). Long-term effect of fibre supplement and reduced energy intake on body weight and blood lipids in overweight subjects. *Acta Medica (Hradec Kralove) / Universitas Carolina, Facultas Medica Hradec Kralove, 43*(4), 129-132.

Birketvedt, G. S., Shimshi, M., Erling, T., & Florholmen, J. (2005). Experiences with three different fiber supplements in weight reduction. *Medical science monitor : international medical journal of experimental and clinical research, 11*(1), PI5-8.

Bravo, L. (1998). Polyphenols: chemistry, dietary sources, metabolism, and nutritional significance. *Nutrition reviews, 56*(11), 317-333.

Brighenti, F. (2007). Dietary fructans and serum triacylglycerols: a meta-analysis of randomized controlled trials. *The Journal of nutrition, 137*(11 Suppl), 2552S-2556S.

Brown, L., Rosner, B., Willett, W. W., & Sacks, F. M. (1999). Cholesterol-lowering effects of dietary fiber: a meta-analysis. *The American Journal of Clinical Nutrition, 69*(1), 30-42.

Butcher, J. L., & Beckstrand, R. L. (2010). Fiber's impact on high-sensitivity C-reactive protein levels in cardiovascular disease. *Journal of the American Academy of Nurse Practitioners, 22*(11), 566-572.

Buttriss, J. L., & Benelam, B. (2010). Nutrition and health claims: the role of food composition data. *European journal of clinical nutrition, 64 Suppl 3*, S8-13.

Champ,M., Kozlowski,F. and Lecannu,G. (2001). In-vivo and in-vitro methods for resistant starch measurement. In McCleary,B., Prosky,L., *Advanced dietary fibre technology*.(pp. 106-119)Blackwell Science, Oxford.

Champ,M., Langkilde,A.M., Brouns,F., Kettlitz,B. and Le Bail Collet,Y. (2003). Advances in dietary fiber characterization. 1. Definition of dietary fiber, physiological relevance, health benefits and analytical aspects. *Nutrition Research Reviews*, 16, 71-82.

Chandalia, M., Garg, A., Lutjohann, D., von Bergmann, K., Grundy, S. M., & Brinkley, L. J. (2000). Beneficial effects of high dietary fiber intake in patients with type 2 diabetes mellitus. *The New England journal of medicine, 342*(19), 1392-1398.

Cho, S., DeVries, J. and Prosky, L. (1997). Dietary fiber analysis and applications. *AOAC International*, Gaithersburg, Maryland.

Craig, W. J. (1997). Phytochemicals: guardians of our health. *Journal of the American Dietetic Association, 97*(10 Suppl 2), S199-204.

Crim, K. C. et al. (2008). Upregulation of p21Waf1/Cip1 expression in vivo by butyrate administration can be chemoprotective or chemopromotive depending on the lipid component of the diet. *Carcinogenesis, 29*(7), 1415-1420.

Cummings, J. H., & Macfarlane, G. T. (1991). The control and consequences of bacterial fermentation in the human colon. *The Journal of applied bacteriology, 70*(6), 443-459.

de Castro, T. G., Gimeno, S. G., Ferreira, S. R., Cardoso, M. A., & Japanese-Brazilian Diabetes Study Group. (2006). Association of dietary fiber with temporal changes in serum cholesterol in Japanese-Brazilians. *Journal of nutritional science and vitaminology, 52*(3), 205-210.

de Munter, J. S., Hu, F. B., Spiegelman, D., Franz, M., & van Dam, R. M. (2007). Whole grain, bran, and germ intake and risk of type 2 diabetes: a prospective cohort study and systematic review. *PLoS medicine, 4*(8), e261.

Edwards, C. A., & Parrett, A. M. (2003). Dietary fibre in infancy and childhood. *The Proceedings of the Nutrition Society, 62*(1), 17-23.

EFSA (European Food Safety Authority). (2007). Statement of the Scientific Panel on Dietetic Products, Nutrition and Allergies related to dietary fibre.

EFSA Panel on Dietetic Products, Nutrition, and Allergies (NDA). (2010). Scientific Opinion on Dietary Reference Values for carbohydrates and dietary fibre. *8(3)*, 1462.

Elmadfa, I. (2009). European Nutrition and Health Report 2009. Preface. *Forum of nutrition, 62*, vii-viii.

Englyst, H. N., Wiggins, H. S., & Cummings, J. H. (1982). Determination of the nonstarch polysaccharides in plant foods by gas- liquid chromatography of constituents sugars as alditol acetates. *107*, 307-318.

Englyst, H.N. and Hudson, G.J. (1996). The classification and measurement of dietary carbohydrates. *57*, 15-21.

Englyst, K. N., & Englyst, H. N. (2005). Carbohydrate bioavailability. *The British journal of nutrition, 94*(1), 1-11.

Englyst, K. N., Liu, S., & Englyst, H. N. (2007). Nutritional characterization and measurement of dietary carbohydrates. *European journal of clinical nutrition, 61 Suppl 1*, S19-39.

Esposito, K. et al. (2004). Effect of a mediterranean-style diet on endothelial dysfunction and markers of vascular inflammation in the metabolic syndrome: a randomized trial. *JAMA : the journal of the American Medical Association, 292*(12), 1440-1446.

Estruch, R. et al. (2009). Effects of dietary fibre intake on risk factors for cardiovascular disease in subjects at high risk. *Journal of epidemiology and community health, 63*(7), 582-588.

FAO. INFOODS Food Composition Database for Biodiversity, Available from: <http://www.fao.org>

FAO/WHO (Food and Agriculture Organization/World Health Organization). (1998). Carbohydrates in human nutrition. Report of a Joint FAO/WHO expert consultation.

Fung, T. T. et al. (2002). Whole-grain intake and the risk of type 2 diabetes: a prospective study in men. *The American Journal of Clinical Nutrition, 76*(3), 535-540.

Fung, T. T., Willett, W. C., Stampfer, M. J., Manson, J. E., & Hu, F. B. (2001). Dietary patterns and the risk of coronary heart disease in women. *Archives of Internal Medicine, 161*(15), 1857-1862.

Gao, X., Bermudez, O. I., & Tucker, K. L. (2004). Plasma C-reactive protein and homocysteine concentrations are related to frequent fruit and vegetable intake in Hispanic and non-Hispanic white elders. *The Journal of nutrition, 134*(4), 913-918.

Giacco, R. et al. (2000). Long-term dietary treatment with increased amounts of fiber-rich low-glycemic index natural foods improves blood glucose control and reduces the number of hypoglycemic events in type 1 diabetic patients. *Diabetes care, 23*(10), 1461-1466.

Hall, J., Hammerich, K., & Roberts, P. (2010). New paradigms in the management of diverticular disease. *Current problems in surgery, 47*(9), 680-735.

He, J., & Whelton, P. K. (1999). Effect of dietary fiber and protein intake on blood pressure: a review of epidemiologic evidence. *Clinical and experimental hypertension (New York, N.Y.: 1993), 21*(5-6), 785-796.

Howarth, N. C., Saltzman, E., & Roberts, S. B. (2001). Dietary fiber and weight regulation. *Nutrition reviews, 59*(5), 129-139.

Hu, F. B. et al. (2001). Diet, lifestyle, and the risk of type 2 diabetes mellitus in women. *The New England journal of medicine, 345*(11), 790-797.

Hu, F. B., Rimm, E. B., Stampfer, M. J., Ascherio, A., Spiegelman, D., & Willett, W. C. (2000). Prospective study of major dietary patterns and risk of coronary heart disease in men. *The American Journal of Clinical Nutrition, 72*(4), 912-921.

Hu, F. B., & Willett, W. C. (2002). Optimal diets for prevention of coronary heart disease. *JAMA : the journal of the American Medical Association, 288*(20), 2569-2578.

IoM (Institute of Medicine). (2005). Dietary reference intakes for energy, carbohydrate, fiber, fat, fatty acids, cholesterol, protein, and amino acids.

Jacobs, D. R.,Jr, Meyer, K. A., Kushi, L. H., & Folsom, A. R. (1998). Whole-grain intake may reduce the risk of ischemic heart disease death in postmenopausal women: the Iowa Women's Health Study. *The American Journal of Clinical Nutrition, 68*(2), 248-257.

Jacobs, D. R., Pereira, M. A., Meyer, K. A., & Kushi, L. H. (2000). Fiber from whole grains, but not refined grains, is inversely associated with all-cause mortality in older women: the Iowa women's health study. *Journal of the American College of Nutrition, 19*(3 Suppl), 326S-330S.

Jenkins, D. J., Kendall, C. W., Axelsen, M., Augustin, L. S., & Vuksan, V. (2000). Viscous and nonviscous fibres, nonabsorbable and low glycaemic index carbohydrates, blood lipids and coronary heart disease. *Current opinion in lipidology, 11*(1), 49-56.

Jenkins, D. J. et al. (2003). Effects of a dietary portfolio of cholesterol-lowering foods vs lovastatin on serum lipids and C-reactive protein. *JAMA : the journal of the American Medical Association, 290*(4), 502-510.

Jenkins, D. J. et al. (2008). Effect of a low-glycemic index or a high-cereal fiber diet on type 2 diabetes: a randomized trial. *JAMA : the journal of the American Medical Association, 300*(23), 2742-2753.

Jones, P. J., Leitch, C. A., & Pederson, R. A. (1993). Meal-frequency effects on plasma hormone concentrations and cholesterol synthesis in humans. *The American Journal of Clinical Nutrition, 57*(6), 868-874.

Juntunen, K. S., Laaksonen, D. E., Poutanen, K. S., Niskanen, L. K., & Mykkanen, H. M. (2003). High-fiber rye bread and insulin secretion and sensitivity in healthy postmenopausal women. *The American Journal of Clinical Nutrition, 77*(2), 385-391.

Kasim-Karakas, S. E., Tsodikov, A., Singh, U., & Jialal, I. (2006). Responses of inflammatory markers to a low-fat, high-carbohydrate diet: effects of energy intake. *The American Journal of Clinical Nutrition, 83*(4), 774-779.

King, D. E., Egan, B. M., & Geesey, M. E. (2003). Relation of dietary fat and fiber to elevation of C-reactive protein. *The American Journal of Cardiology, 92*(11), 1335-1339.

Koh-Banerjee, P. et al. (2004). Changes in whole-grain, bran, and cereal fiber consumption in relation to 8-y weight gain among men. *The American Journal of Clinical Nutrition, 80*(5), 1237-1245.

Krishnan, S. et al. (2007). Glycemic index, glycemic load, and cereal fiber intake and risk of type 2 diabetes in US black women. *Archives of Internal Medicine, 167*(21), 2304-2309.

Kromhout, D., Bloemberg, B., Seidell, J. C., Nissinen, A., & Menotti, A. (2001). Physical activity and dietary fiber determine population body fat levels: the Seven Countries Study. *International journal of obesity and related metabolic disorders : journal of the International Association for the Study of Obesity, 25*(3), 301-306.

Lairon, D. (2007). Dietary fiber and control of body weight. *Nutrition, metabolism, and cardiovascular diseases : NMCD, 17*(1), 1-5.

Lau, C. et al. (2005). Dietary glycemic index, glycemic load, fiber, simple sugars, and insulin resistance: the Inter99 study. *Diabetes care, 28*(6), 1397-1403.

Liese, A. D. et al. (2005). Dietary glycemic index and glycemic load, carbohydrate and fiber intake, and measures of insulin sensitivity, secretion, and adiposity in the Insulin Resistance Atherosclerosis Study. *Diabetes care, 28*(12), 2832-2838.

Liu, S. (2003). Whole-grain foods, dietary fiber, and type 2 diabetes: searching for a kernel of truth. *The American Journal of Clinical Nutrition, 77*(3), 527-529.

Liu, S., Buring, J. E., Sesso, H. D., Rimm, E. B., Willett, W. C., & Manson, J. E. (2002). A prospective study of dietary fiber intake and risk of cardiovascular disease among women. *Journal of the American College of Cardiology, 39*(1), 49-56.

Liu, S., Manson, J.E., Stampfer, M.J., Rexrode, K.M., Hu, F.B., Rimm, E.B. & Willett, W.C. (2000). Whole grain consumption and risk of ischemic stroke in women: A prospective study. *JAMA : the journal of the American Medical Association, 284*(12), 1534-1540.

Ludwig, D. S. et al. (1999). Dietary fiber, weight gain, and cardiovascular disease risk factors in young adults. *JAMA : the journal of the American Medical Association, 282*(16), 1539-1546.

Maki, K. C., Davidson, M. H., Witchger, M. S., Dicklin, M. R., & Subbaiah, P. V. (2007). Effects of high-fiber oat and wheat cereals on postprandial glucose and lipid responses in healthy men. *International journal for vitamin and nutrition research.Internationale Zeitschrift fur Vitamin- und Ernahrungsforschung.Journal international de vitaminologie et de nutrition, 77*(5), 347-356.

Manas, E., & Saura-Calixto, F. (1995). Dietary fibre analysis: methodological error sources. *European journal of clinical nutrition, 49 Suppl 3*, S158-62.

Mann, J. (2007). Dietary carbohydrate: relationship to cardiovascular disease and disorders of carbohydrate metabolism. *European journal of clinical nutrition, 61 Suppl 1*, S100-11.

Marlett, J. A. (1992). Content and composition of dietary fiber in 117 frequently consumed foods. *Journal of the American Dietetic Association, 92*(2), 175-186.

McMillan-Price, J. et al. (2006). Comparison of 4 diets of varying glycemic load on weight loss and cardiovascular risk reduction in overweight and obese young adults: a randomized controlled trial. *Archives of Internal Medicine, 166*(14), 1466-1475.

Meyer, D., & Stasse-Wolthuis, M. (2009). The bifidogenic effect of inulin and oligofructose and its consequences for gut health. *European journal of clinical nutrition, 63*(11), 1277-1289.

Meyer, K. A., Kushi, L. H., Jacobs, D. R.,Jr, Slavin, J., Sellers, T. A., & Folsom, A. R. (2000). Carbohydrates, dietary fiber, and incident type 2 diabetes in older women. *The American Journal of Clinical Nutrition, 71*(4), 921-930.

Miller, W. C., Niederpruem, M. G., Wallace, J. P., & Lindeman, A. K. (1994). Dietary fat, sugar, and fiber predict body fat content. *Journal of the American Dietetic Association, 94*(6), 612-615.

Morgan, L. M., Tredger, J. A., Shavila, Y., Travis, J. S., & Wright, J. (1993). The effect of non-starch polysaccharide supplementation on circulating bile acids, hormone and metabolite levels following a fat meal in human subjects. *The British journal of nutrition, 70*(2), 491-501.

Mozaffarian, D., Kumanyika, S. K., Lemaitre, R. N., Olson, J. L., Burke, G. L., & Siscovick, D. S. (2003). Cereal, fruit, and vegetable fiber intake and the risk of cardiovascular disease in elderly individuals. *JAMA : the journal of the American Medical Association, 289*(13), 1659-1666.

Murakami, K., Okubo, H., & Sasaki, S. (2005). Effect of dietary factors on incidence of type 2 diabetes: a systematic review of cohort studies. *Journal of nutritional science and vitaminology, 51*(4), 292-310.

National Academies Press, Available from: <www.nap.edu>

Newby, P. K., Maras, J., Bakun, P., Muller, D., Ferrucci, L., & Tucker, K. L. (2007). Intake of whole grains, refined grains, and cereal fiber measured with 7-d diet records and associations with risk factors for chronic disease. *The American Journal of Clinical Nutrition, 86*(6), 1745-1753.

North, C. J., Venter, C. S., & Jerling, J. C. (2009). The effects of dietary fibre on C-reactive protein, an inflammation marker predicting cardiovascular disease. *European journal of clinical nutrition, 63*(8), 921-933.

Oh, K. et al. (2005). Carbohydrate intake, glycemic index, glycemic load, and dietary fiber in relation to risk of stroke in women. *American Journal of Epidemiology, 161*(2), 161-169.

Oliveira, A., Rodriguez-Artalejo, F., & Lopes, C. (2009). The association of fruits, vegetables, antioxidant vitamins and fibre intake with high-sensitivity C-reactive protein: sex and body mass index interactions. *European journal of clinical nutrition, 63*(11), 1345-1352.

Pereira, M. A. et al. (2002). Effect of whole grains on insulin sensitivity in overweight hyperinsulinemic adults. *The American Journal of Clinical Nutrition, 75*(5), 848-855.

Pereira, M. A., & Ludwig, D. S. (2001). Dietary fiber and body-weight regulation. Observations and mechanisms. *Pediatric clinics of North America, 48*(4), 969-980.

Pereira, M. A. et al. (2004). Dietary fiber and risk of coronary heart disease: a pooled analysis of cohort studies. *Archives of Internal Medicine, 164*(4), 370-376.

Pittler, M. H., & Ernst, E. (2001). Guar gum for body weight reduction: meta-analysis of randomized trials. *The American Journal of Medicine, 110*(9), 724-730.

Prosky, L. (1999). Inulin and oligofructose are part of the dietary fiber complex. *Journal of AOAC International, 82*(2), 223-226.

Prosky, L., Asp, N. G., Schweizer, T. F., DeVries, J. W., & Furda, I. (1988). Determination of insoluble, soluble, and total dietary fiber in foods and food products: interlaboratory study. *Journal - Association of Official Analytical Chemists, 71*(5), 1017-1023.

Rimm, E. B., Ascherio, A., Giovannucci, E., Spiegelman, D., Stampfer, M. J., & Willett, W. C. (1996). Vegetable, fruit, and cereal fiber intake and risk of coronary heart disease among men. *JAMA : the journal of the American Medical Association, 275*(6), 447-451.

Roberfroid, M. et al. (2010). Prebiotic effects: metabolic and health benefits. *The British journal of nutrition, 104 Suppl 2*, S1-63.

Rodriguez-Moran, M., Guerrero-Romero, F., & Lazcano-Burciaga, G. (1998). Lipid- and glucose-lowering efficacy of Plantago Psyllium in type II diabetes. *Journal of diabetes and its complications, 12*(5), 273-278.

Roy, S., Freake, H. C., & Fernandez, M. L. (2002). Gender and hormonal status affect the regulation of hepatic cholesterol 7alpha-hydroxylase activity and mRNA abundance by dietary soluble fiber in the guinea pig. *Atherosclerosis, 163*(1), 29-37.

Salas-Salvado, J., Bullo, M., Perez-Heras, A., & Ros, E. (2006). Dietary fibre, nuts and cardiovascular diseases. *The British journal of nutrition, 96 Suppl 2*, S46-51.

Salas-Salvado, J. et al. (2008). Effect of two doses of a mixture of soluble fibres on body weight and metabolic variables in overweight or obese patients: a randomised trial. *The British journal of nutrition, 99*(6), 1380-1387.

Salmeron, J., Manson, J. E., Stampfer, M. J., Colditz, G. A., Wing, A. L., & Willett, W. C. (1997). Dietary fiber, glycemic load, and risk of non-insulin-dependent diabetes mellitus in women. *JAMA : the journal of the American Medical Association, 277*(6), 472-477.

Saura-Calixto F. (1988). Effect of condensed tannins in the analysis of dietary fiber in carob pods. *53*, 1769-1771.

Saura-Calixto, F., Garcia-Alonso, A., Goni, I., & Bravo, L. (2000). In vitro determination of the indigestible fraction in foods: an alternative to dietary fiber analysis. *Journal of Agricultural and Food Chemistry, 48*(8), 3342-3347.

Schulze, M. B., Schulz, M., Heidemann, C., Schienkiewitz, A., Hoffmann, K., & Boeing, H. (2007). Fiber and magnesium intake and incidence of type 2 diabetes: a prospective study and meta-analysis. *Archives of Internal Medicine, 167*(9), 956-965.

Sievenpiper, J. L. et al. (2009). Effect of non-oil-seed pulses on glycaemic control: a systematic review and meta-analysis of randomised controlled experimental trials in people with and without diabetes. *Diabetologia, 52*(8), 1479-1495.

Slavin, J. L. (2005). Dietary fiber and body weight. *Nutrition (Burbank, Los Angeles County, Calif.), 21*(3), 411-418.

Slavin, J. L., Martini, M. C., Jacobs, D. R.,Jr, & Marquart, L. (1999). Plausible mechanisms for the protectiveness of whole grains. *The American Journal of Clinical Nutrition, 70*(3 Suppl), 459S-463S.

Slavin, J. L., Savarino, V., Paredes-Diaz, A., & Fotopoulos, G. (2009). A review of the role of soluble fiber in health with specific reference to wheat dextrin. *The Journal of international medical research, 37*(1), 1-17.

Sola, R. et al. (2007). Effects of soluble fiber (Plantago ovata husk) on plasma lipids, lipoproteins, and apolipoproteins in men with ischemic heart disease. *The American Journal of Clinical Nutrition, 85*(4), 1157-1163.

Spieth, L. E. et al. (2000). A low-glycemic index diet in the treatment of pediatric obesity. *Archives of Pediatrics & Adolescent Medicine, 154*(9), 947-951.

Streppel, M. T., Arends, L. R., van 't Veer, P., Grobbee, D. E., & Geleijnse, J. M. (2005). Dietary fiber and blood pressure: a meta-analysis of randomized placebo-controlled trials. *Archives of Internal Medicine, 165*(2), 150-156.

Streppel, M. T., Ocke, M. C., Boshuizen, H. C., Kok, F. J., & Kromhout, D. (2008). Dietary fiber intake in relation to coronary heart disease and all-cause mortality over 40 y: the Zutphen Study. *The American Journal of Clinical Nutrition, 88*(4), 1119-1125.

Thomas, D., & Elliott, E. J. (2009). Low glycaemic index, or low glycaemic load, diets for diabetes mellitus. *Cochrane database of systematic reviews (Online), (1)*(1), CD006296.

Todd, S., Woodward, M., Tunstall-Pedoe, H., & Bolton-Smith, C. (1999). Dietary antioxidant vitamins and fiber in the etiology of cardiovascular disease and all-causes mortality: results from the Scottish Heart Health Study. *American Journal of Epidemiology, 150*(10), 1073-1080.

Toeller, M., Buyken, A. E., Heitkamp, G., de Pergola, G., Giorgino, F., & Fuller, J. H. (1999). Fiber intake, serum cholesterol levels, and cardiovascular disease in European individuals with type 1 diabetes. EURODIAB IDDM Complications Study Group. *Diabetes care, 22 Suppl 2*, B21-8.

Trowell, H. (1972). Ischemic heart disease and dietary fiber. *The American Journal of Clinical Nutrition, 25*(9), 926-932.

Trowell, H., Southgate, D. A., Wolever, T. M., Leeds, A. R., Gassull, M. A., & Jenkins, D. J. (1976). Letter: Dietary fibre redefined. *Lancet, 1*(7966), 967.

Truswell, A. S. (2002). Cereal grains and coronary heart disease. *European journal of clinical nutrition, 56*(1), 1-14.

Tucker, L. A., & Thomas, K. S. (2009). Increasing total fiber intake reduces risk of weight and fat gains in women. *The Journal of nutrition, 139*(3), 576-581.

USDA. National Nutrient Database for Standard Reference, Release 23, Available from: <http://www.ars.usda.gov>

van Dam, R. M., Grievink, L., Ocke, M. C., & Feskens, E. J. (2003). Patterns of food consumption and risk factors for cardiovascular disease in the general Dutch population. *The American Journal of Clinical Nutrition, 77*(5), 1156-1163.

van Dam, R. M., Hu, F. B., Rosenberg, L., Krishnan, S., & Palmer, J. R. (2006). Dietary calcium and magnesium, major food sources, and risk of type 2 diabetes in U.S. black women. *Diabetes care, 29*(10), 2238-2243.

Venn, B. J., & Mann, J. I. (2004). Cereal grains, legumes and diabetes. *European journal of clinical nutrition, 58*(11), 1443-1461.

Weickert, M. O. et al. (2006). Cereal fiber improves whole-body insulin sensitivity in overweight and obese women. *Diabetes care, 29*(4), 775-780.

Willett, W. C. et al. (1995). Mediterranean diet pyramid: a cultural model for healthy eating. *The American Journal of Clinical Nutrition, 61*(6 Suppl), 1402S-1406S.

Wilson, A. J. et al. (2010). Apoptotic sensitivity of colon cancer cells to histone deacetylase inhibitors is mediated by an Sp1/Sp3-activated transcriptional program involving immediate-early gene induction. *Cancer research, 70*(2), 609-620.

Wolever, T. M. et al. (2008). Low glycaemic index diet and disposition index in type 2 diabetes (the Canadian trial of carbohydrates in diabetes): a randomised controlled trial. *Diabetologia, 51*(9), 1607-1615.

Wolever, T. M., Spadafora, P. J., Cunnane, S. C., & Pencharz, P. B. (1995). Propionate inhibits incorporation of colonic [1,2-13C]acetate into plasma lipids in humans. *The American Journal of Clinical Nutrition, 61*(6), 1241-1247.

Wong, J. M., de Souza, R., Kendall, C. W., Emam, A., & Jenkins, D. J. (2006). Colonic health: fermentation and short chain fatty acids. *Journal of clinical gastroenterology, 40*(3), 235-243.

Wu, H., Dwyer, K. M., Fan, Z., Shircore, A., Fan, J., & Dwyer, J. H. (2003). Dietary fiber and progression of atherosclerosis: the Los Angeles Atherosclerosis Study. *The American Journal of Clinical Nutrition, 78*(6), 1085-1091.

25

Mediterranean Diet and Gene-Mediterranean Diet Interactions in Determining Intermediate Cardiovascular Disease Phenotypes

Mercedes Sotos Prieto
University of Valencia, Department of Preventive Medicine and Public Health and CIBER Fisiopatología de la Obesidad y Nutrición, Spain

1. Introduction

Currently, cardiovascular diseases (CVD) are one of the most important problems in the world. In fact, CVD are the first cause of death all over the world and, according to the World Health Organization (WHO), it is expected to remain so over coming years due to aging population and the increase of prevalence of CVD in countries with fewer resources.

According to European statistics, 2008 for CVD, the leading causes of death in Europe are coronary heart disease and stroke. In Europe, deaths from these diseases are 4.3 million each year. Nearly half (48%) of all deaths are due to CVD (54% of deaths in women and 43% of deaths in men). Regional variations in cardiovascular mortality have been observed both between and within countries in Europe (Sans et al., 1997; Müller et al., 2004). Coronary heart disease mortality patterns showed a clear north-east to south-west gradient in CVD mortality (1990-1992; 45-74 years age-adjusted) with the lowest rates for both men and women in France, Spain, Switzerland, and Italy (Sans et al., 1997). Many factors could be related to the different distribution (eating behaviours, life style, and genetics).

To begin with the development of this chapter it is necessary to consider firstly the health determinants to better understand and focus the aim of this chapter.

The model of health fields proposed by Laframboise in 1973 and developed in Lalonde Report in 1974 (Lalonde 1974) has revolutionized contemporary public health due to the approaching and explaining of the health levels in the populations and therefore, the way of formulating health policies. Marc Lalonde proposed a new "health field" concept that can be broken up into four broad elements: Human biology, Environment, Lifestyle, and Health Care Organization".

Of the four determinants of health, the one which is most susceptible to be modified is lifestyle. Apart from not smoking, the most important lifestyle determinants of good health are what we eat and how active we are. A healthy diet helps to maintain or improve our health. However, as we said before, the CVD are increasing all over the word, and authorities view it as one of the most serious Public Health problems in the 21st century.

CVD are complex and the risk factors that contribute to the development of CVD can be classified into different categories depending on whether they are modified or not (Posner et al., 1991, Haskell et al., 2003) and how they contribute to the development of CVD (Linton et al., 2003). Thus, on the one hand, we have not modifiable factors such as age, sex, family history and genetics. With regard to genetics, we inherit the genetic risk to develop CVD, but this risk can be modulated by other modifiable factors. In this chapter we will deeply discuss the relation between genes and environmental factors (especially diet) in the prevention of CVD (Figure 1).

On the other hand, we also have factors that are susceptible to be modified such as cholesterol concentrations, hypertension, smoking, diabetes, type of diet, obesity, sedentary lifestyle, stress and consumption of oral contraceptives. The more risk factors a person has, the higher risk of developing CVD. Some risk factors can be changed, treated or modified, and some others not. But controlling the largest possible number of risk factors through changes in lifestyle and/or drugs can reduce cardiovascular risk. Among the environmental factors associated with CVD, and as a part of one of the health determinants proposed by Lalonde, diet has a great impact on lipid metabolism, oxidative stress and the development of the atherosclerotic process (Ordovas et al., 2004) (Figure 1). Changes in eating behaviours have contributed to the growing epidemic of chronic diseases. These changes are characterized by an unbalanced diet consisting of food with a high density of energy rich in saturated fatty acids (SAF) as well as a decrease in physical activity. This process is called nutritional transition. Given these facts, researchers are trying to elucidate the best diet to prevent CVD. However, there is a widespread of controversy. Different proposals have been considered such as low-fat diet, diet low in carbohydrates and high in proteins, among others, all promoted by the acquisition of knowledge, fashion or business interests (Ordovas et al., 2004).

Traditionally, the American Heart Association (AHA) has based dietary recommendations for primary care of cardiovascular risk in a low-fat diet (Krauss MR et al, 2000). This diet is also based on reducing all types of fat so that the contribution of total fat calories should be less than 30% (of which SAF are less than 10%) and cholesterol intake less than 300 mg daily. This type of diet causes a decrease in total cholesterol (TC) and LDL-C, and a decrease or not variation in HDL-C and increases or unchanged triglycerides (TG) concentrations (Obarzanek et al., 2001; Lichtensein et al., 2002, Howard et al., 2006). Later on, in 2005, a new version of USDA pyramid in which food groups are presented in vertical and which incorporates the concept that the diet should be tailored to individual needs came up (USDA, 2005).

After the AHA recommendations, other types of diets have been proposed such as diets rich in protein, low carb, Mediterranean diet, etc. Mediterranean diet has attracted the most interest by its great relevance regarding the protective role in primary and secondary care of CVD.

The aim of this chapter is to analyse the role of the Mediterranean diet in determining intermediate CVD phenotypes. We also review one of the most emerging topics currently: the role of gene-Mediterranean diet interactions on CVD.

2. Mediterranean diet

Due to the great incidence of CVD, Mediterranean diet has gained a considerable popularity during the last decades. The Mediterranean area is a sociocultural construction built on the countries bordering the Mediterranean Sea. Food habits have been consolidated over the centuries and are the result of geographical and climatic factors, as well as cultural, political and religious factors of Mediterranean people. Mediterranean area is identified by characteristics based on agriculture (natural grain, olives, wine and vegetables), fishing and consumption of poultry instead of other meats.

Furthermore, Mediterranean diet includes food and cooking techniques typical of Mediterranean countries which have been gradually abandoned by western patterns.

The Mediterranean diet has been described as a model from a nutritional point of view due to the good balance that provides its food items (micronutrients, vitamins, antioxidants). Nevertheless, as well as the cooking techniques have been abandoned, in the last few years changes in lifestyle have triggered a move away from the recommended intakes in relation to several nutrients. All these changes make it even more difficult to ensure adequate intakes of vitamins and minerals. This problem could affect more to certain risk groups such us women, the elderly, children, gestating and lactating women and ill people. Knowing the extent of this reality it seems worthy to inform people and society in general about the necessary changes in the diet and about the characteristics of the Mediterranean diet which are being lost and should be restored.

2.1 Definition of the Mediterranean diet

The concept of the Mediterranean diet originated from several observational studies in the 1950s, being the most known the Seven Countries Study initiated by Ancel Keys (Ancel Keys 1970). Subsequently, several studies have associated increased longevity, lower mortality and morbidity to Mediterranean diet (Keys et al., 1986; de Lorgeril et al., 1999; Singh et al., 2002; Trichopoulou et al., 2003; Knoops et al., 2004). Taken as a whole, these studies showed that, despite a high fat intake, these populations had low rates of coronary heart disease and other vascular diseases, cancer, inflammatory and degenerative diseases, resulting in a long life expectancy. The Mediterranean dietary pattern was considered to be largely responsible for the good health observed in these regions (Keys et al., 1986). Currently, there is a great number of clinical and epidemiological studies that have shown the benefits of the Mediterranean diet. However, these effects are attributed to the traditional Mediterranean diet and not to the Westernized patterns that nowadays characterize the South European countries (Serra-Majem et al., 2004).

Although there are several variations of the Mediterranean diet, the main characteristics include high consumption (daily consumption) of vegetables, fruit, whole grain cereals and low fat dairy products; weekly consumption of fish, poultry, tree nuts and legumes; relatively low consumption of red meat (approximately twice a month) as well as moderate daily consumption of alcohol (preferably in the form of wine) normally with meals (keys et al., 1986) (Figure 1).

Most of the articles published so far on Mediterranean diet are observational studies. However, there is a lack of intervention studies that demonstrate causal relationship. Although there are few randomized controlled trials of dietary intervention with Mediterranean Diet, we have recently strong data from one large randomize control trial supporting the beneficial effects of Mediterranean diet on CVD prevention (Estruch et al., 2006).

2.2 Principal studies that focus on Mediterranean diet and cardiovascular diseases

In general, there is a predominance of observational studies related to Mediterranean Diet compared to clinical trials in the study of CVD. Thus, most of the studies are cross-sectional studies with a level III of evidence (based on the quality of evidence according to the 2nd edition of the U.S. Task Force (Harris et al., 2001)). The *ATTICA* study is the most remarkable (Pitsavos et al., 2003) and it was conducted on a representative sample of Greek men and women recruited from May 2001 to December 2002 in order to analyze cardiovascular risk factors, establish associations with lifestyle, socioeconomic factors, psychological characteristics, and assess their impact on CVD over a year, five and ten years. Several studies found a positive association between Mediterranean Diet and CVD (Tzima et al., 2007; Panagiotakos et al., 2006; Pitsavos et al., 2007).

Two other large European cohort studies (evidence level II-2) include the Greek cohort within *EPIC* (European Prospective Investigation into Cancer) (Trichopoulou et al., 2003, Slimani et al., 2002). They study the relationship between nutrition and cancer in 519,978 participants from 23 centers located in 20 European countries.

Another cohort study is the *HALE* (Knoops et al., 2004) (Healthy Ageing: Longitudinal Study in Europe). This project analyzed age-related changes and the determinants of healthy aging in terms of mortality and morbidity, and physical, mental, cognitive and social functionality in 13 European countries. Results from this study suggest that a high adherence to Mediterranean diet is associated with a reduction in both overall mortality and cardiovascular mortality.

Regarding intervention studies (level I of scientific evidence), two of the most known studies analyzing Mediterranean Diet are *PREDIMED* study (Prevention with Mediterranean diet) (Estruch et al., 2006) and *Medi-RIVAGE* study (Mediterranean Diet, Cardiovascular Risks and Gene Polymorphism) (Vincent-Baudry et al., 2005).

PREDIMED study is a multicenter, prospective, randomized, controlled trial whose goals are to assess the efficacy and safety of a Mediterranean diet in primary care of CVD. It was designed in 2002 and it is the first long-term clinical trial that recruits high-risk patients (around 7,000 participants from different regions in Spain) to follow a Mediterranean diet supplemented with virgin olive oil (VOO) (1 liter a week) or nuts (30 g per day of which 15 g almonds and 15 g walnuts).

Medi-RIVAGE study is a randomized clinical trial conducted in France on 212 women and men with at least one cardiovascular risk factor. The aims of the study are to evaluate the effect of two types of diet in the prevention of CVD and to investigate biological mechanisms and genetic polymorphisms related to metabolism. On the one hand, they study the traditional Mediterranean diet (35-38% of total energy from fat: 50% monounsaturated fatty acids (MUFA), 25% polyunsaturated fatty acids (PUFA), 25% SFA) and on the other hand, a low fat diet based on the AHA (30% of total energy from fat: 33% MUFA, 33% PUFA, 33% SFA).

With regard to studies that analyze final cardiovascular risk phenotypes, two of the most outstanding studies (level I of scientific evidence) are the Lyon Diet Heart Study and the Indio-Mediterranean Diet Heart study.

The *Lyon Diet Heart Study* (de Lorgeril et al., 1999), a randomized, controlled trial with free-living subjects (half of 600 men and women in France), tested the effectiveness of a Mediterranean-type diet (consistent with the new AHA Dietary Guidelines) on composite measures of the coronary recurrence rate after a first myocardial infarction during 46 months. Subjects in the experimental group were instructed by cardiologists and dietitians to adopt a Mediterranean-type diet. They demonstrated the effectiveness of Mediterranean diet in the secondary care of CVD. However, the intervention group with Mediterranean diet received margarine rich in alpha-linolenic fatty acid, fact that distorted the interpretation of results, as margarine is not a component of traditional Mediterranean diet. Something similar happens with the Indo-Mediterranean Diet Heart Study (Singh et al., 2002).

The *Indo Mediterranean Diet Heart* study is a randomized, single-blind trial in 1000 patients with angina pectoris, myocardial infarction, or surrogate risk factors for CVD. 499 patients were allocated to a diet rich in whole grains, fruits, vegetables, walnuts, and almonds. 501 controls consumed a local diet similar to the step I National Cholesterol Education Program (NCEP) prudent diet. They showed that an Indo-Mediterranean diet, that is rich in a-linolenic acid, might be more effective in primary and secondary prevention of CVD than the conventional step I NCEP prudent diet. However, as in the Lyon Diet Heart Study, the intervention group with Mediterranean diet increased the consumption of alpha-linolenic fatty acid from soybean and mustard oil, which are not typical from Mediterranean countries.

3. Mediterranean diet in determining intermediate cardiovascular disease phenotypes

There is a great number of studies analysing the effect of the consumption or adherence to Mediterranean diet and intermediate CVD phenotypes. In the following sections we review the studies analysing Mediterranean diet and obesity, lipid metabolism, glucose concentrations, blood pressure and inflammation. Table 1 shows the effect of Mediterranean diet on the aforementioned phenotypes.

3.1 Mediterranean diet and obesity

Currently, it is not known which is the best diet is to lose weight (low-carb, high protein, low fat diet, etc.). Consumption of nuts, and high fat diets (rich in MUFA), characteristics of the Mediterranean diet, have been traditionally associated with an increased body weight by its high contain in fats. However, recent scientific evidence does not support these data. Adherence to Mediterranean diet was inversely associated with BMI and obesity in a cross-sectional survey carried out in the northeast of Spain (Schröder et al., 2004). Obesity risk decreased in both men and women with increasing adherence to the traditional Mediterranean diet.

Results from epidemiological studies on large populations indicate that subjects who usually consume nuts have lower BMI than those who do not consume (Bes-Rastrollo et al, 2009, Garcia-Lorda et al, 2003; Schroder et al, 2004). In addition, the SUN cohort (Seguimiento Universidad de Navarra) (follow-up University of Navarra) evaluated 11,895 participants and found an inverse association between consumption of nuts and weight gain per year (Martinez-Gonzalez & Bes-Ballostro, 2011). Similarly, a recent study carried out in EPIC-PANACEA project showed that individuals with high adherence to Mediterranean diet, according to the score based on a questionnaire of adherence to Mediterranean diet (11-18 points), showed in a weight change of 20.16 kg (95% CI :20,2-20, 7 kg) 5 years and they were also 10% less likely to become overweight and obese compared with individuals with lower adherence (0-6 points) (Romaguera et al., 2010). Furthermore, a study that evaluated 497,308 individuals aged between 25-70 years in 10 European countries found that high adherence to the Mediterranean diet is associated with lower abdominal adiposity, using waist circumference as a measure (Romaguera et al., 2009).

With respect to intervention studies, it has been shown that subjects that consume daily tree nuts in their diet are less likely to gain weight (Li et al., 2010). A study evaluating the intake of almonds (42-72 g daily) in 81 patients over 6 months found that there was no significant weight gain (Fraser et al., 2002). Similarly, García-Londa et al, (2003) found that in the short term, the addition of tree nuts to diet, in amounts up to 50 g daily, does not increase weight. After one year of intervention in the PREDIMED study, beneficial effects on waist circumference were shown (Martinez-Gonzalez & Bes-Ballostro, 2011).

Finally, a meta-analysis regarding Mediterranean diet and weight loss analyzing randomize controlled trials has been recently published (Esposito et al., 2011), and it concludes that Mediterranean diet does not cause weight gain, which removes the objection to its relatively high fat content. Mediterranean diet could be a strategy to help people lose weight.

Some of the proposed mechanisms that might explain these facts are that the absorption of nuts may be incomplete, thus some of its fat content may not be absorbed by the body and would be excreted in the feces. Moreover, the consumption of nuts may have a satiating effect, producing a decrease in consumption of other foods and helping to control total energy intake. Although it still has not been proved, there may be an adaptation of the metabolism, so that energy consumption could be more efficient and get the body burn more energy, thus avoiding an accumulation of body fat (Brennan et al., 2010; Garcia-Lorda et al., 2003; Rajaram & Sabaté, 2006).

3.2 Mediterranean diet and lipid metabolism

Mediterranean diet has been largely studied in relation to lipid metabolism because of its beneficial effect on CVD. However, different results have been shown regarding a variety of studies, designs, and sample sizes. Cross-sectional studies with similar characteristics, with a sample size between 1762 and 2032 participants in Greece (ATTICA study), evaluated the adherence to Mediterranean diet and lipid profile. Thus, Tzima et al (2007) reported that subjects who are overweight (BMI 25-29.9) or obese (BMI $\geq$ 30) in the highest tertile of the Mediterranean diet score had lower total cholesterol (TC) (-13 %, $P = 0.001$) after adjusting for age, sex and BMI compared to the first tertile. However, there were no significant differences in triglycerides (TG) and HDL-C. This increase in the adherence to Mediterranean diet was also associated with lower total cholesterol ($p < 0.001$) in a study carried out by Panagiotakos et al (2006). In addition to that, individuals with abdominal obesity and less physically active had lower adherence to Mediterranean diet ($p = 0.008$) with lower HDL-C ($p < 0.05$) (Pitsavos et al., 2007).

Moreover, seven studies of 29 clinical trials with 3,822 subjects (2,202 assigned to Mediterranean diet and 1,903 assigned to a control diet) reported beneficial effects of adherence to Mediterranean diet on HDL-C (Papadaki & Scott, 2008; Esposito et al., 2004; Estruch et al., 2006; Esposito et al., 2003; Esposito et al., 2009; Athryros et al., 2011). A recent meta-analysis (Kastorini et al., 2011) showed that, overall, adherence to Mediterranean diet was associated with higher HDL-C levels as compared with a control diet.

Benefits in TC have also been shown in some randomized controlled trials (Estruch et al., 2006; Vincent-Baudry et al., 2005; Ambring et al., 2004). In this sense, Estruch et al., (2006) carried out a study of 3 months with individuals who had diabetes mellitus or one or more cardiovascular risk factors, which were assigned to three intervention groups (n = 257-8 / group) (2 Mediterranean diet (one supplemented with VOO and another one with 15g of almonds+15g walnuts/day) and one control diet low in fats). Regarding the lipid profile, both Mediterranean diets showed significant increase in HDL-C levels ($p = <0.001$ and $p = 0.006$, respectively) and a significant reduction ($p <0.001$ and $p = 0.002$, respectively) in the atherogenic index (TC/HDL-C) in contrast to the control group. However, only Mediterranean diet supplemented with nuts showed a significantly reduction in TC ($p = 0.040$) and TG ($p = 0.022$), compared to control. Neither of the Mediterranean diets significantly reduced LDL-C compared to the control diet (low fat diet).

Concerning TG, three observational studies reported a beneficial effect of Mediterranean diet (Chrysohoou et al., 2004; Tzima et al., 2007; Barzi et al., 2003) as compared with low adherence to Mediterrenean diet. Five interventional studies showed beneficial effects of Mediterranean diet on TG concentrations (Shai et al., 2008; Esposito et al., 2004; Estruch et al., 2006; Esposito et al., 2009; Elhayany et al., 2011), whereas other studies did not find significant differences (de Lorgeril et al., 1994; Castro et al., 2000; Michalsen et al., 2006).

Moreover, results from a crossover study during 4 weeks for each intervention (22 healthy people (12H/10M)) found an improvement in lipid profile to compare a Mediterranean diet (rich in omega 3) with a Swedish standard diet (Ambring et al., 2004). The results showed a significant decrease in TC, LDL-C, TG (17%, 22%, and 17%) in the group with Mediterranean diet. On the other hand, one non-randomize control trial carried out in Italy (47 obese women) during 4-month with an hypoenergetic Mediterranean diet together with a program of physical exercise showed a significant decrease in total cholesterol and TG concentrations. Levels of LDL-C decreased ($p <0.001$) after 4 months of intervention, whereas HDL-C increased (Andreoli et al., 2008). However, another study carried out in 71 healthy Canadian found a significant decrease in TC at 6 weeks of intervention ($p <0.05$), whereas no significant changes were observed after 12 weeks. Levels of HDL-C, LDL-C and TG were not affected after 6 or 12 weeks of intervention (Goulet et al., 2003). Different characteristics of the recruitment of individuals can influence the final results of the studies.

The relationship between nut consumption and reduced risk of CVD has been established in numerous epidemiological studies. Thus, Ros et al (2004), in a crossover study carried out in hypercholesterolemia subjects in Spain, determined whether a diet containing nuts (18% of energy) could improve markers related to endothelial function against another typical Mediterranean diet with similar energy intake, fat, protein, carbohydrates, but not MUFA intake, after 4 weeks. Estruch et al (2006) also found a significant decrease in TC ($p = 0.017$) and LDL-C ($p = 0.010$). However, no differences were found in TG concentrations and HDL-

C. Pooled analysis in 25 clinical trials to evaluate nut consumption in blood lipids showed that the most important finding is that the cholesterol-lowering effects of nut consumption are dose related and are more pronounced in subjects with higher baseline LDL-C or lower BMI. Nut consumption also lowered TG levels in subjects with hypertriglyceridemia (Sabate et al., 2010).

3.3 Mediterranean diet and glucose concentrations

The increasing incidence of type 2 diabetes throughout the world is also linked to westernized dietary patterns. Lifestyle changes are effective measures to prevent diabetes. The Mediterranean diet has also shown beneficial effects on diabetes risk and glucose concentrations.

Two observational studies reported a beneficial effect of close adherence to Mediterranean diet as compared with a control diet in lowering fasting glucose (FG) levels (Tzima et al., 2007; Panagiotakos et al., 2007).

Furthermore, Estruch et al., 2006 found that participants in the intervention group with Mediterranean diet supplemented with VOO or nuts, showed a significant reduction in FG compared with the control group (-0.39 mmol / L and -0.30 mmol / L, respectively).

In this sense, in another randomized controlled trial (Vincent-Baudry et al., 2005) with Mediterranean diet or low-fat diet, after 3 months of intervention, both diets significantly reduced blood glucose, insulinemia, insulin resistance and HOMA-IR index. Insulin levels remained significant after adjusting for BMI. However, there was no interaction between time and type of diet for any of the variables. Negative results were shown in a study that compared the intervention with Mediterranean diet rich in omega 3 versus the standard Swedish diet (Ambring et al., 2004). Recently, results from PREDIMED study also reported that, after a median follow-up of 4 years, diabetes incidence was lower in the groups with Mediterranean diet as compared with control group (10,1% in Mediterranean diet with VOO, 11% in Mediterranean diet with nuts, 17,9% in control group) (Salas-Salvado et al., 2011).

In conclusion, overall adherence to Mediterranean diet is associated with lower FG levels as compared with the control diet (Kastorini et al., 2011). Among the mechanisms associated with that decrease in glucose levels are the properties of the components of Mediterranean diet. Fiber delays gastric emptying, antioxidants increase oxidative capacity and moderate alcohol could have a role in adiponectin. As a consequence, it ends in the prevention of insulin resistance and, finally, in prevention of type 2 diabetes (Schröder, 2007).

3.4 Mediterranean diet and blood pressure

Nutritional factors and dietary patterns have been associated with hypertension. Hypertensive individuals can remarkably reduce their blood pressure through nutritional changes. Mediterranean diet has also shown beneficial effects in the prevention and control of blood pressure.

Cross-sectional studies associate the consumption of Mediterranean diet with lower systolic blood pressure (SBP). Higher adherence to Mediterranean diet was associated with lower SBP ($p<0.001$) (Tzima et al., 2007; Panagiotakos et al., 2006) as well as with 70% of decrease of prevalence of hypertension (Alvarez-León et al., 2006). In contrast, lower adherence was associated with increased blood pressure (BP) (Pitsavos et al., 2007). However, one study showed higher SBP in the group more closely following the Mediterranean diet in the SUN cohort in young individuals after a median follow-up of 4.2 years (Nunez-Cordoba et al., 2009). Most of the effects of the Mediterranean diet on blood pressure have been attributed to the consumption of olive oil, fruits, nuts and vegetables. Psaltopoulou et al (2004) in the Greek-EPIC cohort studied whether Mediterranean diet together or olive oil in particular reduced blood pressure in 20,343 people without a diagnosis of hypertension. In this study, the Mediterranean diet score was inversely and significantly associated with both, SBP and diastolic blood pressure (DBP), as well as the intake of olive oil, fruits and vegetables. However, Giuseppe et al (2008) found a significant and positive association of BP with the rate of adaptation to the Mediterranean diet. However, we have to consider that the study was carried out in older women (> 60 years). In the Italian EPIC Florence cohort, which include more than 10,000 non-hypertensive women aged 35-64 years, consumption of olive oil was inversely associated with DBP (Masala et al., 2008). However, with regard to DBP and Mediterranean diet as a whole, observational studies did not found significant associations (Kastorini et al., 2011).

Regarding randomized clinical trials (level I scientific evidence) in a meta-analysis, it was found that the overall adherence to Mediterranean diet was associated with lower SBP and DBP as compared with control diet (Kastorini et al., 2011). In the PREDIMED study, results showed a significant decrease in both SBP and DBP in the two groups with Mediterranean diet (one supplemented with VOO and another with nuts) as compared with control group (Estruch et al., 2006). Finally, in a non-randomized clinical trial whose aim was to evaluate the effect of a moderately hypoenergetic Mediterranean diet with an exercise program in women with overweight-obesity, DBP decreased significantly ($p < 0.001$) after two months of intervention, while the SBP was not changed significantly after four months of intervention (Andreoli et al., 2008).

In conclusion, as we mention before, the beneficial effects of the Mediterranean diet on blood pressure have been attributed to a synergy of its components, especially to fruits, vegetables, nuts and olive oil. These components are low in sodium and rich in minerals (magnesium, potassium and calcium), antioxidant, fiber, PUFA and MUFA, all of them with potentially protective properties against hypertension.

3.5 Mediterranean diet and inflammation

Obesity and other related diseases associated with CVD are caused or related to inflammation. Three of five cross-sectional studies, showed a significant decrease in inflammation markers with higher adherence to Mediterranean diet (Sotos-Prieto et al., 2010). Thus, Panagiotakos et al (2006) found significant negative association between adherence to Mediterranean diet and protein C reactive (CRP) ($p < 0.001$). Also, the highest score in the AHEI index (Alternate Healthy Eating Index) and AMED (alternate mediterranean diet index) was associated with lower inflammation biomarkers concentrations (IL-6 and CRP) (24% and 16% respectively). This study was carried out in 690 nurses, in the Nurses' Health Study (Fung et al., 2005). Moreover, subjects in the highest tertile of adherence to Mediterranean diet had 20 % lower CRP levels ($p = 0.015$) and 17% IL-6 ($p = 0.025$) (Chrysohoou et al., 2004), while the lower adherence to Mediterranean diet was associated with higher levels of CRP (> 3.0 mg / ml) (Pitsavos et al., 2007).

Salas-Salvado et al (2008), in a study that included subjects with high cardiovascular risk (339H/433M, 55-80 years), found an association between consumption of certain foods that characterized the Mediterranean pattern (fruits, cereals, VOO and nuts) with lower concentrations of inflammatory markers, especially those related to endothelial function (ICAM-1 and VCAM-1). However, participants with higher adherence to a Mediterranean diet showed no significant decrease in the inflammatory biomarkers' concentrations (CRP, IL-6, ICAM-1 and VCAM-1), although there was a statistical trend in the case of ICAM-1 and VCAM-1 (p <0.1).

In two randomized controlled trials, CRP levels decreased only in the group with Mediterranean diet supplemented with VOO (-0.54 mg / L) compared with the control group (low-fat). The IL-6 decreased in both groups with Mediterranean diet (VOO and nuts), whereas it increased in the group with low-fat diet. Similarly, Esposito et al (Esposito et al., 2004), in a study conducted in Italy with 180 people with metabolic syndrome (99H, 81M), observed a significant decrease in CRP (p = 0.01) and IL-6 (p = 0.04) in the intervention group (instructed to follow a Mediterranean diet) compared with the control group (prudent diet with fat percentage <30%) after two years. By contrast, Michalsen et al (2006) found no changes in CRP levels, although there were some limitations in the study.

In a non-randomized clinical trial, plasma levels of CRP decreased significantly (6%, P <0.02) after two hours of Mediterranean diet rich in MUFA intake (Blum et al., 2006).

In conclusion, Mediterranean diet is characterized by a high consumption of fruit and vegetables. This adds other mechanistic benefits provided by their polyphenolic content to its high antioxidant content that could be linked with the prevention of inflammation. Other components of the Mediterranean diet such as VOO and red wine gather antioxidants and anti-inflammatory actions that may contribute to the healthy effects of this diet on inflammation.

	Decrease	**Increase**	**No significant**
BMI (kg/m^2)	Scröder et al., 2004 Romaguera et al., 201 Bes-Ballostro et al., 2009; Garcia-Londa et al., 2003 Martinez-Gonzalez & Bes-Ballostro, 2011		
Weight gain	Fraser et al., 2002 Martinez-Gonzalez & Bes-Ballostro, 2011		
Waist circumference	Romaguera et al., 2002 Martinez-Gonzalez & Bes-Ballostro, 2011		
TC	Estruch et al.,2006 Vicent-Baudry et al., 2005 Ambring et al., 2004		
LDL-C	Vicent-Baudry et al., 2005 Ambring et al., 2004 Ros et al., 2004 Andreoli et al., 2008		Michalsen et al., 2006 Goulet et al., 2003 Estruch et al., 2006

	Decrease	Increase	No significant
HDL-C	Pitsavos et al., 2007	Estruch et al, 2006 Andreoli et al.,2008 Papadaki & Scott, 2008 Esposito et al., 2004; Esposito et al., 2003; Esposito et al., 2009; Athryros et al., 2011 Ambring et al., 2004	Michalsen et al., 2006 Goulet et al., 2003
TG	Estruch et al.,2006 Vicent-Baudry et al., 2005 Ambring et al., 2004 Ros et al., 2004 Chrysohoou et al., 2004; Tzima et al., 2007; Barzi et al., 2003 Shai et al., 2008 Esposito et al., 2004 Esposito et al., 2009 Elhayany et al., 2011 Sabate et al., 2010		Michalsen et al., 2006 de Lorgeril et al., 1994 Castro et al., 2000 Goulet et al., 2003
Glucose	Estruch et al., 2006 Vicent-Baudry et al., 2005 Andreoli et al.,2008 Panagiotakos et al., 2007 Tzima et al., 2007 Salas-Salvado et al., 2011		Ambring et al., 2004
SBP	Estruch et al., 2006 Tzima et al., 2007 Psaltopoulou et al., 2004 Panagiotakos et al., 2006	Giussepe et al., 2008 Nunez-Cordoba et al., 2009	Andreoli et al., 2008
BP	Estruch et al., 2006 Andreoli et al., 2008 Alvarez-Leon et al., 2006 Psaltopoulou et al., 2004 Pitsavos et al., 2007 Masala et al., 2008		
CRP	Estruch et al., 2006 Esposito et al., 2004 Blum et al., 2006 Fung et al., 2005 Chrysohoou et al., 2004 Panagiotakos et al., 2006	Pitsavos et al., 2007	Michalsen et al., 2006 Salas-Salvado et al., 2008
IL-6	Estruch et al., 2006 Esposito et al., 2004		Salas-Salvado et al., 2008

BMI: Body mass index; TC: Total Cholesterol; LDL-C: Low density lipoprotein cholesterol
HDL: High density lipoprotein cholesterol; TG: Triglycerides; SBP: Systolic blood pressure; BP: Blood pressure; CRP: Protein C reactive; IL-6: Interleukin 6

Table 1. Studies that analyze Mediterranean diet and variation (decrease, increase, no significant) in intermediate cardiovascular disease phenotypes.

4. Nutritional genomics

Current changes in lifestyle, in part promoted by the nutritional transition, have contributed to the development of CVD, cancer and other non-comunicable diseases.

Since the Human Genome Project finished in April 2003, we have the information about the complete genome. However, we still unknown the role of the majority of genes involved in the development of CVD. For that reason, currently, considering diet as one of the most important environmental factor, the molecular nutrition begins with the approach to better understand the mechanism involved in the gene-diet interaction and to personalize the diet with the aim to prevent common diseases, among them, CVD. Since Human Genome Project finished, the classic candidate gene approach and the new genome-wide association studies have identified genetic variants that predispose people to CVD.

In this sense, it was shown that human genome is sensitive to nutritional environment in two ways: nutrients may regulate genes and genes also influence the effect of diet (Loktionov, 2003). Nutritional health is dependent on the interaction between the environmental aspects of dietary components and the genetically controlled aspects (Figure 1). The concept of gene-diet interaction describes the modulation of the effect of a dietary component on a specific phenotype (plasma lipid concentrations, obesity, etc.) by a genetic polymorphism (Ordovas & Corella, 2004). A better understanding of these interactions has the potential to support disease prevention and will lead to different requirements between individuals via modification of dietary recommendations. This research has led to the development of concepts that study the effect of genetic variation on the interaction between diet and specific phenotypes known as *nutrigenetics*.

The goal of nutrigenetics is to generate personalized recommendations regarding the genetic susceptibility of each individual. It is also known as *personalized nutrition*.

On the other hand, the study of the characterization of gene products and the physiological function and interactions of these products is known as *nutrigenomics* (Figure 1). The unifying term "*nutritional genomics*" refers to nutrigenomics and nutrigenetics (Ordovas & Corella, 2004). The term Nutrigenetics was named for the first time by Brennan in 1975 in his book "Nutrigenenetics: New concepts for Relieving Hypoglycemia", while nutrigenomics was used in 1999 by DellaPenna when he studied the plant genomics field. The new technology research together with the knowledge of the human genome sequence have led in the study of the new "omics" to better understand the molecular basis of the disease development. They are the disciplines known as:

- *Transcriptomic*: to quantify the level of gene expression by using techniques to analyse thousands of mRNA molecules at the same time by using a technique based on microarrays.
- *Proteomic*: large-scale study of proteins (particularly their structure and function) is possible to identify proteins that can diagnose disease or predict the evolution of it.
- *Metabolomics:* to study techniques dedicated to complete a system composed of a series of molecules that are metabolic intermediates, metabolites, hormones and other signal molecules, and secondary metabolites, which can be found in a biological system.
- *Systems Biology*: integration of proteomic data, genetic, metabolomics.
- *Bioinformatics*: to interpret the data to provide biological mechanisms to explain the experimental observations.

Following these new concepts, other related terms have emerged: *nutritranscriptomic* (the study of messenger RNA expression at the cellular level under some nutritional conditions), *nutriproteomic* (large-scale analysis of the structure and function of the protein, as well as protein-protein interactions in a cell to identify molecular targets of dietary components) or *nutrimetabolomic* (measuring all metabolites in response to stimuli nutritional body) (Panagiotou & Nielsen, 2009).

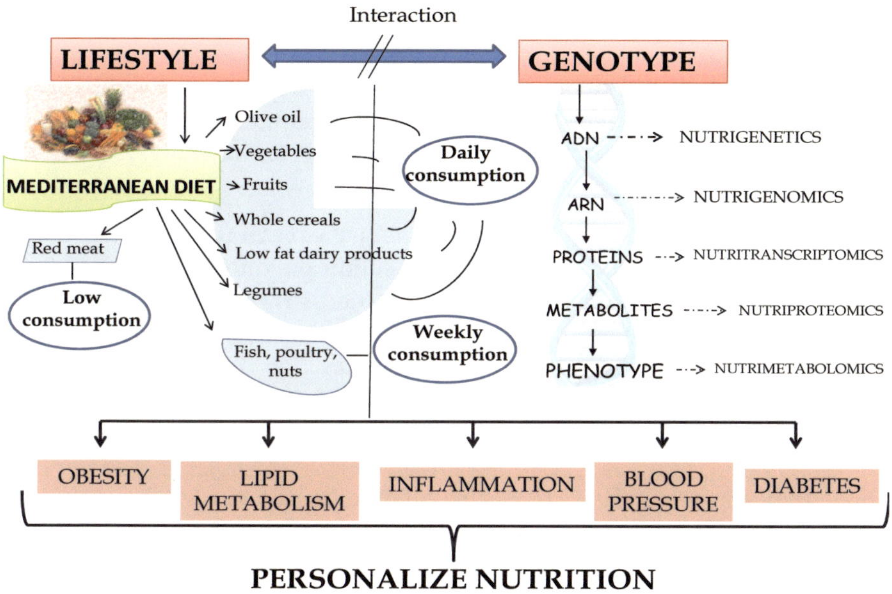

Fig. 1. Personalized Nutrition. As part of health determinants, lifestyle interacts with genetic susceptibility to modulate obesity risk, lipid metabolism, inflammation, blood pressure and diabetes. Among lifestyle factors, diet, and especifically, Mediterrranean diet, has an important role in gen-diet interactions. On the other hand, with the new technology research together with the knowledge of human genome sequence have led in the study of the nutrigenetics and nutrigenomics (nutritional genomics) to better understand the molecular basis of the disease development, they are the disciplines knows as: transcriptomic, proteomic, metabolomic that allow us to know phenotypes characteristics. These interactions between Mediterranean diet and genetic susceptibility will contribute to create personalized diets.

5. Gene-Mediterranean diet interaction in intermediate cardiovascular diseases phenotypes

In the following sections we are going to review some studies analyzing nutrigenetics and nutrigenomics effects on CVD.

5.1 Nutrigenetics in the prevention of cardiovascular diseases

In the last decades the eating pattern has changed considerably towards less healthy habits with excessive intake of calories and SFA. Considering this as a risk factor of CVD these changes are contributing to the increase of CVD. As a result, researchers are wondering which could be the best diet to prevent CVD and related phenotypes. Different opinions have emerged about the virtues of low-carbohydrate diets, low fat diets, high-protein diets or Mediterranean dietary pattern in the control of body weight and factors related to CVD (Shai et al., 2008, Larsen et al., 2010, Sacks et al., 2009).

Given the great diversity that exists with regard to dietary recommendations and their effects, several authors insist on the fact that there is no perfect diet. Diet will be different depending on individual characteristics. The response to the same diet has not the same effectiveness on different two people. While some people appear to have no response to dietary intervention (hiporesponders), others have a high response (hiperresponders) (Katan MB et al., 1986). It has been suggested that this inter-individual variability to dietary modification is determined by genetic factors, especially for phenotypes related to lipid metabolism (Loktionov, 2003).

Most of the studies carried out to determine whether genetic factors could explain these differences are based on the study of single nucleotide polymorphisms (SNPs) as well as dietary factors, particularly those that characterize Mediterranean Diet. The table 2 shows some studies conducted to assess genetic modulations according to different types of diets or macronutrients. In the following paragraphs we describe the results from intervention studies and observational studies that analyze gene-diet interactions on CVD.

Results from intervention studies

Intervention studies in which subjects receive a controlled dietary intake provide the most valuable information for the study of gene-nutrient-phenotype association. However, intervention studies have some limitations, such as the low number of participants. The sample size is important in nutrigenetic studies because otherwise, there is a lack of statistical power to assess the main associations. Something similar happens with the study of some genetic variants. Prevalence of certain polymorphisms is small and requires a large sample size to study these associations. Another limitation is the short duration of these interventions. A review conducted by Masson et al, (2003) concluded that there is evidence to suggest that variations in the *APOA1, APOA4, APOB* and *APOE* genes contribute to the heterogeneity of the lipid response to dietary interventions, and that these genes are directly or indirectly regulated by PPAR or other nuclear receptors. New examples that confirm the importance of gene-diet interaction in the field of nutrigenetics are the study of the perilipin gene (*PLIN*) (Corella D et al., 2005, Smith CE et al., 2010) and *SR-BI* (Perez-Martinez P et al., 2005).

Recently, some studies investigating the genetic modulation of the Mediterranean diet in PREDIMED study have been published. Thus, a study examining a polymorphism in the *FTO* gene (associated with obesity) shows that the A allele of the polymorphism rs9939609 in the FTO gene was not associated with baseline body weight, but after 3 years of nutritional intervention with Mediterranean diet carriers of A allele had a lower body weight gain than subjects with the ancestral allele (Razquin C et al., 2010 A).

Another example carried out in the PREDIMED study showed that CC subjects for the polymorphism-174G / C in the *IL-6* gene had a lower weight gain after three years only in those subjects who followed a Mediterranean diet supplemented with nuts and olive oil (Razquin et al., 2010 B)

Results from observational studies

Observational studies have the advantage of incorporating a large number of participants and the ability to estimate dietary habits. They also have the advantage that the distribution of genetic variants in the population is independent of eating behaviors by the principle of Mendelian randomization. Although nowadays the number of studies examining gene-diet interactions is increasing, few studies have investigated the interaction between SNPs in candidate genes and cardiovascular risk factors analyzing the consumption of Mediterranean diet or intake of MUFA, PUFA or SFA.

One of the most studied genes has been the Pro12Ala polymorphism in the *PPARG* gene and its interaction with MUFA intake. Obese subjects with the Ala12 allele have higher HOMA index when they eat low amounts of MUFA. Another example analyzing MUFA intake and body weight depending on variation in *APOA5* gene is one carried out in the Framingham study. They found a significant interaction between the promoter polymorphism -1131T>C in the *APOA5* gene and fat intake, particularly MUFA, regulating body weight (Corella D et al., 2007). The study of C677T polymorphism in the gene for methylenetetrahydrofolate reductase (*MTHFR*) is another example of modulation of LDL oxidation by the Mediterranean diet (Pitsavos et al., 2006). Recently, we published a significant gene-diet interaction in a variant of the promoter of *APOA2* gene. This study included 3462 volunteers from three different populations and it studied the interaction between the polymorphism-265T>C in the *APOA2* gene, food intake, and BMI. Carriers of the variant allele which had higher intake of SFA had a higher prevalence of obesity while this was not showed if the source of fat was MUFA or PUFA. These results were replicated for the first time in three independent populations (Corella et al., 2009). Subsequently, the authors replicated this interaction in Mediterranean and Chinese populations (Corella et al., 2011) confirming the importance of genetic modulation by dietary factors, and also the need to replicate gene-diet interactions to increase the scientific evidence and finally to contribute to personalize diet based on genetic susceptibility.

Author	Phenotype		Gene	Gen-diet interaction
Lopez-Miranda et al., 1994	Lipid metabolism	LDL-C	-75G>A APOA1	They studied the influence of the LDL-C postprandial response to MUFA intake. After high MUFA intake carriers of A allele had higher LDL-C but not the GG.
Jansen et al., 1997		LDL-C	Thr347Ser APOA4	347Ser carriers had lower LDL-C postprandial response when they switched from a diet rich in SFA to a diet based on NCEP.
Campos et al., 2001		VLDL, HDL-C	APOE	Higher VLDL and lower HDL-C in E2 with a high SFA intake.
Corella et al., 2001		LDL-C	APOE	E2 carriers had lower LDL-C in those with moderate alcohol consumption than in non-consumers. However, carriers of E4 allele that had a moderate alcohol consumption had higher LDL-C.
Brown et al., 2003		TC and LDL-C	T455C y T625 *APOC3*	In -45T and -625T homozygous subjects, SFA intake was associated with higher LDL-C.
Tai et al., 2005		TG and APOCIII	L162V *PPARA*	Carriers of 162V allele had higher TG concentrations and APOC3 levels only in that subjects with a low PUFA consumption.

Author	Phenotype		Gene	Gen-diet interaction
Robitaille et al., 2007		Lipids	Leu72Met Grelina	Interaction with fat intake modulating TG concentrations.
Ordovas, 2002		HDL-C	-514C>T *LIPC*	T alelle was associated with higher HDL-C in subjects that had an intake of fat < 30% of total energy.
Luan et al., 2001	Antropometric variables	BMI	Pro12Ala PPARG	AlaPPARG carriers had higher BMI than ProPPRG, but when the ratio PUFA:SFA was high, opposite results were shown.
Memisoglu et al., 2003		BMI	Pro12Ala PPARG	Among ProPro subjects, those with higher fat intake of had higher BMI compared to those with lower intake . No association was shown for 12Ala.
Robitaille et al., 2007		WC	Pro12Ala PPARA	Interaction Pro12Ala with the intake of fat modulating waist circunference.
Corella et al., 2009		BMI and Obesity	-265 T>C APOA2	C carriers that had high SFA intake had higher prevalence of obesity.
Corella et al., 2011		BMI and obesity	-265 T>C APOA2	Interaction of -265CC with SFA intake modulating risk of obesity.
Corella et al., 2010		BMI and obesity	rs9939609 FTO	Interacction of rs9939609 with educational level. A carriers had higher risk of obesity and BMI only in those without uneversity studies.
Razquin et al., 2010 (A)		Weight	rs9939609 FTO	A allele was associated with higher weight at the beginnung of the study. After three years of intervention with Mediterranean diet, A carriers had a lower weight gain.
Razquin et al., 2010 (C)		Weight	+45T/G, +276G/T Adiponectin	Genotype GG (+45T/G) was associated with higher weight gained during three years of intervention. TT (+276G/T) was associated with higher weight gain in men. Mediterranean diet suplemented with VOO and nuts reverted this effects.
Razquin et al., 2010 (B)		Weight	-174G/C IL-6	CC subjects that followed Mediterranean diet suplemented with VOO had lower weight gain after three years of intervention.

LDL-C: Low density lipoprotein cholesterol; VLDL: Very low density lipoprotein cholesterol
HDL: High density lipoprotein cholesterol; TC: Total cholesterol; BMI: Body mass index
WC: Waist circumference

Table 2. Nutrigenetics studies analysing gene-diet interactions.

5.2 Nutrigenomics in the prevention of cardiovascular diseases

As we explained in the previous section, there is increasing evidence that Mediterranean diet, whose emblematic component is virgin olive oil (VOO), has a beneficial effect on diseases associated with CVD and other diseases (neurodegenerative diseases, cancer).

VOO is a functional food containing high levels of MUFA and a number of minor components (bioactive components). These components are known as phenolic compounds. These phenolic compounds have a key role in plasma lipid concentrations and oxidative damage (that is related to CVD). It is believed that the benefits from the consumption of VOO are due to the interaction of its nutrients and minor components with genes. Several studies have shown changes in gene expression mediated by the consumption of VOO. In table 3 some studies analyzing changes in gene expression of some genes related to CVD by Mediterranean diet or its components are shown.

Autor	N / duración	Intervención	Cambios de expresión	Ruta implicada
Konstantinidou et al., 2010	N=90 (20-50 years) 3 months	1. MD +VOO 2. MD+ VOO 3. Control	INF-y ARHGAP15 IL7R ADRB2 POLK	Inflammation Oxidative stress
Konstantinidou et al., 2009	N=6 Postprandial study (0-6h)	50 ml VOO (26082 genes)	USP48 OGT AKAP13 IL10 DCLRE1C POLK	Cellular process Inflammation DNA damage
Khymenets et al., 2009	N= 6 H(262-28 years; 4 M (20-44) 3 weeks	VOO (25 ml/day)	ADAM17, ALDH1A, BIRC1, ERCC5, LIAS, OGT,PPARBP, TNFSF10, USP48, XRCC5	Mechanism involved in atherosclerosis
Camargo et al., 2010	N=20 with MS (56 years, 9 H, 11 M) Postprandial state	Breakfast with VOO (40 ml).	EGR1 IL1B, IL6 CCL3 CXCL1 CXCL2 CXCL3 CXCR4 TRIB1, NFKBIA	Inflammation
Llorente-Cortes et al., 2009	N=48 (55-80 years)	MD+VOO MD+nuts Control group	COX-2 LRP1 MCP-1 CD36 TFPI	Inflammation, foam cell formation, thrombosis
De Mello VD et al., 2008	34overweight MS 33 weeks	Weight reduction (n=24) Control group (n=10)	TLR4 TLR2 CCL5 TNFRSF1A IKBKB	Related to insulin sensitivity
Crujeiras et al., 2008	12 Obese (37,7 years) 8 weeks	Hypocaloric diet	SIRT1 SIRT2 NDUFS2	

MD: Mediterranean diet; VOO: Virgin olive oil; MS: Metabolic Syndrome

Table 3. Nutrigenomics studies

6. Conclusions and future directions

Current results of the studies analyzing the effect of Mediterranean diet on CVD suggest that adherence to the Mediterranean dietary pattern was associated with lower CVD phenotypes. Mediterranean diet has a beneficial effect on abdominal obesity, lipids levels, glucose metabolism, blood pressure and inflammation. The antioxidant and anti-inflammatory effects of the Mediterranean diet as a whole, and also the effects of the individual components, specifically VOO, fruits, vegetables, whole grains and fish could offer an explanation for the aforementioned beneficial effects of the Mediterranean diet.

These results are of considerable public health importance because this dietary pattern can be easily adopted by all population groups and various cultures, and they cost effectively serve for the primary and secondary prevention of CVD.

On the other hand, the current evidence from nutrigenetics studies is not enough to begin implementing specific personalized information. However, there is a large number of examples of common SNPs modulating the individual response to Mediterranean diet and other components as proof of concept of how gene-diet interactions can influence lipid metabolism, BMI, or other disorders, and it is expected that in the near future we will be able to harness the information contained in our genomes by using the behavioural tools to achieve successful personalized nutrition. In order to achieve that, it is recommended that future advises on nutrition will be based on studies using the highest level of epidemiological evidence and supported by mechanistic studies within the Nutritional Genomics and Systems biology. However, we have to take into account that in order to forget successful results in personalized nutrition through genetic variation, health professionals need to be prepared to learn and interpret genetic knowledge about their patients.

7. References

Alvarez León, EE., Henríquez, P., & Serra-Majem, L. (2006). Mediterranean diet and metabolic syndrome: a cross-sectional study in the Canary Islands. *Public Health Nutr*; 9(8A):1089-98.

Ambring, A., Friberg, P., Axelsen, M., Laffrenzen, M., Taskinen, MR., & Basu, S. (2004). Effects of a Mediterranean-inspired diet on blood lipids, vascular function and oxidative stress in healthy subjects. *M Clin Sci*; 106(5):519-25.

Andreoli, A., Lauro, S., Di Daniele, N., Sorge, R., Celi, M., & Volpe, SL. (2008). Effect of a moderately hypoenergetic Mediterranean diet and exercise program on body cell mass and cardiovascular risk factors in obese women. *Eur J Clin Nutr*;62(7):892-7.

Athyros, VG., Kakafika, AI., Papageorgiou, AA., Tziomalos, K., Peletidou, A., Vosikis, C., Karagiannis, A., & Mikhailidis, DP. (2011). Effect of a plant stanol ester-containing spread, placebo spread, or Mediterranean diet on estimated cardiovascular risk and lipid, inflammatory and haemostatic factors. *Nutr Metab Cardiovasc Dis*;21(3):213-21.

Barzi, F., Woodward, M., Marfisi, RM., Tavazzi, L., Valagussa, F., & Marchioli, R. (2003). Mediterranean diet and all-causes mortality after myocardial infarction: results from the GISSI-Prevenzione trial. *Eur J Clin Nutr*; 57(4):604-11.

Bes-Rastrollo, M., Wedick, NM., Martinez-Gonzalez, MA., Li, TY., Sampson, L., & Hu, FB. (2009). Prospective study of nut consumption, long-term weight change, and obesity risk in women. *Am J Clin Nutr*; 89(6):1913-9.

Blum, S., Aviram, M., Ben-Amotz, A., & Levy, Y. (2006). Effect of a Mediterranean meal on postprandial carotenoids, paraoxonase activity and C-reactive protein levels. *Ann Nutr Metab*; 50(1):20-4.

Brennan, AM., Sweeney, LL., Liu, X., & Mantzoros, CS. (2010). Walnut consumption increases satiation but has no effect on insulin resistance or the metabolic profile over a 4-day period. *Obesity (Silver Spring)*;18(6):1176-82.

Brennan, RO. (1975) Nutrigenetics: new concepts for relieving hypoglycemia. New York: M. Evans and Co.

Brown, S., Ordovás, JM., Campos, H. (2003) Interaction between the APOC3 gene promoter polymorphisms, saturated fat intake and plasma lipoproteins. *Atherosclerosis*; 170(2):307-13.

Camargo, A., Ruano, J., Fernandez, JM., Parnell, LD., Jimenez, A., Santos-Gonzalez, M. et al. (2010). Gene expression changes in mononuclear cells in patients with metabolic syndrome after acute intake of phenol-rich virgin olive oil. *BMC Genomics*; 11:253.

Campos, H., D'Agostino, M., & Ordovás, JM. (2001). Gene-diet interactions and plasma lipoproteins: role of apolipoprotein E and habitual saturated fat intake. *Genet Epidemiol*; 20(1):117-128.

Castro, P., Miranda, JL., Gómez, P., Escalante, DM., Segura, FL., Martín, A., et al. (2000). Comparison of an oleic acid enriched-diet vs NCEP-I diet on LDL susceptibility to oxidative modifications. *Eur J Clin Nutr*; 54(1):61-7.

Chrysohoou, C., Panagiotakos, DB., Pitsavos, C., Das, UN., & Stefanadis, C. (2004). Adherence to the Mediterranean diet attenuates inflammation and coagulation process in healthy adults: The ATTICA Study. *J Am Coll Cardiol*; 44(1):152-8.

Corella, D., Carrasco, P., Sorlí, JV., Coltell, O., Ortega-Azorín, C., Guillén, M., et al. (2010). Education modulates the association of the FTO rs9939609 polymorphism with body mass index and obesity risk in the Mediterranean population. Nutr Metab Cardiovasc Dis. 2010 Dec 24. [Epub ahead of print]

Corella, D., Lai, CQ., Demissie, S., Cupples, LA., Manning, AK., Tucker, KL., & Ordovas, JM. (2007). APOA5 gene variation modulates the effects of dietary fat intake on body mass index and obesity risk in the Framingham Heart Study. *J Mol Med (Berl)*; 85(2):119-28.

Corella, D., & Ordovas, JM. (2005). Integration of environment and disease into 'omics' analysis. *Curr Opin Mol Ther*; 7(6):569-76.

Corella, D., Peloso, G., Arnett, DK., Demissie, S., Cupples, LA., Tucker, K., et al. (2009). APOA2, dietary fat, and body mass index: replication of a gene-diet interaction in 3 independent populations. *Arch Intern Med*; 169(20):1897-906.

Corella, D., Tai, ES., Sorlí, JV., Chew, SK., Coltell, O., Sotos-Prieto, M., et al. (2011). Association between the APOA2 promoter polymorphism and body weight in Mediterranean and Asian populations: replication of a gene-saturated fat interaction. *Int J Obes (Lond)*; 35(5):666-75.

Corella, D., Tucker, K., Lahoz, C., Coltell, O., Cupples, LA., Wilson, et al. (2001). Alcohol drinking determines the effect of the APOE locus on LDL-cholesterol concentrations in men: the Framingham Offspring Study. *Am J Clin Nutr*; 73(4):736-45.

Crujeiras, AB., Parra, D., Goyenechea, E., Abete, I., González-Muniesa, P., & Martínez, JA. (2008). Energy restriction in obese subjects impact differently two mitochondrial function markers. *J Physiol Biochem*; 64(3):211-9.

de Lorgeril, M., Renaud, S., Mamelle, N., Salen, P., Martin, JL., Monjaud, I., et al. (1994). Mediterranean alpha-linolenic acid-rich diet in secondary prevention of coronary heart disease. *Lancet*; 343(8911):1454-9.

de Lorgeril, M., Salen, P., Martin, JL., Monjaud, I., Delaye, J., & Mamelle, N. (1999). Mediterranean diet, traditional risk factors, and the rate of cardiovascular complications after myocardial infarction: final report of the Lyon Diet Heart Study. *Circulation*; 99(6):779-85.

de Mello, VD., Kolehmainen, M., Pulkkinen, L., Schwab, U., Mager, U., Laaksonen, DE., et al. (2008). Downregulation of genes involved in NFkappaB activation in peripheral blood mononuclear cells after weight loss is associated with the improvement of insulin sensitivity in individuals with the metabolic syndrome: the GENOBIN study. *Diabetologia*; 51(11):2060-7

DellaPenna, D. 1999. Nutricional genomics: manipulating plant micronutrients to improve human health. *Science*; 285:375-79

Elhayany, A., Lustman, A., Abel, R., Attal-Singer, J., & Vinker, S. (2010). A low carbohydrate Mediterranean diet improves cardiovascular risk factors and diabetes control among overweight patients with type 2 diabetes mellitus: a 1-year prospective randomized intervention study. Diabetes Obes Metab;12(3):204-9.

Esposito, K., Kastorini, CM., Panagiotakos, DB., & Giugliano, D. (2011). Mediterranean diet and weight loss: meta-analysis of randomized controlled trials . *Metab Syndr Relat Disord*; 9(1):1-12.

Esposito, K., Maiorino, MI., Di Palo, C., Giugliano, D., & Campanian. (2009). Postprandial Hyperglycemia Study Group. Adherence to a Mediterranean diet and glycaemic control in Type 2 diabetes mellitus. *Diabet Med*; 26(9):900-7.

Esposito, K., Marfella, R., Ciotola, M., Di Palo, C., Giugliano, F., Giugliano, G., et al. (2004) Effect of a mediterranean-style diet on endothelial dysfunction and markers of vascular inflammation in the metabolic syndrome: a randomized trial. *JAMA*; 292(12):1440-6.

Esposito, K., Pontillo, A., Di Palo, C., Giugliano, G., Masella, M., Marfella, R., & Giugliano, D. (2003). Effect of weight loss and lifestyle changes on vascular inflammatory markers in obese women: a randomized trial. *JAMA*; 289(14):1799-804.

Estruch, R., Martínez-González, MA., Corella, D., Salas-Salvadó, J., Ruiz-Gutiérrez, V., Covas, MI., et al, (2006). Effects of a Mediterranean-style diet on cardiovascular risk factors: a randomized trial. *Ann Intern Med*;145(1):1-11.

Fraser, GE., Bennett, HW., Jaceldo, KB., & Sabaté, J. (2002). Effect on body weight of a free 76 Kilojoule (320 calorie) daily supplement of almonds for six months. *J Am Coll Nut*; 21(3):275-83.

Fung, TT., McCullough, ML., Newby, PK., Manson, JE., Meigs, JB., Rifai, N., et al. (2005). Diet-quality scores and plasma concentrations of markers of inflammation and endothelial dysfunction. *Am J Clin Nutr*; 82(1):163-73.

García-Lorda, P., Megias Rangil, I., & Salas-Salvadó, J. (2003). Nut consumption, body weight and insulin resistance. *Eur J Clin Nutr*; 57 Suppl 1:S8-11.

Giuseppe, RD., Bonanni, A., Olivieri, M., Castelnuovo, AD., Donati, MB., Gaetano, GD., et al. (2008). Adherence to Mediterranena diet and anthropometric and metabolic parameters in an observational study in the "Alto Molise" region: The MOLI-SAL project. *Nutr Metab Cardiovasc Dis*; 18(6):415-21.

Goulet, J., Lamarche, B., Nadeau, G., & Lemieux, S. (2003). Effect of a nutritional intervention promoting the Mediterranean food pattern on plasma lipids, lipoproteins and body eight in healthy French-Canadian women. *Atherosclerosis*; 170(1):115-24.

Harris, RP., Helfand, M., Woolf, SH., Lohr, KN., Mulrow, CD., Teutsch, SM., et al. (2001). Third U.S. Preventive Services Task Force. Current methods of the U.S. Preventive Services Task Force: a review of the process. *Am J Prev Med*; 20(3S):21-35.

Haskell, WL. (2003). Cardiovascular disease prevention and lifestyle interventions: effectiveness and efficacy. *J Cardiovasc Nurs*; 18:245-55

Howard, BV., Van Horn, L., Hsia, J., Manson, JE., Stefanick, ML., Wassertheil-Smoller, S., Kuller, LH., et al. (2006). Low-fat dietary pattern and risk of cardiovascular disease: the Women's Health Initiative Randomized Controlled Dietary Modification Trial. *JAMA*; 295(6):655-66.

Jansen, S., Lopez-Miranda, J., Salas, J., Ordovas, JM., Castro, P., Marin, C., et al. (1997). Effect of 347-serine mutation in apoprotein A-IV on plasma LDL cholesterol response to dietary fat. Arterioscler *Thromb Vasc Biol*; 17(8):1532-8.

Kastorini, CM., Milionis, HJ., Esposito, K., Giugliano, D., Goudevenos, JA., & Panagiotakos, DB. (2011). The effect of Mediterranean diet on metabolic syndrome and its components: a meta-analysis of 50 studies and 534,906 individuals. *J Am Coll Cardiol*; 57(11):1299-313.

Katan MB, Beynen AC, de Vries JH, Nobels A. (1986). Existence of consistent hypo- and hyperresponders to dietary cholesterol in man. *Am J Epidemiol*; 123(2):221-34.

Keys, A. (1970). Coronary Heart Disease in Seven Countries. *Circulation*; 41(1):1-211.

Keys, A., Menotti, A., & Karoven, MI. (1986). The diet and the 15-year death rate in the Seven Countries Study. *Am J Epidemiol*; 124:903-915.

Khymenets, O., Fitó, M., Covas, MI., Farré, M., Pujadas, MA., Muñoz, D., Konstantinidou, V., & de la Torre, R. (2009). Mononuclear cell transcriptome response after sustained virgin olive oil consumption in humans: an exploratory nutrigenomics study. *OMICS*; 13(1):7-19

Knoops, KT., de Groot, LC., Kromhout, D., Perrin, AE., Moreiras-Varela, O., Menotti, A., et al. (2004). Mediterranean diet, lifestyle factors, and 10-year mortality in elderly European men and women: the HALE project. *JAMA*; 292(12):1433-9.

Konstantinidou, V., Covas, MI., Muñoz-Aguayo, D., Khymenets, O., de la Torre, R., Saez, G., et al. (2010). In vivo nutrigenomic effects of virgin olive oil polyphenols within the frame of the Mediterranean diet: a randomized controlled trial. *FASEB J*; 24(7):2546-57.

Konstantinidou, V., Khymenets, O., Fito, M., De La Torre, R., Anglada, R., Dopazo, A., & Covas, MI. (2009). Characterization of human gene expression changes after olive oil ingestion: an exploratory approach. *Folia Biol (Praha)*; 55(3):85-91

Krauss, RM., Eckel, RH., Howard, B., Appel, LJ., Daniels, SR., & Deckelbaum, RJ. (2000). AHA Dietary Guidelines: revision 2000: A statement for healthcare professionals from the Nutrition Committee of the American Heart Association. *Stroke;* 31(11):2751-66.

Lalonde, M. (1974). A new perspective on the health of canadians: a working document. Ottawa: Department of Health and Welfare.

Larsen, TM., Dalskov, SM., van Baak, M., Jebb, SA., Papadaki, A., Pfeiffer, AF., et al. (2010). Diet, Obesity, and Genes (Diogenes) Project. Diets with high or low protein content and glycemic index for weight-loss maintenance. *N Engl J Med;* 363(22):2102-13.

Li, Z., Song, R., Nguyen, C., Zerlin, A., Karp, H., Naowamondhol, K., et al. (2010). Pistachio nuts reduce triglycerides and body weight by comparison to refined carbohydrate snack in obese subjects on a 12-week weight loss program. *J Am Coll Nutr;* 29(3):198-203.

Lichtenstein, AH., Ausman, LM., Jalbert, SM., Vilella-Bach, M., Jauhiainen, M., McGladdery, S., et al. (2002). Efficacy of a Therapeutic Lifestyle Change/Step 2 diet in moderately hypercholesterolemic middle-aged and elderly female and male subjects. *J Lipid Res;*43(2):264-73.

Linton MF, Fazio S, National Cholesterol Education Program (NCEP)- the third Adult Treatment Panel (ATP III). (2003). A practical approach to risk assessment to prevent coronary artery disease and its complications. *Am J Cardiol;* 92(1A):19i-26i.

Llorente-Cortés V, Estruch R, Mena MP, Ros E, González MA, Fitó M, et al. (2010). Effect of Mediterranean diet on the expression of pro-atherogenic genes in a population at high cardiovascular risk. . *Atherosclerosis;* 208(2):442-50

Loktionov, A. (2003) Common gene polymorphisms and nutrition: emerging links with pathogenesis of multifactorial chronic diseases (review). *J Nutr Biochem;*14(8):426-51.

Lopez-Miranda J, Ordovas JM, Mata P, Lichtenstein AH, Clevidence B, Judd JT, Schaefer EJ. (1994). Effect of apolipoprotein E phenotype on diet-induced lowering of plasma low density lipoprotein cholesterol. *J Lipid Res;* 35(11):1965-75.

Luan, J., Browne, PO., Harding, AH., Halsall, DJ., O'Rahilly, S., Chatterjee, VK., & Wareham NJ. (2001). Evidence for gene-nutrient interaction at the PPARgamma locus. *Diabetes;* 50(3):686-9.

Martínez-González, MA., & Bes-Rastrollo, M. (2011). Nut consumption, weight gain and obesity: Epidemiological evidence. *Nutr Metab Cardiovasc Dis;*21 Suppl 1:S40-5.

Martínez-González, MA., Fuente-Arrillaga, CD., Nunez-Cordoba, JM., Basterra-Gortari, FJ., Beunza, JJ., Vazquez, Z., et al. (2008). Adherence to Mediterranean diet and risk of developing diabetes: prospective cohort study. *BMJ;* 336(7657):1348-51.

Masala, G., Bendinelli, B., Versari, D., Saieva, C., Ceroti, M., Santagiuliana, F., et al. (2008). Anthropometric and dietary determinants of blood pressure in over 7000 Mediterranean women: the European Prospective Investigation into Cancer and Nutrition-Florence cohort. *J Hypertens;* 26(11):2112-20.

Masson, LF., McNeill, G., & Avenell, A. (2003). Genetic variation and the lipid response to dietary intervention: a systematic review. *Am J Clin Nutr;* 77(5):1098-111.

Memisoglu, A., Hu, FB., Hankinson, SE., Manson, JE., De Vivo, I., Willett, WC., & Hunter, DJ. (2003). Interaction between a peroxisome proliferator-activated receptor gamma gene polymorphism and dietary fat intake in relation to body mass. *Hum Mol Genet*; 12(22):2923-9.

Michalsen, A., Lehmann, N., Pithan, C., Knoblauch, NT., Moebus, S., Kannenberg, F., et al. (2006). Mediterranean diet has no effect on markers of inflammation and metabolic risk factors in patients with coronary artery disease. *Eur J Clin Nutr*; 60(4):478-85.

Müller-Nordhorn, J., Rossnagel, K., Mey, W., & Willich, SN. (2004). Regional variation and time trends in mortality from ischaemic heart disease: East and West Germany 10 years after reunification. *J Epidemiol Community Health*; 58:481–485.

Núñez-Córdoba, JM., Valencia-Serrano, F., Toledo, E., Alonso, A., & Martínez-González, MA. (2009). The Mediterranean diet and incidence of hypertension: the Seguimiento Universidad de Navarra (SUN) Study. *Am J Epidemiol*; 169(3):339-46.

Obarzanek, E., Sacks, FM., Vollmer, WM., Bray, GA., Miller, ER3rd., Lin, PH., et al. DASH Research Group. (2001). Effects on blood lipids of a blood pressure-lowering diet: the Dietary Approaches to Stop Hypertension (DASH) Trial. *Am J Clin Nutr*; 74(1):80-9.

Ordovas, JM., Corella, D., Demissie, S., Cupples, LA., Couture, P., Coltell, O., et al. (2001). Dietary fat intake determines the effect of a common polymorphism in the hepatic lipase gene promoter on high-density lipoprotein metabolism: evidence of a strong dose effect in this gene-nutrient interaction in the Framingham Study. *Circulation*;106(18):2315-21.

Ordovas, JM., & Corella, D. (2004). Nutritional genomics. *Annu Rev Genomics Hum Genet*; 5:71-118

Ordovas JM, Mooser V. (2004). Nutrigenomics and nutrigenetics. *Curr Opin Lipidol*; 15(2):101-8.

Panagiotakos, DB., Pitsavos, C., Arvaniti, F., & Stefanadis, C. (2007). Adherence to the Mediterranean food pattern predicts the prevalence of hypertension, hypercholesterolemia, diabetes and obesity, among healthy adults; the accuracy of the MedDietScore. *Prev Med*; 44(4):335-40.

Panagiotakos, DB., Pitsavos, C., & Stefanadis, C. (2006). Dietary patterns: a Mediterranean diet score and its relation to clinical and biological markers of cardiovascular disease risk. *Nutr Metab Cardiovasc Dis*; 16(8):559-68.

Panagiotakos, DB., Tzima, N., Pitsavos, C., Chrysohoou, C., Zampelas, A., Toussoulis, D., et al. (2007). The association between adherence to the Mediterranean diet and fasting indices of glucose homoeostasis: the ATTICA Study. *J Am Coll Nutr*; 26(1):32-8.

Panagiotou, G., Nielsen J. (2009). Nutritional systems biology: definitions and approaches. *Annu Rev Nutr*; 29:329-39.

Papadaki, A., Scott JA. (2008). Follow-up of a web-based tailored intervention promoting the Mediterranean diet in Scotland. *Patient Educ Couns*; 73(2):256-63.

Pérez-Martínez, P., Pérez-Jiménez, F., Bellido, C., Ordovás, JM., Moreno, JA., Marín, C., et al. (2005). A polymorphism exon 1 variant at the locus of the scavenger receptor class B type I (SCARB1) gene is associated with differences in insulin sensitivity in healthy people during the consumption of an olive oil-rich diet. *J Clin Endocrinol Metab*; 90(4):2297-300.

Pitsavos, C., Panagiotakos, D., Trichopoulou, A., Chrysohoou, C., Dedoussis, G., Chloptsios, Y., et al. (2006). Interaction between Mediterranean diet and methylenetetrahydrofolate reductase C677T mutation on oxidized low density lipoprotein concentrations: the ATTICA study. *Nutr Metab Cardiovasc Dis*; 16(2):91-9.

Pitsavos, C., Panagiotakos, DB., Chrysohoou, C., & Stefanadis, C. (2003). Epidemiology of cardiovascular risk factors in Greece: aims, design and baseline characteristics of the ATTICA study. *BMC Public Health*; 3:32-40.

Pitsavos, C., Panagiotakos, DB., Tzima, N., Lentzas, Y., Chrysohoou, C., Das, UN-, et al. (2007). Diet, exercise, and C-reactive protein levels in people with abdominal obesity: the ATTICA epidemiological study. *Angiology*;58(2):225-33.

Polychronopoulos, E., Panagiotakos, DB., Polystipioti. (2005). A.Diet, lifestyle factors and hypercholesterolemia in elderly men and women from Cyprus. *Lipids Health Dis*; 6;4:17

Posner, BM., Cobb, JL., Belanger, AJ., et al. (1991). Dietary lipid predictors of coronary heart disease in men. The Framingham Study. *Arch Intern Med*; 151:1181-7.

Psaltopoulou, T., Naska, A., Orfanos, P., Trichopoulos, D., Mountokalakis, T., Trichopoulou, A. (2004). Olive oil, the Mediterranean diet, and arterial blood pressure: the Greek European Prospective Investigation into Cancer and Nutrition (EPIC) study. *Am J Clin Nutr*;80(4):1012-8.

Rajaram, S., & Sabaté, J. Nuts, body weight and insulin resistance. Br J Nutr. 2006;96 Suppl 2:S79-86.

Razquin, C., Martinez, JA., Martinez-Gonzalez, MA., Bes-Rastrollo, M., Fernández-Crehuet, & J., Marti, A. (2010 A). A 3-year intervention with a Mediterranean diet modified the association between the rs9939609 gene variant in FTO and body weight changes. *Int J Obes (Lond)*; 34(2):266-72.

Razquin, C., Martinez, JA., Martinez-Gonzalez, MA., Fernández-Crehuet, J., Santos, JM., & Marti, A. (2010 B). A Mediterranean diet rich in virgin olive oil may reverse the effects of the -174G/C IL6 gene variant on 3-year body weight change. *Mol Nutr Food Res*;54 Suppl 1:S75-82.

Razquin, C., Martínez, JA., Martínez-González, MA., Salas-Salvadó. J-, Estruch, R., & Marti, A. (2010 C). A 3-year Mediterranean-style dietary intervention may modulate the association between adiponectin gene variants and body weight change. *Eur J Nutr*; 49(5):311-9.

Robitaille, J., Pérusse, L., Bouchard, C., & Vohl, MC. (2007). Genes, fat intake, and cardiovascular disease risk factors in the Quebec Family Study. *Obesity (Silver Spring)*;15(9):2336-47.

Romaguera, D., Norat, T., Vergnaud, AC., Mouw, T., May, AM., Agudo, A., et al. (2010). Mediterranean dietary patterns and prospective weight change in participants of the EPIC-PANACEA project. *Am J Clin Nutr*; 92(4):912-21.

Ros, E., Núñez, I., Pérez-Heras, A., Serra, M., Gilabert, R., Casals, E., et al. (2004). A walnut diet improves endothelial function in hypercholesterolemic subjects: a randomized crossover trial. *Circulation*; 109(13):1609-14.

Sabaté, J., Oda, K., & Ros, E. (2010). Nut consumption and blood lipid levels: a pooled analysis of 25 intervention trials. *Arch Intern Med*; 170(9):821-7.

Sacks, FM., Bray, GA., Carey, VJ., Smith, SR., Ryan, DH., Anton, SD., et al. (2009). Comparison of weight-loss diets with different compositions of fat, protein, and carbohydrates. *N Engl J Med*; 360(9):859-73.

Salas-Salvadó, J., Bulló, M., Babio, N., Martínez-González, MÁ., Ibarrola-Jurado, N., Basora, J., et al. PREDIMED Study Investigators. (2011). Reduction in the incidence of type 2 diabetes with the Mediterranean diet: results of the PREDIMED-Reus nutrition intervention randomized trial. *Diabetes Care*; 34(1):14-9.

Salas-Salvadó, J., Garcia-Arellano, A., Estruch, R., Marquez-Sandovalm F., Corellam D., Fiol, M., et al. (2008). Components of the mediterranean-type food pattern and serum inflammatory markers among patients at high risk for cardiovascular disease. *Eur J Clin Nutr*, 62(5):651-9.

Sans, S., Kesteloot, H., & Kromhout, D. (1997). The burden of cardiovascular diseases mortality in Europe. Task Force of the European Society of Cardiology on Cardiovascular Mortality and Morbidity Statistics in Europe. *Eur Heart J*; 18:1231–1248.

Schröder, H., Marrugat, J., Vila, J., Covas, MI., & Elosua, R. (2004). Adherence to the traditional mediterranean diet is inversely associated with body mass index and obesity in a Spanish population. *J Nutr*; 134(12):3355-61.

Schröder H. (2007). Protective mechanisms of the Mediterranean diet in obesity and type 2 diabetes. *J Nutr Biochem*; 18(3):149-60.

Serra-Majem, L., Trichopoulou, A., Ngo de la Cruz, J., Cervera, P., García Alvarez, A., La Vecchia, C., et al. (2004). Does the definition of the Mediterranean diet need to be updated? *Public Health Nutr*; 7(7):927-9.

Serrano-Martínez M, Martínez-González MA. (2007). Effects of Mediterranean diets on plasma biomarkers of inflammation. *Eur J Clin Nutr*; 61(8):1035-6; author reply 1036.

Shai, I., Schwarzfuchs, D., Henkin, Y., Shahar, DR., Witkow, S., & Greenberg, I.; Dietary Intervention Randomized Controlled Trial (DIRECT) Group. (2008). Weight loss with a low-carbohydrate, Mediterranean, or low-fat diet. *N Engl J Med*; 359(3):229-41.

Singh, RB., Dubnov, G., Niaz, MA., Ghosh, S., Singh, R., Rastogi, SS., et al. (2002). Effect of an Indo-Mediterranean diet on progression of coronary artery disease in high risk patients (Indo-Mediterranean Diet Heart Study): a randomised single-blind trial. *The Lancet*; 360(9344):1455-61.

Slimani, N., Kaaks, R., Ferrari, P., Casagrande, C., Clavel-Chapelon, F., Lotze, G., et al. (2002). European Prospective Investigation into Cancer and Nutrition (EPIC) calibration study: rationale, design and population characteristics. *Public Health Nutr*; 5(6B):1125-45.

Smith, CE., Arnett, DK., Corella, D., Tsai, MY., Lai, CQ., Parnell, LD., et al. (2010). Perilipin polymorphism interacts with saturated fat and carbohydrates to modulate insulin resistance. *Nutr Metab Cardiovasc Dis*. 2010 Dec 30. [Epub ahead of print].

Sotos-Prieto, M., Zulet, MA., & Corella, D. (2010). Scientific evidence of the mediterranean diet effects in determining intermediate and final cardiovascular disease phenotypes. *Med Clin (Barc)*;134(1):22-9

Tai, ES., Collins, D., Robins, SJ., O'Connor, JJ., Bloomfield, HE., Ordovas, JM., et al. (2006). The L162V polymorphism at the peroxisome proliferator activated receptor alpha locus modulates the risk of cardiovascular events associated with insulin resistance and diabetes mellitus: the Veterans Affairs HDL Intervention Trial (VA-HIT). *Atherosclerosis*; 187(1):153-60.

Trichopoulou, A., Costacou, T., Bamia, C., & Trichopoulous, D. (2003). Adherente to a Mediterranean diet and survival in a Greek population. *N Eng J Med*; 348:2599-2608.

Tzima, N., Pitsavos, C., Panagiotakos, DB., Skoumas, J., Zampelas, A., Chrysohoou, C., et al. (2007). Mediterranean diet and insulin sensitivity, lipid profile and blood pressure levels, in overweight and obese people; the Attica study. *Lipids Health Dis*; 6:22.

Vincent-Baudry, S., Defoort, C., Gerber, M., Bernard, MC., Verger, P., Helal, O., et al. (2005). The Medi-RIVAGE study: reduction of cardiovascular disease risk factors after a 3-mo intervention with a Mediterranean-type diet or a low-fat diet. *Am J Clin Nutr*; 82(5):964-71.